Care of People with Diabetes

This book is dedicated to all people with diabetes and their families who continue to be a source of inspiration; valued research colleagues and participants, and to all the health professionals who shared their wisdom and experience with us.

Care of People with Diabetes

A Manual for Healthcare Practice

5th Edition

Professor Trisha Dunning AM
RN, MEd, PhD, CDE, FACN (DLF)
Registered Nurse and credentialed Diabetes Educator
Chair in Nursing at Barwon Health and Deakin University Partnership in Geelong
Victoria, Australia

Professor Alan Sinclair
MSc, MD, FRCP
Director of the Foundation for Diabetes Research in Older People (FDROP) at Diabetes Frail
Visiting Chair in Diabetes Care, King's College London
London, UK

WILEY Blackwell

Registered Office(s)
John Wiley & Sons, Inc., 111 River Street, Hoboken, NJ 07030, USA
John Wiley & Sons Ltd, The Atrium, Southern Gate, Chichester, West Sussex, PO19 8SQ, UK

Editorial Office
9600 Garsington Road, Oxford, OX4 2DQ, UK

For details of our global editorial offices, customer services, and more information about Wiley products, visit us at www.wiley.com.

Wiley also publishes its books in a variety of electronic formats and by print-on-demand. Some content that appears in standard print versions of this book may not be available in other formats.

Library of Congress Cataloging-in-Publication Data

Names: Dunning AM, Trisha, author. | Sinclair, Alan (Alan J.), author.
Title: Care of people with diabetes : a manual for healthcare practice /
  Professor Trisha Dunning, Professor Alan Sinclair.
Description: 5th edition. | Hoboken, NJ : Wiley-Blackwell, 2020. | Includes
  bibliographical references and index.
Identifiers: LCCN 2019024442 (print) | ISBN 9781119520856 (paperback) |
  ISBN 9781119520863 (adobe pdf) | ISBN 9781119520870 (epub)
Subjects: MESH: Diabetes Mellitus
Classification: LCC RC660 (print) | LCC RC660 (ebook) | NLM WK 810 |
  DDC 616.4/620231–dc23
LC record available at https://lccn.loc.gov/2019024442
LC ebook record available at https://lccn.loc.gov/2019024443

Cover Design: Wiley
Cover Image: © Robert Kneschke/Shutterstock

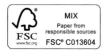

Contents

Foreword   xiii
Preface   xv
Acknowledgments   xvii
List of Abbreviations and Symbols   xix

1   Diagnosing and Classifying Diabetes   1
    Key points   1
    What is diabetes mellitus?   2
    Prevalence of diabetes   2
    Classification of diabetes   3
    Overview of normal glucose homeostasis   3
    Brain-centric model of glucose homeostasis   10
    Metabolic syndrome in children and adolescents   13
    Types of diabetes   14
    Diagnosing diabetes   22
    Preventing diabetes   26
    Managing diabetes mellitus   29
    Key points   29
    Complications of diabetes   36
    Aims and objectives of diabetes care   38
    Technology and diabetes management   40
    A sobering final comment   42
    References   43

2   Holistic Personalised Diabetes Care   49
    Key points   49
    Rationale   49
    Shared decision-making (SDM)   50
    Holistic diabetes care   51
    Communication and the power of language   52
    Reading fiction to improve empathy and communication skills   53
    Care models   53
    Characteristics of an holistic health history   55
    References   58

3   Assessing and Monitoring People with Diabetes   61
    Key points   61
    Rationale   61
    Key issues to consider in comprehensive assessments   62
    Monitoring glucose levels   62
    Monitoring 1: Blood glucose   64
    Key points   64

Insulin pumps   75
Monitoring 2: Urine glucose   76
Key points   76
Monitoring 3: Additional assessment   78
Self-care   82
The annual review   83
Summary   83
References   83

4 Nutrition and Weight Management   87
Key points   87
Rationale   87
The importance of good nutrition   88
Malnutrition and undernutrition   88
Method of screening for dietary characteristics and problems   90
Principles of dietary management for people with diabetes   92
Goals of dietary management   95
Overweight and obesity   95
Methods of measuring weight   99
Managing obesity and diabetes   100
Dietary management: overweight and obesity   101
Factors associated with making dietary changes   103
Key points   104
Alcohol   107
Exercise/activity   107
References   108
Further reading   112

5 Medicine Management   113
Key points   113
Introduction   114
QUM   114
QUM and diabetes   114
GLM   117
Medicine interactions   129
Combining GLMs and insulin   130
When should insulin be initiated in Type 2 diabetes?   131
Challenges to initiating insulin therapy   134
Some strategies to overcome the barriers   135
Insulin therapy   136
Types of insulin available   136
Storing insulin   139
Injection sites and administration   140
Mixing short/rapid acting- and intermediate-acting insulins   141
Commonly used insulin regimens   141
Interpreting morning hyperglycaemia   143
CSII   143
Continuous blood glucose sensors   144
Subcutaneous insulin sliding scales and top-up regimens   145
Uses of insulin infusions   147
Insulin allergy   149
Pancreas transplants   150
Stabilising diabetes   150
Stabilising diabetes in hospital   150
Community and outpatient insulin stabilisation   151

Lipid-lowering agents	153
Monitoring lipid medicines	157
Antihypertensive agents	158
Antiplatelet agents	159
Medication safety, adherence, and medication self-management	161
Enhancing medication self-care	163
Example protocol for outpatient stabilisation onto insulin	166
References	167

6 Hypoglycaemia **175**

Key points	175
Rationale	175
Introduction	176
The counter-regulatory response	178
Definition of hypoglycaemia	179
Recognising hypoglycaemia	182
The brain and glucose homeostasis	183
Causes of hypoglycaemia	183
Preventing and managing hypoglycaemia	184
Hypoglycaemic unawareness	185
Prevalence of HU	186
Nocturnal hypoglycaemia	187
Relative hypoglycaemia	189
Medicine interactions	189
Objectives of care	190
Treatment	190
Prolonged hypoglycaemia	191
Patients most at risk of hypoglycaemia	192
Psychological effects of hypoglycaemia	193
Guidelines for administering glucagon	194
Adverse reactions	195
References	196

7 Hyperglycaemia, Acute Illness, Diabetic Ketoacidosis (DKA), Hyperosmolar Hyperglycaemic States (HHS), and Lactic Acidosis **199**

Key points	199
Rationale	200
Prevention: proactively managing intercurrent illness	200
Self-care during illness	202
Hyperglycaemia	202
Diabetic ketoacidosis (DKA)	204
Brittle diabetes and hyperglycaemia	211
Euglycaemic DKA	211
Hyperosmolar hyperglycaemic states	212
Lactic acidosis	214
References	216

8 Long-Term Complications of Diabetes **219**

Key points	219
Introduction	220
Diabetes and complexity	220
Pathophysiology of diabetes complications	221
Cardiovascular disease and diabetes	223
Key points	223
Cerebrovascular disease	236

Diabetes and eye disease   237
Diabetes and renal disease   243
Peripheral and autonomic neuropathy   255
Autonomic neuropathy   266
References   270

9   Management in Hospital, Surgery, and Investigations   279
Emergency department   279
Key points   279
Surgical procedures   280
Key points   280
Preoperative care   284
Postoperative care   289
Guidelines for informing people with diabetes about what they should do
    prior to surgical procedures   290
Insulin pump therapy in patients undergoing surgery   292
Emergency procedures   292
Bariatric surgery   293
Investigative procedures   293
Key points   293
The objectives of care   294
General management   294
Eye procedures   295
Complementary medicines and other therapies during surgery
    and investigative procedures   298
Preoperative phase   298
Postoperative phase   299
Implications for care   299
References   300
Example Information 2(a): Instructions for people with diabetes
    on oral glucose-lowering medicines having procedures as outpatients under
    sedation of general anaesthesia   301
Example Instruction Sheet 2(b): Instructions for people with diabetes
    on insulin having procedures as outpatients under sedation
    or general anaesthesia   302

10   Conditions Associated with Diabetes   303
Key points   303
Introduction   303
Enteral and parenteral nutrition   304
Diabetes and cancer   309
Smoking, alcohol, and illegal drug use   315
Brittle or labile diabetes   326
Oral health and diabetes   328
Diabetes and liver disease   329
Haemochromatosis   332
Diabetic mastopathy   333
Diabetes and coeliac disease   334
Cystic fibrosis–related diabetes   336
Incontinence   338
Sleep disturbance and diabetes   340
Diabetes and tuberculosis   341
Diabetes and HIV/AIDS   342
Diabetes and hearing loss   343

Diabetes, musculoskeletal disease, and osteoporosis 345
Corticosteroid medications and diabetes 347
Key points 347
Diabetes and driving 350
Diabetes and fasting for religious observances 359
Education and counselling 359
References 360

11 Sexual and Reproductive Health 371
Key points 371
Rationale 371
Sexual health 372
Sexual development 373
Sexual problems 374
Possible causes of sexual difficulties and dysfunction 374
Sexuality and older people 375
Women 376
Men 377
Sexual counselling 380
Role of the clinician 383
References 383

12 Diabetes and Older People 385
Key points 385
Rationale 386
Introduction 386
Determining functional status 392
Geriatric syndromes 394
Cognitive functioning and dementia 395
Depression and older people with diabetes 400
Dementia 400
Caring for older people with diabetes 401
Education approaches 408
Self-care 409
Factors that can affect metabolic control 410
Overall care strategies 417
References 418

13 Diabetes in Children and Adolescents 425
Key points 425
Rationale 425
Introduction 426
Impact of hyper- and hypoglycaemia on brain development and function 429
Managing children and adolescents with diabetes 430
Aspects of care that apply to both type 1 and type 2 diabetes in children
    and adolescents 430
Managing type 1 diabetes 431
Managing type 2 diabetes 433
Medicine self-management 436
Other conditions associated with diabetes 436
Strategies for enhancing adherence during adolescence 437
Ketoacidosis in children 438
Complementary therapy use in children 438
References 439

14   Women, Pregnancy, and Gestational Diabetes   443
     Key points   443
     Rationale   443
     Polycystic ovarian syndrome   444
     Contraception options for women with diabetes   447
     Pregnancy   449
     Gestational diabetes   455
     Menopause and diabetes   459
     References   462

15   Psychological and Quality of Life Issues Related to Having Diabetes   467
     Key points   467
     Rationale   468
     Introduction   468
     Clinician factors   469
     Adjustment and spirituality   472
     Diabetes: reputation and myths   473
     Diabetes-related distress   474
     Quality of life   474
     Diabetes and depression   476
     Mental health and type 1 diabetes   480
     Mental health and type 2 diabetes   480
     Psychological distress and cardiovascular disease   481
     Psychiatric disorders, diabetes, and antipsychotic medicines   482
     Diabetes conversations and language   483
     References   486
     Further reading   490

16   Diabetes Education   491
     Key points   491
     Rationale   492
     Introduction   492
     Learning styles   495
     Education and other theories/models   497
     Communication – having good conversations   500
     Teaching: an art and a process   503
     Health literacy   504
     Survival skills   507
     Empowerment   508
     Special issues   509
     The clinicians' role in diabetes education   509
     Documenting diabetes education   512
     Evaluating diabetes education   515
     References   517
     Further reading   521

17   Managing Diabetes at the End of Life   523
     Key points   523
     Introduction   524
     Explanation of terms: values, life limiting illness, palliative care,
         terminal care, and end-of-life care   524
     Palliative care   525
     General management considerations for managing diabetes at the end of life   531
     Diabetes-specific considerations   532

Medicine management   534
Type 1 diabetes   534
Nutrition and hydration   536
Diabetogenetic medicines   537
Supporting family/carers   538
Withdrawing treatment   539
Diabetes education   539
References   540

18 Complementary Medicine   543
Key points   543
Rationale   543
Introduction   544
CAM philosophy   546
Integrating complementary and conventional care   547
Can Complementary Therapies Benefit People with Diabetes?   549
Spirituality   552
CM and surgery   552
Herb/medicine interactions   556
How can CM be used safely?   556
Clinician responsibilities   560
Identifying quality health information on the internet   561
Recommended resources   563
References   563

Index   567

Foreword

Diabetes is a serious and complex condition.

No one chooses to get diabetes, but for those living with the condition, there is no respite – diabetes is 24/7 through all ages and stages.

Within a generation, there have been unprecedented advances in our approach to diabetes – in its treatment and management and more broadly. For example, new technologies (both approved and DIY) have greatly diminished the need to constantly draw blood to check glucose levels; insulin and metformin are on the cusp of being replaced as first-line oral therapies; we now better appreciate that diabetes is both a physical as well as a psycho-social challenge; and we strive to use and encourage health professionals and the media in particular to use, nonjudgemental language when referring to diabetes.

Faced with this degree of change, it's not surprising that this important manual of healthcare practice has now been updated for the fifth time in 25 years.

I congratulate Professors Trisha Dunning AM and Alan Sinclair, along with all their expert advisors, for their unstinting efforts in helping those who care for people living with diabetes to navigate this rapidly changing environment. The breadth of issues highlighted in the 18 chapters of this manual reflects the often complex daily challenges faced by people living with diabetes, as well as by those health professionals advising them. From first symptoms to end-of-life care and all the phases in between, what shines through all these pages is empathy, compassion, and a desire to help those people living with this relentless condition to lead long, dignified, healthy, and productive lives – all of which are truly universal aspirations. In updating this manual, Professors Dunning and Sinclair have tapped into their extensive Australian and UK networks and have also been well supported by diabetes colleagues working elsewhere in the world – an impressive and very commendable collaboration.

I hope future editions will document even more progress, reflecting our greater understanding of all types of diabetes resulting from the simply breathe-taking quality and quantity of research currently underway in so many centres across the world. Perhaps we will finally learn how to prevent type 2 diabetes as well as some of its serious complications; be clearer about whether type 2 diabetes can ever be reversed; and one day find a cure for type 1 diabetes and other similar autoimmune conditions.

On behalf of an organisation that strives to support, empower, and campaign for all those affected by, or at risk of, diabetes, I'm optimistic.

Craig Bennett
Melbourne, Australia

Craig Bennett is a health economist by training; the CEO of Diabetes Victoria; and an Adjunct Professor at Deakin University.

Preface

It is humbling to be preparing the fifth edition of *Care of People with Diabetes: a Manual of Nursing Practice* and to change the title to *Care of People with Diabetes; A Manual for Healthcare Practice* to reflect the broad range of readers it attracts.

It is certainly an honour to have my dear friend and colleague, Professor Alan Sinclair, co-edit this edition with me. Alan brings with him a wealth of experience as an acknowledged world expert in diabetes care. The book has evolved a great deal since the first edition was published in 1994. Many readers will not know that the first edition was *volume 2* of my Master of Education degree. It originated from comments given by the nursing staff from St. Vincent's Hospital Melbourne who suggested, 'It would be good to have some guidance about nursing care for "diabetics" besides the guidelines, which are mostly medical'.

I developed a draft based on their suggested topics, and they used those draft versions to guide care and then provided feedback about the usefulness, clinical relevance, and ease of use. We developed several iterations before we reached consensus about the content and presentation of the information. The evaluation process became *volume 1* of my thesis and the information became *volume 2*, and ultimately the first edition of *Care of People with Diabetes: a Manual of Nursing Practice.*

Readers will find much that is the same in this fifth edition. Obviously, there are changes that reflect new research and technological and philosophical changes. Therefore, there are some new text and references. There is emerging global interest in 'the language of diabetes', and its impact on outcomes, which were mentioned in the preface to the fourth edition. The fifth edition continues to advocate for shared decision-making and personalised (person-centred/tailored) integrated care plans developed *with* the individual, and holistic care.

These include the increasing prevalence of type 1, type 2, and gestational diabetes, population ageing, the focus on prevention and the need to maximise value while containing the spiraling cost of diabetes care. The need to proactively plan for end of life care is emerging globally and represents a challenge for many clinicians. Obviously, there are differences among countries, even within countries, but these are common global trends.

The book was designed to support clinical practice guidelines, not replace them. It is impossible to include 'everything' in any publication: we hope readers will find something of value that will help them improve the care they plan for people with diabetes.

Trisha Dunning AM and Alan Sinclair

Acknowledgments

We sincerely thank Blackwell for supporting the first edition of the book published in 1994 and Wiley for supporting subsequent editions. We especially thank Mr James Watson, Commissioning Editor for Wiley, for commissioning the 5th edition, Ms Yogalakshmi Mohanakrishnan, project editor, for her collaboration and advice and for taking such good care of our work, and Ms Monisha Swaminathan for the fine editing that went into this project.

We both work in supportive teams of doctors, nurses, and allied health professionals, and with wonderful academic colleagues. Our special thanks go to them for their friendship and critical comment on various aspects of the book. We especially thank those people who reviewed the book and gave very useful feedback, most of which has been incorporated in this edition.

We acknowledge the generosity of the Australian Commonwealth Department of Health and Ageing for permission to reproduce the figure depicting how the Quality Use of Medicines framework can be applied to diabetes management that appears in Chapter 5. We acknowledge colleagues Dr Sally Savage, Nicole Duggan, and Professor Peter Martin for giving permission to include our hypoglycaemia risk assessment tool in Chapter 7. We thank Natalie Whischer, Heather Hart, Kate Marsh, and Jennifer Hunter for comments about Chapters 2, 14, 4, and 19, respectively, and especially Professor Jane Speight for her advice and contribution to Chapter 15 on psychological and quality of life issues.

We sincerely thank Virginia Dicson-Smith and Tara Watts for assistance with checking the references and Dr Joan Ostakiewictz for her interest and ongoing support during the revision process.

We are in awe of the people who undertook the research and critical thinking cited in this edition and other researchers and clinicians who contribute so much information about diabetes that challenge, inform, and inspire us. As Isaac Newton said: *"If I* [we] *have seen further it is by standing on the shoulders of Giants."*

We both learned, and continue to learn, a great deal about diabetes from the people with diabetes and their families whom we teach and care for/with, and who participate in our research as participants, advisors, and co-researchers, as well as their families. It is a privilege to be with them and share information and their stories: they inspire us.

We sincerely thank Mr Craig Bennett, CEO of Diabetes Victoria, for agreeing to write the foreword for this edition.

Finally, and most importantly, we thank our respective families for their support and understanding, not just during the revision of this book but over the years.

A very special thank you and our love go to John Dunning and Caroline Sinclair 'for everything', and our furry four-legged family, Flora Weadora Dunning and Posey and Pippen Sinclair.

List of Abbreviations and Symbols

↑	Increased
↓	Decreased
≤	Equal to, or less than
<	Less than
≥	Equal to, or greater than
>	Greater than
ACEI	Angiotensin-converting enzyme (ACE) inhibitor
ADA	American Diabetes Association
ADDQoL	Audit of Diabetes-Dependent Quality of Life
ADL	Activities of daily life
AE	Adverse effect
AMA	American Medical Association
ASQHS	Australian Commission on Safety and Quality in Health Care
ADS	Australian Diabetes Society
AGS	American Geriatrics Society
ARB	Angiotensin II receptor blocker
BG	Blood glucose
BGAT	Blood glucose awareness training
BGM	Blood glucose monitoring
BMI	Body mass index
BP	Blood pressure
BUN	Blood urea nitrogen
CAM	Complementary and alternative medicine
CAPD	Continuous ambulatory peritoneal dialysis
CCF	Congestive cardiac failure
CCU	Coronary care unit
CDA	Canadian Diabetes Association
CM	Complementary medicine
COPD	Chronic obstructive pulmonary disease
CVD	Cardiovascular disease
CSII	Continuous subcutaneous insulin infusion
DA	Diabetes Australia
DAFNE	Dose adjustment for normal eating
DEXA	Dual-energy X-ray absorptiometry
DKA	Diabetic ketoacidosis
DSM-V	*Diagnostic and Statistical Manual of Mental Disorders, 5th edition*
DUK	Diabetes UK
ECG	Electrocardiogram
EMA	European Medicines Agency

EN	Enteral nutrition
euDKA	Euglycaemic diabetic ketoacidosis
FFA	Free fatty acids
GDM	Gestational diabetes mellitus
GIK	Glucose, insulin, and potassium
GIT	Gastrointestinal tract
GLM	Glucose-lowering medicines
HbA1c	Glycosylated haemoglobin (often written as HBA_{1c})
HDL	High-density lipoproteins
HHS	Hyperosmolar hyperglycaemic states
HIV	Human immunodeficiency virus
HLA	Human leukocyte antigen
HU	Hypoglycaemic unawareness
IAPO	International Alliance of Patient Organisations
ICU	Intensive care unit
IADL	Instrumental activities of daily living
IDF	International Diabetes Federation
IV	Intravenous therapy
LADA	Latent autoimmune diabetes in adults
LFT	Liver function test
LDL	Low-density lipoproteins
MAO	Monoamine oxidase inhibitor
MI	Myocardial infarction
MODY	Maturity onset diabetes of the young
NAFLD	Nonalcoholic fatty liver disease
NDSS	National Diabetes Supply Scheme
NICE	National Institute of Clinical Excellence
NSAIDs	Nonsteroidal anti-inflammatory drugs
OHAs	Oral hypoglycaemic agents
OGTT	Oral glucose tolerance test
PADL	Physical activities of daily living
PCOS	Polycystic ovarian syndrome
QoL	Quality of life
SGLT-2	Sodium glucose cotransporter inhibitor -2
SIGN	Scottish Intercollegiate Guidelines Network
SMBG	Self-monitoring blood glucose
SSRI	Selective serotonin reuptake inhibitor
STI	Sexually transmitted infection
TPN	Total parenteral nutrition
TPR	Temperature, pulse, and respiration
TZD	Thiazolidinediones
UTI	Urinary tract infection
WHO	World Health Organization

The acronyms are generally spelled out the first time they appear in the text, often spelled out the first time used in a chapter. All abbreviations are internationally accepted and recognised.

Chapter 1
Diagnosing and Classifying Diabetes

Cancer, diabetes, and heart disease are no longer diseases of the wealthy. Today they hamper the people and economies of the poorest populations ... this represents a health emergency in slow motion.

(Ban Ki Moon, Secretary General of the United Nations)

Key points

- Diabetes is the modern pandemic. It represents a considerable global economic and social burden for the person with diabetes, families, and for health services.
- The prevalence of the metabolic syndrome, type 1, type 2 and gestational diabetes (GDM) is increasing.
- The greatest increase in diabetes prevalence is occurring in Africa, the Middle East, and South East Asia.
- The overlapping mechanisms by which obesity leads to the metabolic syndrome and type 2 diabetes are complex and still evolving.
- Not everybody who is obese has insulin resistance or diabetes.
- Central obesity plays a key role in the progression to insulin resistance and type 2 diabetes.
- Lean people may be at higher risk of morbidity and mortality than obese people.
- Primary prevention and early detection are essential to reduce the personal and community burden associated with the metabolic syndrome and diabetes and their complications.
- Type 2 diabetes is a progressive disease, and complications are often present at diagnosis. Thus, early diagnosis is essential. Insulin will eventually be necessary in most people with type 2 diabetes.
- The prevalence of obesity, the metabolic syndrome, and type 2 diabetes in children are increasing.

What is diabetes mellitus?

Diabetes mellitus is a metabolic disorder in which the body's capacity to utilise glucose, fat, and protein is disturbed due to insulin deficiency or insulin resistance or both. Both states lead to hyperglycaemia, lipid abnormalities, and glycosuria.

The body is unable to utilise glucose in the absence of insulin and mobilises fat and protein stores in an effort to supply fuel for energy. Insulin is necessary for the complete metabolism of fats, however, and when carbohydrate metabolism is disordered fat metabolism is incomplete and intermediate products (ketone bodies) can accumulate in the blood leading to ketosis, especially in type 1 diabetes. Protein breakdown also occurs and leads to weight loss and weakness and contributes to the development of hyperglycaemia and lethargy.

The different types of diabetes have different underlying causal mechanisms and clinical presentation: in general, young people are insulin-deficient (type 1 diabetes), whilst older people usually secrete sufficient insulin in the early stages but demonstrate resistance to insulin action (type 2 diabetes). In the early stages of type 2, hyperinsulinaemia might be present. Type 2 is a progressive disease with slow destruction of the insulin-producing beta cells and, consequently, insulin deficiency.

There appear to be differences in insulin sensitivity and beta cell function between young people and adults with prediabetes and type 2 diabetes (Rise Consortium 2018). Clamp studies show young people are more resistant to insulin and have hyper-responsive beta cells. The TEDDY study suggests beta cell function declines at a faster rate with early onset type 2 diabetes and the beta cells do not respond well to glucose lowering medicines (GLMs) (Rewers et al. 2018). Complications appear at an early age, which leads to higher rates of morbidity and mortality. Potential contributing factors are puberty-related insulin resistance and obesity.

Some people diagnosed with type 2 diabetes have evidence of transient autoimmunity before they are diagnosed (Turner et al. 1997; ADA 2019). They are usually younger than people with negative autoantibodies and have evidence of reduced beta cell function such as lower fasting C-peptide, worse metabolic control and are more symptomatic (Sørgjerd et al. 2018). This group of people could represent a heterogeneous phenotype of type 2 diabetes distinct from Latent Autoimmune Diabetes in Adults (LADA). Thus, diabetes is a complex disease of evolving aetiology and increasing prevalence. Type 2 diabetes is the most common, accounting for about 90% of diagnosed cases and type 1 accounts for about 10% of diagnosed cases.

Prevalence of diabetes

Diabetes is a global health problem affecting about 451 million people aged 18–99 years worldwide in 2017 (International Diabetes Federation [IDF] 2018) and an estimated 49.7% or people with diabetes are undiagnosed and an estimated 374 million have impaired glucose tolerance (prediabetes) (IDF 2017). More than 187 million are unaware they have diabetes. The prevalence is expected to increase to 693 million by 2045 unless the epidemic can be halted. In addition, almost 21.3 million live births were to women affected by some form of hyperglycaemia. Significantly, 5 million deaths in people aged 20–99 were attributable to diabetes worldwide.

The Australian Institute of Health and Welfare (AIHW 2005) shows that diabetes prevalence is escalating and rates are higher amongst males, Indigenous Australians, and socioeconomically disadvantaged people. This accounts for about 1.2 million people, about 6%, and 16 400 deaths in 2015. Most have type 2 diabetes (AIHW 2005). In the United Kingdom, an estimated 3.7 million people have diabetes, and up to another 12.3 million are at increased risk of type 2 diabetes: thus, 4.6 million people in the United Kingdom are living with diabetes (Diabetes UK 2014). The US Centers for Disease Control (CDC) estimated that 30.3 million Americans had diabetes and 84.1 million had prediabetes (CDC 2017).

The reason for the increasing global prevalence of type 2 diabetes is due to many interrelated factors, including genetic predisposition, environmental factors, and the ageing population. Type 2 is the most common type, accounting for 80–90% of cases. Significantly, and worrying, the prevalence of type 2 diabetes in children is increasing.

There is wide variation in the incidence rates of newly diagnosed type 1 diabetes in children in different populations. However, type 1 in children and adolescents is increasing, particularly in developed countries (EURODIAB 2000; Soltesz et al. 2006; The DIAMOND Project Group 2006). The incidence of type 1 diabetes in children <15 years on the Western Australian Children's Database has increased gradually over the past 25 years but occurs in peaks and troughs rather than in a linear progression (Haynes et al. 2012). For example, peak years were 1992, 1997, and 2003 in Australia. The incidence of type 1 appears to fluctuate in five-year cycles and might be influenced by circulating viruses, especially enterovirus infections or other environmental factors (Haynes et al. 2012).

The association between ingesting cow's milk in infancy and pathogenesis of type 1 diabetes is discussed in Chapter 13. IRE1α may have a role in inducing thioredoxin-interacting protein to activate the NLRP3inflammasome and promote programmed pancreatic cell death (Lerner et al. 2012). The researchers stated that the findings suggest dietary modification could extend the honeymoon period in type 1 diabetes or possibly prevent diabetes.

Thus, the economic burden of diabetes and health-care costs are high to society and individuals and their families. The proportion of people with diabetes admitted to the hospital is increasing, and they mostly have longer lengths of stay (ADS 2012). Some people not known to have diabetes develop hyperglycaemia in the hospital. Hyperglycaemia is associated with increased morbidity and mortality, independent of diabetes (Chapter 7).

It is not clear whether hyperglycaemia in people without a diabetes diagnosis is due to undiagnosed diabetes/IGT or whether it is an indicator of underlying critical illness. However, because in-hospital hyperglycaemia in nondiabetics may represent undiagnosed diabetes or risk of future diabetes, these people should receive education and be followed up.

Classification of diabetes

Diabetes is broadly classified into type 1 and type 2 diabetes and several other types. An overview of the types of diabetes, pathophysiology diagnostic criteria and management are shown in Table 1.1. Having a broad understanding of glucose normal homeostasis is important to understanding the pathophysiologic changes associated with the different types of diabetes and management strategies.

Overview of normal glucose homeostasis

Blood glucose regulation (glucose homeostasis) relies on a delicate balance between the fed and fasting states and is dependent on several simultaneously operating variables including hormones, nutritional status, especially liver and muscle glucose stores, exercise, tissue sensitivity to insulin, and the type of food consumed. Figure 1.1 shows the key features of the fed and fasting states.

Insulin release occurs in two phases. The first phase is important to controlling the postprandial blood glucose rise and is lost early in the progression to type 2 diabetes. Postprandial glucose >7.8 mmol/l is associated with cardiovascular events and plays a role in the development of other co-morbidities (IDF 2011). Insulin action is mediated via two protein pathways: Protein 13-kinase through insulin receptors and influences glucose uptake into the cells; and MAP-kinase, which stimulates growth and mitogenesis.

The interaction between insulin and its primary binding site on the insulin receptor and the conformational switch in insulin once it engages with the receptor is well known (Menting et al. 2013). Conformational switching is unusual in the tyrosine receptor kinases. The clinical significance of the finding is not yet clear but it could influence the development of future insulin analogues.

Table 1.1 Overview of the classification, underlying pathophysiology, and diagnosis of common types of diabetes. Diabetes type and time of diagnosis have implications for disease treatment and disease progression.

Diabetes type	Pathophysiology	Diagnostic criteria	Management	Considerations
Prediabetes Individuals who have blood glucose above the normal range but do not meet diagnostic levels.	It signifies increased risk of type 2 diabetes and cardiovascular disease. It is associated with abdominal obesity, dysglycaemia, hypertriglyceridaemia >2.82 mmol/l, and/or low HDL <0.90 mmol/l and hypertension. BP >140/90 mmHg. BMI >25 kg/m² or 23 kg/m² in Asian and African peoples.	Meets criteria on valid risk screening tools and FPG between 5.6 and 6.9 mmol/l (100–125 mg/dl) and two hour. FPG 7 mmol/l (126 mg/dl) is provisionally diabetes and needs to be confirmed with and OGTT using 75 g anhydrous glucose 2 hour PG 7.8–11.1 mmol/l (140–199 mg/dl impaired fasting glucose and 11.1 mmol/l (>200 mg/dl) diagnosis of diabetes	Annual risk screening Lifestyle counselling and weight management. Rescreen at changes in health and/or functional status. Regular screening for diabetes and CVD including managing lipid abnormalities and hypertension. Early diagnosis and treatment. Relevant general healthcare.	Proactive screening in at-risk populations and individuals is important in primary and secondary prevention. Valid screening tools such as the ADA Type 2 Diabetes Risk and Australian AUSDRISK tools, and diagnostic procedures should be used. Screen tests should begin at age 45 for at risk individuals and repeated as indicated: minimum every 3 years. People with type 2 diabetes can have complications before diagnosis. Thus, screening for cardiovascular and other risk factors is also important. The WHO and some other diabetes organisations use 6.1 mmol/l as the upper cut point level. Deedwania et al. (2014) suggested there is no independent association between prediabetes, heart failure, cardiovascular events, and mortality in community dwelling older people in contrast to younger and middle-aged adults. Risk factors for people with myocardial infarction and/or coronary revascularisation include smoking and not participating in cardiac rehabilitation programmes (Munkhaugen et al. (2018).

Type 1

Two main types are describe immune-mediated and idiopathic type 1 diabetes.

People with type 1 usually have absolute insulin deficiency

Autoimmune B-cell destruction usually leading to absolute insulin deficiency indicated by low or no C-peptide in blood.

Persistent presence of two or more autoantibodies increases the risk in individual and first-degree relatives.

Hyperglycaemia and high HbA1c can be present before symptoms occur and diabetes is diagnosed.

Immune-mediated diabetes is due to autoimmune destruction of the pancreatic beta-cells and accounts for 5–10% of diabetes.

Autoimmune markers include islet cell autoantibodies, GAD 65 autoantibodies and autoantibodies to insulin and the tyrosine phosphatases A-2, A-2B, and ZnTB.

Idiopathic type 1 occurring for no known reason. Insulin levels are permanently low and people are prone to DKA.

It is rare, and most people with idiopathic type 1 are from African or Asian backgrounds. It is strongly inherited.

Insulin requirements may be intermittent.

The following tests are used to screen for and diagnose diabetes and prediabetes:

Presence of multiple autoantibodies

Dysglycaemia: IFG and/or IGT

FPG 5.6–6.9 mmol/l

HbA1c >6.5% performed using standardised laboratory techniques.

PPG >11.1 mmol/l after fasting (no calories ingested for 8 hours before the test) or 2 hours after ingesting 75 g anhydrous glucose during a glucose tolerance test performed under test conditions.

Insulin, which should not be stopped, except under medical advice and e.g. fasting for a procedure, when an IV infusion is indicated to prevent DKA.

Diabetes self-management education including DAFNE, if indicated, and educating parents.

Regular blood glucose monitoring.

Complication screening.

Developing strategies to transfer to adult diabetes services when indicated.

Recommended childhood vaccinations.

Heterogeneous: clinical presentation and progression can vary.

Can occur at any age. Children usually present with polydipsia, polyuria, and weight loss: about 33% present with DKA.

The presentation is variable in adults.

The rate of progression depends on age when antibodies are first detected, the number of antibodies present and their specificity and the titre.

Point of care HbA1c testing is subject to tester inaccuracies and may not use NGSP standard assay techniques.

Likewise, HbA1c is an indirect measure of the average blood glucose and can be affected by a range of factors such as haemoglobinopathies, anaemia, age, and pregnancy.

(Continued)

Table 1.1 (Continued)

Diabetes type	Pathophysiology	Diagnostic criteria	Management	Considerations
Type 2 Insulin resistance and usually have relative rather than absolute insulin deficiency, initially and throughout their lifetime for some people. They do not need insulin treatment to survive, usually continuing to produce enough insulin to prevent DKA except in overwhelming stress states. They can develop hyperglycaemic hyperosmolar states, which can be life threatening.	Progressive loss of beta-cell mass and insulin secretion and/or insulin resistance with relative insulin deficiency.	FPG 5.6–6.9 mmol/l HbA1c > 6.5% performed using standardised laboratory techniques. PPG >11.1 mmol/l after fasting (no calories ingested for eight hours before the test) or two hours after ingesting 75 g anhydrous glucose during a glucose tolerance test performed under test conditions. Two abnormal plasma glucose levels are required from the same or two separate samples.	Follow prescribing algorithms for GLMs but consider medicine burden, potential medicine interactions and self-care capability when prescribing additive GLMs or other medicines. Initiate insulin when indicated. Regular complication screening and management and geriatric and palliative care assessment when indicated. Diabetes self-management education including DESMOND when relevant. Relevant vaccination and other screening programmes such as for cancer and periodontal disease. Advance care planning for palliative and end of life care.	Heterogeneous: clinical presentation and progression can vary. Can occur at any age. Children usually present with polydipsia, polyuria and weight loss: about 33% present with DKA. The presentation is variable in adults. Some people with type 2 have transient evidence of autoimmunity before diagnosis. These people are younger at diagnosis and present with characteristics indicative of reduce beta cell function (lower fasting C-peptide, higher HbA1c, and more symptoms). The transient autoantibody appears to indicate earlier onset type 2 and may occur in ~3% individuals with type 2. (Sørgjerd et al. 2018). Point of care HbA1c testing is subject to tester inaccuracies and may not use NGSP standard assay techniques. Likewise, HbA1c is an indirect measure of the average blood glucose and can be affected by a range of factors such as haemoglobinopathies, anaemia, age, and pregnancy. General healthcare is important.

Latent Autoimmune Diabetes in Adults (LADA) LADA presents in various ways and is often misdiagnosed as type 2 or type 1 diabetes and may not be managed appropriately, which could lead to faster progression of beta cell loss, increased risk of complications and the need for insulin. It can present at any age.	Heterogeneous condition and shares characteristics of type 1 and type 2 diabetes. Beta cell destruction is highly variable and individuals have varying degrees of insulin resistance and autoantibodies. Some people have elevated GADA (glutamic acid decarboxylase), often low C-peptide and are prone to ketosis, sometimes called LADA 1. LADA 2 have more abdominal obesity, hypertension, and cardiovascular risk. They do not have GADA but have islet cell autoantibodies (Pozilli and Pieralice 2018).	Consider a diagnosis of LADA. Measure blood glucose, HbA1c, GADA, and islet cell antibodies to determine the likely pathophysiology.	There are no specific management guidelines for LADA. Treat early to preserve beta cell function and reduce complication risk, e.g. DPP-4 may help preserve C-peptide. Insulin may be needed early in the course of LADA. Some research that Sulphonylureas should not be used (Pozilli and Pieralice 2018). Regular complication screening and managing cardiovascular risk. Personalised diabetes education.	Taking a careful history assessment and investigations helps identify LAD, enables appropriate treatment to be decided and helps reduce rates of misdiagnosis and improve outcomes, especially complications.
Gestational diabetes Refers to diabetes first diagnosed during pregnancy usually in trimester 2 or 3. GDM usually resolves after delivery but women are at increased risk of developing GDM in subsequent pregnancies. Confers increased risk of type 2 diabetes in later life for the mother and the child is at increased risk of type diabetes in late adolescence and early adulthood. It also increases the likelihood of adverse outcomes for the mother and baby.	GDM could represent an early stage in the progression to T2DM caused by the stresses of pregnancy (Law and Zhang 2017). The exact pathophysiology is unclear. Low grade obesity-induced inflammation that induces xanthurenic acid could play a role. It is associated with the development of prediabetes, T2DM and GDM.	OGTT using recommended protocols at 24–28 weeks. Test is diagnostic if FPG 5.1–6.9 mmol/l or >10.0 mmol/l after one hour and >8.5 mmol/l after 2 hours. (International Association of Diabetes and Pregnancy Study Groups)	Educate the woman and her family and introduce blood glucose monitoring, healthy diet and regular activity. Commence insulin if indicated. Collaboration between the diabetes team. Obstetrician and paediatrician are essential to holistic care.	Follow recommended guidelines. Test for diabetes at the first prenatal visit in women with risk factors or prediabetes and then at 24–28 weeks. Retest at 4–12 weeks post-partum and then lifelong screening. Follow up monitoring is essential to detect diabetes early. Ensure general health and obstetric care are provided. Encourage breast feeding. Educate the family about the risk of T2DM.
Cystic fibrosis (CF) and pancreatitis-related are diseases of the exocrine pancreas. Diabetes is the most common comorbidity in people with CF and occurs in approximately 20% of adolescents and 40–50% adults with CF.	Insulin insufficiency is the most common but genetics and inflammatory IRS can also contribute.	HbA1c is not recommended as a diagnostic test in people with CF. Screening before age 10 can identify diabetes risk progression but no specific criteria for weight, height, BMI, or lung function are currently available.	Follow the Clinical Care Guidelines for Cystic Fibrosis-related Diabetes: a Position Statement of the American Diabetes Association (ADA) and/ or the International Society for Paediatric and Adolescent Diabetes (2014).	Screen children with CF annually from age 10 if they do not have an existing diagnosis of diabetes. CF-related diabetes is associated with inadequate nutritional status and worse inflammatory lung disease and higher mortality

(Continued)

Table 1.1 (Continued)

Diabetes type	Pathophysiology	Diagnostic criteria	Management	Considerations
Post transplantation diabetes Several names are used in the literature for post transplantation diabetes, including new onset diabetes in people with no existing diagnosis of diabetes. People with diabetes also have transplants.	Hyperglycaemia is common in the first few weeks after organ transplantation. It is often stress or steroid-induced and usually resolves over time. People with risk factors for diabetes are most at risk because they enhance the risk of hyperglycaemia associated with immunosuppressive treatment.	Screen for hyperglycaemia after organ transplantation once the person is stable on immunosuppression therapy.	Screen the individual for diabetes risk pretransplant. Optimise weight and lifestyle. Insulin therapy is generally recommended, especially in the early stages. Monitor blood glucose. Revise diabetes self-management behaviours and provide other relevant education.	After organ transplantation. Immunosuppressive treatment regimens likely to achieve the best outcomes for the individual should be used and the person monitored for diabetes.
Monogenic syndromes Maturity Onset Diabetes of the Young (MODY) Neonatal diabetes occurring before 6 months of age: 80–85% have an underlying monogenetic cause. Neonatal diabetes can be temporary or permanent. These types of diabetes are rare only occurring in <5% of people with diabetes.	There are three common forms of MODY: GCK-MODY, HNF1A-MODY and HNF-AA MODY	MODY and neonatal diabetes are diagnosed on the basis of genetic testing.	Most people with MODY require specialist care. Treatment depends on the specific genetic abnormality, e.g. sulphonylureas are first line treatment for HNF1A-MODY and HNF-AA MODY. Currently there is no specific treatment for GCK-MODY. Genetic counselling is important.	Children diagnosed with diabetes in the first 6 months of life and those diagnosed with diabetes that does not fit the criteria for type 1 or type 2 diabetes should have genetic testing for MODY. Screen family members. Genetic counselling and support might be required.
Medicine-induced diabetes Medicines such as thiazides, glucocorticoids and antipsychotics cause hyperglycaemia	Various changes to glucose homeostasis depending on the class of medicine and individual medicines within the class. Some interfere with insulin production or secretion, some interfere with insulin action, and some cause hyperglycaemia independent of insulin action. May precipitate insulin resistance.			People with prediabetes are more at risk. Screen for prediabetes before commencing these medicines.

Diabetes associated with diseases of or injury to the exocrine pancreas; and other endocrine disorders such as acromegaly, Cushing Syndrome Phaeochromocytoma.	Any process or trauma that cause extensive injury to the pancreas can cause diabetes. For example, infection, pancreatectomy, pancreatic cancer, cystic fibrosis (see this table) and haemochromatosis. Adenocarcinomas that only involve a small part of the pancreas can contribute to diabetes.	Consider diabetes and monitor blood glucose and relevant hormone levels, especially in people with diabetes risk factors.	Palliative and end of life care planning might be indicated. Some endocrine disorder requires lifelong hormone replacement therapy and monitoring, e.g. acromegaly and Cushing's syndrome. Diabetes usually resolves when the hormone excess is resolved.
Ketosis-Prone Diabetes type 2 diabetes (Flatbush diabetes)	Recognised since 1984. Mostly occurs in African American, Afro-Carribbean, sub-Saharan African, Asian, Indian and Hispanic peoples, however, there are differences in the syndrome depending on the ethnic background. The clinical course is similar to type 2 diabetes. Underlying causes are unknown but inability of blood glucose to stimulate insulin secretion is a central abnormality and leads to severe hyperglycaemia.	Usually present with acute onset of significant hyperglycaemia with ketoacidosis requiring hospital admission and treatment with insulin and fluid replacement. They are GAD and islet cell antibody negative.	After several months, insulin may no longer be required and some can be managed with lifestyle diet and exercise: some people require GLMs. Sulphonylurea can prolong periods of glycaemic control. The role of newer GLMs is unclear.

Source: Information derived from ADA (2009, 2019), Oeedwania et al. (2013), Deedwania et al. (2014), Ferreira et al. (2018), Lecte et al. (2018), Lebowitz and Banerji (2018), Munkhaugen et al. (2018), Zhang and Pollin (2018).

Type 1 and type 2 diabetes have various underlying genetic predispositions that interact with environmental factors and result in progressive loss of B-cell mass and/or function that lead to hyperglycaemia. Hyperglycaemia and the accompanying inflammatory process increase the risk of tissue and organ damage and diabetes complications. Treatment should be decided with the individual and personalised to their diabetes type, health status, values, goals, and health status.

DKA: diabetic ketoacidosis.

DAFNE: dose Adjustment for Normal Eating.

HHS Hyperosmolar Hyperglycaemic State.

IPG: impaired plasma glucose,

FPG – fasting plasma glucose.

PPG: Post-prandial plasma glucose.

IGT: Impaired glucose tolerance.

IRS: insulin resistance syndrome.

OGGT: Oral glucose tolerance test.

NSGP: National glycohemoglobin Standardisation Program (NGSP) Certified Assays and Laboratories (NSGP www.ngsp.org).

Anabolism (fed state)	Catabolism (fasting state)
• Driven by insulin and the incretin hormones • Insulin release stimulated by the rise in blood glucose • Two-phase response • Facilitates glucose uptake • Reduces hepatic glucose output	• Driven by a variety of hormones, e.g. catecholamines, cortisol, growth hormone, glucagon • Increases endogenous glucose output: 80% liver, 20% kidney • Induces insulin resistance • Reduces glucose utilisation • Insulin output reduced • Protective during hypoglycaemia

– Fasting state 12–16 hours after an overnight fast and is an important determinant of day-long glycaemia
– Postprandial (fed) state–dynamic regulated by insulin and glucagon especially in the first 30–60 minutes
– Insulin is secreted in two phases and regulates the rate of glucose entry into cells and removal from the circulation:
  • Post prandial blood glucose rise is usually transient
  • Peaks 60–90 minutes
  • Usually returns to normal within 3 hours
  • Usually there is very little diurnal variation in the blood glucose level
  • Isolated post-prandial hyperglycaemia occurs in IGT

Figure 1.1   Overview of glucose homeostasis showing the key factors operating during the fed and fasting states. Usually the blood glucose is maintained within the normal range by the interplay of the anabolic and catabolic hormones, which are, in turn, influenced by other hormones and a number of factors such as nutritional status and intake.

Brain-centric model of glucose homeostasis

The brain-centric model of glucose homeostasis suggests the brain also has a key role in glucose homeostasis, but it is not clear whether the effects are important in day-to-day blood glucose regulation, which does not require active participation from the brain (Schwartz et al. 2013, Deem et al. 2017). The brain can influence the biologically defended level of circulating glucose: partly through rapid highly coordinated adjustment of insulin sensitivity and insulin secretion. Research shows the brain responds to humoral signals including blood glucose, amino acids, and free fatty acids (FFAs) and the nutritionally relevant hormones leptin, ghrelin, and GLP-1 to influence key determinants of glucose homeostasis: glucose production and utilisation (Deem et al. 2017).

Glucose regulatory neurocircuits are involved in the response to hypoglycaemia, Control of food intake and social behaviours. A subset of neurons in the parabrachial nucleus are involved in glucose counter-regulation. Pharmacologic activation of these neurons increases blood glucose by activating the response to hypoglycaemia: secretion of glucagon and corticosterone and inhibition of glucose-induced insulin secretion (Garfield et al. 2014). Less is known about neurocircuits involved when hypoglycaemia is not present.

However, other research shows that the brain can normalise diabetic hyperglycaemia through the action of fibroblast growth factors. Intracerebroventricular injections of PGF1 induced remission in rodent models of T2DM (Scarlett et al. 2016). It is possible that defects in the brain-centric glucoregulatory system could have a primary or secondary causal role in beta cell dysfunction in T2DM, which involves gradual progressive inability of the brain to sense and respond to signals pertaining to the blood glucose level. This regulatory dysfunction is similar to the pathogenesis of obesity (Deem et al. 2017). These findings could have implications for future treatments and explanatory models of diabetes.

Prediabetes and the metabolic syndrome

Prediabetes/metabolic syndrome is outlined in Table 1.1. The metabolic syndrome consists of a cluster of risk factors for cardiovascular disease and type 2 diabetes. Several researchers and organisations continue to explore the factors that predict diabetes risk. These include the World Health Organization (WHO), International Diabetes Federation (IDF), Diabetes Epidemiology Collaborative Analysis of Diagnostic Criteria in Europe (DECODE), Epidemiology Study on the

Insulin Resistance Syndrome (DESIR), US National Cholesterol Education Programme Adult Treatment Panel (NCEP ATP 111), and the European Group for the Study of Insulin Resistance: Relationship Between Insulin Sensitivity and Cardiovascular Disease Risk (EGIR-RISC). Their work produced a number of diabetes risk assessment tools used in prevention programmes and clinical care to identify T2DM early.

A range of studies concerning epigenetic factors associated with type 1 and type 2 diabetes continually add to our knowledge of this complex disease. Epigenetics refers to a group of mechanisms concerning gene expression and gene regulation that consist of heritable changes in DNA but that do not alter the DNA sequence (Zhang and Pollin 2018). Epigenetic changes are often specific to various developmental life stages that include regulation of cell differentiation and are often tissue specific (e.g. beta cells in the pancreas).

Normal growth and development of the human body depends on good nutrition and the neuroendocrine system (Ferreira et al. 2018). It is also influenced by poverty and other factors. Exposure to environmental compounds, behaviours, placental insufficiency in utero, and inadequate maternal nutrition or metabolic abnormalities can epigenetically program susceptibility to various diseases in the first and sometimes subsequent generations (Ferreira et al. 2018).

The period from birth to age two represents an important phase to promote healthy habits because nutritional damage at this time can determine structural, metabolic, and functional changes that predispose the child to chronic diseases in adulthood. Significantly, obesity/abdominal obesity, hypertension, and dyslipidemia, significant cardiovascular risk factors and mortality, are more prevalent in children who were undernourished in early life (Ferreira et al. 2018). Overweight and obesity contribute to the development of insulin resistance, including during puberty. Thus, risk screening for prediabetes or T2DM should begin at puberty in at risk adolescents (ADA 2019). T2DM with onset in young people leads to faster rate of beta cell destruction and reduced responsiveness to GLMs (TODAY Study Group 2012).

Key features of the metabolic syndrome

- The metabolic syndrome appears to be a result of genetic predisposition and environmental factors, which include high-saturated-fat diets, inactivity, smoking, hormone imbalances contributing to metabolic stress, maternal obesity, age, and some medicines (Bruce and Byrne 2009). These factors represent a cumulative risk and most are largely modifiable.
- Central obesity, waist circumference: Europeans >94 cm in men and >80 cm in women; South Asian and Southeast Asian men >90 cm, women >80 cm: (Zimmet et al. 2005); childhood/adolescent body mass index (BMI) 25–29 overweight, >30 obese. Interestingly, Carnethon et al. (2012) reported that overweight people diagnosed with diabetes live longer than leaner people with diabetes in a prospective study to identify cardiovascular risk factors (n = ~2600). The death rate was 1.5 in overweight people compared to 2.8 in lean people after accounting for cardiovascular risk factors such as age, hypertension, hypercholesterolaemia, and smoking. The authors acknowledged the limitations of the study. They also noted Asian people are more likely to be normal weight at diagnosis and stressed the need for extra vigilance in leaner people. Significantly, not all obese people develop the metabolic syndrome. See also Chapter 4.
- Raised serum triglycerides >1.7 mmol/l.
- Low serum HDL-c: <1.03 mmol/l males, <1.29 mmol/l women.
- Hypertension: systolic >130 mmHg or diastolic >85 mmHg in women.
- IFG: >5.6 mmol/l or previously diagnosed diabetes (e.g. GDM). IFG is associated with a 20–30% chance of developing type 2 diabetes within 5–10 years. The chance increases if high-fasting glucose (FPG) is also present.

Other key features include:

- Increasing age.
- Insulin resistance. High serum levels of sugar metabolites, amino acids, and chlorine-containing phospholipids are associated with reduced insulin sensitivity and insulin secretion and higher

risk of type 2 diabetes (Floegel et al. 2013). A small study suggests people who sleep for <4 hours are 30% more insulin resistant than those who sleep longer (Cappuccio and Miller 2012). However, the sample size was a small one and only one participant was female, which could be important because men and women respond to sleep deprivation differently. Thus, research is continuing.

- Genetic predisposition and the Developmental Origins of Adult Health and Disease (DOHaD) hypothesis. Maternal obesity at conception alters gestational metabolism and affects placental, embryonic, and foetal growth and development (King 2006) and increases the susceptibility of the child to components of the metabolic syndrome (Taylor and Poston 2007; Bruce and Byrne 2009; Armitage et al. 2008; Nakamura and Omaye 2012). Epigenetic changes occur during early foetal development when mothers suffer malnutrition during pregnancy. Their children are more likely to develop metabolic syndrome, diabetes, obesity, and cardiovascular disease. In addition, the grandchildren of malnourished mothers are more likely to be low weight at birth, regardless of the nutritional status of their mothers (www. themedicalbiochemistrypage.org 1996–2012). In addition, undernutrition in early life is associated with increased likelihood the child will develop other chronic conditions besides diabetes (Ferreira et al. 2018). It also increases susceptibility to infection and micro-and macronutrient deficiencies. Conversely, undernutrition can also lead to obesity. Overnutrition leads to obesity, immunoactivation, and susceptibility to inflammatory diseases such as diabetes and other chronic diseases (Dandona et al. 2010). Likewise, *Helicobacter pylori* may predispose individuals to diabetes (Jeon et al. 2012). Jeon et al. followed 800 Latino nondiabetic adults over age 60 for 10 years; 144 developed diabetes. People who tested positive for *Helicobacter pylori* were 2.7 times more likely to develop diabetes compared to other infections.
- Hyperinsulinaemia, which occurs in the presence of insulin resistance and exaggerates the proliferative effects of the MAP-kinase pathway.
- Procoagulent state: elevated plasma fibrinogen and plasminogen activator inhibitor-1 (PAI-1).
- Vascular abnormalities include increased urinary albumin excretion and endothelial dysfunction, which affect vascular permeability and tone.
- Both overnutrition and infection induce inflammation. Dietary fats and sugars can induce inflammation by activating an innate immune receptor, Toll-like receptor 4 (TLR4) (Nakamura and Omaye 2012). Recent research suggests 'good' intestinal bacteria have a preventative role and pre- and probiotics help maintain healthy gut and immune systems (www. themedicalbiochemistrypage.org 1996–2012; Nakamura and Omaye 2012). Inflammatory markers such as cytokines, Interleukin, adhesion molecules and TNF-alpha alter endothelial function. C-reactive protein is a significant predictor of cardiovascular disease and possibly depression, and there is an association amongst diabetes, cardiovascular diseases, and depression. In fact, some experts suggest depression could be an independent risk factor for type 2 diabetes (Loyd et al. 1997) and accelerates the progression of coronary artery disease (Rubin 2002). Depression is associated with behaviours such as smoking, unhealthy eating, lack of exercise, and high alcohol intake, which predisposes the individual to obesity and type 2 diabetes. Peripheral cytokines induce cytokine production in the brain, which activates the hypothalamic–pituitary–adrenal axis and the stress response, which inhibits serotonin and leads to depression. Inflammation appears to be the common mediator amongst diabetes, cardiovascular disease, and depression (Lesperance and Frasure-Smith 2007; Bruce and Byrne 2009).
- Hyperuricaemia. More recently, liver enzymes such as sustained elevations of alanine aminotransferase (ALT) and gamma-glutamyl transferase (GGT), which are associated with nonalcoholic fatty liver disease and low adiponectin, have been associated with diabetes and cardiovascular disease. Therefore, the relationship is complex. Conversely, normal testosterone levels appear to be protective against diabetes in men, and low testosterone levels in men with diabetes are associated with a significantly increased risk of death (Jones 2011). In women, high testosterone indicates greater risk of developing diabetes: high oestradiol levels confer increased diabetes risk in both men and women (American Diabetes Association 2007).

Consequences of the metabolic syndrome include:

- A fivefold increased risk of type 2 diabetes
- A two- to threefold increased risk of cardiovascular disease (myocardial events, stroke, and peripheral vascular disease)
- Increased mortality, which is greater in men but women with type 2 diabetes have a greater risk than nondiabetic women
- Increased susceptibility to conditions such as:
  - GDM
  - Foetal malnutrition
  - Polycystic ovarian syndrome (PCOS)
  - Fatty liver
  - Gallstones
  - Periodontal disease
  - Asthma
  - Sleep problems
  - Some forms of cancer

The risk of developing cardiovascular disease and type 2 diabetes increases significantly if three or more risk factors are present (Eckel et al. 2005; ADA 2019).

Metabolic syndrome in children and adolescents

The prevalence of metabolic syndrome in children and adolescents is usually extrapolated from adult definitions and may not be accurate. However, it is vital that children and adolescents at risk of developing the metabolic syndrome be identified early. Future risk appears to be influenced in utero and early childhood by factors such as GDM, low birthweight, feeding habits in childhood, genetic predisposition, and socioeconomic factors (Burke et al. 2005; Nakamura and Omaye 2012).

The IDF proposed that the metabolic syndrome should not be diagnosed before age 10, but children at risk should be closely monitored, especially if there is a family history of metabolic syndrome, diabetes, dyslipidaemia, cardiovascular disease, hypertension and obesity, and preventative strategies should be implemented (Weiss and Caprio 2005; Zimmet et al. 2007).

In the 10- to 16-year-old age range, diagnostic features are waist circumference >90th percentile, triglycerides >1.7 mmol/l, HDL-c > 1.03 mmol/l, glucose >5.6 mmol/l (oral glucose tolerance test (OGGT) is recommended), systolic blood pressure > 130 mmHg and diastolic >85 mmHg. Adult criteria are recommended for adolescents over 16 years. The long-term impact on morbidity and mortality will emerge as young people with the metabolic syndrome become adults. However, heart disease may be apparent in children as young as 10 and early onset of type 2 diabetes in adolescents is associated with more rapid progression of complications than occurs in type 1 (Sørgjerd et al. 2018).

Management of the metabolic syndrome in children and adults consists of primary prevention through population-based strategies aimed at early detection, regular follow-up of at-risk individuals and personalised education. Primary prevention encompasses at least annual monitoring for risk factors using tools such as AUSDRISK, UK Know Your Risk, and the ADA Risk Test, which all monitor similar parameters. Those at high risk (HbA1c 5.7–6.4% (39–47 mmol/mol), impaired glucose tolerance or impaired fasting glucose) should be referred to prevention programmes and assessed for conditions associated with diabetes. These programmes focus on lifestyle and behaviour changes to manage weight, increase exercise, and eat a healthy diet (ADA 2019). Technology interventions such as apps to monitor activity and coaching can be helpful.

Secondary prevention concentrates on preventing the progression to diabetes and cardiovascular disease. Therefore, early detection is imperative because many people with type 2 diabetes have complications at diagnosis. Lasting effects demonstrating reduced cardiovascular and type 2 diabetes risk have been demonstrated in studies such as the Diabetes Prevention Program (DPP), the Finnish Diabetes Prevention Study (DPS), and the Da Quing IGT and Diabetes Study. These studies showed the importance of multidisciplinary team care, modifying lifestyle factors that contribute to obesity by improving diet and activity levels to reduce weight (10% body weight in the long term), and stopping smoking. Some programmes include health coaching, but it has not been demonstrated that the benefits outweigh the costs of such programmes (Twigg et al. 2007). The Transformational Model of Change is frequently used to implement preventative strategies.

Medicines might be required for secondary prevention – for example, to control blood glucose and lower lipids, antihypertensives such as statins, and weight management medicines in addition to lifestyle modification. Several medicines have been shown to reduce the incidence of diabetes in people with the metabolic syndrome. These include Metformin 850 mg, which showed a 31% risk reduction in the DPP; 100 mg of Acarbose TDS by 25% after three years (STOP-NIDDM). Rosiglitazone reduced the risk of prediabetes progressing to diabetes by 60% over three years in the DREAM study, but it has since been associated with increased risk of MI. Poiglitizone might increase the risk of bladder cancer; the risk appears to be higher with long duration of use (NPS 2012) (see Chapter 5). Orlistat, an intestinal lipase inhibitor taken TDS, reduced the risk of progression to diabetes in obese adults with metabolic syndrome by 37% over four years (XENDOS study). However, compliance with Orlistat is low due to the side effects; see Chapter 5.

The macrovascular risk factors need to be managed proactively and screening programmes are imperative, so abnormalities are identified and treated early; see Chapter 8. A 75 g OGGT may be performed initially to diagnose the metabolic syndrome and repeated after 12 months to determine whether glucose tolerance changed. Then the test interval can be increased to every two to three years (WHO 1999). If an individual demonstrates significant weight gain and their random blood glucose is high when fasting, these parameters may be diagnostic; however, OGGT still may be performed earlier. Increasingly, random and fasting blood glucose levels of HbA1c are used to screen for risk with a relevant diabetes risk assessment tool.

The Consensus Development Conference on Antipsychotic Drugs and Obesity and Diabetes (American Diabetes Association et al. 2004) recommended monitoring people on antipsychotic medicines, including:

- BMI at baseline and every visit for six months, then quarterly, and treat if weight increases by one BMI unit.
- Blood glucose and lipids at baseline; if weight increases by 7%, then annually.
- HbA$_{1c}$ four months after starting antipsychotic medicines and then annually in people with metabolic syndrome or diabetes risk factors.

Types of diabetes

Type 1 diabetes

Type 1 diabetes is a disease of absolute insulin deficiency that usually affects children and young adults but can occur in older people, where it usually manifests as LADA, see the following section. Recent research has indicated that insulin resistance is also a feature in lean people with uncomplicated type 1 diabetes (Donga et al. 2013). However, Donga et al.'s sample was small, eight people using insulin pumps and eight healthy controls matched for age, gender, and BMI; thus, the clinical relevance of the finding is not clear.

The symptoms usually occur over a short space of time (two to three weeks) following a subclinical prodromal period of varying duration where the beta cells are destroyed. The precipitating event may have occurred many years prior to the development of the symptoms. Type 1 diabetes can be due to an autoimmune or idiopathic process. Various researchers have demonstrated that exogenous factors play a role in the development of type 1 diabetes on the basis that

<10% of susceptible people develop diabetes and <40% of monozygotic twins both develop diabetes, the >10-fold increase in the incidence of type 1 diabetes in European Caucasians in the last 50 years, and migration studies that show the incidence of type 1 has risen in people who migrated from low- to high-incidence regions (Knip et al. 2005). This is known as the trigger-bolster hypothesis. Seasonal variations in incidence of new diagnosis occur.

The EURODIAB sub-study 2 study group researchers (EUROBIAB 1999) suggested low plasma 25-hydroxyvitamin D may be implicated in the development of type 1 diabetes (1999). Later, Stene and Joner (2003) suggested there was no link between vitamin D supplementation and lower rates of type 1 diabetes. A systematic review and meta-analysis of observational studies and a meta-analysis of cohort studies undertaken in 2008 suggest vitamin D supplementation in early childhood might reduce the risk of type 1 diabetes by 30% (Zipitis and Akobeng 2008). A recent prospective study in Spain identified a significant inverse association between vitamin D and risk of type 2 diabetes (Gonzalez-Molero et al. 2012). However, randomised controlled trials are required to clarify whether there is a causal link and the optimal vitamin D dose, duration of treatment, and the best time to begin using vitamin D supplements.

As indicated earlier in this chapter, and in Chapter 13, a range of other environmental triggers has been implicated in the development of type 1 such as potatoes, cow's milk, and various viruses. Thus, the cause of type 1 diabetes appears to be multifactorial due to a combination of genetic predisposition and a diabetogenic trigger that induces an immune response, which selectively destroys pancreatic beta cells. Islet cell antibodies (ICA), glutamic acid carboxylase (GAD), or tyrosine phosphatase (IA-2A) antibodies are present in 85% of cases.

Type 1 diabetes in children usually presents with the classic symptoms of diabetes mellitus, shown below, but can present differently in older people:

- Polyuria
- Polydipsia
- Lethargy
- Weight loss
- Hyperglycaemia
- Glycosuria
- Blood and urinary ketones

In severe cases, the person presents with diabetic ketoacidosis (DKA) (see Chapter 7). Bed-wetting may be a consequence of hyperglycaemia in children (and older people). Classically, insulin secretion does not improve after treatment, but tissue sensitivity to insulin usually does.

Figure 1.2 is a schematic representation of the progression of type 1 diabetes. It shows the progressive relentless destruction of the beta cells from the time of the initial triggering event. Of first-degree relatives of people with type 1 diabetes, 5–10% have beta cell antibodies, usually with normal glucose tolerance, and some progress to diabetes.

Research suggests early infant feeding could be associated with the development of type 1 diabetes-related autoantibodies such as GAD, 1A-2A with a male preponderance, and is more common in children of mothers with type 2 diabetes or coeliac disease and with short-term breastfeeding (Ziegler et al. 2003; Wahlberg et al. 2006) (Chapter 13).

Latent autoimmune diabetes (LADA)

LADA is a genetically linked autoimmune disorder that occurs in about 10% of people who are often initially diagnosed with type 2 diabetes. LADA prevalence varies amongst ethnic groups (www.actionlada.org). LADA has some features of both types 1 and 2 diabetes. The UKPDS (1998) identified that 1 in 10 adults aged between 25 and 65 presumed to have type 2 diabetes were GADAb positive, and these findings have been evident in other studies (Zinman et al. 2004). LADA often presents as type 2 but has many of the genetic and immune features of type 1 (see the previous section and Table 1.2).

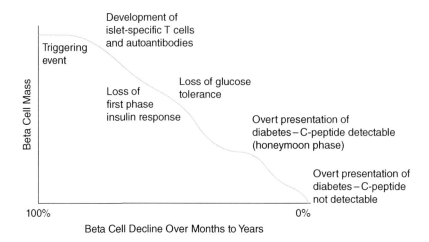

Figure 1.2   Schematic representation of the slow progressive loss of beta cell mass following the initial trigger event in type 1 diabetes.

Table 1.2   Classification of single gene mutations resulting in Maturity Onset Diabetes of the Young (MODY).

Genetic variety	Prevalence: % of overall MODY gene mutations depending on the populations studied	Features
HNFIA	30–50%	Common mutation
		Progressive beta cell failure
		> 5 mmol/l BG rise at two hours on OGTT (75 g)
		Sensitive to sulphonylureas
GCK	30–50%	Common mutation
		Elevated fasting BG with small, <3 mmol/l, rise at 2 hours on OGTT (75 g) Mild hyperglycaemia and may not require treatment
HNF-4A	5%	Similar presentation to HNF1A Associated with higher birthweight Transient neonatal hyperglycaemia Progressive beta cell failure Sensitive to sulphonylureas
HNF1B	5%	Associated with renal disease Urogenital tract abnormalities in girls
ᵃINS	< 1%	Varied clinical presentation Usually present with neonatal diabetes but can present in childhood and early adulthood
ᵃIPF1	< 1%	Average age at diagnosis 35 years
ᵃNUEROD1	< 1%	Vary rare
		Similar to type 2 diabetes
		Onset mid-20s Development of beta cell failure and reduced insulin production May be overweight
ᵃCEL	< 1%	Very rare Due to exocrine pancreatic dysfunction but pathophysiology is unknown
		Adult onset about age 36
ᵃPAX4	< 1%	Vary rare

Source: Data from Rice et al. (2012).
ᵃ fewer than five families reported with the genes.

People with LADA had a different clinical course from type 2 diabetes: in a six-year follow-up in the UKPDS, 84% of people with GADA required insulin compared to 14% of antibody-negative people. LADA is primarily an insulin deficiency state, where type 2 has a long progression to insulin and is characterised by insulin resistance. The clinical features also resemble type 1 in that people with LADA are not usually obese, are often symptomatic, and do not have a family history of type 2 diabetes.

However, GADA appears to have a bimodal distribution in LADA identifying two LADA subgroups with different, distinct clinical, autoimmune, and genetic features. People with high GADA titers are younger, leaner, insulin deficient, have lower C-peptide and high HbA1c, higher prevalence of other diabetes-specific autoantibodies, or other autoimmune diseases such as thyroid disease, and lower prevalence of metabolic syndrome than people with LADA and low GADA titers (Buzzetti et al. 2007).

There are no current guidelines for managing LADA (Cermea et al. 2003), although an expert panel convened by the ADA suggested C-peptide response is an appropriate measure of beta cell function and response to treatment. Management depends on the GADA titers and clinical presentation and should be individualised. Management considerations include the following:

- Lean people presenting with type 2 diabetes are tested for autoantibodies, especially GADA and C-peptide to correctly diagnose LADA, which is treat appropriately with insulin to prevent episodes of ketoacidosis (Niskanen et al. 1995; Cermea et al. 2003).
- Insulin is introduced early to support insulin secretion and protect the remaining beta cells (Cernea et al. 2003). Sulphonylureas appear to achieve similar or worse glycaemic control than insulin alone and lead to the early need for insulin. Thus, sulphonylureas are not recommended as first-line treatment (Cremea et al. 2003).
- Thiazolidediones may have a beta cell protective/augmentative effect, but their benefit in LADA has not been demonstrated and the contraindications need to be considered.
- Metformin may be contraindicated because insulin resistance is not always a feature of LADA and because of the potential risk of lactic acidosis in susceptible people (Chapter 5).
- Diet and exercise are relevant to the individual and the treatment mode.
- Stress management and regular complication screening and mental health assessment are necessary (as per types 1 and 2 diabetes).
- Appropriate education and support are vital.

Type 2 diabetes

Type 2 diabetes is not 'just a touch of sugar' or 'mild diabetes'. It is a *serious*, insidious progressive disease that is often diagnosed late when complications are present. Therefore, population screening and preventative education programmes are essential. Type 2 diabetes often presents with an established long-term complication of diabetes such as neuropathy, cardiovascular disease, or retinopathy. Alternatively, diabetes may be diagnosed during another illness or on routine screening. The classic symptoms associated with type 1 diabetes are often less obvious in type 2 diabetes. However, once diabetes is diagnosed and treatment instituted, people often state they have more energy and are less thirsty. Other subtle signs of type 2 diabetes, especially in older people, include recurrent candida and urinary tract infections, incontinence, constipation, symptoms of dehydration, and cognitive changes, particularly in information processing speed and executive function (Spauwen et al. 2013). As indicated, insulin resistance often precedes type 2 diabetes.

Insulin resistance is the term given to an impaired biological response to both endogenous and exogenous insulin that can be improved with weight loss and exercise. Insulin resistance is a stage in the development of impaired glucose tolerance. When insulin resistance is present, insulin production is increased (hyperinsulinaemia) to sustain normal glucose tolerance; however, the hepatic glucose output is not suppressed and fasting hyperglycaemia and decreased postprandial glucose utilisation results in postprandial hyperglycaemia.

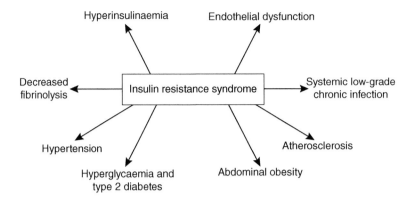

Figure 1.3   Some consequences of the insulin resistance syndrome. These factors lead to increased morbidity and mortality unless diabetes is diagnosed early treatment commenced.

Insulin resistance is a result of a primary genetic defect and secondary environmental factors (Turner and Clapham 1998). When intracellular glucose is high, FFAs are stored. When it is low, FFAs enter the circulation as substrates for glucose production. Insulin normally promotes tryglyceride synthesis and inhibits postprandial lipolysis. Glucose uptake into adipocytes is impaired in the metabolic syndrome, and type 2 diabetes and circulating FFAs as well as hyperglycaemia have a harmful effect on hepatic glucose production and insulin sensitivity. Eventually, the beta cells do not respond to glucose (glucose toxicity). Loss of beta cell function is present in over 50% of people with type 2 diabetes at diagnosis (United Kingdom Prospective Study [UKPDS] 1998) (Figure 1.2). Figure 1.3 depicts the consequences of insulin resistance.

Insulin is secreted in two phases: an effective first phase is essential to limit the postprandial rise in blood glucose. The first phase is diminished or lost in type 2 diabetes, leading to elevated postprandial blood glucose levels (Dornhorst 2001; IDF 2011). Postprandial hyperglycaemia, >7.8 mmol/l two hours after a meal, contributes to the development of atherosclerosis, hypertriglyceridaemia and coagulant activity, endothelial dysfunction, and hypertension, is a strong predictor of cardiovascular disease, and contributes to the development of other diabetes complications (Ceriello 2003; IDF 2011).

Interestingly, the beta cells do respond to other secretagogues, in particular sulphonylurea medicines.

The net effect of these abnormalities is sustained hyperglycaemia as a result of:

- Impaired glucose utilisation (IGT)
- Reduced glucose storage as glycogen
- Impaired suppression of glucose-mediated hepatic glucose production
- FPG
- Reduced postprandial glucose utilisation leading to postprandial hyperglycemia

Various tools and risk calculators are used to detect type 2 diabetes. They encompass some or all of the following risk factors (Abassi et al. 2012; Australian Government Department of Health 2010; ADA 2019):

- Individuals have the metabolic syndrome.
- Abdominal obesity, increased BMI, and high waist-hip ratio (>1.0 in men and >0.7 in women) are all risk factors. The limitations of the waist circumference in some ethnic groups are outlined later in the chapter. Elevated FFAs inhibit insulin signalling and glucose transport (see Figure 1.4) and are a source of metabolic fuel for the heart and liver. Binge eating precedes type 2 diabetes in many people and could be one of the causes of obesity; however, the prevalence of eating disorders is similar in types 1 and 2 diabetes (Herpertz et al. 1998).

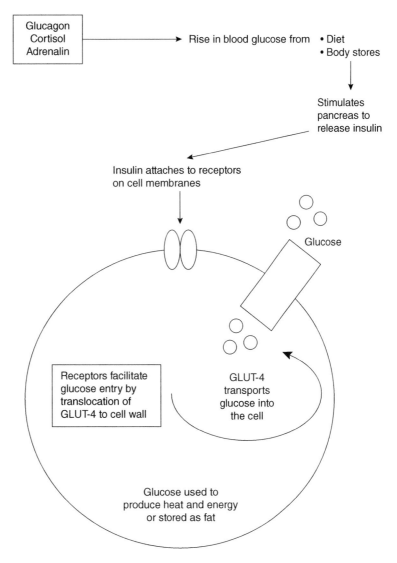

Figure 1.4 Simplistic diagrammatic representation of insulin binding, insulin signalling, translocation of GLUT-4 and glucose entry into the cell. GLUT-4 is a glucose transporter contained in vesicles in the cell cytoplasm. Once insulin binds to an insulin receptor GLUT-4 moves to the cell membrane and transports glucose into the cell. During fasting GLUT-4 is low and increases in response to the increase in insulin. Failure of GLUT-4 translocation could explain some of the insulin resistance associated with type 2 diabetes. The effects of insulin are mediated by two protein pathways: P13-kinase through the insulin receptors (glucose uptake) and MAP-kinase, which stimulates growth and mitogenesis.

- Risk increases for people over 40 years of age, but note the increasing prevalence in younger people (see also Chapter 13).
- Individuals are closely related to people with diabetes.
- Women who have had GDM or who had large babies in previous pregnancies are at greater risk.
- The children of a woman who had GDM, maternal obesity or maternal malnutrition are at greater risk.
- High levels of sedentary time is associated with 117% increase in the relative risk of type 2 diabetes and 147% increase in the risk of cardiovascular disease and 49% increased risk of all-cause mortality (Wilmot et al. 2012). Occupational sitting time also represents increased risk of type 2 diabetes (van Ufelen et al. 2010).

Other metabolic syndrome-associated risk factors for type 2 diabetes include active and former smoking and acanthosis nigricans, which is associated with hyperinsulinaemia (Kong et al. 2007). Baseline and progressive hypertension are independent predictors of type 2 diabetes (Conen et al. 2007). Insulin lack might be partly due to the enzyme PK Cepsilon (PKCe), which is activated by fat and reduces insulin production. Future medicines may target this deficiency and restore normal insulin function (Biden 2007).

Swedish researchers Mahdi et al. (2012) demonstrated that people with high serum secreted frizzled-related protein 4 (SFRP4) have a fivefold increased risk of developing diabetes in the following five years. SFR4 plays a role in the inflammatory process, and its release from islet cells is stimulated by interleukin-1β. High-serum SFRP4 reduces glucose tolerance. SFRP4 is elevated several years before type 2 diabetes is diagnosed, indicating it could be a useful risk marker for type 2 diabetes independent of other risk factors.

Vitamin D deficiency may also be a risk factor for diabetes independent of other risk factors in longititudinal studies such as the Australian Obesity and Lifestyle (AusDiab) study (Gagnon et al. 2011). Given the increasing information about the complexity of type 2 diabetes pathophysiology, it is unlikely that any single intervention will prevent or treat the disease effectively; thus, it is not clear whether vitamin D supplementation is likely to modify diabetes risk. Vitamin D deficiency is very common and is also a marker of general health status and may be indicated to manage other concomitant conditions such as osteoporosis.

The characteristics of type 1 and type 2 diabetes are shown in Table 1.3.

Table 1.3 Generally agreed characteristics of type 1 and type 2 diabetes mellitus. However, type 2 is a very heterogeneous disease and can occur at any age, and type 1 diabetes can be first diagnosed in older age.

	Type 1	Type 2
Age at onset	Usually <30 years[a]	Usually >40 years. But increasing prevalence in children and adolescents
Speed of onset	Usually rapid	Usually gradual and insidious
Body weight	Normal or underweight; often recent weight loss	80% are overweight
Heredity	Associated with specific human leukocyte antigen (HLA-DR3 or 4)[b]	No HLA association
		Genetic predisposition, which is complex and only beginning to be understood
	Autoimmune disease and environmental triggers	Environmental and lifestyle factors contribute
Insulin	Early insulin secretion	Often preceded by the metabolic syndrome (see section on the metabolic syndrome).
	Impaired later; may be totally absent	Insulin resistance is reversible if appropriate diet and exercise regimens are instituted.
		Type 2 is associated with slow, progressive loss of beta cell function.
Ketosis	Common	Rare
Symptoms	Usually present	Often absent, especially in the early stages. Acanthosis nigricans is common in some ethnic peoples.
Frequency	~15% of diagnosed cases	~85% of diagnosed cases
Complications	Common but not usually present at diagnosis	Common, often present at diagnosis
Treatment	Insulin, diet, exercise, stress management, regular health and complication assessment	Diet, GLM, exercise, insulin, stress management, regular health, and complication assessment

[a] Increasing incidence of the metabolic syndrome and type 2 diabetes in children and adolescents.
[b] Occurs in older people; see LADA.

Management is discussed in Chapter 2. The majority of people with type 2 diabetes require multiple therapies to target the multiple underlying metabolic abnormalities and achieve and maintain acceptable blood glucose and lipid targets over the first nine years after diagnosis (UKPDS 1998). Between 50% and 70% eventually require insulin, which is often used in combination with other GLMs, which means diabetes management becomes progressively more complicated for people with type 2 diabetes, often coinciding with increasing age when their ability to manage may be compromised, which increases the likelihood of nonadherence and the costs of managing the disease for the patient and the health system.

Type 2 diabetes in indigenous children and adolescents

Type 2 diabetes in children and adolescents is discussed in Chapter 13, but it is a significant problem in indigenous children and adolescents. Indigenous Australians, like other indigenous peoples, are at high risk of type 2 diabetes, especially when they live in remote communities, and it develops at a younger age (Mingea et al. 2011). Onset is often in early adolescence and frequently asymptomatic. Indigenous children and adolescents with diabetes usually have a family history of type 2 diabetes, are overweight, and have signs of hyperinsulinaemia and acanthosis nigricans. There is a high prevalence of misrovascular and macrovascular complications and the associated morbidity and mortality (Azzopardi et al. 2012).

A number of causative factors are implicated including intrauterine exposure to risk during maternal pregnancy, obesity, physical inactivity, genetic predisposition, and socioeconomic and environmental factors. Consequently, experts recommend screening Aboriginal and Torres Strait Islander children over age 10 for metabolic syndrome and diabetes. The IDF (2011) criteria for diagnosing type 2 diabetes in indigenous children and adolescents are:

- Random laboratory venous blood glucose (BG) >10 mmol/l and polyuria and polydipsia especially when the symptoms occur at night; OR
- Fasting laboratory venous BG > 7 mmol/l performed after fasting for at least eight hours; OR
- Random laboratory plasma BG 0.11.1 mmol/l on at least two separate occasions.

Oral glucose tolerance tests (OGTT) are not practical in many remote indigenous communities. Point-of-care HbA1c might be an alternative, but no clear diagnostic recommendations are available for children. Ketones should be checked in newly diagnosed indigenous children to ensure treatment is appropriate. Management should be individualised, taking into account the psychosocial factors that influence adherence.

Gestational diabetes

Diabetes occurring during pregnancy is referred to as GDM. GDM occurs in about 5% of all pregnancies (Rice et al. 2012). The incidence of GDM is increasing with the global obesity epidemic. GDM refers to carbohydrate intolerance of varying degrees that first occurs or is first recognised during pregnancy. Several factors have been implicated in the development of GDM including diet and lifestyle, smoking, some medicines, older age, genetic background, ethnicity, number of previous pregnancies and recently, short stature (Langer 2006).

People at risk of GDM should be screened for diabetes using standard diagnostic criteria at the first prenatal visit. High-risk women have impaired fasting glucose (5.6–6.9 mmol/l) and/or impaired glucose tolerance (2-hour OGTT 7.8–11.0 mmol/l). Women with HbA1c 5.7–6.4% are also at increased risk (Rice et al. 2012). For more information about GDM, refer to Chapter 14.

Maturity onset diabetes of the young (MODY)

MODY is a rare heterogeneous group of disorders that result in beta cell dysfunction. MODY can develop at any age up to 55. It has a genetic basis and at least nine different genes that result in the MODY phenotype, which suggests MODY is a single entity. MODY accounts for 1–2% of people diagnosed with diabetes, but the prevalence could be underestimated because population-based screening programmes have not been performed (Gardner and Tai 2012). The different genetic aetiologies vary in age at onset, hyperglycaemia pattern, response to treatment, and extra-pancreatic manifestations. The varieties of MODY are shown in Table 1.2.

People with MODY often have a strong family history of diabetes, insulin independence, no insulin autoantibodies and evidence of endogenous insulin production, low insulin requirement, and generally do not become ketotic (McDonald et al. 2011). However, there are distinct phenotypes that might present differently. Treatment depends on the MODY type but generally includes GLMs, diet, and exercise, although insulin might eventually be required. HNFIA individuals are very sensitive to sulphonylureas.

MODY can be difficult to recognise and the diagnosis missed or delayed (Appleton and Hattersley 1996). This can have implications for the individual and their family in commencing appropriate treatment for the specific type of MODY. Genetic counselling is also advisable.

Practice points

(1) MODY is a different disease process from type 2 diabetes that occurs in young people and has a different genetic and inheritance pattern from type 2.
(2) The prevalence of type 2 diabetes in children is increasing and is associated with obesity and insulin resistance (Sinha et al. 2002).
(3) MODY has been misdiagnosed as type 1 diabetes and insulin commenced unnecessarily.
(4) MODY has also been diagnosed instead of type 1 diabetes in the United Kingdom (Health Service Ombudsman 2000).
(5) Type 2 diabetes is a serious, insidious life-threatening disease.

These points demonstrate the importance of taking a careful clinical history and undertaking appropriate diagnostic investigations.

Diagnosing diabetes

Urine glucose tests should not be used to diagnose diabetes; if glycosuria is detected, the blood glucose should be tested. When symptoms of diabetes are present, an elevated blood glucose alone is often sufficient to confirm the diagnosis. See Table 1.4 for diagnostic criteria.

If the person is asymptomatic, abnormal fasting blood glucose values of >7 mmol/l should be demonstrated on at least two occasions before the diagnosis is made (note that some guidelines suggest >6.5 mmol/l). Random plasma glucose >11.1 mmol/l and symptoms are diagnostic of type 2 diabetes. An OGTT using a 75 g glucose load may be indicated to determine the presence of glucose intolerance if results are borderline. The criteria for diagnosing diabetes according to the WHO are shown in Table 1.3. A protocol for preparing the patient and performing an OGTT are outlined later in the chapter. However, some experts suggest 75 g may be too high a load for some ethnic groups such as Vietnamese.

Abnormal plasma glucose identifies a subgroup of people at risk of diabetes-related complications. The risk data for these complications is based on the two-hour OGTT plasma glucose level. However, the fasting glucose of >7.8 mmol/l does not equate with the two-hour level used to diagnose diabetes. Recently, the ADA and the WHO lowered the fasting level to 7.0 mmol/l to more closely align it to the two-hour level.

WHO continues to advocate routine OGTT screening in at-risk individuals to identify people at risk of complications early, in order for early treatment to be instituted. The ADA does not advocate routine OGTT use because it believes that the revised fasting level is sensitive enough to detect most people at risk. Therefore, there could be differences internationally about the

Table 1.4 Diagnostic criteria for non-pregnant adults with diabetes based on the World Health Organization (WHO) and the American Diabetes Association (ADA) Guidelines.

Stage	Fasting plasma glucose	Random plasma glucose	Oral glucose tolerance test (OGTT)
Normal	< 6.1 mmol/l		2-hour plasma glucose <7.8 mmol/l
Impaired glucose tolerance	Impaired fasting glucose – fasting glucose ≥6.1 and <7.0 mmol/l		Impaired glucose tolerance – 2-hour plasma glucose ≥7.8 and <11.1 mmol/l
Diabetes	≥ 7.0 mmol/l	≥ 11.1 mmol/l and symptoms	2-hour plasma glucose >11.1 mmol/l

Note: In this table venous plasma glucose values are shown. Glucose in capillary blood is about 10–15% higher than venous blood. HbA1c can be used to make the diagnosis instead of or as well as venous blood glucose; >6.5% in a laboratory using certified assay method standardised to DCCT criteria.

routine use of the OGTT. The ADA and WHO do agree on how the test should be performed. Australia supports the continued use of the OGTT when the diagnosis is equivocal and to detect GDM (Hilton et al. 2002; Twigg et al. 2007). However, OGTT may not always be practical in remote communities (Azzopardi et al. 2012).

A recent study suggested untrained people could perform self-administered OGTT in the community setting using a specific device (*n* = 18 people without diabetes and 12 with type 2) OGTT were performed unaided in the home twice, unaided but observed in the clinic and one OGGT/participant was perfumed by a nurse. The results were verified with simultaneous laboratory values of the 0 and 120-minute samples (Bethel et al. 2013). A data recorder attached to the test device recorded information about the test. Device failures meant 0 and 120 minutes BG was only available for 141/180 OGTTs independent of the test setting. Self-performed and laboratory values were similar and reproducible. The clinical implications are unclear at this time.

Other prevention measures include providing the public with information about screening and health maintenance programmes, and self-risk assessment lists, such as checklists from the Agency for Healthcare Research and Quality (AHRQ). Checklists can be downloaded from the Internet (http://www.ahrq.gov/ppip/healthywom.htm or http://www.ahrq.gov/ppip/helthymen.htm). The information is based on the US Preventative Services Task Force recommendations.

HbA1c has an accepted place in monitoring metabolic control in people with diabetes. In addition, the WHO, IDF, and the American Diabetes Association (ADA) recommend using HbA1c as screening test for type 2 diabetes. The Australian Diabetes Society (ADS), Royal College of Pathologists of Australasia, and the Australasian Association of Clinical Biochemists released a position statement in 2012 that recommended HbA1c be used to diagnose diabetes, if the analysis is performed in a laboratory that meets external quality assurance standards and recommended HbA1c >6.5% (48 mmol/mol) as the diagnostic cut point.

Point-of-care HbA1c tests are useful clinical decision-making tools, but they are not recommended for diagnosing diabetes. The ADS noted that HbA1c <6.5% (48 mmol/mol) does not exclude a diagnosis of diabetes based on existing fasting BG or OGTT criteria. The latter remain the diagnostic tests of choice for GDM, type 1 diabetes, and when people have conditions that affect the HbA1c result (d'Emden et al. 2012). In November 2012 a Medicare Consultation paper was released in Australia proposing a rebate of $16.90 when HbA1c was performed as a diagnostic test, but the rebate would be limited to one test per year per person; an additional confirmatory test would be covered if the result was ≥6.5% (48 mmol/mol). The rate of screening in primary care might increase if the rebate is introduced.

Advantages of HbA1c as a diagnostic test are that people do not need to fast before blood is collected and the test can be performed at any time of the day. HbA1c measures chronic glycaemia and HbA1c levels are strongly associated with retinopathy, macrovascular outcomes, and mortality (d'Emden et al. 2012). HbA1c assays are standardised and generally reliable in most countries. However, errors associated with nonglycaemic factors such as haemoglobinopathies and anaemia that affect HbA1c (increase or decrease) need to be considered when interpreting the findings (Saudek et al. 2008; Banerjee 2014).

Other markers of hyperglycaemia and diabetes risk include fructosamine, glycated albumin, and 1,5 anhydroglucitol (1,5-AG), which are associated with the development of diabetes independent of baseline HbA1c and fasting glucose (Juraschek et al. 2012). It is not clear what place these markers have in diagnosing or monitoring diabetes as yet, but they could be useful when HbA1c is not reliable, such as haemoglobinopathies. In fact, fructosamine is recommended in the latter situation.

Other experts suggests the combination of HbA1c 5.7–6.4% (39–46 mmol/mol) and fasting plasma glucose 5.6–6.9 mmol/l are likely to reduce the likelihood of missing a diagnosis of diabetes and be more likely to identify people with prediabetes (fasting plasma glucose 6.1–6.9 and HbA1c 6.0–6.4% (42–46 mmol/mol) who are likely to progress to diabetes (Heianza et al. 2012). Abikshyeet et al. (2012) suggested salivary glucose could be a useful noninvasive diagnostic and monitoring test for diabetes but acknowledged more research is needed before salivary glucose testing is adopted.

Most prediction models for the risk of developing type 2 diabetes appear to identify individuals at high and low risk of developing diabetes but extended models that include conventional biomarkers perform better. Some models overestimate risk (Abassi et al. 2012). Thus, it could be important to ensure the screening parameters such as BMI and glycaemic targets are relevant to the target population.

Oral glucose tolerance test (OGTT)

An OGTT is used to diagnose diabetes:

- When fasting and random blood glucose results are equivocal
- When there is a strong family history of diabetes, especially during pregnancy
- If the suspicion of diabetes is high but blood glucose tests are normal/equivocal

An OGTT should not be performed when the person:

- Is febrile
- Is acutely ill – for example, postoperatively or uraemic
- Has been immobilised for more than 48 hours
- Has symptoms of diabetes or an elevated blood glucose before commencing the test

Rationale for OGTT
Early diagnosis and treatment of diabetes reduces the morbidity and mortality associated with the hyperglycaemia.

Preparing the patient for an OGTT
(1) Follow test protocol in the place of work.
(2) Give specific oral and written instructions to the patient. A sample is given in Example Instruction Sheet 1 below.
(3) Ensure the diet contains at least 200 g/day carbohydrate for at least three to five days before the test.
(4) If possible, stop medicines that can influence the blood glucose levels three days before the test: some of these will need to be reduced gradually, e.g. corticosteroids (Chapter 10). People should be informed about the consequences of stopping their medicines and when to resume taking them after the test:
   - Thiazide diuretics
   - Antihypertensive medicines
   - Analgesic and anti-inflammatory medicines
   - Antineoplastic medicines
   - Corticosteroids

(5) Fast from 12 midnight, the night before the test.
(6) Avoid physical/psychological stress for one hour prior to, and during, the test.
(7) Avoid smoking for at least one hour prior to the test.
(8) Allow the patient to relax for 30 minutes before beginning the test.

Example Information Sheet for People Requiring and an OGTT

Date of test: **Name**:
Time: **I.D. label**

Location Where Test Will Take Place

(1) Please ensure that you eat high-carbohydrate meals each day for three days before the test. Carbohydrate foods are: breads, cereals, spaghetti, noodles, rice, dried beans and pulses, vegetables, fruit. These foods should constitute the major part of your diet for the three days.
(2) Have nothing to eat or drink after 12 midnight on the night prior to the test day, except water.
(3) Specific information about managing medicines: ....
(4) Bring a list of all the medications you are taking with you when you come for the test.
(5) Do not smoke for at least one hour before the test.

The Test

The test is performed in the morning. You are required to rest during the test, which will take approximately three hours to complete. A small needle will be inserted into an arm vein for blood sampling. The needle will stay in place until the test is completed. You will be given 300 ml of glucose to drink. This is very sweet but it is important to drink it all over the five minutes, so that the results of the test can be interpreted correctly. Water is permitted. You will be given a drink and something to eat when the test is finished. The doctor will discuss the results with you.

Information for clinicians: OGGT test protocol
(1) The person should rest during the test to avoid dislodging the cannula.
(2) Insert a cannula into a suitable vein for blood sampling, e.g. the cubical fossa.
(3) The blood glucose should be tested before commencing the test. If elevated, clarify with the doctor ordering the test before proceeding. Collect two millilitres of blood in fluoride oxalate tubes for laboratory analysis at each test time point.
(4) Flush the cannula with normal saline between samples to prevent clots forming in the cannula. One to two millilitres of blood should be withdrawn and discarded before collecting each sample to avoid contaminating the sample with saline left in the tubing.
(5) Collect blood samples at the following times. However, sometimes only a baseline (0) and a two-hour sample are collected:

minutes: −10
　　　　　　0
　　　　　　⇒　　75 g glucose, consumed over 5 minutes. Water can be given after the glucose is all consumed. It is very sweet and some people find it difficult to drink.
　　　　+30
　　　　+60
　　　+120

The glucose used for an OGTT is prepacked in 300 ml bottles containing exactly 75 g of glucose.
(6) Ensure the person has a follow-up appointment with the referring doctor whose responsibility it is to explain the test results and commence or arrange for appropriate management and education.

Screening for diabetes

Because of the insidious nature and increasing incidence and prevalence of type 2 diabetes, many countries have instituted population-based education and screening and/or case detection programmes in at-risk populations. Finger-prick blood glucose tests are not generally used to diagnose diabetes; see Table 1.3 for the diagnostic criteria. Many programmes also involve checking for obesity and cardiovascular risk factors. At-risk groups include:

- Age >55 years
- High-risk ethnic groups such as indigenous people, Southeast Asians, Indians from the subcontinent
- Women with PCOS
- Previous GDM
- Family history of diabetes
- People with symptoms, but symptoms are often absent in type 2 diabetes
- Older people > 65 years, but classic symptoms are often absent
- People with known diabetes complications such as cardiovascular disease, erectile dysfunction, and renal disease
- Active smokers (Willi et al. 2007)

Screening for type 1 diabetes is not usually necessary because it presents differently and has a more rapid onset and symptoms are usually present. First-degree relatives of people with type 1 diabetes can be tested for risk markers (autoantibodies) for diabetes, but the preventative strategies applicable to type 2 diabetes do not apply.

An example of one screening and preventative model of care is shown in Figure 1.5.

Practice point

Hyperglycaemia often occurs as a stress response to serious intercurrent illness such as cardiovascular disease, and it may be difficult to diagnose diabetes in such circumstances. However, controlling the blood glucose during the illness is important and leads to better outcomes, including in nondiabetics (Chapters 7 and 9).

Preventing diabetes

Preventing type 2 diabetes

A number of clinical trials have demonstrated that it is possible to prevent type 2 diabetes and may, in turn, prevent the associated morbidity from long-term complications. Most prevention trials were conducted amongst people with IGT because it is a strong predictor of type 2 diabetes. These programmes include the Da Qing Study (Pan et al. 1997), the Oslo Diet and Exercise Program, the Diabetes Prevention Program (DPP) (2002), and the Finnish Diabetes Prevention Study (DPS) (Lindström et al. 2003), which showed a 58% reduction in the progression to diabetes in people who followed a healthy lifestyle. The effects were still present at the four-year follow-up (Tuomilehto et al. 2001). The DPS was stopped early because the intervention was so successful, but the researchers continued to follow people who did not develop diabetes for up to 10 years. The intervention group achieved a reduction of about 40% compared to controls.

Elements of these programmes have been adapted and implemented in many countries since the findings were first published, especially the DPP. Examples include *Go for Your Life* and the Life Programme in Australia. However, a Cochrane review (Nield et al. 2008) stated, 'There is no

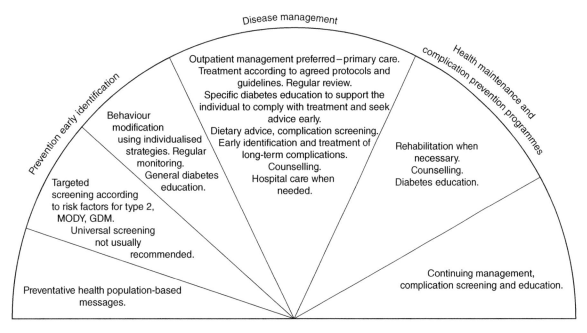

Figure 1.5   Example of a screening and preventative model of healthcare.

high quality data on the efficacy of dietary intervention for the prevention of type 2 diabetes'. Since causes of the metabolic syndrome and type 2 diabetes are complex and multifactorial, it is not surprising that dietary interventions in isolation are ineffective.

Key features of the DPS are weight reduction (~5%), reducing fat intake to <30%, with <10% coming from saturated fats, fibre intake of >15 g per 1000 cal and >30 minutes of moderate exercise per day. In the DPS, weight loss and exercise appeared to be more important than dietary goals in preventing diabetes. Achieving weight loss and making dietary changes is difficult, and only 2% of participants in the DPS achieved four or five targets but no participant who did so developed diabetes compared to 50% of the control group. Weight management strategies are discussed in Chapter 4.

Studies concentrating on increasing fibre and magnesium to prevent type 2 diabetes show inconsistent results despite current guidelines to increase the total fibre intake. The type of fibre consumed may be important in that soluble fibre may enhance gastric emptying and reduce the postprandial glucose rise. A meta-analysis revealed lower diabetes risk with increased intake of cereal fibre but no significant association with fruit and vegetable fibre. Thus, including whole grain foods is important in diabetes prevention diets (Krishnan et al. 2007) and, as indicated, pre- and probiotics are emerging as important considerations for gut health and preventing immune- and inflammatory-related diseases such as diabetes. An example of a screening and prevention model is shown in Figure 1.5.

Vegetarians appear to have reduced risk of metabolic syndrome and reduced risk of type 2 diabetes. Likewise, Mediterranean diets, whilst not strictly vegetarian, are generally high in fibre. Prebiotics and whole grains and are associated with reduced risk of type 2 diabetes. Avoiding liquid calories such as those in sugar-sweetened beverages, fruit juice, and alcohol appears to be important. These liquids also lead to dental caries. Rice is the staple food in many countries such as China where white rice is consumed at three to four times per day. The Glycaemic Index of white rice is higher than other whole grains and basmati type rice. Studies suggest the relative risk of developing diabetes is 1.11 for every serving of white rice consumed per day (Hu et al. 2012).

Many existing public health screening and prevention models fall into five main categories (Lang and Rayner 2012):

- Sanitary-environmental model.
- Biomedical model that can be individual or population focused.
- Social behavioural model, which rivals the biomedical model. It might not take account of who has the strongest influence on behaviour, which may be companies like Coca-Cola.
- Technoeconomic model, which views health as depending on economic growth and knowledge development.
- Ecological model, which focuses on interactions amongst factors that impact on health, including climate change, and integrates elements of the other four models. Climate change impacts on factors such as food security/availability, extreme weather events, which displace people and affect their lifestyle and social circumstances (IDF 2012).

The relative merits of these models have not been tested but current policies do not appear to be halting the exponential rise in the prevalence of the metabolic syndrome and diabetes. In fact, Simmons et al. (2012) suggested screening for diabetes does not reduce deaths. The researchers followed a cohort of nearly 12 000 people at high risk of diabetes for 10 years and found they were no more likely to have died than 4000 people who were not screened, and there were no significant differences between the two groups for deaths specifically attributable to diabetes. Interestingly, benefits for microvascular disease were not analysed. It is unlikely that screening alone *would* reduce risk unless relevant prevention strategies were used and early diagnosis and management incorporated into the model. Likewise, population-wide prevention may not reduce health-care spending because it does not reduce the risk of serious illness or premature death, because of the number of people who need to receive a particular preventive treatment to prevent a single illness (Begley 2013). Targeted prevention programmes that incorporate environmental and social factors and collaborating with local government and religious institutions and other key stakeholders need to be part of prevention programmes.

Two European projects DE-PLAN and IMAGE are addressing implementation processes for DPPs and developing a toolkit to help people develop and implement programmes for preventing type 2 diabetes. The kit includes a practical guideline that targets everybody who could have a role in prevention, such as health professionals, teachers, traditional healers, and politicians, it explains key aspects of financial management, how to identify people at risk, as well as educating and training key personnel, and monitoring and quality assurance processes that need to be addressed. It will be interesting to determine whether the toolkit makes a difference in actual practice, since many prevention programmes already encompass all the elements in the toolkit, including education.

One important factor that might lead to changes is the Global Monitoring Framework (GMF) for noncommunicable disease, which was agreed in November 2012 between the WHO and national governments. The GMF is ambitious and has been dubbed '25 by 25' in recognition of the first target, which is to reduce NCD-related deaths by 25% by 2025. Other targets include reducing the:

- increase in diabetes and obesity;
- prevalence of inactivity by 10%;
- harmful use of alcohol by 10%;
- consumption of salt by 30%;
- prevalence of tobacco use by 30%;
- prevalence of hypertension by 25%.

Signatory countries to the agreement will be required to report their performance against the agreed targets in 2013. The targets reflect metabolic syndrome risk factors such as hypertension, inactivity, and smoking. Importantly, one target is to halt the increasing prevalence of diabetes and premature mortality from noncommunicable diabetes. Important proposed strategies to help meet the Global Framework is to ensure essential medicines and self-management preventative education are available (IDF 2012).

Research into the genetics that predispose people to insulin resistance and type 2 diabetes is ongoing and can help predict the risk for diabetes and better target prevention and management strategies. Significant progress has been made in identifying the variations in DNA sequence involved in the development of diabetes as part of the genome-wide study (GWAS). Sixty-five regions of the human genome associated with diabetes have been identified (Morris 2012); however, the effects of the variants are too subtle to be used as risk predictors at present.

Research to determine how beta cells and insulin-responsive tissues normally develop and function are also progressing, e.g. discovering the relationship between the FTP gene and obesity. Animal studies are underway to determine the mechanisms that affect appetite and metabolism and predispose to obesity. Genetic studies are increasing our understanding of the relationship between SHBG levels and diabetes risk. SHBG is a binding protein produced in the liver that transports testosterone, and to oestrogen to some extent, to target tissues. SHBG levels are often low in people with type 2 diabetes. Previously, researchers assumed that insulin resistance lowered SHBG, however genetic studies suggest low SHBG may have a causal role in type 2 diabetes (Ding et al. 2009).

Preventing type 1 diabetes

Research for the elusive cure for type 1 diabetes continues. Approaches include:

- Immune intervention using monoclonal antibodies to prevent the immune system destroying beta cells. People diagnosed early enough to still have some functioning beta cells receive a combination of medicine such as Teplizumab and Otelixizumab. The medicines protect the remaining beta cells and people may need less insulin. The results of clinical trials vary amongst countries. For example, in Europe and America young, slim people appear to benefit from the medicines; however, people from Asia derive less benefit. Genetic differences, age, and BMI might account for the different responses.
- Stem cells. Blood stem cells have been used in a similar way to treatment for leukaemia in Brazil. Radiation is used to destroy the immune system and fresh blood stem cells are infused to calm the immune system so it no longer destroys beta cells. Early clinical studies show 'promise'. The following is more specifically treatment, but it is relevant to stem cell research. In Australia, researchers have isolated stem cells in the adult pancreas and developed a technique to transform the stem cells into insulin-producing beta cells that release insulin in response to glucose. The hope is that people with type 1 diabetes may be able to regenerate their own beta cells if the immune attack that initially caused diabetes can be prevented.
- Reprogrammed liver cells are being researched in animal studies in Israel.

Managing diabetes mellitus

Key points

- The person with diabetes undertakes >90% of their diabetes management; thus, they are experts in *their* diabetes and their lives.
- Collaborative interdisciplinary team care is essential.
- Visits to health professionals occur at regular intervals and mostly concern assessing physical, psychological, and metabolic status and making treatment recommendations.
- Diabetes education is the cornerstone of management. The phrase generally refers to people with diabetes BUT it applies equally, if not more so to the health professionals who provide education and care for people with diabetes.
- It is essential to personalise care plans and develop them with the individual concerned.

Management strategies for specific aspects of care are discussed in almost every chapter of the book. This section deals with general management information.

Many 'diabetes care models' have been developed as the framework within which to provide diabetes care. These include the Chronic Disease Model and its derivations such as the Flinders Model used in some Australian states. Research suggests effective diabetes care models need to enable early diagnosis and coordinate diagnosis, treatment and ongoing management, and educate people with diabetes and their health professionals (Renders et al. 2012). Effective components of management programmes appear to be high frequency of contact with people with diabetes and ability for the people managing the disease (primarily the person with diabetes) to adjust their medicines and are more effective for people with inadequate glycaemic control (HbA1c >8% at baseline) (Pimouguet et al. 2010).

Diabetes education is an essential component of diabetes management and the benefit seems to apply equally to groups and individual education and combinations of both (Pimouguet et al. 2010) (Chapter 16).

The interdisciplinary diabetes team

Effective diabetes management depends on having a collaborative interdisciplinary healthcare team. The person with diabetes is the central player in the team. Good communication amongst team members is vital and information the individual with diabetes receives must be consistent between and within hospital departments, health services, and clinicians to ensure smooth transition amongst services and avoid confusing the individual with inconsistent information. The team usually consists of some or all of the following:

- Diabetologist
- Diabetes nurse specialist/diabetes educator and/or diabetes nurse practitioner
- Dietitian
- Podiatrist
- Social worker
- Psychologist
- General practitioner

Other professionals who contribute regularly to the diabetes management:

- Opthalmologist
- Optometrist
- Pharmacist
- Specialists such as geriatricians, vascular, and orthopaedic surgeons, neurologists, dentists/periodontists, urologists, dentist, palliative care experts, and audiologists
- Cultural/traditional health workers, for example, Aboriginal health workers in Australia and traditional healers in Canada and Africa
- Exercise physiologists
- Physiotherapists

The ward staff who care for the person in hospital and the community clinicians also become team members during presentations to hospital and emergency departments and care in home settings.

It is easy to understand why people with diabetes can be confused about health professional roles and responsibilities and about their own role and responsibilities in diabetes care if they receive conflicting information from health professionals.

Managing diabetes consists of dietary modification, regular exercise/activity, and in some cases, insulin or GLMs. Diabetes education and regularly assessing metabolic control and complication status is essential. In addition, general healthcare is very important and includes dental checks, mammograms, prostate checks, and preventative vaccinations, such as fluvax, and pneumovax. As indicated many times in this book, it is essential to personalise the care plan and individualise management targets to suit the person's risk status, social situation, and capabilities. Repetition is one important education strategy. Politicians and marketers also use it! Helping people manage their diabetes requires clinicians to be effective marketers, politicians, and communicators.

Aims of management

Diabetes management should be determined within the Quality Use of Medicine framework; see Chapter 4. Management aims for Australia are defined in the National Diabetes Strategy and a number of other specific guidelines such as those described in the ADS Position Statements, and Clinical Management Guidelines for Diabetes in General Practice. A range of other guidelines produced by various countries and diabetes associations such as the United Kingdom, Scotland, the United States, and the IDF, some of which are listed in this and other chapters in the book.

The aim of diabetes management is to maintain quality of life and keep the person free from the symptoms of diabetes, and the blood glucose and blood lipids within an acceptable range to prevent complications. The blood glucose range needs to be determined on an individual basis, usually between 4.0 and 6.0 mmol/l for 90% of tests, especially during acute illness and surgery, young people and during pregnancy and HbA1c <7% (Diabetes Australia [DA] and Royal Australian College of General Practitioners [RACGP] 2011/12), Table 1.5. However, higher targets might be more appropriate for people at risk of hypoglycaemia (Chapter 6), older people (Chapter 12), and children (Chapter 13). The aim is to obtain results as near as possible to the target blood glucose range, but there must be a balance between the food plan, medication (insulin/GLMs), and exercise/activity. Maintaining emotional well-being is essential (Chapter 1). General management goals (target ranges) are shown in Table 1.4.

The regimen should affect the person's lifestyle as little as possible, although some modification is usually necessary. People with type 1 require insulin in order to survive. Obese people with type 2 can sometimes be treated effectively with a combination of diet and exercise, but research suggests that people managed with diet are not as rigorously monitored and have more hyperglycaemia and hypertension than those on medicines (Hippisley-Cox and Pringle 2004). Many people with type 2 diabetes require GLMs and usually eventually insulin due to the progressive loss of beta cell function.

In the current person-centred empowerment model of diabetes care, the person with diabetes is the pivotal person in the management team. Forming a therapeutic partnership with the individual and accepting their choices is essential to achieving optimal outcomes. Putting the person at the centre of care means respecting their choices, even when the individual elects not to follow advice after receiving adequate information (informed decision-making). Not following advice

Table 1.5 Diabetes management targets; but note most current guidelines recommend targets be individualised according to specific microvascular, macrovascular, and hypoglycaemia risk (ADS 2012, 2019; DA/RACPG 2011/12).

Glucose: Fasting blood glucose 6–8 mmol/l; and 8–10 post prandial HbA$_{1c}$ <7% (53 mmol/mol)) up to 8% (64 mmol/mol) in older people with high risk of hypoglycaemia.

Lipids: LDL-c < 2.5 mmol/l; triglycerides <1.5 mmol/l; HDL-c > 1.3 mmol/l, total cholesterol <4.0 mmol/l

Blood pressure: 130/80 mmHg; 125/75 mmHg if proteinuiria exceeds 1 g/day: 140/90 if over 65 years and 130/90 if high risk of cardiovascular disease.

BMI <25 kg/m^2 (ideal); waist circumference women <80 cm, men <94 cm.

Renal function: Urine albumin excretion 20 mm/min in timed overnight collection; <20 mm/min spot collection; albumin–creatinine ratio < 3.5 mg/mmol in women, <2.5 mg/mmol men eGFR.

Alcohol intake: Women, 1 standard drink/day, men, 2 standard drinks/day.

No smoking

Exercise/activity: >150 minutes/week; at least 30 minutes brisk walking or equivalent/day or on at least 3–5 days/week

should not be labelled 'noncompliant or nonadherent'. Accepting the person's decision does not mean the health professional does not continue to provide information and advice. It does mean *they* might need to change the way they do things and try new strategies.

Clinical observation

Diabetes is a balancing act. The individual's physical, psychological, spiritual, and social and relationship needs must be balanced to enable people to undertake the necessary self-management to achieve management targets (optimal physical health). In fact, the emphasis should be on balance rather than control. Spirituality, resilience, and positive thinking, in particular, are important but neglected aspects of current diabetes management strategies and are key to being able to manage life changes (turning/tipping points), self-empowerment, and self-determination (Parsian and Dunning 2008).

Management involves educating the person with diabetes and other family members and carers in order to help them:

- Understand diabetes, be involved in deciding their care plan and adopt relevant self-care strategies necessary to maintain optimal health and meet glycaemic targets.
- Manage the impact of diabetes on their physical, psychological, and spiritual functioning to maintain an acceptable quality of life.
- Achieve and maintain an acceptable weight.
- Achieve acceptable blood glucose levels and HbA1c.
- Achieve a normal blood lipid profile.
- Relieve symptoms of diabetes (polyuria, polydipsia, and lethargy). This involves helping the person recognise and manage relevant signs and symptoms associated with diabetes and any concomitant condition/s.
- Prevent and/or manage hypolycaemia.
- Manage intercurrent illnesses (sick days).
- Prevent complications of diabetes and of treatment.
- Maintain a healthy, independent lifestyle where the person is able to manage the necessary self-care tasks to achieve acceptable glycaemic control and have a good quality of life.
- Understand social and legal responsibilities and entitlements such as driving, insurance, and National Diabetes Supply Scheme (in Australia).
- Plan for life transitions, including stopping driving, moving to supported or aged-care facilities, and end-of-life care.

Table 1.5 described the management targets. Table 1.6 provides some glycaemic information to consider when assessing metabolic control. *HbA1c is only part of the overall picture and should NOT be considered in isolation.*

A suggested model for managing diabetes is shown in Figure 1.6. The model is divided into phases and indicates that management, education, and counselling are required for life.

Exercise/activity

Exercise plays a key role in the management of type 1, type 2 diabetes, and GDM as well as people without diabetes (including health professionals). It increases tissue sensitivity to insulin aiding in the uptake and utilisation of glucose during exercise and for several hours afterwards. The energy sources during exercise are depicted in Figure 1.7.

Table 1.6 Guidelines for assessing the patient's blood glucose testing pattern.

% Haemoglobin A1c	Glucose (mmol/l)		Control
	Fasting	*Two hours after food*	
4.0–6.0 (~ 31–48 mmol/mol)	4	<7	Excellent or 'too good' high risk of hypoglycaemia a, especially older people on insulin and some other GLMs[a]
6.0–7.4 (48–58 mmol/mol)	7	9	Upper limit of target range
7.5–9.4 (58–75 mmol/mol)	10	14.5	Increased short- and long-term complication risk.
>9.5 (> 75 mmol/mol)	14	20	Increased short- and long-term complication risk

The results should be considered as part of the overall situation not as isolated pieces of data. The general target HbA$_{1c}$ is <7%(53 mmol/mol) (<6.5%i(48 mmol/mol) in some countries) but up to 8% (64 mmol/mol) in older people at high risk of hypoglycaemia.
Note the HbA1c mmol/mol values are the closest approximations to the HbA1c percentage values. The general target is ≤7% (53 mmol/mol), but must be individualised.
[a] If fasting glucose is high, postprandial glucose is often also high. Postprandial glucose is affected by first phase insulin response, glucagons secretion, muscle and live glucose stores, fat tissue sensitivity to insulin, food intake and digestion, and absorption of food from the gut. Both affect the HbA1c level. Fasting and postprandial have the same effect on HbA1c when the HbA1c is 7.3–8.4%. Fasting glucose has a greater effect when the HbA1c is >8.5%. The higher the HbA1c the greater the effect fasting glucose has on HbA1c.

In addition, regular exercise may have beneficial effects on the risk factors that contribute to the development of diabetes complications especially cardiovascular disease (Boule et al. 2001). Exercise provides the following benefits:

- Increases cardiovascular efficiency
- Reduces blood pressure
- Reduces stress
- Aids in weight reduction and appetite control
- Promotes a sense of well-being
- Aids in blood glucose control
- Improves strength and reduces the risk of falls in older people, which helps them remain independent (anaerobic exercise)

All of these factors also reduce the risk of developing the long-term complications of diabetes. People are advised to have a thorough physical check-up before commencing an exercise programme; in particular, the cardiovascular system, eyes, nerves, and feet should be examined. Food, fluid, and clothing should be suitable for the type of exercise and the weather.

Insulin/GLM doses might need to be adjusted. Where the duration of the exercise is <30 minutes adjustments are generally not required. Adjustments are often necessary where the duration of the exercise exceeds 30 minutes (Perlstein et al. 1997). Exercise should be decided in consultation with the individual and suited to their preferences and physical capabilities. It is advisable that the person tests blood glucose before and after exercising and has some carbohydrates available during exercise in case of hypoglycaemia. Infrequent exercise is not advisable; the aim should be to begin with 10–15 minutes exercise and progress to 30–60 minutes of moderate intensity three to five times per week, daily if possible.

Footwear and clothing should be appropriate to the type of exercise and feet should be inspected after exercising. Exercise is not recommended in extremes of temperatures or at periods of hyperglycaemia, especially if ketones are present in the urine or blood. People should discuss their exercise plans with the diabetes team and/or exercise physiologist in order to plan an appropriate routine, adequate carbohydrate intake, and appropriate medication doses. Ensure adequate fluid intake to replace water loss, especially in hot weather.

In general, anaerobic exercise (e.g. weightlifting) does not significantly enhance glucose utilisation. It does build muscle mass and improve strength but does not improve cardiovascular

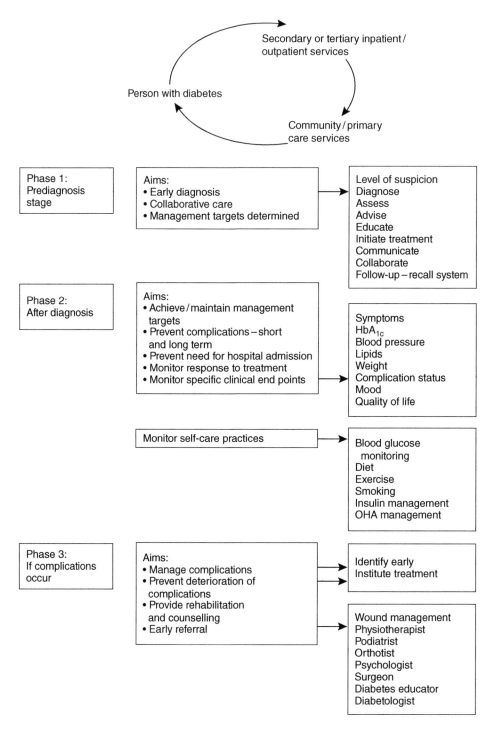

Figure 1.6 Suggested diabetes management model. Most diabetes management occurs in primary care settings in collaboration with secondary and tertiary care services.

fitness and may reduce falls risk in older people. Anaerobic exercise is unlikely to cause an increase in blood glucose. Aerobic exercise (e.g. running, cycling, swimming) uses glucose as the major fuel source and hypoglycaemia can occur. It also confers cardiovascular benefits. Chapter 12 discusses exercise in older people. Falls risks must be considered in older people.

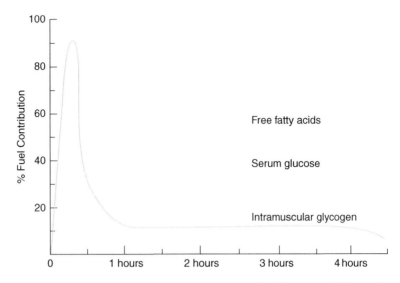

Figure 1.7 Normal energy sources during exercise. *Note*: At rest free fatty acids (FFAs) are the major energy source. As exercise begins muscle glycogen is utilised as the predominant energy source. As exercise continues the blood glucose is utilised, reverting to free fatty acids as the major energy source if exercise is prolonged. Blood glucose is maintained by hormonal regulation of hepatic glucose output and lipolysis.

Practice point

Hypoglycaemia can occur several hours after vigorous or prolonged aerobic exercise due to continuing glucose uptake by muscles. People need to be informed about adequate carbohydrate intake and medication dose adjustment as well as recognising and treating hypoglycaemia before and after exercise; see Chapter 5.

Specific advice about medications and food intake needs to be tailored to the individual. The relationship between hypoglycaemia and exercise is generally well recognised. Hyperglycaemia can also occur if insulin levels are low when exercising. In this situation, the counter-regulatory hormones predominate and increase the blood glucose, and extra medicine doses might be needed. Insulin is easier to titrate in such circumstances.

Exercise for the person in hospital

When someone with diabetes is in the hospital, note these five guidelines:

(1) Encourage as much mobility/activity as the person's condition allows.
(2) Increase movement and activity gradually after a period of being confined to bed.
(3) Consider postural hypotension and differentiate it from hypoglycaemia to ensure correct management is instituted.
(4) Consult the physiotherapy department for assistance with mobility, chair, or hydrotherapy exercises.
(5) Consider having the occupational therapist undertake a home assessment to ensure safety at home, for example, following a stroke.

Practice point

Be aware that resuming normal activity after a period of prolonged inactivity, for example in rehabilitation settings, constitutes unaccustomed exercise and can result in hypoglycaemia, especially if the person is on insulin/GLM and is not eating well or is malnourished. Exercise/activity increases the basal energy requirement by about 20%.

Diabetes education

Diabetes education is an integral part of diabetes management. Regular support and contact with the diabetes care team assists people to self-manage their diabetes by providing advice and support when necessary. For more details see Chapter 16.

Practice points

(1) People with type 2 diabetes do not become type 1 when insulin is needed to control blood glucose. The current accepted term is insulin-treated or insulin-requiring diabetes. The basic underlying pathophysiology does not change and usually enough endogenous insulin is produced to prevent ketosis occurring, except during severe intercurrent illness.
(2) Type 2 diabetes is characterised by progressive beta cell destruction, and insulin is eventually required by >50% of people (UKPDS 1998).
(3) People with LADA often require insulin soon after diagnosis, because they are insulin deficient, not insulin resistant.

Complications of diabetes

Many people with diabetes are admitted to hospital because they have an active diabetes complication. The presence of a diabetic complication can affect the duration of the admission and the patient's ability to care for him or herself. Hence, diabetic complications contribute to the overall cost of healthcare for these patients. In addition, they represent significant physical and mental lifestyle costs to the person with diabetes and their family.

Complications can be classified as acute or long term. Acute complications can occur during temporary excursions in blood glucose levels. Long-term complications occur with long duration of diabetes and persistent hyperglycaemia, especially in the presence of other risk factors. In type 2 diabetes, long-term complications are frequently present at diagnosis. Often there are few symptoms and both the diagnosis of diabetes and the coexisting complication/s can be overlooked (Chapter 8).

Acute complications

(1) Hypoglycaemia (refer to Chapter 6).
(2) Hyperglycaemia:
   • DKA (refer to Chapter 7)
   • Hyperosmolar states (refer to Chapter 7).
(3) Infections can occur if blood glucose control is not optimal. Common infections include dental disease, candidiasis, and urinary tract infections.
(4) Fat atrophy/hypertrophy and insulin allergy occur very rarely with modern highly purified insulins and correct injection site rotation.

Long-term complications

Two important studies, the DCCT in 1993 and the UKPDS in 1998 (DCCT 1993; UKPDS 1998), demonstrated the relationship between the development and progression of the long-term complications of type 1 and type 2 diabetes, respectively. In addition, the UKPDS demonstrated the importance of controlling blood pressure to reduce the risk of cardiovascular disease. Diabetes management guidelines and metabolic targets are regularly revised as new evidence emerges. Long-term complications are discussed in Chapter 8.

Current management targets are shown in Table 1.5. The following are possible long-term complications:

(1) Macrovascular disease or disease of the major blood vessels, for example:
   • Myocardial infarction
   • Cerebrovascular accident
   • Intermittent claudication
(2) Microvascular disease or disease of the small blood vessels associated with thickening of the basement membranes of the small blood vessels; for example:
   • Retinopathy
   • Nephropathy
(3) Neuropathy: diabetes can also cause damage to the central and peripheral nerves:
   • *Peripheral*: decreased sensation in hands and particularly the feet, which can lead to ulcers, Charcot's arthropathy, and amputation
   • *Autonomic*: erectile dysfunction, atonic bladder, gastroparesis, mononeuropathies
(4) Complications of pregnancy: diabetes during pregnancy carries risks for both mother and baby:
   • *Mother*: toxaemia, polyhydramnous intrauterine death, and Caesarean section
   • *Baby*: congenital malformations, prematurity, respiratory distress, hypoglycaemia at birth

A number of other factors might play a role in the development of diabetic complications. For example, studies are under way to determine the role of free radicals or reactive oxygen species (ROS), advanced glycated end products (AGE), changes in cellular signalling, and endothelial humoral components that determine coagulation status and the tendency to form microthrombi. It is the responsibility of all health professionals involved in providing care to comprehensively assess the patient including the presence of complications to determine their self-care potential and devise an appropriate achievable management plan in consultation with the individual, and to be involved in preventative teaching about reducing risk factors for the development of diabetic complications. Health professionals need to be proactive about identifying opportunities for health screening and education.

Practice points

(1) Hyperglycaemia and insulin resistance commonly occur in critically ill patients, even those who do not have diabetes (van den Berghe et al. 2007; ADS 2012).
(2) It is important to control these states in people with diabetes during illness because of the extra stress of the illness and/or surgery, and their compromised insulin response. Elevated blood glucose in these situations in people without diabetes will require decisions to be made about the diagnosis of diabetes after the acute episode resolves.

Aims and objectives of diabetes care

Rationale

Early diagnosis of diabetes and monitoring for short- and long-term complications enables early treatment and improved outcomes. If clinicians understand the pathophysiology and classification of diabetes and its complications and the individual's values and goals, they are more likely to be able to provide holistic personalized care.

Aims

The aim is to formulate an individual management plan so that the person recovers by primary intention, maintains their independence, dignity, and quality of life as far as possible and does not develop any complications of treatment, and, in some cases, help them prepare for a peaceful death.

Recognise the importance of support from the family and other key people (and often pets) to the individual's well-being, self-care capacity, and ability to take responsibility for their diabetes.

Effectively plan for discharge and/or transfer amongst services.

Objectives

(1) Establish a therapeutic relationship based on respect, equality, and trust. The therapeutic relationship is essential to healing, shared decision-making, and personalised care.
(2) Assess the person's:
   - Usual care plan
   - Physical, mental, and social status
   - Usual glycaemic control
   - Ability to care for themselves
   - Knowledge about diabetes and its management
   - Presence of any diabetes-related complications, including lowered mood and depression
   - Acceptance of the diagnosis of diabetes
   - Presence of concomitant disease processes
   - Medicine regimen, including complementary medicines use
(3) Encourage independence as far as the physical condition allows, even in the hospital (monitor own blood glucose, administer own insulin/manage their insulin pump, select own meals).
(4) Obtain and maintain an acceptable blood glucose range that minimises hypoglycaemia or hyperglycaemia and keeps the person free from distressing symptoms and fluctuating blood glucose levels.
(5) Prevent complications occurring as a result of hospitalisation (e.g. falls associated with hypo- and hyperglycaemia and a range of other factors).
(6) Observe an appropriate management plan in order to achieve these objectives.
(7) Inform appropriate health professionals promptly of the patient's admission, e.g. diabetes nurse specialist/diabetes educator, dietitian, or podiatrist.
(8) Ensure the patient has the opportunity to learn about diabetes and its management, particularly self-management and particularly when their usual care changes and new medicines are commenced.
(9) Plan appropriately for surgical procedures and other investigations, transfer amongst services and discharge, including managing medicines and undertaking or referring the person for a home medicine review if they meet the criteria and ensuring they have the equipment necessary to manage their diabetes (medicines, blood glucose meter, insulin devices).
(10) Prevent further hospitalisations and adverse events as a result of diabetes.
(11) Evaluate outcomes of care and clinician performance.

Care of people with diabetes while in the hospital

Being hospitalised is more common for people with diabetes than those without, and they are more likely to stay longer (ADA 2019). Current diabetes management guidelines are heavily weighted towards screening and primary care management, but recently, the ADS (2019) and other diabetes professional associations released guidelines for managing people with diabetes in hospital, and these guidelines should be used to guide care. Specific nursing care is described in most other chapters of the book.

Factors that complicate diabetes management during illness

- The presenting health issue and health status at the time.
- Age.
- Gender.
- Type and duration of diabetes.
- Presence of diabetes complications.
- Nutritional status.
- Potentially erratic insulin absorption, especially in type 1.
- Haemodynamic changes in blood flow.
- Counter-regulatory stress response to illness, hospitalisation, treatment, pain, psychological stress, and fear.
- Timing of meals and snacks as well as during TPN, fasting and renal dialysis. This is especially important in relation to medicine administration.
- Duration of time between insulin administration and meals.
- Effect of medications on the gut, especially narcotics for pain relief. Glucose requirements may need to be increased to compensate for slow transit times, to supply sufficient energy and prevent hypoglycaemia.
- Increased white cell count and impaired leukocyte function as a result of hyperglycaemia might not indicate the presence of infection.
- 'Silent' disease such as MI, UTI, and few classic symptoms of type 2 diabetes, hypoglycaemia, or hyperglycaemia are often present, especially in older people.
- Delayed wound healing and strength of healing tissue.
- Increased risk of thrombosis.
- Development of ketoacidosis and/or hyperosmolar states can result if hyperglycaemia is not reversed.
- Impaired cognitive function and lowered mood can make problem-solving, self-care, and learning difficult.
- Depression.

Personal stories

(1) People with diabetes worry that hospital staff will make mistakes, especially with their medication doses and administration times and managing hypoglycaemia.
(2) They dislike being made to feel incompetent and not trusted by staff who 'take over' the self-care tasks they usually perform for themselves, and who do not believe what they say.
(3) Conversely, some people prefer the nurses to take on diabetes self-care tasks because it is an opportunity to 'let go of' the responsibility for a short time.
(4) They find judgmental attitudes about eating sweet things demeaning, especially when they are accused of dietary indiscretions when their blood glucose is high.
(5) They dislike being labelled noncompliant or uncooperative, if they have difficulty learning and remembering information.

Technology and diabetes management

Technology such as insulin pens, blood glucose meters/sensors, and insulin pumps are well established. Technology increasingly supports diabetes management, self-care, and clinician learning in other ways. Electronic health records, electronic media such as the internet, and mobile platforms (mHealth) enable users to retrieve, exchange, and store information by participating in virtual communities and networks of practice and communicate with the people they care for (Harno 2013). For example, health information services, peer communities, practice guidelines, risk assessment tools, self-management tools, research publications, and counselling are available online.

In addition, electronic media enable clinicians to monitor and advise people with diabetes remotely, which facilitates information exchange such as blood glucose data and more timely management changes. Remote monitoring can be further supported by telehealth consultations, where the person with diabetes can discuss their health with diabetes specialists and/or other clinicians using a laptop, tablet, or smart phone connected to the internet. Electronic monitoring can be highly motivating, especially when it is used with interactive discussions and decision-support tools (Shea et al. 2002).

Research suggests a nurse-led multidisciplinary team can manage a group of people with diabetes using online disease management programmes (Tang et al. 2012), and patients are generally satisfied with electronic monitoring (Mehrotra et al. 2013). Some systems use a combination of health coaching as well as artificial intelligence (AI) and other technologies to support the person with diabetes.

Chatbots, or bots, are of great interest in the health-care technology space. Bots combine AI, machine learning (ML), and natural language processing (NLP) to provide interactions that sound like a normal conversation but are human-like in their nature. The chatbot can incorporate data from connected devices and use the information to tailor feedback specific to the individual, based on pre-set specifications and pattern recognition (Centre for Advanced Hindsight 2019).

The increasing use of AI, including other forms of ML, is a ubiquitous part of life. It powers systems such as navigation services on smartphones, personalises what information is seen during online searches and social media feeds, and is increasingly being used in healthcare. A growing range of diabetes-based systems that use a combination of AI and ML help people with diabetes avoid episodes of hypoglycaemia. Furthermore, there is a growing range of glucose meters, apps, and closed-loop systems that combine data from exercise, dietary intake, and current and past blood glucose patterns to provide personalised self-management feedback and insulin dosing recommendations.

An increasing range of sensors, physiological signals, and home environment monitoring are available to assist the safety and comfort of people living in their home. Video-based sensing, pattern analysis, and Bluetooth-enabled devices can notify clinicians, relatives, and carers about changes or abnormalities in people at home, which aids early intervention (Chen et al. 2016). Additionally, these systems often have the option for telehealth connections that enable immediate or timely follow-up. Medication reminders, automated systems to order medicines, and other useful health apps are also available on a number of these remote home monitoring systems.

Online support and peer-to-peer communication are valuable tools that connect people with diabetes to health services, self-management, and emotional well-being (Browne et al. 2016). Gamification, the application of gaming techniques to activities, is often used online to improve engagement. Gamification is used in various apps for diabetes and other health conditions and positively assists learning and behaviour re-enforcement (Miller et al. 2014; Von Bargen et al. 2014).

Robots are continuing to emerge in various health and medical fields beyond the characteristic surgical and rehabilitation settings (Dahl and Boulos 2014). A number of studies investigated how robots can assist children with diabetes and older people with diabetes and dementia. Robots using natural language, modelling, and memory assist in the development of a genuine rapport and relationships felt by the child, which, in turn, support the child to learn to undertake diabetes self-care behaviours (Belpaeme et al. 2012). They enhance independence, communication, and mobility, reduce isolation, and improve safety in older people living at home. These technologies include humanoid robots, exoskeletons, and rehabilitation robots (Pilotto 2018).

Specific diabetes management technology includes the following:

- A range of increasingly sophisticated blood glucose meters. Some of these have connectivity to other electronic systems such as mobile phones and insulin pumps, and some have inbuilt management algorithms.
- Insulin delivery systems include devices such as pumps.
- Automated support algorithms adjust medicine doses and carbohydrate intake.
- Noninvasive devices detect blood glucose levels and nocturnal hypoglycaemia.
- Automated, portable systems can control blood glucose overnight in people with T1DM.
- The *artificial pancreas* refers to a system designed to match the way a pancreas functions. There are different forms, but they all work by releasing insulin in response to the prevailing blood glucose. A recent version is connected to a smartphone app that is wirelessly connected to a continuous blood glucose monitor (CGM) (Delpande et al. 2019). Delpande et al. demonstrated improved time spent the target blood glucose range (3.9–10 mmol/l, 70–180 mg/dl) and a significant reduction in time spent in hypoglycaemia. However, only six people participated in the trial.
- Hybrid closed-loop systems can monitor blood glucose levels and regulate insulin delivery. They can be monitored by smart phone and remotely by clinicians.
- Health behaviour tracking systems can monitor steps taken, the number of stairs climbed, and kilojoules burned, some of which link to smartphones. They can be used like a personal trainer, encouraging and reminding the user of goals.
- Diabetes-specific and general health apps can assist with the person to record, share, and track their blood glucose levels, exercise, and food intake and decide insulin doses. For example, the OptimAAPP enables insulin doses to be calculated for all the macronutrients, protein, fat, and carbohydrates to prevent hyperglycaemia when consuming foods such as pizza (Smart 2019); see Chapter 4. Fat and protein cause delayed hyperglycaemia and have an additive impact on blood glucose.
- Some apps offer gamification that engage and reinforce positive behaviours and activities.
- Electronic decision-support tools are available for people with diabetes and clinicians, including computer-generated reminders.

There is no doubt that more exciting technological advances will emerge and enhance the care of, for, and by people with diabetes. However, like most health-care options, there are risks and benefits. Some risks to consider include:

- Not all information on the internet is accurate or appropriate. People with diabetes need help to identify reliable sites such as the websites of diabetes organisations such as Diabetes UK, Diabetes Australia, the ADA, and service providers such as authorised government websites and sites that display the HonCode symbol.
- Internet information may improve knowledge but it may not change behaviours (Chapter 16) or health professional practice because social, cultural, and behavioural context are not part of the learning process (Kinson 2012), although socialisation might be a feature of online group activities and support groups.
- Applications that offer a combination of education about how to use management guidelines, decision support tools, and patient registers can lead to improved outcomes for people with type 2 diabetes in general practice settings (Barlow 2013).
- Adequate backup and data management systems need to be in place so important data are not lost or accessible to people not involved in the individual's care. That is, stringent, monitored security systems must be in place wherever confidential information is stored, including on mobile phones.

- Medicolegal issues such as breaches of privacy and confidentiality, such as storing personal patient information, including research data on smartphones. There are significant implications for individuals whose data are not protected and for the health professional concerned if the smartphone is lost or stolen.
- Patient information cannot be used without consent, including in telehealth/video health professional management conferences, case discussions, publications, and presentations.

Barriers and issues to consider

- *A potential barrier to any new health technology tool is the cost.* In addition, the smartphone, tablet or computer, apps, and access to data all cost money.
- *Internet access can be limited in rural and remote regions.* The cost of data can be prohibitive in developing countries.
- *Despite growing enthusiasm for the range of digital tools to support diabetes self-management, the evidence demonstrating safety, cost-effectiveness, and efficacy remains largely unknown.* Many studies concerning health-related technologies are underpowered and/or of limited duration and thus are unable to fully demonstrate meaningful and statistical evidence (Pal et al. 2014).
- *Technology needs to be fit for purpose.* Not all technology is useful or appropriate, even when there is strong evidence for its benefits.

Interoperability continues to be a problem in healthcare. Regulatory and data security restrictions, although important, make linking information additionally challenging. Electronic health records and patient-held information offer promise but face challenges in gaining widespread trust in the community.

Medical assistance dogs

An increasing number of medical assistance dogs provide a range of type of assistance, as well as companionship and love. Recent research shows appropriately trained glycaemia dogs improve the life of people with T1DM but vary in sensitivity to out-of-range blood glucose. Median sensitivity to hypoglycaemia was 83% (range 66–94%) and 67% (range: 17–91%) (*n* = 27 dogs). On average, 81% of alerts occurred when the blood glucose was outside the target range (Rooney et al. 2019). Importantly, the individual characteristics of the dog, the dog–human partnership, and the household were significantly associated with performance. Careful selection of the dog to suit the individual and good initial training are important for optimal companionship (Rooney et al. 2019).

A sobering final comment

OPTIMISE, the Optimal Type 2 Diabetes Management Including Benchmarking and Standard Treatment Trial (Hermans et al. 2013), compared physician's individual performance with a peer group to determine whether benchmarking and assessing change in three quality indicators of vascular risk: HbA1c, LDL-C, and systolic blood pressure improved the quality of type 2 diabetes care in primary care settings (*n* = 3980). The findings show HbA1c targets were only met in 52.2%; 34.9% for LDL-C and 27.3% for systolic blood pressure. Other studies show older physicians are less likely to follow guidelines or use new medicines (Tung 2011) and nurses have inadequate diabetes knowledge (Livingston and Dunning 2010), including about medicines and in aged care settings (Dunning et al. 2012).

These findings are very concerning, even allowing for the many confounding variables that affect the ability of people with diabetes to meet targets. As suggested in Chapters 2 and 16, patient-related targets may not be the best measure of health professional performance, and more appropriate measures should be considered. If they *are* the best measure of clinician performance, clinicians must examine their care practices, behaviours and attitudes, and the care systems in which they operate, to determine whether/how these factors affect their performance. For example, general practitioners identified treatment costs to the patient and reluctance to commence insulin as barriers to their ability to achieve optimal management targets in a cluster randomised trial in Asia-Pacific that involved educating doctors about how to use diabetes guidelines (Reutens et al. 2011).

A great deal of time and money is spent on clinician education; if clinicians are ineffective more than 50% of the time, we need to determine whether education programmes adequately train clinicians to deliver diabetes education and care, and/or are delivered in a manner suitable to their learning needs. Another consideration is inherent weaknesses in the literature and varying interpretations of the same literature base. For example, most guidelines are developed using the same literature but recommendations often differ. In addition, the exclusive nature of randomised trials means the findings might not be relevant in all clinical practice settings.

References

Abassi, A., Peelen, L., Corpeleinj, E. et al. (2012). Prediction models for risk of developing type 2 diabetes: a systematic literature search and independent external validation study. *British Medical Journal* **345**: e5900. https://doi.org/10.1136/bmj.e5900.

Abikshyeet, P., Ramesh, V., and Oza, N. (2012). Glucose estimation in the salivary secretion of diabetes mellitus patients. *Diabetes Metabolic and Obesity Targets and Therapies* **25**: 149–154.

American Diabetes Association (2007). Preventing Diabetes. http://www.diabetes.org/diabetes-basics/preven-tion (accessed June 2019).

American Diabetes Association (2009). Diagnosis and classification of diabetes. *Diabetes Care* **32** (S1): S62–S67.

American Diabetes Association (2019). Prevention or delay of type 2 diabetes: standards of medical care in diabetes-2019. *Diabetes Care* **42** (suppl-1): 529–533. https://doi.org/10.2337/dc19-S003.

American Diabetes Association, American Psychiatric Association, American Association of Clinical Endocrinologists, and North American Association for the Study of Obesity (2004). Consensus development conference on antipsychotic drugs and obesity and diabetes. *Diabetes Care* **27**: 596–601.

Appleton, M. and Hattersley, A. (1996). Maturity onset diabetes of the young: a missed diagnosis. *Diabetic Medicine* (Suppl. 2): AP3.

Armitage, J., Poston, L., and Taylor, P. (2008). Developmental origins of obesity and the metabolic syndrome. *Frontiers of Hormone Research* **36**: 73–84.

Australian Diabetes Society (2012). *Guidelines for Routine Glucose Control in Hospital*. Canberra: Australian Diabetes Society.

Australian Institute of Health and Welfare (2005). *Costs of Diabetes in Australia, 2000–01*. Cat. No. CVD 26. Canberra: Australian Institute of Health and Welfare (AIHW).

Australian Government Department of Health (2010). *The Australian Type 2 Diabetes Risk Assessment Tool (AUSDRISK)*. Canberra: Australian Government Department of Health https://www.health.gov.au/internet/main/publishing.nsf/Content/chronic-diab-prev-aus/$File/austool5.pdf (accessed June 2019).

Azzopardi, P., Brown, A., Fahy, R. et al. (2012). Type 2 diabetes in young indigenous Australians in rural and remote areas: diagnosis, screening, management and prevention. *Medical Journal of Australia* **187** (2): 32–36.

Banerjee, S. (2014). HbA1c result, does it depend upon the testing methods? *Journal of the Association of Physicians of India* **62**: 9–12.

Barlow, J. (2013). Improving management of type 2 diabetes: findings of the Type2Care clinical audit. *Medical Journal of Australia* **42** (12): 57–60.

Begley, S. (2013). *Think Preventative Medicine Will Save Money? Think Again*. New York: Thomson Reuters https://www.reuters.com/article/us-preventive-economics-idUSBRE90S05M20130129 (accessed June 2019).

Belpaeme, T., Baxter, P., Read, R. et al. Multimodal child-robot interaction: building social bonds. *Journal of Human Robot Interaction* **1**: 33–53.

Bethel, M., Price, H., Sourij, H. et al. (2013). Evaluation of self-administered oral glucose tolerance test. *Diabetes Care* **36** (3): 1483–1488.

Biden, T. (2007). Major breakthrough in understanding type 2 diabetes. *Nursing Review* **6**: 10.

Boule, N., Haddard, E., Kenny, G. et al. (2001). Effects of exercise on glycaemic control and body mass index in type 2 diabetes mellitus: a meta-analysis of controlled clinical trials. *Journal of the American Medical Association* **286**: 1218–1227.

Browne, J.L., Bennet, A., Halliday, J.A. et al. (2016). *Diabetes Peer Support in Australia: A National Survey'*. Melbourne: Diabetes Victoria.

Bruce, K. and Byrne, C. (2009). The metabolic syndrome: common origins of a multifactorial disorder. *Postgraduate Medical Journal* **85**: 614–621.

Burke, V., Beilin, U., and Simmer, K. (2005). Predictors of body mass index and associations with cardiovascular risk factors in Australian children: a prospective cohort study. *International Journal of Obesity* **29**: 15–23.

Buzzetti, R., Di Pietro, S., Giaccari, A. et al. (2007). Non-insulin requiring autoimmune diabetes study group. High titer autoantibodies to GAD identifies a specific phenotype of adult-onset autoimmune diabetes. *Diabetes Care* **30**: 932–936.

Cappuccio, F. and Miller, M. (2012). A new challenge to widely held views on the role of sleep. *Annals of Internal Medicine* **157** (8): 593–594.

Carnethon, M., De Chavez, P., Biggs, M. et al. (2012). Association of weight status with mortality in adults with incident diabetes. *Journal American Medical Association* **308** (6): 581.

Ceriello, A. (2003). The postprandial state and cardiovascular disease: relevance to diabetes mellitus. *Diabetes Metabolism Research Reviews* **16**: 125–132.

Cermea, S., Buzzetti, R., and Pozilli, P. (2003). ß-cell protection and therapy for latent autoimmune diabetes in adults. *Diabetes Care* **32** (S2): S546–S5262.

Chen, M., Ma, Y., Song, J. et al. (2016). Smart clothing: connecting human with clouds and big data for sustainable health monitoring. *Mobile Networks and Applications* **21** (5): 825–845. https://doi.org/10.1007/s11036-016-0745-1.

Conen, D., Ridker, P., Mora, S. et al. (2007). Blood pressure and risk of developing type 2 diabetes mellitus: the Women's health study. *European Heart Journal* **28** (23): 2937–2943.

Dahl, T.S. and Boulos, M.N.K. (2014). Robots in health and social care: a complementary technology to home care and Telehealthcare? *Robotics* **2** (3): 1–21.

Dandona, P., Ghanim, A., Chaudhuri, A. et al. (2010). Macronutrient intake induces oxidative and inflammatory stress: potential relevance to atherosclerosis and insulin resistance. *Experiential Molecular Medicine* **42**: 245–253.

DCCT (Diabetes and Control and Complications Trial Research Group) (1993). The effect of intensive insulin treatment on the development and progression of long term complications of insulin dependent diabetes. *New England Journal of Medicine* **329**: 977–986.

Deedwania, P., Patel, K., Fonarow, G.C. et al. (2014). Prediabetes is not an independent risk factor for incident heart failure, other cardiovascular events or mortality in older adults: findings from a population-based cohort study. *International Journal of Cardiology* **168** (4): 3616–3622. https://doi.org/10.1016/j.ijcard.2013.05.038.

Deem, J., Muta, K., Scarlett, J. et al. (2017). How should we think the role of the brain in glucose homeostasis? *Diabetes* **66** (7): 1758–1765. https://doi.org/10.2337/dbi16-0067.

Delpande, S., Pinsker, J., Zavitjanou, S. et al. (2019). Research and clinical evaluation of the interoperable artificial pancreas (iAPS) smartphone: interoperable components with modular design for progressive artificial pancreas research and development. *Diabetes Technology and Therapeutics* **21** (1) https://doi.org/10.1089/dia.2018.0278.

d'Emden, M., Shaw, J., Colagiuri, S. et al. (2012). The role of HbA1c in the diagnosis of diabetes mellitus in Australia. *Medical Journal of Australia* **197** (4): 220–221.

Diabetes Australia (DA) and Royal Australian College of General Practitioners (RACGP) (2011/12). *Diabetes Management in General Practice: Guideline for Type 2 Diabetes*. Canberra: DA and RACGP http://www.racgp.org.au/ (accessed July 2019).

Diabetes Prevention Program (DPP) Research Group (2002). The Diabetes Prevention Program (DPP): description of lifestyle intervention. *Diabetes Care* **25** (12): 2165–2171.

Diabetes UK (2014). *Diabetes Prevalence 2014 (June 2015)*. London: Diabetes UK https://www.diabetes.org.uk/professionals/position-statements-reports/statistics/diabetes-prevalence-2014 (accessed July 2019).

Ding, E., Song, Y., and Manson, J. (2009). Sex hormone-binding globulin and risk of type 2 diabetes in women and men. *New England Journal of Medicine* **361**: 1152–1163.

Donga, E., van Dijk, M., Hoogma, R.P.L. et al. (2013). Insulin resistance in multiple tissues in patients with type 1 diabetes mellitus on long-term continuous subcutaneous insulin infusion therapy. *Diabetes/Metabolism Research and Reviews* **29** (1): 33–38.

Dornhorst, A. (2001). Insulinotrophic meglitinide analogues. *Lancet* **358** (9294): 1709–1716.

Dunning, T., Savage, S., Rasmussen, B., and Wellard, S. (2012). Managing diabetes medicines in residential aged care facilities: Balancing competing challenges. Proceedings OEC 42, IDF Western Pacific Region Congress, Kyoto, Japan.

Eckel, R.H., Grundy, S.M., and Zimmet, P.Z. (2005). The metabolic syndrome. *The Lancet* **365** (9468): 1415–1428.

EURODIAB ACE Study Group (2000). Variation and trends in incidence of childhood diabetes in Europe. *Lancet* **355**: 873–876.

EURODIAB Substudy 2 Study Group (1999). Vitamin D supplement in early childhood and risk for type 1 (insulin-dependent) diabetes mellitus. *Diabetologia* **42** (1): 51–54.

Ferreira, H., Xavier, A., Assuncao, M. et al. (2018). Developmental origins of health and disease: a new approach for the identification of adults who suffered. Undernutrition in early life. *Metabolic Syndrome and Obesity Targets and Therapy* **11**: 543–551.

Floegel, A., Stefan, N., Yu, Z. et al. (2013). Identification of serum metabolites associated with risk of type 2 diabetes using a targeted metabolomic approach. *Diabetes* **62** (2): 639–648.

Gagnon, C., Lu, Z.X., and Magliano, D. (2011). Serum 25-hydroxyvitamin D, calcium intake and risk of type 2 diabetes after 5 years results from a national population-based prospective study (the Australian diabetes, obesity and lifestyle study). *Diabetes Care* **34**: 1133–1138.

Gardner, D. and Tai, E. (2012). Clinical features and treatment of maturity onset diabetes of the young (MODY). *Diabetes, Metabolic Syndrome and Obesity* **25**: 101–108.

Garfield, A., Shah, B., Madara, J. et al. (2014). A parabrachial-hypothalamic cholecystokinin neurocircuit controls counterregulatory responses to hypoglycaemia. *Cell Metabolism* **20**: 1030–1037.

Gonzalez-Molero, I., Rojo-Martinez, G., Gauterrez-Repiso, C. et al. (2012). Vitamin D incidence of diabetes: a prospective cohort study. *Clinical Nutrition* **31** (4): 571–573.

Harno, K. (2013). The advance of health information technology: traveling the internet superhighwayChapter 12. In: *Diabetes Education: Art, Science and Evidence* (ed. T. Dunning), 200–214. Chichester: Wiley Blackwell.

Haynes, A., Bulsars, M., Bower, C. et al. (2012). Cyclical variation in the incidence of childhood type 1 diabetes in Western Australia (1985–2010). *Diabetes Care* **35** (11): 2300–2302. https://doi.org/10.2337/dc12-0205.

Health Service Ombudsman (2000). *Errors in the Care and Treatment of a Young Woman with Diabetes*. London: The Stationery Office https://assets.publishing.service.gov.uk/government/uploads/system/uploads/attachment_data/file/235530/0013.pdf (accessed July 2019).

Heianza, Y., Arase, Y., Fujihara, K. et al. (2012). Screening for pre-diabetes to predict future diabetes using various cut-off points for HbA1c and impaired fasting glucose: the Toranomon Hospital Health Management Centre study 4. *Diabetic Medicine* **29**: 279–285. https://doi.org/10.1111/j.1464-5491.2012.03686.x.

Hermans, M.P., Brotons, C., Elisaf, M. et al. (2013). Optimal type 2 diabetes mellitus management: the randomised controlled OPTIMISE benchmarking study: baseline results from six European countries. *European Journal of Preventive Cardiology* **20** (6): 1095–1105.

Herpertz, S., Albus, C., and Wagener, R. (1998). Cormorbidity of eating disorders. Does diabetes control reflect disturbed eating behaviour? *Diabetes Care* **21** (7): 1110–1116.

Hilton, D., O'Sourke, P., Welbourn, T., and Reid, C. (2002). Diabetes detection in Australian general practice: a comparison of diagnostic criteria. *Medical Journal of Australia* **176**: 104–107.

Hippisley-Cox, J. and Pringle, M. (2004). Prevalence, care, and outcomes for patients with diet-controlled diabetes in general practice: cross sectional survey. *The Lancet* **364** (9432): 423–428.

Hu, E., Pan, A., Malik, V., and Sun, O. (2012). White rice consumption and risk of type 2 diabetes: meta-analysis and systematic review. *British Medical Journal* **344**: 1454. https://doi.org/10.1136/bmj.e1454.

International Diabetes Federation (IDF) (2011). *Guideline for Management of Post-Meal Glucose in Diabetes*. Brussels: IDF https://www.idf.org/e-library/guidelines/82-management-of-postmeal-glucose.html (accessed June 2019).

International Diabetes Federation (IDF) (2012). *Diabetes and Climate Change Report*. Brussels: IDF https://ncdalliance.org/sites/default/files/rfiles/IDF%20Diabetes%20and%20Climate%20Change%20Policy%20Report.pdf (accessed July 2019).

International Diabetes Federation (IDF) (2017). *IDF Diabetes Atlas*, 8e. Brussels: International Diabetes Federation. http://www.diabetesatlas.org (accessed July 2019).

Jeon, C.Y., Haan, M.N., Cheng, C. et al. (2012). Helicobacter pylori infection is associated with an increased rate of diabetes. *Diabetes Care* **35** (3): 520–525.

Jones, H. (2011). Increase in deaths in men with type 2 diabetes and testosterone deficiency may be prevented by testosterone replacement. *ScienceDaily* (April 14, 2011). https://www.sciencedaily.com/releases/2011/04/110413090030.htm (accessed July 2019).

Juraschek, S., Steefes, M., Miller, E., and Selvin, E. (2012). Alternative markers for hyperglycaemia and risk of diabetes. *Diabetes Care* **35**: 2265–2270.

King, J.C. (2006). Maternal obesity, metabolism, and pregnancy outcomes. *Annual Review of Nutrition* **26**: 271–291.

Kinson, J. (2012). Lecture presented at the Diabetes UK Annual Professional Conference, Glasgow. *Practical Diabetes* **29** (6): 247–251.

Knip, M., Veijola, R., Virtanen, S. et al. (2005). Environmental triggers and determinants in type 1 diabetes. *Diabetes* **54** (S2): s125–s126.

Kong, A., Williams, R., Smith, M. et al. (2007). Acanthosis nigricans and diabetes risk factors: prevalence in young persons seen in southwestern US primary care practices. *Annals of Family Medicine* **5** (3): 202–208.

Krishnan, S., Rosenberg, L., Singer, M. et al. (2007). Glycaemic index, glycaemic load and cereal fiber intake and risk of type 2 diabetes in US black women. *Archives of Internal Medicine* **167** (21): 2304–2309.

Lang, T. and Rayner, G. (2012). Ecological public health: the 21st century's big idea. *British Medical Journal* **345**: 17–20.

Langer, O. (2006). Management of gestational diabetes: pharmacological treatment options and glycaemic control. *Endocrinology Metabolic Clinics of North America* **35**: 53–78.

Law, K. and Zhang, H. (2017). The pathogenesis and pathophysiology of gestational diabetes mellitus: deductions from a three-part longitudinal metabolomics study in China. *Clinical Chim Acta* **468**: 60–70. https://doi.org/10.1016/j.cca.2017.02.008.

Lerner, L., Upton, J.P., Praveen, P. et al. (2012). IRE11α induces Thioredoxin-interacting protein to activate the NLRP3 inflammasome and promote programmed cell death under irremediable stress. *Cell Metabolism* 16 (2): 250–264.

Lesperance, F. and Frasure-Smith, N. (2007). Depression and heart disease. *Cleveland Clinic Journal of Medicine* 74 (S1): S63–S66.

Lindström, J., Louheranta, A., Mannelin, M. et al. (2003). The Finnish Diabetes Prevention Study (DPS): Lifestyle intervention and 3-year results on diet and physical activity. *Diabetes Care* 26 (12): 3230–3236.

Livingston, R. and Dunning, T. (2010). Practice nurses' role and knowledge about diabetes management within rural and remote Australian general practice. *European Diabetes Nursing* 7: 55–61.

Loyd, C., Wilson, R., and Forrest, K. (1997). Prior depressive symptoms and onset of coronary heart disease. *Diabetes* 46: 3A.

Mahdi, T., Hanzelmann, S., Salehi, A. et al. (2012). Secreted frizzled-related protein 4 reduces insulin secretion in type 2 diabetes. *Metabolism* 18: 625–633.

McDonald, T., Coldclough, K., and Brown, R. (2011). Islet autoantibodies and discriminate maturity-onset diabetes of the young (MODY) from type 1 diabetes. *Diabetic Medicine* 28 (9): 1028–1035.

Mehrotra, A., Paone, S., Maritch, D. et al. (2013). A comparison of e-visits and physician office visits for sinusitis and urinary tract infections. *Journal of International Medicine* 173 (1): 72–74.

Menting, J., Whittaker, J., Margetts, M. et al. (2013). How insulin engaged its primary binding site. *Nature* 493: 241–245.

Miller, A.S., Cafazzo, J.A., and Seto, E. (2014). A game plan: gamification design principles in mHealth applications for chronic disease management. *Health Informatics Journal* 22 (2): 184–193. https://doi.org/10.1177/1460458214537511.

Mingea, K., Zimmet, P., and Magliano, D. (2011). Diabetes prevalence and determinants in indigenous Australian populations: a systematic review. *Diabetes Research and Clinical Practice* 93: 139–149.

Morris, A. (2012). Large scale association analysis provides insight into the genetic architecture and pathophysiology of type 2 diabetes. *National Genetics* 44: 981–990.

Munkhaugen, J., Hjelmeseath, J., Otterstad, J. et al. (2018). Managing patients with prediabetes and type 2 diabetes after coronary events: individual tailoring needed – a cross-sectional study. *BMC Cardiovascular Disease* 18: 160. https://doi.org/10.1186/s12872-018-0896-z.

Nakamura, Y. and Omaya, S. (2012). Metabolic diseases and pro-and prebiotics: mechanistic insights. *Nutrition & Metabolism* 9 (1): 60.

National Prescribing Service (NPS) (2012). *Type 2 Diabetes Drug Table*. Canberra, Australia: NPS http://www.nps.org.au.

Nield, L., Summerbell, C., Hooper, L. et al. (2008). Dietary advice for the prevention of type 2 diabetes mellitus in adults (review). *Cochrane Database of Systematic Reviews* 3: CD004097. https://doi.org/10.1002/14651858.CD004097.pub4.

Niskanen, L., Tuomi, T., Groop, L., and Uusitupa, M. (1995). GAD antibodies in NIDDM. Ten-year follow-up from diagnosis. *Diabetes Care* 18 (12): 1557–1565.

O'Brien, J.D. (2019). Chatbots for Diabetes Self Management. Centre for Advanced Hindsight. https://advanced-hindsight.com/wp-content/uploads/2018/08/Chatbots-for-Diabetes-Self-Management-.pdf (accessed July 2019).

Pal, K., Eastwood, S.V., Michie, S. et al. (2014). Computer-based interventions to improve self-management in adults with type 2 diabetes: a systematic review and meta-analysis. *Diabetes Care* 37: 1759–1766.

Pan, X., Li, G., Hu, Y. et al. (1997). Effects of diet and exercise in preventing NIDDM in people with impaired glucose tolerance. The Da Qing IGT and diabetes study. *Diabetes Care* 20: 537–544.

Parsian, N. and Dunning, T. (2008). Spirituality and coping in young adults with diabetes. *Diabetes Research and Clinical Practice* 79: S121–S122.

Perlstein, R., McConnell, K., and Hagger, V. (1997). *Off to a Flying Start*. Melbourne: International Diabetes Institute.

Pilotto, A. (2018). Technology in geriatrics. *Age Ageing* 47 (6): 771–774.

Pimouguet, C., Le Goff, M., Thiebaut, R. et al. (2010). Effectiveness of disease self-management programs for improving diabetes care: a meta-analysis. *Canadian Medical Association Journal* 183 (2): 115–127. https://doi.org/10.1503/cmaj.091786.

Pozilli, P. and Pieralice, S. (2018). Latenet autoimmune diabetes in adults: current status and new horizons. *Endocrinology and Metabolism* 33 (2): 147–149. https://doi.org/10.3803/EnM.2018.33.2.147.

Renders, C., Valk, G., Griffin, S. et al. (2012). Interventions to improve the management of diabetes mellitus in primary care outpatient and community settings. *Cochrane Database of Systematic Reviews* (1): CD001481.

Reutens, A., Hutchinson, R., van Binh, T. et al. (2011). The GIANT study: a cluster-randomised controlled trial of efficacy of education of doctors about type 2 diabetes mellitus management guidelines in primary care practice. *Diabetes Research and Clinical Practice* 98 (1): 38–45.

Rewers, M., Hyöty, H., Lernmark, Å. et al. (2018). The Environmental Determinants of Diabetes in the Young (TEDDY) study: 2018 update. *Current Diabetes Reports* 18 (12): 136.

Rice, G., Illanes, S., and Mitchell, M. (2012). Gestational diabetes mellitus: a positive predictor of type 2 diabetes? *International Journal of Endocrinology* https://doi.org/10.1155/2012/721653.

RISE Consortium (2018). Metabolic contrast between youth and adults with impaired glucose tolerance or recently diagnosed type 2 diabetes: observations using th hyperglycaenic clamp. *Diabetes Care* **41**: 1696–1706.

Rooney, N., Guest, C., Swanson, L., and Morant, S. (2019). How effective are trained dogs at alerting their owners to changes in blood glycaemic levels? Variations in performance of glycaemia alert dogs. *PLOS ONE* https://doi.org/10.1371/journal.pone.0210092.

Rubin, R. (2002). Was Willis right? Thoughts on the interaction of depression and diabetes. *Diabetes Metabolism Research Reviews* **18**: 173–175.

Saudek, C., Herman, W., Sacks, D. et al. (2008). A new look at screening and diagnosing diabetes mellitus. *Journal of Clinical Endocrinology and Metabolism* **93** (7): 2447–2453.

Scarlett, J., Rojas, M., Matsen, M. et al. (2016). Central injection of fibroblast growth factor 1 induces sustained remission of diabetic hyperglycaemia in rodents. *Nat Medicine* **22**: 800–806.

Schwartz, M., Seeley, R., Tschop, M. et al. (2013). Cooperation between brain and islet in glucose homeostasis and diabetes. *Nature* **503**: 59–66.

Shea, S., Starren, J., Weinstock, R.S. et al. (2002). Columbia University's Informatics for Diabetes Education and Telemedicine (IDEATel) project: rationale and design. *Journal of the American Medical Informatics Association* **9** (1): 49–62.

Simmons, R., Echouffo-Tcheugui, J., Sharp, J. et al. (2012). Screening for type 2 diabetes and population mortality over 10 years (ADDITION-Cambridge): a cluster-randomised controlled trial. *The Lancet* **380** (9855): 1741–1748.

Sinha, R., Fisch, G., Teague, B. et al. (2002). Prevalence of inpaired glucose tolerance among children and adolescents with marked obesity. *New England Journal of Medicine* **346** (11): 802–810.

Smart, C. (2019). App goes beyond carb counting. *The Limbic* (January 30) https://thelimbic.com/endocrinology/app-goes-beyond-carb-counting/ (accessed July 2019).

Soltesz, G., Patterson, C., and Dahlquist, G. (2006). Global trends in childhood obesity. In: *Diabetes Atlas*, 3e, 154–190. Brussels: International Diabetes Federation (IDF).

Sørgjerd, E.P., Åsvold, B.O., Thorsby, P.M., and Grill, V. (2018). Individuals Fulfilling Criteria for Type 2 Diabetes Rather Than LADA Display Transient Signs of Autoimmunity Preceding Diagnosis With Possible Clinical Implications: The HUNT Study. *Diabetes Care* **41** (12): e161–e163.

Spauwen, P.J., Köhler, S., Verhey, F.R. et al. (2013). Effects of type 2 diabetes on 12-year cognitive change: results from the Maastricht Aging Study. *Diabetes Care* **36** (6): 1554–1561.

Stene, L. and Joner, G. (2003). Use of cod liver oil during the first year of life is associated with lower risk of childhood-onset type 1 diabetes: a large, population-based, case-control study. *The American Journal of Clinical Nutrition* **78** (6): 1128–1134.

Tang, P., Overhage, M., Chan, S. et al. (2012). Online disease management of diabetes: engaging and motivating patients online with enhanced resources-diabetes (EMPOWERE_D): a randomized controlled trial. *Journal of the American Medical Association* **20** (3): 526–534. https://doi.org/10.1136/amiajnl-2012-001263.

Taylor, P.D. and Poston, L. (2007). Developmental programming of obesity in mammals. *Experimental Physiology* **92** (2): 287–298.

The DIAMOND Project Group (2006). Incidence and trends of childhood type 1 diabetes worldwide 1990–1999. *Diabetic Medicine* **23**: 857–866.

TODAY Study Group (2012). A clinical trial to maintain glycaemic control in youth with type 2 diabetes. *New England Journal Medicine* **366**: 2247–2256.

Torgerson, J., Hauptman, J., Boldrin, M., and Sjostrom, L. (2004). XENical in the prevention of diabetes in obese subjects (XENDOS) study: a randomized study of orlistat as an adjunct to lifestyle changes for the prevention of type 2 diabetes in obese patients. *Diabetes Care* **27**: 155–161.

Tung, A. (2011). The mystery of guideline non-compliance: why don't doctors do the right thing? *Anaesthesiology* **503**: 3–10.

Tuomilehto, J., Eriksson, J., and Valle, T. (2001). Prevention of type 2 diabetes mellitus by changes in lifestyle among subjects with impaired glucose tolerance. *New England Journal of Medicine* **344**: 1343–1350.

Turner, N. and Clapham, C. (1998). Insulin resistance, impaired glucose tolerance and non-insulin-dependent diabetes pathologic mechanisms and treatment: current status and therapeutic possibilities. *Progress in Drug Research* **51**: 33–94.

Turner, R., Stratton, I., Horton, V. et al. (1997). UKPDS 25 autoantibodies to islet cell cytoplasm and glutamic acid carboxylase for prediction of insulin requirement in type 2 diabetes. UKPDS Study group. *Lancet* **350**: 1288–1293.

Twigg, S., Kamp, M., Davis, T. et al. (2007). Prediabetes: a position statement from the Australian Diabetes Society and Australian diabetes educators association. *Medical Journal of Australia* **186** (9): 461–465.

UKPDS (United Kingdom Prospective Diabetes Study) (1998). Intensive blood glucose control with sulphonylureas or insulin compared with conventional treatment and risk of complications in patients with type 2 diabetes (UKPDS 33). *Lancet* **352**: 837–853.

van den Berghe, G., Wouters, P., Weekers, F. et al. (2007). Intensive insulin therapy in critically ill patients. *New England Journal of Medicine* **345** (19): 1359–1367.

van Ufelen, J., Wong, J., and Chau, J. (2010). Occupational sitting and health risks: a systematic review. *American Journal of Preventative Medicine* **39**: 379–388.

von Bargen, T., Zientz, C., and Haux, R. (2014). Gamification for mHealth – a review of playful mobile healthcare. *Studies in Health Technology and Informatics* **202**: 225–228.

Wahlberg, J., Vaarala, O., Ludvigsson, J., and ABIS-study group (2006). Dietary risk factors for the emergence of type 1 diabetes-related autoantibodies in 2 1/2 year-old Swedish children. *British Journal of Nutrition* **95** (3): 603–608.

Weiss, R. and Caprio, S. (2005). The metabolic consequences of childhood obesity. *Best Practice & Research Clinical Endocrinology & Metabolism* **19** (3): 405–419.

Willi, C., Bodenmann, P., Ghali, W. et al. (2007). Active smoking and the risk of type 2 diabetes: a systematic review and meta-analysis. *Journal of the American Medical Association* **298**: 2654–2664.

Wilmot, E., Edwardson, C., Achana, A. et al. (2012). Sedentary time in adults and the association with diabetes, cardiovascular disease and death: systematic review and meta-analysis. *Diabetologia* **55** (11): 2895–2905. https://doi.org/10.1007/s00125-012-2677-z.

World Health Organization (WHO) (1999). *Definition, Diagnosis and Classification of Diabetes Mellitus and its Complications: Report of a WHO Consultation. Part 1: Diagnosis and Classification of Diabetes Mellitus.* Geneva: WHO https://apps.who.int/iris/handle/10665/66040 (accessed July 2019).

Zhang, H. and Pollin, T. (2018). Epigenetics variation and pathogenesis in diabetes. *Current Diabetes Reports* **18**: 121.

Ziegler, A.G., Schmid, S., Huber, D. et al. (2003). Early infant feeding and risk of developing type 1 diabetes–associated autoantibodies. *Jama* **290** (13): 1721–1728.

Zimmet, P., Alberti, G., and Shaw, J. (2005). Mainstreaming the metabolic syndrome: a definitive definition. *Medical Journal of Australia* **183** (4): 175–176.

Zimmet, P., Alberti, G., Kaufman, F. et al. (2007). The metabolic syndrome in children and adolescents – an IDF consensus report. *Paediatric Diabetes* **8**: 299–306.

Zinman, B., Kahn, S., Haffner, S. et al. (2004). Phenotypic characteristics of GAD antibody-positive recently diagnosed patients with type 2 diabetes in North America and Europe. *Diabetes* **53** (12): 3193–3200.

Zipitis, C.S. and Akobeng, A.K. (2008). Vitamin D supplementation in early childhood and risk of type 1 diabetes: a systematic review and meta-analysis. *Archives of Disease in Childhood* **93** (6): 512–517.

Chapter 2

Holistic Personalised Diabetes Care

Every person who requires healthcare has a unique set of values, goals, and needs.

Key points

- An holistic diabetes assessment, education, and management plan must:
  - Encompass the cultural, religious, physical, emotional, spiritual, family, social, and environmental factors relevant to the individual and be developed in collaboration with them and significant family members and carers.
  - Respect the individual's dignity, personhood, and support their autonomy.
  - Include general nursing and health-care needs as well as diabetes management.
- Incorporate diabetes-specific factors likely to affect self-care, health professional care, and outcomes.
- Collaboratively develop individual care plans based on the best available evidence using shared-decision-making and communicate them to other relevant health professionals, family and carers, keeping in mind the individual's right to privacy.
- Evaluate outcomes relevant to the overall management goals, agreed metabolic target ranges as well as short-term goals formulated within the overall plan for a specific episode of care such as an admission to hospital.
- Discharge planning and transitional care amongst health services should be part of the care plan.
- Providing holistic diabetes care requires clinicians to be reflective practitioners who can combine art and science.

Rationale

Best-practice diabetes education and care relies multidisciplinary team care, a combination of the best available evidence, intuition, and clinical judgement, effective communication skills, and, importantly, the informed participation of the person with diabetes. Careful assessment enables physical, psychological, spiritual, cultural, religious, and social issues that affect care to

Care of People with Diabetes: A Manual for Healthcare Practice, Fifth Edition. Trisha Dunning and Alan Sinclair.
© 2020 John Wiley & Sons Ltd. Published 2020 by John Wiley & Sons Ltd.

be identified and incorporated into management and discharge/transition plans. Life balance, coping with significant life transitions, and emotional well-being are essential to achieving optimal diabetes-related outcomes.

Significantly, many care standards now include person-centred and family-centred care. It is a key aspect of the Australian Commission on Safety and Quality in Health Care (2017) Health service standards, The UK Department of Health (2006), the US Institute of Medicine (IOM) (2001) and The American Diabetes Association (2019). Patient-centeredness is variously defined and described using various terms. I prefer *person-centred* or personalised to *patient-centred* because the word 'patient' suggests a hierarchy and does not apply in all settings where care is delivered.

The move towards person-centred care reflects the focus on respecting individuals and their values and goals and involving them in decisions about their care. The IOM defined person-centeredness as:

Providing care that is respectful of and responsive to individual patient preferences, needs, and values and ensuring that patient values guide all clinical decisions.

However, the degree to which an individual wants to be involved, and has the capacity to be involved, varies amongst individuals, the same individual at different times and during different consultations and the issue at the time. Thus, whilst there is commitment and support for person-centred care there is a great deal of uncertainty associated with applying the concepts/philosophy in the real-world, day-to-day practice.

As well as the focus on person-centred care, there is a global shift towards managing health and wellbeing using an holistic, predictive approach and from extending life to improving quality of life, and taking a life course approach to healthy, active ageing. Engaging with consumers and sharing in decision making are essential to achieving these aims. There is also emerging interest in 'uncertainty tolerance' and its effect on various health outcomes (Strout et al. 2018). Diagnostic uncertainty is a large contributor to diagnostic errors in most medical specialties. It leads to more hospital admissions and referrals, ordering more diagnostic investigations and higher health-care costs (Alam et al. 2017). Uncertainty tolerance is an individual characteristic and affects the way clinicians respond to diagnostic, prognostic, and therapeutic decision, many of which are not straightforward and can create uncertainty (Han et al. 2011).

Hillen et al. (2017) defined uncertainty tolerance as 'a set of negative and positive psychological responses-cognitive, emotional, and behavioral-provoked by the conscious awareness of ignorance about particular aspect of the world.' It also encompasses ethical factors (Alam et al. 2017). The definition by Hillen et al. (2017) denotes the breadth of potential responses to uncertainty and applies to people with diabetes and clinicians; both groups respond to uncertainty in different ways. Some may feel vulnerable and avoid making a decision (negative); others see opportunity and hope and seek information, decide on a solution and make a decision (positive). Tolerance of uncertainty is a balance between the two, and may differ in different contexts and with different issues. Understanding these issues can help clinicians communicate effectively with people with diabetes to achieve personalised diabetes care.

Shared decision-making (SDM)

SDM is a key aspect of good clinical practice as well as an 'ethical imperative' (Australian Commission on Quality and Safety in Health Care [ACSQHC] 2017) and is increasingly incorporated into policies and guidelines. SDM refers to a communication process where a clinician/s and individual participate in making a decision. It is also a process for bringing evidence into care discussions to aid decisions as well as a way of resolving the differences between clinicians' and people with diabetes' different estimations of benefits and risks (Hoffman et al. 2014). If done well, it can reduce unnecessary investigations, referrals and possibly health costs.

In many cases, decisions do not have to be made all at once, such as developing an advance care plan (Chapter 18) (Legare et al. 2013; Hoffman et al. 2014; Elwyn et al. 2017). The process encompasses equal respect between the parties to enable collaborative discussion about the issue/s being discussed, the various management options, their risks and benefits, the veracity of the information, and clinicians providing information in a format that suits the individual's learning style, health literacy, and numeracy and preference for making a decision. Culture can also be important. People from some cultural groups, especially older people, prefer to be told what to do.

Some experts describe the need to activate such people, called *patient activation*. The term has patriarchal and judgmental connotations. Nevertheless, patient activation can be measured using the Patient Activation Measure (PAM), although its validity has been questioned. Sadly, there is not a clinician activation measure, although experts suggest training in SDM is essential for clinicians (Legare et al. 2012), which could be a form of activation! Many clinicians believe 'they do shared decision-making,' often because they do not actually know what it is, yet observational studies show low levels of clinician behaviours that indicate they actually involve people in making decisions (McCaffery et al. 2013).

A range of decision aids with various content and formats are available and can be used in SDM, but it is not essential to use a decision aid. Decision aids can be used in various ways, such as during a consultation and/or provided to the person with diabetes/family to consider before the consultation. Plain language evidence summaries, guidelines, and policies are commonly used decision aids for clinicians. SDM models can also help clinicians collaborate with individual and their families. These include the three-talk model (Elwyn et al. 2017), which encompasses active listening and inclusive language, and depends on clinicians having good communication skills. It consists of:

(1) Team talk – work together as a team to make a decision.
(2) Option talk – compare the various options.
(3) Decision talk – agree on a decision. That meets the individual's needs and values.

Personal stories

Identifying the issues that give meaning and purpose to a person's life (their values) can be very useful to SDM and other aspects of emotional health, as well as end of life care. Ask the individual to name three to five things that are very important to them and monitor changes at annual complication screening and any change in function or psychological health status. A simple Likert scale can be used.

Holistic diabetes care

Holistic care aims to heal the whole person using art and science to support the individual to mobilise their innate healing potential: that is, to become empowered. Healing occurs when the individual embraces and transforms traumatic life events and is open to and/or recognises his or her potential (Dossey et al. 1995, p. 40). Transcending traumatic life events such as the diagnosis of diabetes or a diabetes complication is part of the spiritual journey to self-awareness, self-empowerment, and wholeness. Significantly, spirituality is not the same as religion, although it may encompass religion (Dossey et al. 1995, p. 6; Parsian and Dunning 2008; Dunning 2013).

Thus, in order to achieve holistic care, nurses must consider the individual's beliefs and attitudes because the meaning people attach to their health, diabetes, and treatment, including medicines, affects their self-care behaviour, and health outcomes. At least eight broad interpretations of illness have been identified: challenge, enemy, punishment, weakness, relief, irreparable loss/damage, value adding, and denial (Lipowski 1970; Dunning 1994; Dunning and Martin 1998). In addition, the author has identified other explanatory models during routine clinical care: diabetes is an opportunity for positive change; and diabetes is a visitation from God.

Holistic diabetes care encompasses respect for the person's dignity, including dignity of risk, and is a key aspect of quality care (Barclay 2016). People have dignity when they have respect and clinicians do not transgress their standards and values (Killmister 2010). Many encounters in healthcare, including diabetes care, can make people feel vulnerable and humiliated. For example, some conditions such as incontinence and exposing parts of the body are regarded as shameful. Defining dignity is challenging, but the term generally refers to an individual's right to autonomy to make choices and self-determination. Two forms are described: human dignity and social dignity (Jacobson 2009). Importantly, dignity belongs to individuals and to collectivities.

Violations to people's dignity increase or create vulnerability. Repeated violations lead to a spiral of damage and loss and suboptimal outcomes. Dignity therapy programmes are emerging in a range of settings, including for people with a serious illness, those at the end of life, people living in aged care homes, and for family members of such people. Dignity therapy might not have been evaluated in diabetes care as yet; however, individuals with diabetes, and families with diabetes in them, are highly likely to benefit from being treated with respect.

Communication and the power of language

Good communication using appropriate language is essential to achieve holistic, personalised care and SDM. The influence of the language and diabetes dialect have gained prominence over the past few years (Dickinson et al. 2017; Dunning 2013; Diabetes Australia 2016; Dunning et al. 2017; American Diabetes Association 2019; Diabetes UK – Hendrieckx et al. 2019). All of these publications recommend clear, nonjudgemental language in spoken and written materials. Clear language and avoiding jargon are also important from a health literacy perspective.

> To write jargon is like perpetually shuffling around in the fog and cotton wool of abstract terms.
> (Sir Arthur Quiller-Couch 1916)

Clinicians use a lot of jargon during clinical encounters and diabetes education session, which often creates a lot of fog for people with diabetes. Unless clinicians check for understanding using probes and clarifying questions and teach back methods individuals can shuffle around in the fog for long periods and the clinicians might not even be aware the fog exists (Dunning 2013). Miscommunication is more likely when the clinician and person with diabetes speak different languages and/or have different literacy and numeracy skills, goals values, and experiences. Clinicians need excellent communication skills to achieve shared understanding.

Language is powerful. Most health-related critical incidents and complaints about health clinicians arise from ineffective communication (McCreaddie, Benwell, and Gritti 2018). Inappropriate language can contribute to inadequate diabetes self-care and suboptimal outcomes, and can inhibit the capacity to provide informed consent and reduce morbidity and mortality (Flores et al. 2002). People with diabetes are often under stress and vulnerable during education and clinical encounters, especially during hospital admissions and in aged-care facilities.

Factors that lead to miscommunication include:

- Not listening
- Incorrect assumptions about knowledge, competence, attitudes, and behaviours amongst people engaged in the conversation
- Sensory defects such as sight and hearing
- The way information is structured and presented (design as well as the words used)
- How the speaker signals connections amongst the pieces of information and with the listener
- Whether the information flows logically
- The setting and the number of distractions

Reading fiction to improve empathy and communication skills

Researchers have been exploring the importance of reading fiction to social intelligence for over 25 years. The findings suggest that stories are a type of simulation that helps readers understand the characters in the book, their relationships and social situations, and human characters, generally. They build the theory of mind (Djikic et al. 2013; Mar, Tackett, and Moore 2010; Oatley 2011). Theory of mind describes the capacity to understand other people's perspectives, develop mental models of others and understand that people can have different attitudes, beliefs, and intentions from one's self. People begin to develop a theory of mind about age four years. Development continues throughout life. These are key skills that clinicians need to provide holistic personalised diabetes care and education. Social skills are essential to developing theory of mind.

Reading fiction improves social skills (social intelligence), capacity for empathy, and the ability to appreciate other people's point of view (Oatley 2011). The more fiction people read, the more they are able to make mental models of other people (Djikic et al. 2013). Significantly, people who read good-quality fiction perform better on social reasoning tests than people who read the same information in a nonfiction format (Mar, Tackett, and Moore 2010), which suggests fiction primes people to think more about the social world and that fiction readers are better able to develop a theory of mind. These notions are consistent with narrative medicine programmes in health professional teaching. Narrative medicine courses were developed based on the philosophy that 'the effective health care requires narrative competence' (Charon 2001). Narrative competence refers to the capacity to identify people's stories and concerns and to acknowledge, interpret, and act on their stories.

Care models

There is considerable international variation amongst diabetes care models, although most are based on similar philosophies. Model variation is necessary to address the specific context and other factors in specific countries and settings and is consistent with current implementation science models that stress the importance of considering context and co-developing services and models with end users. Interestingly, Lenzen et al. (2018) developed a conversation approach (model) to enhance practice nurses' capacity to engage in shared decision making in primary care. It encompasses the three-talk model (Elwyn et al. 1999; Elwyn, Tilburt, and Montori 2014) and goal setting and planning.

The essential elements of quality diabetes services encompass the following:

- Evidence-based planned care including management guidelines and policies.
- Appropriate service and practice design that encompasses interdisciplinary team care, prevention, and early detection programmes and expedites referral and communication amongst services.
- Systems to support self-management.
- Process to ensure clinicians are knowledgeable and competent, collaborate and communicate effectively, have sufficient time to provide individual care, and are supported to do so and where their roles are clearly defined and complementary.
- Clinical information systems that enable disease registries to be maintained, outcomes to be monitored, relevant reminders to be sent to patients, and performance to be evaluated (Wagner, Austin, and ConKorff 1996a).
- Processes for assess individual's health status as well as process for assessing the performance of the service and the clinicians providing services. For example, the Australian National Diabetes Audit (Department of Health 2017).

Many current diabetes management models such as the Lorig and Flinders models, the Group Health Cooperative Diabetes Roadmap, Kaiser-Permanente in Colorado, nurse led case management, and various shared care models including computer programmes (Interactive Health Communication Applications [IHCA]) encompass these elements and improve people with diabetes adherence to management strategies and satisfaction with care. However, their application is still limited by time and resource constraints, including timely access to health professionals.

Research suggests Internet-based support can improve patient-practitioner communication and collaboration, and enhance a patient's sense of being valued and secure (Ralston et al. 2004). However, more research is needed to determine the best way to use these programmes and their effects in specific patient groups (Murray et al. 2005). Generally, patients have a better understanding of what is expected of them if they receive both written and verbal information (Johnson et al. 2003). The font size, colour, and language level of any written material provided, including instructions for procedures and appointments and health professional contact details, must be appropriate to the age, education level, and culture of the individual concerned (see Chapter 16).

In addition, clinicians must clearly promote a patient-centred approach to care (National Managed Care Congress 1996) that is evident within the service. For example, patients are involved in decisions about their care and see the same doctor each time they attend an appointment. They should also be involved in service planning and deciding what constitutes quality care and what metrics to use to measure quality (Jones 2013). Most patients want to be cared for by knowledgeable, competent, and caring health professionals who are approachable and expert communicators; yet these issues, that are so important to patients, are not always included in quality metrics.

Patient satisfaction surveys fall short of demonstrating person-centred care, although such surveys often seek information to help them make services more patient friendly. They often reflect selection bias and contain multiple confounders, and many are not validated in any appropriate way. In addition, patient satisfaction does not reflect person-centred care or quality care.

Although person-centred care is difficult to define and achieve, often because it is a subjective concept and, as indicated, because of time constraints, it generally refers to steps such as the following:

- Personalise care rather than using one target fits all: diabetes management guidelines are beginning to encompass individualised management targets (European Alliance for Personalized Medicine 2016; Green-Thompson et al. 2017).
- Ensure that care considers the individual's social, mental, physical, and social situation as well as their goals, explanatory models, capability (physical, mental, spiritual, and linguistic), and health and general beliefs, experiences, religion, and culture.
- Deliver care that is culturally sensitive and relevant to the individual but that is also family-centred (The Joint Commission 2010).
- Use effective communication strategies that account for any disabilities the individual might have and use translators sensitively. Effective communication is a two-way process in which messages are negotiated until the information is correctly understood by everybody involved in the communication.
- Develop strategies to help the patient trust their health professionals (Wagner et al. 1996a) and vice versa!
- Help people acquire the information they need to make informed decisions (McCulloch et al. 1998).
- Improve people's adherence to management recommendations (Wagner et al. 1996b): also see Chapters 15 and 16.
- Make collaborative decisions with the patient and communicate them to relevant people.

Kleinman et al. (1978) suggested that the following simple questions could help create shared understanding between people with diabetes and clinicians. The questions are still relevant; in fact, they were recommended by the Joint Commission roadmap for hospitals concerning advocacy and person- and family-centred care (2010):

- What do you think caused your illness/problem/s?
- Why do you think the problem started when it did?
- How is the problem affecting you?
- How serious do you think the problem is?
- What sort of treatment do you think will help?

- What do you want the treatment to do (outcomes)?
- What are your main concerns about the problem?
- How can I/we help?

Obviously, the questions should not be used as a tick list, and they should be supplemented with clarifying questions and by checking assumptions.

Specific programmes that train health professionals how to deliver person-centred care improve patient trust in doctors (Lewin et al. 2001; McKinstry, Colthart, and Walker 2006) and the delivery of information (Kinnersley et al. 2007). In addition, people may need specific education about how to ask relevant questions during consultations and how to participate in making management decisions. Both parties may need education about how to negotiate the complex nature of SDM to balance the imperative for evidence-based care with the need to incorporate the individual's values and preferences. In order to assist the process, the Foundation for Informed Decision-Making in the USA (2007) developed a series of interactive videos and written materials for patients about a range of common medical conditions.

Clinicians need to undertake a thorough assessment, using appropriate questions and clinical reasoning to identify the patient's needs and management guidelines to determine whether the recommended treatment is likely to benefit the individual, whether the benefits outweigh the risks, and whether the individual can/will adhere to the recommendations, including their self-care capacity, and then decide appropriate treatment options to the individual.

Characteristics of an holistic health history

The nursing/medical history is actually the individual's story: clinicians are privileged to learn part of that story. The art of story listening is essential to compiling a useful patient history:

- The history/story includes demographic data (age, gender, social situation, culture, religion).
- Units of information about past and current individual and family health, and family and social relationships (see Figure 2.1) are collected to enable individual care plans to be co-decided considering the person's values, goals, and expectations:
  - Obtain baseline information about the person's physical and mental status before and after and the presenting illness.
  - Collect information about the person's general health and diabetes-related beliefs and attitudes and the meaning they attach to and the importance they place on symptoms.
- The story should be concise to enable information to be collected in a short time.
- Focus should be on maintaining the person's dignity and independence whilst they are in hospital (e.g. allowing them to monitor their own blood glucose and administer their insulin).

The findings should be documented in the medical record (think about that term – does it reflect personalised care and the person's story?) and communicated to the appropriate caregivers. There is an increasing trend towards electronic data collection and management process that enables information to be easily and rapidly transferred amongst health professionals. Some systems enable patients to access their health information. Most modern electronic blood glucose meters have a facility for marinating a record of blood glucose test results that can be downloaded into computer programmes. These systems have the capacity to significantly improve healthcare; however, consideration must be given to the privacy and confidentiality of all personal information and appropriate access and storage security mechanisms should be maintained according to the laws of the relevant country.

Assessing the person with diabetes does not differ from assessing people with any other disease process. Assessment should take into account social, physical, and psychological factors in order to co-develop an appropriate care plan, including a plan for diabetes education and discharge/transitions amongst services. Any physical disability the patient has could affect their ability to self-manage their diabetes (inject insulin, care for their feet, monitor blood glucose). Impaired sight, hearing, and psychological distress and mental illness may preclude people attending group education programmes. Management and educational expectations may need to be modified to accommodate such disabilities.

If the person has diabetes, however, metabolic derangements may be present or could develop as a consequence of hospitalisation. Therefore, careful assessment enables potential problems to be proactively identified, alerts to be flagged if necessary, a coordinated collaborative care plan to be developed, and appropriate referral to other health professionals (medical specialist, podiatrist, diabetes nurse specialist/diabetes educator, dietitian, geriatrician, palliative care expert, and psychologist) to take place. A health problem list that ranks care issues in order of priority can also help clinicians plan individualised care that addresses immediate and future management goals. The first step in any assessment is to document a comprehensive health history.

Diabetes-specific assessment and screening processes and target ranges are discussed in relevant chapters throughout the book. They are also described in regularly updated guidelines such as the ADS Standards of Medical care (2019), The UK National Institute for Health and Care Excellence (NICE). They all advocate for person centred, interdisciplinary team care and prevention and early detection.

Documenting in the health record

Documentation is an essential part of health management. Alternative methods of documenting care are emerging – for example, charting by exception, where only events outside the normal expected progress are recorded. This form of charting requires supportive documentation in the form of guidelines, flowcharts, care plans, and care maps. They can avoid duplication and streamline documentation. The use of care pathways is becoming increasingly common in Australia and in the United Kingdom (O'Brien and Hardy 2000).

Other ways of documenting holistic care incorporate genomaps and ecomaps (see Figure 2.1), which can effectively convey a great deal of information about the social relationship and support base aspects of an individual's life (Cluning 1997). They are particularly useful for

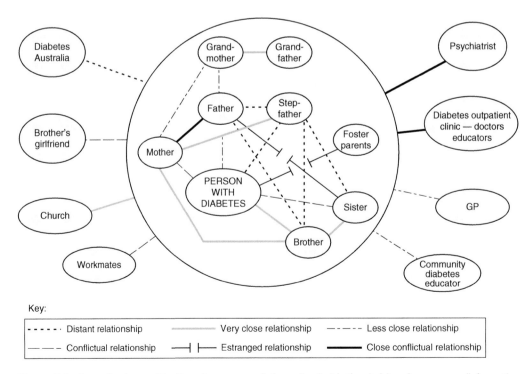

Figure 2.1 Example of a combination of a genomap (information inside the circle) and an ecomap (information outside the circle) of a 50-year-old woman with type 2 diabetes and a history of childhood molestation and sexual abuse. It shows a great deal of conflict within and outside the family and identifies where her support base is.

long-term chronic diseases such as diabetes where these factors affect management outcomes; see Chapters 15 and 16. They also record information that is often passed on anecdotally during handover or in the 'corridor,' which means vital information that could assist in planning care is not available or is misinterpreted.

Genograms illustrate how an individual relates to other people in the family and ecomaps place the family in the context of the wider social situation in which they live. Ecograms and ecomaps can be simple or convey complex and detailed information. Together, they give a great deal of information about the following:

- The individual's environment
- Their relationships with people in their environment
- Family structure
- Family and extended support
- Family health history
- Family functioning
- Health service utilisation
- Social orientation

This information helps determine how social support and other networks influence the person's life generally, self-management, and the assistance they can rely on, for example, to manage serious hypoglycaemia and intercurrent illness.

Documenting care plans

The employing institution's policy regarding the method of documentation and care pathways should be followed. Good documentation enables the required care to be communicated to all staff. In the future, changes will occur to the methods of documenting care. For example, focus charting and flowcharts may replace narrative notes. Flowcharts are designed to enable all health-care providers to document care on a single care plan, which reduces duplication and may enhance communication. Most services now use some form of electronic data collection, documentation, and communication processes.

Due consideration must be given to data security. Confidential information should be labelled as such in the medical record. Extra care is required with mobile technology such as smart phones, laptops, and palm pilots to ensure patient confidentiality is protected if any patient data are stored and/or communicated via these media.

Nursing/medical notes

Due consideration needs to be given to standard policies for good documentation and the laws governing privacy and confidentiality and people's right to access their medical records. Medical notes are a record of the patient's encounter with a service provider in any setting and hospital admission, the care they received and the outcomes of the care provided, and acts as a guide for discharge planning. Handwritten documentation should be written legibly and objectively. Medical records are not legal documents but can subpoenaed for a court hearing. In such cases, good documentation can help the health professional recall the situation.

Documentation should contain the following:

- The condition of the patient recorded objectively. For example, describe wounds in terms of size and depth.
- Quantification of the patient's condition. Record swelling, oedema, temperature, pulse, and respiration (TPR), and blood pressure (BP) using objective measures.
- All teaching the patient receives. Note instructions that are still required.
- The patient's response to treatment.
- All medications received. Note any associated adverse events.

- Removal of all invasive medical devices (e.g. packs, drains, IV lines).
- Psychological, spiritual, and social factors.

Clinical observation

In some cases, it is possible to refer to standard protocols in medical records if there is a set procedure documented and regularly revised, e.g. there is a standard procedure for performing an oral glucose tolerance test. The documentation could note relevant details such as the time, date, and person's name and then state 'OGGT performed according to the standard protocol'. Where any deviation from the protocol occurred, it should be recorded. If required, the standard protocol could be produced.

Documentation by people with diabetes

People with diabetes also document a great deal of information about their diabetes. They use a variety of written and electronic record-keeping methods including blood glucose monitoring diaries, complication screening records, and other management information such as medication lists and the results of investigative procedures. These records are a vital part of the documentation process. They not only supply written information but also contain a great deal of information about an individual's self-care ability. For example, a blood glucose diary covered with blood smears could mean the person is having difficulty placing the blood on the strip. Discussing the issue with the patient might reveal that they often get the shakes and their vision is blurred due to hypoglycaemia. It is important, however, that all such assumptions are checked.

Importantly, the information in the individual's documents must be valued and used in the clinical encounter. It is a tangible record of the hard work of self-care.

References

Alam, R., Cheraghi-Sohl, S., Panagioti, M. et al. (2017). Managing diagnostic uncertainty in primary care: a systematic critical review. *BMJ Family Practice* **18**: 79. https://doi.org/10.1186/s12875-017-0650-0.

American Diabetes Associations (ADS) (2019). Standards of medical care. *Diabetes Care* **42** (Suppl 1): 182–183. https://doi.org/10.2337/dc19-S016.

Australian Commission on Safety and Quality in Health Care (ACSQHC) (2017). *National Safety and Quality Health Service Standards*, 2e. Sydney, Australia: ACSQHC. https://www.safetyandquality.gov.au/wp-content/uploads/2017/11/National-Safety-and-Quality-Health-Service-Standards-second-edition.pdf (accessed 26 June 2019).

Barclay, L. (2016). In sickness and in dignity: a philosophical account or the meaning of dignity in health care. *International Journal of Nursing Studies*. https://doi.org/10.1016/j.ijnurstu.2016.06.010.

Charon, R. (2001). Narrative medicine: a model for empathy, reflection, profession and trust. *Journal American Medical Association* **286** (15): 1897–1902.

Cluning, T. (1997). Social assessment documentation: genomaps and ecomaps, chapter 7. In: *Nursing Documentation: Writing What we Do* (ed. J. Richmond). Melbourne, Australia: Ausmed Publications.

Department of Health (2017). Australian National Diabetes Audit (ANDA). https://www.health.gov.au/internet/main/publishing.nsf/Content/pq-diabetes-pubs (accessed 26 June 2019).

Diabetes Australia (2016). A new language for diabetes: Improving communications with and about people with diabetes. Position statement – Diabetes Australia. https://static.diabetesaustralia.com.au/s/fileassets/diabetes-australia/f4346fcb-511d-4500-9cd1-8a13068d5260.pdf (accessed 26 June 2019).

Dickison, J., Marynuik, M., O'Brien, C. et al. (2017). The use of language in diabetes care and education. *Diabetes Care* **40**: 1790–1799.

Djikic, M., Oatley, K., and Moldoveanu, M. (2013). Reading other minds: Effects of literature on empathy. *Scientific Study of Literature* **3** (1): 28–47. https://doi.org/10.1075/ssol.3.1.06dji.

Dossey, B., Keegen, L., Guzzetta, C., and Kolkmeier, L. (1995). *Holistic Nursing: A Handbook for Practice*, 20–21. Maryland: Aspen Publishers.

Dunning, P. (1994). Having diabetes: young adult perspectives. *The Diabetes Educator* **21** (1): 58–65.

Dunning, T. (2013). Turning points and transitions: crises and opportunities, chapter 8. In: *Diabetes Education: Art, Science and Evidence* (ed. T. Dunning), 117–131. Chichester: Wiley Blackwell.

Dunning, P. and Martin, M. (1998). Beliefs about diabetes and diabetes complications. *Professional Nurse* **13** (7): 429–434.

Dunning, T., Speight, J., and Bennett, C. (2017). Language, the 'diabetes restricted code/dialect' and what it means for people with diabetes and clinicians. *The Diabetes Educator*. https://doi.org/10.1177/0145721716683449.

Elwyn, G., Edwards, A., Gwyn, R., and Grol, R. (1999). Towards a feasible model for shared decision making: focus group study with general practice registrars. *BMJ* **319** (7212): 753–756. https://doi.org/10.1136/bmj.319.7212.753.

Elwyn, G., Tilburt, J., and Montori, V. (2014). The ethical imperative for shared decision-making. *European Journal Person Centered Healthcare* **1**: 129–131.

Elwyn, G., Durand, M., Song, J. et al. (2017). A three-talk model for shared decision making: multistage consultation process. *British Medical Journal* **359**: J4891. https://doi.org/10.1136/bmj.j4891.

European Alliance for Personalised Medicine (2016). Taking stock: the role of personalized medicine in modern-day healthcare. http://www.euapm.eu (accessed 26 June 2019).

Flores, G., Rabke-Verani, J., Pine, W., and Sabharwal, A. (2002). The importance of cultural and linguistic issues in the emergency care of children. *Pediatric Emergency Care* **18** (4): 271–284.

Foundation for Informed Medical Decision Making (2007). http://www.ihi.org/resources/Pages/OtherWebsites/FoundationforInformedMedicalDecisionMaking.aspx (accessed 26 June 2019).

Green-Thompson, L., McInerney, P., and Woollard, B. (2017). The social accountability of doctors: a relationship based framework for understanding emergent community concepts of caring. *BMC Health Services Research* **17**: 269. https://doi.org/10.1186/s12913-017-2239-7.

Han, P., Klein, W., and Arora, N. (2011). Varieties of uncertainty in health care: a conceptual taxonomy. *Medical Decision Making* **31**: 828–838.

Hendrieckx, C., Halliday, J.A., Beeney, L.J., and Speight, J. (2019). *Diabetes and Emotional Health: A Practical Guide for Healthcare Professionals Supporting Adults with Type 1 and Type 2 Diabetes*, 2e. London, UK: Diabetes UK.

Hillen, M., CuTheil, C., Strout, T. et al. (2017). Tolerance of uncertainty: concept analysis, integrative model and implications for healthcare. *Health Care Society* **14**: 62–67.

Hoffman, T., Legare, F., Simmons, M. et al. (2014). Shared decision making: what do clinicians do clinicians need to know and why should they bother. *Medical Journal of Australia* **201** (1): 35–39.

Institute of Medicine (2001). *Crossing the Quality Chasm: A New Health System for 21st Century*. Washington, DC: National Academy Press. http://www.nationalacademies.org/hmd/Global/News%20Announcements/Crossing-the-Quality-Chasm-The-IOM-Health-Care-Quality-Initiative.aspx.

Jacobson, J. (2009). A taxonomy of dignity: a grounded theory study. *BMC International health and Human Rights* **9**: 3. https://doi.org/10.1186/1472-698X-9-3.

Johnson, A., Sandford, J., and Tyndall, J. (2003). Written and verbal information versus verbal information only for patients being discharged from acute hospital settings to home. *Cochrane Database of Scientific Reviews* (4): Cd003716. https://doi.org/10.1002/14651858.CD003716.

Jones, I. (2013). Health care decision making and the politics of health. In: *Critical Theory and Health* (ed. J. Habermas), 76–93. London, UK: Routledge.

Kinnersley, P., Edwards, A., Hood, K. et al. (2007). Interventions before consultations for helping patients address their information needs. *Cochrane Database of Scientific Reviews* (3): CD 004565. https://doi.org/10.1002/14651858.CD004565.pub2.

Kleinman, A., Eisenberg, L., and Goode, B. (1978). Culture, illness and care: clinical lessons from anthropological and cross cultural research. *Annals of Internal Medicine* **88** (2): 251–258.

Killmister, S. (2010). Dignity: not such a useless concept. *Journal of Medical Ethics* **36** (3): 160–164. https://doi.org/10.1136/jme.2009.031393.

Legare, F., Politi, M., Drolet, R. et al. (2012). Health professionals in shared decision making: an international environmental scan. *Patient Education and Counselling*. **88**: 159–169.

Legare, F., Stacey, D., Briere, N. et al. (2013). Healthcare providers' intention to engage in an interprofessional approach to shared decision-making in home care programs: a mixed methods study. *Journal Interprofessional Care* **27**: 214–222.

Lenzen, S.A., Daniëls, R., van Bokhoven, M.A. et al. (2018). Development of a conversation approach for practice nurses aimed at making shared decisions on goals and action plans with primary care patients. *BMC Health Services Research* **18** (1): 891.

Lewin, S., Skea, Z., Entwistle, V. et al. (2001). Interventions for providers to promote a patient-centred approach in clinical consultations. *Cochrane Database of Systematic Reviews* (4): CDOO 3267. https://doi.org/10.1002/14651858.CD003267.

Lipowski, Z.J. (1970). Physical illness, the individual and the coping processes. *Psychiatry in Medicine* **1** (2): 91–102.

Mar, R.A., Tackett, J.L., and Moore, C. (2010). Exposure to media and theory-of-mind development in preschoolers. *Cognitive Development* **25** (1): 69–78.

McCaffery, K., Holmes-Rovner, M., Smith, S. et al. (2013). Addressing health literacy in patient decision aids. *BMC Medical Information Decision Making* **13** (Suppl2): S10.

McCreaddie, M., Benwell, B., and Gritti, A. (2018). Traumatic journeys: understanding the rhetoric of patients' complaints. *BMC Health Services Complaints* **18** (551). https://doi.org/10.1186/s12913-018-3339-8.

McCulloch, D., Price, M., Hindmarsh, M. et al. (1998). A population based approach to diabetes management in a primary care setting: early results and lessons learned. *Effective Clinical Practice* **1**: 1222.

McKinstry, B., Colthart, I., and Walker, J. (2006). Can doctors predict patients' satisfaction and enablement? A cross-sectional observational study. *Family Practice* **23** (2): 240–245.

Murray, E., Burns, J., See Tai, S. et al. (2005). Interactive health communication applications for people with chronic illness. *Cochrane Database of Systematic Reviews* (4): CDOO4274. https://doi.org/10.1002/14651858.CD004274.pub4.

National Managed Health Care Congress (NHCG) (1996). *The Disease Management Strategic Research Study and Resource Guide.* Washington, DC: NHCG.

Oatley, K. (2011). Fiction and its study as gateways to the mind. *Scientific Study of Literature* **1** (1): 153–164.

O'Brien, S. and Hardy, K. (2000). Impact of a care pathway driven diabetes education programme. *Journal of Diabetes Nursing* **4** (5): 147–150.

Parsian, N. and Dunning, T. (2008). Spirituality and coping in young adults with diabetes. *Diabetes Research and Clinical Practice* **79** (182): S82–S121.

Quiller-Couch, S.A. (1916). *On the Art of Writing: Lectures Delivered in the University of Cambridge, 1913–1914.* Cambridge, UK: University Press www.bartleby.com/190/.

Ralston, J., Revere, D., and Robins, L. (2004). Patients' experience with a diabetes support program based on an interactive electronic medical record: qualitative survey. *British Medical Journal* **328**: 115–162.

Strout, T., Hillen, M., Cutheil, C. et al. (2018). Tolerance of uncertainty: a systematic review of health and health care outcomes. *Patient Education and Counselling* **101** (9): 1518–1537. http://doi.org/10.1016/j.pec2019.03.030.

The Joint Commission (2010). Advancing effective communication, cultural competence and patient- and family-centered care: a road map for hospitals. www.jointcommission.org/Advancing_Effective_Communication.

UK Department of Health (2006). Quality standards for health and social care. http://www.health-ni.gov.uk/articles/quality-standards-health-and-social-care (accessed 26 June 2019).

Wagner, E., Austin, B., and von Korff, M. (1996a). Organizing care for patients with chronic illness. *The Milbank Quarterly* **74** (4): 511–544. https://doi.org/10.2307/3350391.

Wagner, E., Austin, B., and von Korff, M. (1996b). Improving outcomes in chronic illness. *Managed Care Quarterly* **4** (2): 12–25.

Chapter 3

Assessing and Monitoring People with Diabetes

Key points

- Regularly assessing the individual's physical, emotional, social, spiritual, relationship status, and their capacity to perform their usual activities of daily living and self-care is essential to enable proactive personalised management and self-care strategies to be implemented and changed when indicated.
- Structured regular assessment and screening programmes that encompass general health, functional status, mental health, self-care, driving safety, medicine reviews, and education are needed at least annually.
- The health and well-being of family carers need to be considered, especially family caring for children, adolescents, and older people.
- Diabetes education and management programmes/policies should be evaluated and revised regularly to ensure they remain current.
- People with diabetes should be involved in designing and evaluating services, education programmes, education, and other information and research.
- Assessing and monitoring encompasses considering the individual's life story, life and disease trajectories, and whether change is temporarily or represents changing life expectancy and the need to consider palliative and end of life care: see Chapter 18.
- People with diabetes have a responsibility to undertake appropriate self-care to manage their disease.

Rationale

Regular proactive health assessments and risk screening considering the individual's age, social situation, type of diabetes, and self-care capabilities are key aspects of quality diabetes care.

Proactive assessment and monitoring programmes enable the individual's blood glucose and lipid patterns, health and complication status, and self-care capacity to be identified and a management plan tailored for/with the individual. The accuracy of the person's blood glucose self-monitoring (SMBG) technique and appropriate equipment maintenance are important

Care of People with Diabetes: A Manual for Healthcare Practice, Fifth Edition. Trisha Dunning and Alan Sinclair.
© 2020 John Wiley & Sons Ltd. Published 2020 by John Wiley & Sons Ltd.

aspects of safe, quality diabetes care, and they help ensure management decisions are based on the best available data when used in conjunction with laboratory investigations and physical and mental assessments.

Self-monitoring enables people with diabetes to identify the effects of diet, exercise, stress, and other factors on their blood glucose levels and helps them gain insight into and control over their diabetes. It also helps the individual and care providers recognise patterns and cues to changes such as hyper- and hypoglycaemia that could require temporary or permanent changes to their diabetes management.

Monitoring and meeting management targets is also a key quality management activity in many countries. Funding and service accreditation processes often depend on organisations and clinicians providing cost-effective care, value for money, and complying with guidelines and care standards. In addition, health services are expected to demonstrate shared decision-making and person-centred care. These regulatory and budget-based expectations, along with the increasing diabetes prevalence, put pressure on services, service managers, clinicians, clerical staff, and ultimately people with diabetes and their families.

Some guidelines and position statements that address these issues are shown in Table 3.1. It is important to manage risks and enhance the benefits of care. Thus, undertaking proactive personalised risk assessments with the individual for some aspects of care help decide strategies to manage the risk; for example, hypoglycaemia, medicine-related adverse events, hyperglycaemia, falls, and pain.

Key issues to consider in comprehensive assessments

Most guidelines include important factors to assess, recommend relevant metabolic and other target ranges, and the time these assessments/investigations need to be undertaken. Most of these guidelines focus on diabetes: some are beginning to include other important issues such as social issues, technology use, vaccination status, and complementary medicines use. Guidelines for the care of older people with diabetes highlight the need to consider functional status, frailty, falls risk, pain, and screening for concomitant conditions such as cancer, polypharmacy, life expectancy, and advance care planning.

Thus, it is clear that one size assessment does not fit everybody. It is also important to consider the person's story and explanatory models to plan management with them (shared decision-making to personalise care, Chapter 2). Asking people about their past general and diabetes medical history may not elicit important information. Most people, including clinicians, find it difficult to give a sequential health history because memory for specific episodic events (episodic memory) is affected by age and defects in encoding and storage (Kessels 2003).

Likewise, the standard recommendations for when to undertake assessments, initial visit and annually, may not be frequent enough for some people and some health issues. Some need to be assessed at every visit (ADA 2019). Some need to be assessed at every change in health status and major life transition: for adolescents, these include moving to adult care services, leaving home, and starting university. Key life transitions for older people include retiring, stopping driving, and moving into an age-care home. These are all stressful events and are often associated with grief and loss, depression, and isolation. The following information concentrates on monitoring some specific parameters such as blood glucose.

Monitoring glucose levels

Monitoring blood glucose is an important part of diabetes management. The results form the basis for adjusting glucose lowering medicines (GLMs), food intake, and activity levels. Urine glucose is not a reliable method of determining the prevailing blood glucose level. It *might* still be useful for some people and in some countries where no other method is available, provided the individual's renal threshold for glucose is known.

Table 3.1   Some commonly used guidelines concerning care of people with diabetes.

American Diabetes Association (ADA) European Association for the Study of Diabetes (EASD) Guidance on Diabetes https://www.medscape.com/viewarticle/898697

British National Formulary (2018) BNF 75;Ed. 75 https://www.pharmpress.com/assets/docs/bnf%2075.pdf
ADA (2019) Standards of Medical Care in Diabetes http://www.diabetes.org/diabetes
Diabetes Australia (2016) Mastering Diabetes in Schools www.da.com.au/school
Australian Medicines Handbook (2018) (AMH)
https://amhonline.amh.net.au
Diabetes Australia. (2017) Diabetes in Schools.
www.diabetesaustralia.com.au/school
Diabetes UK (2018) End of Life Care www.diabetes.org.uk/professionals/position...management.../end-of-life-care
Dunning T, Martin P, on behalf of the Advisory Group (2019) Guidelines for deciding palliative and end of life care with people with diabetes. Centre for Quality and Patient Safety Research, Barwon Health Partnership, Deakin University, Geelong.
International Diabetes Federation (IDF) (2013) Global Guideline for Managing Older People with Type 2 Diabetes. https://www.idf.org/e-library/ guidelines/79-global-guideline-for-type-2-diabetes
IDF (2018) Clinical Recommendations on the Diabetic Foot (2017)
https://www.idf.org/component/attachments/?task=download&id=1152
KDIGO Guideline on Chronic Kidney Disease http://kdigo.org/wp-content/.../2017/04/KDIGO-CKD-Guideline-Manila_Kasiske.pdf
Management of Type 2 Diabetes (NICE Guideline) | MIMS online
www.mims.co.uk/management-type-2-diabetes-nice-guideline/diabetes/.../8918...
Type 1 diabetes in adults: diagnosis and management...
www.nice.org.uk/guidance/ng17
Type 2 diabetes in adults: management
www.nice.org.uk/guidance/ng28
Diabetes in pregnancy: management from preconception to the delivery NICE
www.nice.org.uk/guidance/ng3
Sinclair, A.J., Ahmed Abdelhafiz, A., Dunning, T. et al. (2018). An International Position Statement on the Management of Frailty in Diabetes Mellitus: Summary of Recommendations 2017. *The Journal of Frailty and Aging* **7**(1): 10–20.
http://www.jfrailtyaging.com/all-issues.html?article=609.
SIGN type 2 diabetes guideline | SIGN guideline | Guidelines
http://www.guidelines.co.uk/diabetes/sign-type-2-diabetes-guideline-/453869.article.
The McKellar Guidelines for Managing Older People with Diabetes in Residential and Other Care Settings...
www.adma.org.au/.../133-the-mckellar-guidelines-for-managing-older-people-...
Tools: Assessment Instruments – Diabetes Initiativehttp://www.diabetesinitiative.org/resources/type/assessmentInstruments.html.
Royal Australian College of General Practitioners /Diabetes Australia (2016) General Practice Management of Type 2 Diabetes 2016–2018.
www.diabetesaustralia.com.au/best-practice-guidelines
Royal Australian College of General Practitioners/Australian Diabetes Society 2018 Emergency management of hyperglycaemia in primary care. www.racgp.org.au/usage/ licence (accessed January 2019).

Table 3.2   Blood ketone levels and potential management.

Blood ketone level (B-OHB)	Potential management
Normal <0.5 mmol/l	
Low/moderate 0.6–1.5 mmol/l	Early warning, implement sick-day-care plan
High 1.6–2,9 mmol/l and blood glucose ≥15 mmol/l	Ketosis risk/impending ketosis; insulin dose may need to be increased. Seek underlying cause, e.g. infection.
	Food intake might be low due to fasting, poor appetite, or anorexia
High/acidosis >3 mmol/l and blood glucose >16 mmol	Ketones established and ketoacidosis risk; medical review required
	Insulin required, possibly as an IV infusion
	Treat underlying cause, e.g. infection or inappropriate withholding insulin. Review sick-day-care plan and organisational policies.

The renal threshold refers to the plasma glucose concentration above which significant glycosuria occurs. Glucose appears in the urine when the glomerulus filters more glucose from the blood than the renal tubule can reabsorb.

Abnormal quantities of glucose in the urine occur when the blood glucose is high and/or the kidney glucose absorption processes are overwhelmed and can be detected using urine test strips or laboratory tests. However, some urine test strips do not detect glycosuria until it is much higher (50–250 mg/dl) (Cowart and Stachura 1990). The individual's renal threshold for glucose is fairly constant, about 10 mmol/l (25 mg/dl), but may be higher in older people and during pregnancy (Sonksen et al. 1998).

Practice point

Urine glucose testing cannot detect hypoglycaemia.

People with diabetes are expected to, and do, manage their diabetes at home; i.e. they make over 90% of diabetes management decisions. Over time, each individual becomes an expert in his/her diabetes and accumulates a great deal of general and diabetes-related knowledge and experience. People should be encouraged to continue to self-monitor their blood glucose in hospital if they are well enough to do so. If clinicians perform the monitoring, they should inform the individual about the result, unless they are too ill to understand the information. Blood glucose monitoring (BGM) times can be used as teaching opportunities and opportunities to assess the individual's SMBG technique. The results of blood and urine monitoring are only useful if they are accurately performed, and importantly, clinicians value self-monitoring and use the information to inform diabetes education and care decisions for the individual.

Monitoring 1: Blood glucose

Key points

- Follow correct procedure when monitoring blood glucose.
- Perform meter control and calibration tests regularly.
- Clean and maintain equipment regularly.
- Record and interpret results according to the clinical situation and with the individual when relevant.

The role of BGM in diabetes management

BGM provides insight into the effectiveness of the diabetes management plan and enables direct feedback to the individual about their prevailing blood glucose and emerging blood glucose patterns. However, there is still debate about the value and cost-efficiency of SMBG in some situations, e.g. people with T2DM who are not using insulin. The DiGEM investigators undertook a randomised control trial involving people with T2DM age 25 treated with diet or GLMs, which showed no statistically significant difference in HbA1c at 12 months but there was a significant change in total cholesterol (Farmer 2007). Subjective parameters such as quality of life and sense of control were not measured. Other research also shows that people who monitor their blood glucose are younger at diagnosis and present with a higher HbA1c than people who do not monitor (Franciosi et al. 2005; Davis and Bruce 2006).

In contrast, the ROSSO study (Schneider et al. 2006) showed metabolic control improved in people with T2DM who monitored their blood glucose frequently. They demonstrated a 51% lower risk of death and a 32% lower risk of microvascular and macrovascular complications. In addition, people who monitored were more aware of their blood glucose levels and sought advice from health professionals sooner. Likewise, Karter et al. (2006) demonstrated improved HbA1c after SMBG.

Other researchers show lower rates of SMBG in men and people with low education level, those who do not have health insurance, in countries where equipment is not subsidised, those not on insulin, those taking GLMs, having less than two annual consultations with the doctor, and not attending diabetes education programmes (Centers for Disease Control and Prevention [CDC] 2007). These studies suggest there may be gender, age, and other differences in the rates of SMBG but the rates are similar amongst different countries. Some studies suggest SMBG is associated with higher rates of depression and increased costs (O'Kane et al. 2008).

The Choosing Wisely campaign, launched in the USA in 2012, has been adopted by service organisations, professional associations, specialty areas, and consumer groups in many countries. It aims to promote conversations between clinicians and consumers to enable informed decisions about medical investigations, treatment and targets, especially when they are not supported by evidence, and especially those that have a high risk of causing harm (www.choosingwisely.org).

Choosing Wisely programmes in several countries recommend people with T2DM not using insulin do not undertake SMBG and that HbA1c be used to guide management and promote healthy eating and regular activity. The Australian government reduced access to subsidised BGM strips for people with T2DM not using insulin in July 2016. People with T2DM on insulin and/or sulphonylureas, corticosteroids, those at high risk of symptomatic hypoglycaemia, those operating heavy machinery, older people, people with renal failure, and pregnant women can obtain subsidised test strips on clinician recommendation. People with T1DM have unrestricted access (Furler et al. 2016, Young et al. 2017).

Other experts state BGM promotes awareness of prevailing blood glucose and emerging patterns and can lead to changes to diet and activity and more timely management changes, especially using modern technology. Thus, research demonstrates mixed findings about SMBG in T2DM. There is considerable variability amongst the study methods used and the outcomes measured, which makes comparisons difficult.

SMBG needs to be tailored to the individual's needs. Structured SMBG; short periods of SMBG up to seven times per day over three days and documenting information about meals, activity, medicine dose and times and other factors that could affect the BG can be a useful way to reduce the monitoring burden and costs. Unstructured SMBG: routine, random and/or low frequency, is less useful (Speight et al. 2015). Structured monitoring enables the BG pattern to be identified. One study showed a statistically significant reduction in HbA1c (−0.3%) using structured SMBG four times per year (Polonsky et al. 2011). The extra attention that occurs when people participate in research is known to have an effect on findings (Hawthorne effect). Likewise, people are more likely to monitor their BG if clinicians acknowledge the work involved and value, discuss, and use the findings.

Most management guidelines continue to recommend SMBG as an integral part of the management plan. Monitoring frequency should be individualised depending on the glycaemic pattern, health status, medicine regimen, type of diabetes, the individual's preferences and self-care and social and financial capacity The American Diabetes Association (ADA) (2019) recommend people using multiple daily injections or using an insulin pump should undertake SMBG or continuous glucose monitoring (CSII) prior to meals and snacks at bedtime, occasionally before exercise, before and after they treat hypoglycaemia and prior to critical behaviours such as driving. The ADA also recommends SMBG be part of diabetes education programmes, used to guide treatment decisions and assessed as part of comprehensive medical assessments. People with diabetes should receive personalised SMBG education at a time and in format they can understand.

Importantly, blood glucose meters must be accurate and well maintained to provide meaningful information. They must meet International Standards Organisation Standards (ISO 15197-2013) and be approved by relevant regulatory authorities. This includes blood glucose meters individual's use for SMBG and those used in hospitals and other care facilities (US Food and Drug Administration 2016). In addition, they must be fit for purpose. For example, people with diabetes who use blood glucose meters vary in age, manual dexterity and vision. Physiological factors can interfere with BG meter accuracy; these include some medicines, temperature, blood oxygen saturation, e.g. meters that use glucosidase reagents were designed for capillary blood and can give false lows if the person is on oxygen therapy or arterial blood is used. False highs can occur in people with hypoxia or in venous blood samples. Meters that use glucose dehydrogenase reagents are not sensitive to blood oxygen levels (Rajendran and Rayman 2014).

SMBG is performed to:

- Monitor the effectiveness of the diabetes management plan and guide adjustments to the food plan, GLMs/insulin dose, exercise/activity, mental well-being, and quality of life; see Chapter 2.
- Achieve blood glucose target ranges, which need to be based on a health and risk assessment, decided with the individual and adjusted when indicated. The aim is to keep the blood glucose as close to the normal range as possible (tight control) when it is safe for the individual. However, tight control increases the risk of hypoglycaemia, Chapter 6.
- Reduce glucose variability, which, like persistent hyperglycaemia is associated with diabetes complications and mortality. Therefore, the aim is to try to achieve a stable blood glucose pattern and avoid/reduce swings (variability) in blood glucose between hyperglycaemia and hypoglycaemia.
- Detect hypoglycaemia, hypoglycaemic unawareness, and nocturnal hypoglycaemia, and monitor recovery from hypoglycaemia. Nocturnal hypoglycaemia can present as sleep disturbances, snoring, restlessness, or bad dreams.
- Detect hyperglycaemia and recovery from episodes of hyperglycaemia, ketoacidosis (DKA), and hyperosmolar states (HHS) (Chapter 7). Detecting persistent hyperglycaemia is important to prevent or delay the onset of long-term complications such as cardiovascular disease (Chapter 8). Long-term complications can be present at diagnosis in people with T2DM (Chapter 1).
- Establish the renal threshold for glucose to determine the reliability of urine testing in those rare cases where people still monitor urine glucose.
- Achieve 'tight' control in pregnancy to decide insulin doses and reduce the risks associated with hyperglycaemia in both mother and baby (Chapter 14).
- Provide continuity of care following hospitalisation.
- Manage intercurrent illnesses at home and when recovering from an illness (sick day care, see Chapter 7).
- Establish the effectiveness of new/adjusted treatment regimens.
- Tailor GLM and/or insulin doses and dose regimen, e.g. for:
  - People with renal failure, autonomic neuropathy, cardiovascular disease, or cerebrovascular insufficiency where hypoglycaemia signs can be masked or not recognised;
  - During investigations such as angiograms and surgical procedures;
  - Detecting actual or potential medicine/medicine or medicine/herb interactions;
  - During travel.

Achieving normoglycaemia (optimal control) is important to prevent or delay the onset of diabetes complications, but is hard, relentless work and often not achieved. The person is usually blamed for not complying with recommendations if they do not achieve optimal control. However, the progressive nature of T2DM and clinical inertia also play a part (Grant et al. 2004). Clinical inertia refers to clinicians recognising a problem but failing to act. Like non-compliance, *clinical inertia* is a derogatory term for a complex phenomenon where behaviours are influenced by many interrelated factors such as competing demands, time constraints, and patients presenting with multiple problems that cannot all be addressed at the same time (Parchman et al. 2007). However, clinician inertia combined with patient nonadherence probably increases the risk of suboptimal control and may be mutually causative. It might also partly explain why many people do not undertake SMBG!

There is increasing emphasis on reducing post prandial hyperglycaemia because it is associated with increased risk of retinopathy, cardiovascular disease, increased risk of cancer, and impaired cognitive function in older people (IDF 2007). Significantly, postprandial hyperglycaemia is present before T2DM is diagnosed and partly explains why cardiovascular complications are frequently present at diagnosis. Managing postprandial hyperglycaemia is discussed in Chapters 5 and 8.

SMBG is used with other investigations such as HbA_{1c} described later in this chapter.

Blood glucose target ranges and monitoring frequency

ADA (2019) generally recommended capillary blood glucose target ranges for most nonpregnant adults with diabetes and those in hospital as follows:

- 4.4–7.2 mmol/l (80–130 mg/dl) preprandial
- 10 mmol/l (180 mg/dl) postprandial

Recommended target ranges for people in hospital are:

- Those on insulin: 7.8–10 mmol/l (140–180 mg/dl)
- Hypoglycaemia alert level 3.9 mmol/l (<70 mg/dl)
- Hyperglycaemia in hospital >7.8 mmol/l (140 mg/dl)

Organisational policies and procedures should support staff to deliver evidence-based care. BGM is performed before meals and before bed (e.g. 7 a.m., 11 a.m., 4 p.m. and 9 p.m.) in many hospitals to obtain a profile and help decide the effectiveness of diabetes management plan. However, these times more likely to reflect work routines than optimal times to monitor BG.

Each person's needs should be assessed and the monitoring schedule tailored to their individual requirements, where work routines and staffing levels allow. One way to achieve an individualised monitoring regimen in hospital and aged-care facilities is to support the individual to perform their own BGM, where their condition permits them to do so. Many people with diabetes are expert at adjusting their insulin doses to account for carbohydrate intake, during illness and exercise. Specific policies might be required to enable self-BGM to occur. Capillary BGM should only be performed by adequately qualified staff or the person with diabetes. Therefore, staff BGM training programmes should be in place to support accurate and timely BGM.

SMBG frequency and target ranges depend on the individual's needs, goals, and safety (ADS 2019). It is particularly important for people using insulin and sulphonylureas to detect asymptomatic hypoglycaemia and hyperglycaemia. People using multiple daily insulin injections (MDI) should monitor their BG before meals and snacks, at bedtime, when they suspect and after treating hypoglycaemia and occasionally after exercise (ADS 2019). More frequent monitoring is required when the person is sick, often every two hours (Chapter 7).

The medicine regimen is often 'intensified' when the individual is in hospital to optimise metabolic control and support recovery. Such intensification is associated with lower 30-day readmission/

emergency presentation risk and lower HbA1c on outpatient follow-up (Wei et al. 2013). However, it can increase the risk of hypoglycaemia. BGM should be performed before meals in people who are in hospital and eating meals. Those who are not eating should be monitored every 4–6 hours, unless they are on an insulin infusion when more frequent monitoring is necessary: every 30 minutes to 2 hours (ADS 2019).

Continuous blood glucose monitoring (CBGM) is becoming widely used, especially by people with T1DM. However, there is limited data about CBGM in hospitals and ICU. ADA (2019) recommended it not be used in adults in hospital until safety and efficacy are established. This could lead to conflict with some people who use CBGM, which clinicians will need to manage. Most clinicians do not have sufficient knowledge to interpret the emerging blood glucose profile. Misinterpreting the information can lead to adverse events, including insulin stacking that can lead to hypoglycaemia.

The BGM regimen in all settings should reflect the action profile of the prescribed insulin/s, the action profile of other GLMs and the time and content of meals see Chapter 5, as well as the specific situation.

- People using insulin pumps and those on IV insulin infusions require more frequent monitoring.
- Many people with T1DM use continuous BGM.
- People in hospital are usually ill and require at least four-hourly BGM. The frequency can often be reduced in rehabilitation, mental health, and care facilities for older people, and in the end stages of life.

Special circumstances include:

(1) Insulin infusion: BGM is usually performed every one to two hours during the infusion and reviewed every two hours. Reduce to three to four hours when blood glucose levels are stable (see Chapter 5).
(2) People on corticosteroid therapy because these medicines induce insulin resistance and increase hepatic glucose output, which might be greater in people who already have insulin resistance and hyperglycaemia and may be a risk factor for hyperos-molar states; see Chapters 7, 10, and 18. Ketones should also be monitored in people with T1DM because some corticosteroids also induce lipolysis and increase the risk of ketoacidosis.
    (a) The effects on blood glucose depend on the formulation, dose, dose frequency and duration of action, and the response of the individual to the particular preparation used. Often, the BG increases during the day and is higher in the afternoon (Diabetes UK 2018).
    (b) Oral preparations have a greater impact on blood glucose than IV preparations, which usually do not cause a significant increase in the blood glucose.
(3) TPN guidelines suggest routine BGM for the first 48 hours: 7 a.m., 11 a.m., 4 p.m., and 9 p.m., until the patient is stable on TPN then develop a personalised BGM plan with the individual/and or family.
(4) Screen people who do not have a diagnosis of diabetes but have diabetes risk factors for hyperglycaemia.

It is important to monitor blood for ketones in all people with T1DM and those with T2DM during severe stress, for example surgery, infection, and myocardial infarction and when the blood glucose is high (Chapter 7). Urine ketone tests might still be used in some places but are an unreliable indicator of the blood ketone level.

Occasionally, urine glucose is measured at these times for 24 hours to establish the renal threshold. As indicated, testing two hours after food, especially in T2DM, may be preferable and provide information about glucose clearance from the blood after a meal as an indicator of cardiovascular risk. BGM may be monitored at 2 a.m. or 3 a.m. for two to three days if the blood glucose is high before breakfast and there is a possibility of nocturnal hypoglycaemia; see Chapter 6.

(1) Food: times of last food intake, quantity, and type of carbohydrate/fibre consumed in relation to meals and activity.

(2) Exercise: timing with respect to food, medication and insulin doses, injection site, type of exercise, and blood glucose level when commencing exercise. Hypoglycaemia can occur several hours after exercise.

(3) Intercurrent illness, for example, influenza, urinary tract infection.

(4) Glucose lowering medicines: GLMs, insulin, and other injectable GLMs; see Chapter 5.

(5) Intercurrent illnesses and stress, including stress due to hospital admissions.

(6) Condition of insulin injection site, the actual site, and injection technique.

(7) Other medicines, for example, corticosteroids, oral contraceptives, beta blockers, and nonprescription medications that contain glucose, ephedrine, pseudoephedrine or alcohol, for example, cold remedies, and glucose-lowering complementary medicines; see Chapters 5 and 18.

(8) Alcohol: type, relationship to food intake, amount consumed.

(9) Complementary medicines/therapies, for example, glucose-lowering herbs, stress management techniques; see Chapter 18.

(10) Emotional (emotional dwelling) and physical stress – not only stress itself but medicines used to treat stress.

(11) Accuracy of SMBG monitoring technique.

(12) Pregnancy in people with diabetes and gestational diabetes.

(13) Childhood: erratic swings in blood glucose levels are common.

(14) Adolescence: hormonal factors during adolescence.

(15) Renal, liver, and pancreatic disease.

(16) Other endocrine disorders, for example, thyroid disease, Cushing's disease, and acromegaly.

(17) Parenteral nutrition.

(18) Obtaining the blood sample from unwashed fingers, for example, after the individual or clinician treated a hypoglycaemic event with oral glucose.

Clinical observation

Insulin absorption can be delayed if insulin is injected into areas of lipodystrophy from repeatedly injecting into the same area, injecting into an oedemateous or ascitic abdomen and when the peripheral circulation is compromised. Delayed absorption can affect insulin onset of action and the blood glucose level. The thigh or upper arm may be preferable sites if the abdomen is oedemateous/ascitic.

Hyperglycaemia in people with and without diabetes in hospital is associated with more morbidity and mortality in general, surgical, ICU, and cardiology settings. Recommended target range for critically ill people with diabetes in hospital is 7.8–10 mmol/l (140–180 mg/dl) and 7.8 mmol/l (140 mg/dl) before meals and random glucose <10 mmol/l (180 mg/dl) for those who are not critically ill (ADA 2019).

Practice point

Never prick the feet of an adult because it can cause trauma and increases the risk of infection. Heel pricks can be performed on babies.

Blood glucose meters are point-of-care devices used to monitor blood glucose in the home and in many health service settings, diabetes prevention screening programmes and in hospital. The first capillary blood glucose meter was introduced in 1974. Over the following decades the

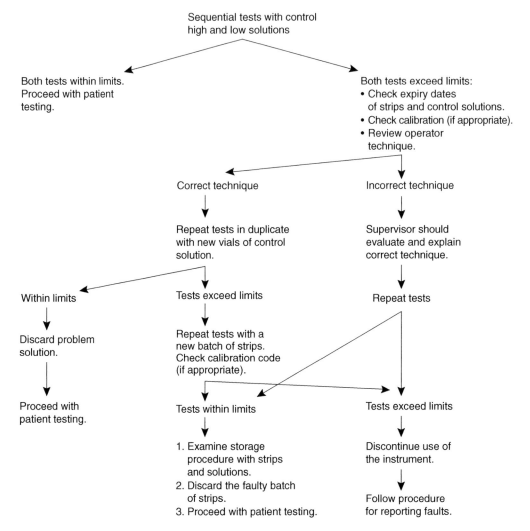

Sequential tests with control high and low solutions

Both tests within limits. Proceed with patient testing.

Both tests exceed limits:
• Check expiry dates of strips and control solutions.
• Check calibration (if appropriate).
• Review operator technique.

Correct technique

Incorrect technique

Repeat tests in duplicate with new vials of control solution.

Supervisor should evaluate and explain correct technique.

Within limits

Tests exceed limits

Repeat tests

Discard problem solution.

Repeat tests with a new batch of strips. Check calibration code (if appropriate).

Proceed with patient testing.

Tests within limits

Tests exceed limits

1. Examine storage procedure with strips and solutions.
2. Discard the faulty batch of strips.
3. Proceed with patient testing.

Discontinue use of the instrument.

Follow procedure for reporting faults.

Figure 3.1   An example of a quality control flow chart for quality control checking blood glucose meters. The meters should be checked at least daily.

technology of both meters and test strips changed rapidly. Staff should become familiar with the current system and related policies used in their place of employment. Consult the diabetes educator/specialist team or manufacturer for specific advice.

Where meters are used, a blood glucose meter quality management programme with a centralised coordinator is a key aspect of quality and safety (Figure 3.1). Such policies could encompass the following information:

• Meters must meet the International Organisation for Standardisation (ISO) standard number 15197:2013 for 95% of blood glucose results:
  ○ Within ±0.83 mmol/l of laboratory results at concentrations <5.6 mmol/l (100 mg/dl)
  ○ Within ±15 mg/dl of laboratory results at concentrations 5.6 mmol/l (100 mg/dl)
  ○ Within ±20% of laboratory results at concentrations >5.6 mmol/l (100 mg/dl) or more
• Individual nurses and other users demonstrate competence to use the system in operation.
• Meters must be subject to regular control testing and calibration according to the manufacturer's recommendations, calibrated as required, and appropriately cleaned and maintained.

The outcomes of control testing should be documented. Inadequate quality control affects the accuracy of the meter: clinical decisions based on inaccurate information can be inappropriate and can cause harm.

- A procedure for dealing with inaccurate results and meter malfunction must be in place.
- The US Food and Drug Administration (2010) recommended that blood glucose meters should not be shared amongst patients in hospital: if dedicated meters for each person in hospital is not possible, meters should be cleaned with disinfectant after every use. Some organisations also recommend that unused BGM strips and other supplies taken to one patient's bedside should not be used for other patients.

Most meters can be programmed to read in mmol/l or mg/dl. The latter is used in the United States. Most meters also store a record of blood glucose results and other information that can be downloaded into computer software programmes that enable the data to be displayed in a range of ways. Increasingly, they include other functions that enable personalised information to be entered, and decision aids to help people with diabetes manage their diabetes.

Modern meters are small and light, easy to operate, and only require a very small amount of blood. Particular meters are designed specifically for particular target audiences such as children and older people, who have different requirements (e.g. large result display screens and talking meters for vision-impaired people). Test strips require a minimal amount of blood. Therefore, many of the systems errors associated with early meters have been eliminated. However, inaccuracies still occur and are mostly due to user technique and inadequate quality control checks.

Meter technology changes rapidly, and health professionals need to be aware that the system in use in the hospital may be different from the system the person uses at home, and should be aware that:

- Although blood glucose readings obtained from the fingertip most closely correlate with arterial glucose, there are usually small differences in test results between capillary and venous blood.
- There are often small differences between blood glucose tests performed on different meters at the same time. Several factors account for the difference, such as squeezing the finger to obtain a second drop of blood. Usually, a difference of ~3% is acceptable. People may need to be reassured that their meter is not at fault. The individual's needs and understanding and likely reaction need to be considered before comparing results on different meters in the presence of the person with diabetes.
- Alternative site testing (from sites other than the fingertip such as the forearm, abdomen and thigh) are available and cause less discomfort but only yield a small quantity of blood ~3 ml. However, blood glucose levels vary amongst different sites. For example, there is a lag in increases and reductions in blood glucose by up to 30 minutes at the forearm compared with the fingertip, which can lead to delay in detecting and treating hypoglycaemia (Jungheim and Koschinsky 2002). Less variation occurs between the palm and ball of the thumb.
- Heat and light affect strip accuracy.

Interpreting different results

Capillary glucose values are likely to differ from laboratory values reported on venous blood. Capillary glucose is ~5% higher than venous glucose. Laboratory values can be affected by glycolysis. Glucose in whole blood decreases by ~5–7% per hour because of the glycolytic enzyme activity in red blood cells. Thus, venous samples should be sent to the laboratory promptly or kept at 4 °C for short periods if it is not possible to transport the sample immediately. Preservatives such as fluoride in blood tubes slow but do not stop glycolysis in blood samples.

Pcople are often confused by the different ways of reporting blood glucose (mmol/l or mg/dl), HbA1c (% and mmol/mol). Meter blood glucose and HbA1c results may not give an accurate indication of the average blood glucose level or of the minute fluctuations that occur

PROCEDURE FOR MONITORING BLOOD GLUCOSE

(1) Assemble materials and prepare environment according to hospital policy and testing system used:
  - Test strip removed from vial and cap replaced immediately or open foil package
  - Dry cotton or rayon ball or tissue to blot the test site if required
  - Disposable finger-pricking device or a device with disposable end cap to avoid the possibility of cross-infection from blood left on the device
(2) Explain procedure to individual.

Obtain a drop of blood

(3) Wash the person's hands with soap and warm water, dry carefully.
(4) Choose a site on any finger, near the side or tip. Avoid using the pad of the finger where nerves and arteries are concentrated: it is more painful.
(5) Prick finger firmly, using a finger prick device.
(6) 'Milk' along the length of the finger to well up blood at the puncture site. Avoid squeezing too hard.
(7) Allow the drop of blood to fall onto the strip or be drawn up by capillary action, depending on the type of meter and strips in use.
(8) Dispose of sharps into an appropriate sharps container.

Document the results

(1) Record test results on diabetes chart and in any other pertinent record.
(2) Communicate results to appropriate person, for example, the doctor and the patient.

Tips

(a) Warm hands bleed more readily.
(b) If peripheral circulation is deficient, obtaining blood can be difficult. Trap blood in fingertip with one hand, by milking the length of the finger and applying pressure with finger before pricking.
(c) Excess squeezing can dilute the red cells with plasma and lead to inaccurate results.
(d) Check with biochemistry result if the result does not match the clinical picture.

minute-by-minute (glucose variability). As indicated, A1c-derived glucose was introduced to make it easier for people with diabetes understand their average blood glucose over time.

Discrepancies between blood glucose meter readings and HbA1c could be used as an opportunity to explore the individual's monitoring technique, other factors that affect the results such as monitoring methods and the individual's feelings about diabetes and its management. The differences may be a sign of underlying stress, especially in adolescents (Rose et al. 2002); see Chapter 13.

Reasons for inaccurate blood glucose results

Inaccurate blood glucose readings from meters or test strips can occur for the following reasons:

- Using the incorrect strip for the meter
- Using the incorrect calibration or code, although several meters no longer need to be coded
- Using an unclean meter
- Low or flat batter
- Inserting the strip incorrectly or facing the wrong way
- Insufficient blood on the strip will give a false low reading with some older meters
- Quality control tests/calibration are not performed
- Strips used after the expiry date
- Failure to wash hands before testing, especially if sweet substances have been handled
- Humidity and high temperatures affect some meters and/or strips

If in doubt, repeat the test or confirm biochemically.

Practice points

- It is not necessary to swab the finger with alcohol prior to testing because it can dry the skin. Alcohol swabbing does not alter the blood glucose results (Dunning et al. 1994).
- The hands should be washed in soap and water and dried carefully before testing, especially if the person has been handling glucose, e.g. in an accident and emergency department/casualty when the person presents with hypoglycaemia.
- Incorrect operator technique, inadequate quality control testing, incorrect meter calibration, and using out-of-date test strips are the major causes of inaccurate results using blood glucose meters.

Glucometer is not a generic term for blood glucose meters. It was the name of a specific meter that has not been available on the market for at least 10 years. A more appropriate term is blood glucose meter or use the name of the particular meter.

Continuous blood glucose monitoring systems (CBGM)

CBGM was initially used to determine blood glucose profiles before using insulin pumps, during GDM, in paediatrics, and to detect unrecognised hypoglycaemia, rather than for routine home monitoring because of the cost. CBGM meters and the associated equipment are still more expensive than other blood glucose meters but the technology has advanced significantly and is moving rapidly towards the ultimate closed-loop system that encompasses continuous BG monitoring, fed to an insulin pump/artificial pancreas, which releases insulin into the blood.

Capillary BGM misses many excursions between hypoglycaemia and hyperglycaemia: CBGM enables real-time BG levels to be identified. Sampling generally occurs from interstitial and tissue sites and enables the trend towards hyperglycaemia or hypoglycaemia (trend analysis) to be monitored and preventative action to be taken.

The original CBGM consisted of a pager-sized glucose monitor, disposable subcutaneous glucose sensor and a cable connecting these two components to a communication system that stores data, which is downloaded into a computer software programme that enables the results to be displayed in graph form. Glucose target ranges can be assigned, the duration and frequency of hypo- and hyperglycaemic episodes and modal time determined using modern software. This provides important information that can help clinicians and people with diabetes recognise their BG patterns, the time they are within their target range, and the frequency of hyper- and hypoglycaemia (glucose variability) (Abraham et al. 2018; Bergenstal et al. 2018).

Current CGM systems show real time BG on the monitor about every five minutes. Many have hypo-and hyperglycaemia alarms. A significant advantage of CBGM is the ability to monitor glucose variability, which enables the individual/clinician to adjust the diabetes management regimen to reduce glucose variability, which is associated with increased risk of complications and mortality; Chapter 8. HbA1c does not measure glucose variability. A range of CBGMs are available, including:

- Flash BGM, e.g. using the Abbott Libre Freestyle meter; the blood glucose is read using a scanning device or a mobile phone and information can be downloaded to a computer, stored in the cloud and transferred to the persons clinicians. It is still important to continue some finger-prick blood glucose tests.
- Dexcom g6.
- Contour Nest One.
- Medtronic.
- Eversense XL.

CBGM is a specialised field: therefore, a competent trained team is essential to help the individual learn how to use the CGM, interpret the wealth of data generated and use it to manage their diabetes. Recent research shows CBGM data over 14 or more days can be used to provide a good estimate of the average blood glucose. The data can be analysed using a standard formula to derive and estimated A1C (eA1C) and can approximate the HbA1c. Although the two do not match closely, eA1C can be a useful guide to diabetes management (Bergenstal et al. 2018). Recently, eA1C was listed as one of the core CGM metrics included in standard CBGM reports (Danne et al. 2017). These developments highlight the speed at which technology is changing diabetes care.

Personal stories

Quincy koala, who lives in San Diego Zoo, was diagnosed with T1DM in 2018. T1DM is very rare in koalas. A group of veterinarians and endocrinologists commenced Quincy on the Dexcom G6 CGMs system, which made life easier for all concerned (zoonooz 2018).

The prevalence of diabetes in pet animals is increasing as it is in humans. Several of the author's colleagues have dogs with T1DM and use CBGM meters. Publications in veterinary journals discuss very similar topics about CBGM in animals as papers in journals about humans!

Monitoring blood ketones

A 10-second capillary blood ketone testing meter is a useful adjunct to BGM for people with T1DM during illness and enables them to detect ketosis and institute treatment or seek a health professional early to prevent ketoacidosis, see Chapter 7. Blood ketone testing is increasingly being used in the clinical setting for the same reasons, as well as giving an indication of the adequacy of the treatment during illness (Wallace et al. 2001; ADS 2012).

Blood ketone monitoring is essential during sustained hyperglycaemia and can reduce attendances at emergency departments, e.g. SIGN (2010) quoted a 50% reduction in the need for a hospital admission for DKA in people testing blood ketones compared with people using urine ketone testing, but the event rates in most trials are small (SIGN 2010). Thus, many guidelines still indicate there is not enough evidence to recommend routine ketone testing in type 1 or type 2 diabetes. However, there is enough expert clinician and individual with diabetes experience to suggest it is warranted in acute illness, including in hospital.

Blood ketones are raised after fasting, in the morning, or during starvation. This might indicate a UTI in nondiabetic patients, after hypoglycaemia not due to excess insulin, some inborn errors of metabolism and ketoacidosis, which is most commonly due to diabetes. Ketosis characteristic of untreated type 1 diabetes can occur in LADA and type 2 diabetes. The main ketone bodies are:

- Acetoacetate, which is an end product of fatty acid metabolism.
- Acetone, which is formed from spontaneous decarboxylation of acetoacetate. Acetone is volatile and is expelled in expired air. It is the ketone responsible for the acetone smell of ketoacidosis.
- Beta-hydroxybutyrate (B-OHB), which is a reduced form of acetoacetate and the major ketone formed in acidosis. It is not detected by urine test strips.

Acetoacetate and B-OHB are important energy substrates for many tissues, especially the brain, particularly during fasting and inadequate food intake. Blood ketone testing for B-OHB is more reliable than urine ketone testing (Fineberg 2000). Currently available urine ketone test strips do not measure B-OHB, and laboratory ketone testing often does not do so either, unless it is specifically requested.

The ketone meter measures capillary B-OHB, which is the most abundant ketone body and the best guide to the patient's metabolic status: Levels >1 mmol/l require further action, e.g. extra insulin, levels >3 mmol/l require medical assessment.

People with T1DM are advised to test for ketones during illness, hyperglycaemia, pregnancy, if polyuria, polydipsia, and lethargy are present and if they have abdominal pain. Abdominal pain is common in ketoacidosis and usually resolves as the ketosis clears. If it persists, it could indicate an abdominal emergency; see Chapter 7. People with T1DM who develop hyperglycaemia and HbA1c > 8.5%, in association with B-OHB, are insulin deficient and at risk of ketosis. Table 3.1 depicts normal and abnormal ketone levels and suggests some management considerations.

Monitoring ketones is important during illness in:

- all people with Type 1 diabetes
- people with Type 2 who are severely ill
- during fasting
- after severe hypoglycaemia:
  ○ severe stress;
  ○ TPN feeds high in glucose or lipids;
  ○ in the pre-, inter-, and post-operative periods.

The rate of fall of B-OHB using blood ketone strips can potentially avoid these situations and improve self-care and enable preventative action to be taken early to avoid ketoacidosis. Blood ketone strips can be used as an indicator of the adequacy of the treatment in acute care settings.

Clinical observation

Lower than actual capillary blood glucose levels can be recorded using some blood glucose meters in the presence of moderate-to-heavy ketosis. The reason for this finding is not clear. As a consequence, clinicians and people with diabetes can underestimate the severity of the hyperglycaemia, miss developing ketoacidosis, and delay appropriate treatment.

Practice points

(1) Ketones are present in people without diabetes during fasting and can be detected in 30% of first-voided morning urine specimens of pregnant women.
(2) Ketone test strips using nitroprusside reagents (used on urine test strips) give false-positive ketone results in the presence of sulphydryl drugs such as captopril.
(3) Insulin replacement corrects the acidosis by facilitating the conversion of B-OHB into acetoacetate and indicates the ketosis is resolving. However, urine ketone tests can indicate the ketones are still high. That is, urine ketone levels lag behind actual blood ketone levels.
(4) Urine ketone test strips give false-negative results when they have been exposed to the air for some time, have passed their expiry date, and if the urine is highly acidic, such as in a person taking large doses of vitamin C.

Insulin pumps

Insulin pumps improve glycaemic outcomes, improve quality of life, and reduce the risk of hypoglycaemia (Abraham et al. 2018). Most research concerns people with T1DM. Managing CBGM and insulin pumps requires significant parental support for children.

Some pumps, used with CGM, known as sensor augmented pumps (SAP), have inbuilt algorithms that suspend insulin during hypoglycaemia and then restart it when the BG returns to the normal range, which reduces the occurrence of severe hypoglycaemia and the related fear and injury risks. Examples of SAPs are:

- MedTrinic MiniMed
- Veo System
- Northbridge

Recently, the move to DIY looping emerged, largely because of the cost. The trend is spreading rapidly through social media and sites such as #WeAreNotWaiting. Four main systems exist and were developed by people with diabetes or families: Nightscout (CGM in the Cloud), Open APS, Android APS, and Loop, which connect to smart phones. There are safety and medicolegal concerns about looping (Diabetes Australia 2018). Specific education and training are needed to help people with diabetes safely use insulin pumps.

Monitoring 2: Urine glucose

Key points

Monitoring urine glucose is not recommended except in countries that do not have ready access to blood glucose meters or for people who cannot afford to buy a blood glucose meter (meters are sometimes supplied without charge in some countries but strips have to be purchased).
  If it is used:
- Establish renal threshold to determine the reliability of urine tests.
- Fluid intake, hydration status, urine concentration, and time since last voiding affect results.
- Double voiding is unnecessary.
- However, a full urinalysis can provide important clinical information, such as the presence of infection, which is often silent in people with diabetes, haematuria, and indicates jaundice.

In the presence of normal kidney function, glycosuria is correlated to the blood glucose concentration. Glycosuria occurs when the tubular maximum reabsorption is exceeded, usually around 8–10 mmol/l blood glucose. The test reflects the average glucose during the interval since the person last voided, rather than the level at the time the test is performed. This is called the renal threshold for glucose and varies within and between individuals. The renal threshold may be changed by:

- Increasing age
- Renal disease
- Long-standing diabetes

Therefore:

- The blood glucose can be elevated without glycosuria being present.
- Traces of glucose in the urine can indicate loss of control.
- The renal threshold can be low in children and glycosuria present when blood glucose is normal.

It is important to establish the renal threshold during a period of good control (normoglycaemia) by simultaneously testing blood and urine glucose, if possible.

Practice points

- Urine glucose monitoring is not an accurate reflection of the blood glucose level. In addition, it does not give warning of impending hypoglycaemia.
- A negative urine glucose finding does not indicate hypoglycaemia.
- Double voiding prior to testing is not necessary.

Indications for urine glucose tests

(1) A person refuses to monitor their blood glucose or cannot afford the equipment.
(2) The aim is to avoid glycosuria.

Monitoring kidney function

Diabetic nephropathy is the leading cause of end-stage renal disease; thus, early identification of declining renal function is imperative; see Chapter 8. Twelve- and 24-hour urine collections are used to monitor kidney function and detect early kidney damage by monitoring creatinine clearance rates and microalbumin excretion rates. Microalbuminuria reflects abnormally elevated albumin level not detectable on urine dipsticks.

Microalbuminuria is the earliest marker of the onset of kidney and cardiovascular damage and predicts deteriorating renal function (Krolewski et al. 1995). Up to 30% of newly diagnosed people with T1DM already have high urine albumin levels; of these, about 75% have microalbuminuria and 25% have overt nephropathy. People with T2DM in the MICRO-Hope study (HOPE 2000) had a 20% risk of progression from normal to microalbuminuria to nephropathy over five years, which is similar to T1DM.

Early diagnosis and treatment can delay the onset by 24 years, reduce the need for dialysis, and increase life expectancy (Borch-Johnsen et al. 1993). Of people with essential hypertension, 17% develop proteinuria despite satisfactory treatment (Ruilope et al. 1990).

Microalbuminuria is diagnosed when the urine albumin level is >30 mg/dl and is expressed as the quantity of albumin excreted in a given time (>20 m/minute) or as a concentration (>20 m/l urine). Most experts prefer the albumin–creatinine ratio because the other tests can be affected by the concentration of the urine.

Methods of screening for microalbuminuria

Several methods are available:

- Timed overnight collections target albumin <20 mg/l.
- Spot urine tests target urine albumin <20 mg/l.
- Urine-to-creatinine-ratio (UACR) women <3.5 mg/mmol and men <2.5 mg/mmol.
- Glomerular filtration rate (GFR). The degree of reduction in the GFR is linked to the development of renal disease. GFR is used as the index to classify the severity of renal disease; see Chapter 8 (Royal Australian College of General Practitioners 2016-18; National Kidney Foundation 2017; ADA 2019).
- Estimated GFR (e-GFR) is calculated using a predictive equation that uses serum creatinine, age, and gender. It is less accurate in Chinese people and possibly other Asian peoples and indigenous Australians (Zuo et al. 2005). In the United States, the Modification of Diet in Renal Disease (MDRD) is a valid method of determining e-GFR and classifying renal disease (National Kidney Foundation 2017). e-GFR may be unreliable in the following situations:
  - Acute changes in kidney function
  - People on dialysis
  - High protein and high vegetable diets and those who take creatinine supplements

○ Skeletal muscle diseases such as paraplegia and amputees
○ Those with high muscle mass
○ In the presence of severe liver disease
○ When the e-gfr is >60 ml/min/1.73 m²
○ Children <18 years
○ Asian peoples
○ Maori and Pacific Islander peoples
○ Aboriginal and Torres Strait Islander peoples

The following tests might still be used in some settings:

- Serum creatinine, used as a surrogate marker of GFR, is relatively inaccurate (Chadban et al. 2003). Significantly, serum creatinine is not reliable in older people; especially those with lean muscle mass who can have creatinine in the normal range despite severely compromised renal disease (Mathew 2003).
- Random urine tests using dipsticks or automated urine analysers measure microalbumin and calculate the microalbumin–creatinine ratio (normal level in males is <2 mg/mmol and <2.8 mg/mmol in women). These tests should be negative for protein (Tobe et al. 2002).
- Micral-Test dipstick tests (Boehringer Mannheim, GmbH Mannheim, Germany) is an immunochemical-based urinary dipstick used to test for microalbuminuria and can be used in the ward situation. Compared to radioimmunoassays, Micral-Test has a sensitivity of 92.2%, specificity of 92.3%, and a positive predictive value of 37.8% in predicting an albumin excretion rate > 20 m/minute (Jerums et al. 1994). However, it is not often used clinically in Australia.

Monitoring 3: Additional assessment

The following issues are important to general health and well-being and are part of holistic care; see Chapter 2.

(1) Psychological and emotional health and well-being (see Chapter 15).
(2) Self-care capacity.
(3) Regular weight checks. Height is also required to calculate BMI. Waist circumference is preferred and sometimes arm circumference in older people.
(4) Regular physical examination, especially:
- Blood pressure (lying and standing to detect any postural drop that could indicate the presence of autonomic neuropathy)
- Eyes (retina) and visual acuity
- Cardiac status
- Feet
- Kidney function
- General health and well-being such as vaccinations, dental care, and cancer screening
- Driving safety, especially in older people
(5) Regular education about:
- Diet
- Self-monitoring techniques
- Injection sites
- General diabetes information, especially new technology and research findings that need to be discussed in the context of the individual (Chapter 16)
- Changes to diabetes care as a result of research

Specific age groups such as children (Chapter 13) and older people (Chapter 12) require additional assessment, such as physical and mental functioning (Chapter 15).

Practice points

Normal ranges for the tests described can differ amongst laboratories, depending on the assay methods used and point-of-care metrics. It is helpful if people attend the same pathology service to have blood and urine tests performed.

People performing point-of-care tests such as HbA1c must be trained and meet relevant competency standards. The meter must meet relevant ISO standards. HbA1c assays must meet glycohaemoglobin standard processes traceable to the DCCT (Banerjee 2014; ADA 2019).

Clinician responsibilities

(1) Have a basic knowledge of the tests in order to be able to explain them to the individual and or family.
(2) Ensure people who are required to fast are given appropriate *written* instructions about their medications and any other preparation required, before the test.
(3) Ensure the correct collection technique, appropriate amount of blood, and correct test tubes are used.
(4) Mix the sample by inverting the tube two or three times if an anticoagulant tube is required. Vigorous shaking causes haemolysis of red blood cells, which affects the results.
(5) Ensure the specimen reaches the laboratory within 30 minutes of collection or is refrigerated to prevent glycolysis occurring and consequent inaccurate results.
(6) Ensure results are available for medical evaluation.
(7) Know the effects of illness and stress on the results of the test.
(8) Ensure the appropriate sterile blood collection technique is used.
(9) Ensure appropriate disposal of used equipment, and to protect themselves from needlestick injury.
(10) Ensure people with diabetes are given their medication and something to eat after completing tests when fasting is required and that they are informed about when to recommence any medications that were temporarily stopped, and what doses to take.

Glycosylated or glycated haemoglobin (HbA1c)

Clinical Points

HbA1c is a marker of the weighted average blood glucose over the preceding three months. It can be used with SMBG but it does not provide information about glucose variability or the blood glucose pattern.

A1c-Derived Average Glucose Equivalent (ADAGE) aims to estimate the person's average blood glucose from their HbA1c. The time/order of glucose values affects the HbA1c. The purpose of using was to report chronic glycaemia (high or low) in the same units as SMBG to make their glycaemic status easier to understand (Treviño 2007).

It is most useful to have the HbA_{1c} result at the time the person is assessed by the doctor/diabetes educator. Blood can be drawn from a vein and measured in the laboratory before the clinic/doctor visit so the result is available at the time of the consultation. Alternatively, blood can be drawn from a finger-prick sample at the time of the visit using point of care devices such as the DCA 2000 (Bayer) analyser.

Circulating blood glucose attaches to the haemoglobin in the red blood cells and undergoes an irreversible non-enzymatic interaction with amino groups of lysine and valine residues in haemoglobin (Amadori reaction) whereby the glucose becomes permanently fixed to the haemoglobin (glycosylation).

The glycosylated haemoglobin, HbA1c can be measured and quantified to give an indication of the average blood glucose concentration over the preceding three months (normal 4–5.9%) and to predict risk of long-term diabetes complications (Bloomgarden 2007; Kilpatrick et al. 2007). Currently, four main assays and about 20 different measurement methods are used that measure different glycated products and report different units (% HbA1c, % HbA1, and total GHb)

(Colman et al. 2008). The four assay methods are: ion-exchange chromatography, electrophoresis, affinity chromatography, and immunoassay.

Fasting prior to obtaining the blood sample for HbA1c is not necessary. Tests are usually performed at least three months apart but can be done sooner to gauge the effect of a treatment modification and in research.

HbA1c is a proxy measure of average blood glucose and can be misleading because individuals are higher or lower glycosylators at specific mean blood glucose levels, which emphasises the importance of considering the individual and the overall clinical picture.

Current assay methods use a mixture of glycated haemoglobins to determine the HbA1c. Representatives from the American Diabetes Association, The European Association for the Study of Diabetes, the International Diabetes Federation, and the International Federation of Clinical Chemistry and Laboratory Medicine (IFCC) regularly discuss ways to standardise HbA1c measurement (Consensus Committee 2007).

Key recommendations were:

- Standardising the method of measuring HbA1c and the reference system used to report results.
- The IFCC reference system is the only currently valid method of measuring HbA1c and should be used as the basis to standardise HbA1c measurements.
- The results should be reported in IFCC units (mmol/mol), and derived national Glyco-haemoglobin. Standardisation Program Units (NGSP) (%) should be calculated using the IFCC-NGSP master equation.
- Laboratories should be able to maintain a CV <3% at HbA1c between 6% and 9%, and manufacturer's assays should have a CV <5% (Colman et al. 2008).
- If the ongoing average plasma glucose study using frequent capillary glucose measurements and continuous glucose monitoring due to be published in early 2008 fulfils its priori-specified criteria, an A1c-derived average glucose value (ADAG) should also be reported (Nathan 2007). The ADAG value is calculated from the individual's HbA1c result to deduce an estimate of their average blood glucose (O'siordan 2007).
- Clinical guidelines should be revised and glycaemic targets be expressed as IFCC units, derived NGSP units, and ADAG.

Glycaemic targets should be considered with other risk factors for complications such as hyperlipidaemia, hypertension and smoking, age, and comorbidities. HbA1c targets differ slightly amongst various guidelines. Generally accepted targets are:

- As low as possible to reduce the likelihood of microvascular complications. Most recommend <6.5% (48 mmol/mol) or < 7% (53 mmol/mol) for most people with T2DM with very low risk of hypoglycaemia.
- Individualised for specific individuals after discussing the risks and benefits with them. For example, children, older and frail people, and those with limited life expectancy might require higher targets (<8%) (64 mmol/mol) and those at very high risk of microvascular complications may need lower targets (range 7–7.5%) (53–58 mmol/mol).
- Avoid adverse events such as frequent hypoglycaemia (ADA 2019).

Practice points

- People who experience frequent hypoglycaemic episodes may have a low HbA1c that might not reflect their complication risk.
- HbA1c results should be evaluated as part of the total clinical picture and not viewed in isolation.
- HbA1c does not represent the blood glucose profile, but gives an average level. It is considered to be the gold standard for monitoring metabolic control.

Table 3.3 lists some factors that might affect HbA1c results.

Table 3.3   Nonglycaemic factors that can affect results of glycosylated haemoglobin assays.

False high	False low
Chronic alcohol abuse	Anaemia
Foetal haemoglobin	Abnormal haemoglobins such as HbS, HbC, HbD found in some ethnic groups
Hyperlipidaemia	
Hyperbilirubinaemia	
Renal failure	Chronic blood loss
Splenectomy	Haemolysis
	Haemorrhage
	Recent blood transfusion

Fructosamines

The fructosamines are a group of glycosylated blood and tissue proteins that reflect the average blood glucose levels within the preceding three weeks. Fructosamine results can be lower in patients with low serum albumin, cirrhosis of the liver, or haemoglobinopathies.

Fructosamine estimations are not performed very often but they are useful for monitoring:

- Diabetes during pregnancy
- Initial response to diabetes medication
- People with chronic anaemia
- People with haemoglobinopathies

Serum Lipids

Serum lipids are usually elevated if the blood glucose is elevated. Three classes of lipids are measured as shown with the target range in brackets:

(1) Cholesterol (<4.0)
(2) Triglycerides (<2.0)
(3) Lipoproteins:
 - low-density lipoprotein (LDL-C) (< 2.0) and non-HDL-C < 2.5 mmol/l
 - high-density lipoprotein (HDL) (>1.0)

Although it is generally accepted that fasting blood lipid levels are most useful, recent research suggests nonfasting levels correlate more closely with cardiovascular risk (Bansal et al. 2007; Varbo et al. 2007). However, there are many forms of hypertriglyc-eridaemia, and more research is needed to determine the exact relationship with atherosclerosis. High lipids, especially elevated triglycerides and LDL, and low HDL is a common lipid profile in people with poorly controlled T2DM, which may be secondary to hyperglycaemia, and is a clinical useful measure of the need for lipid-lowering medications such as fibrates, fish oil concentrates, or nicotinic acid, depending on the type of lipid abnormality present; see Chapter 5.

Alcohol should not be consumed for 24 hours before the blood sample for serum lipid measurements is taken.

C-peptide

C-peptide is the connecting peptide, which determines the folding of the two insulin chains during insulin production and storage in the pancreas. It splits off in the final stages and can be measured in the blood. It is used to measure endogenous insulin production, to determine the type of diabetes (along with various antibodies; see Chapter 1) if it is not clear in the clinical presentation. C-peptide is present in normal or elevated amounts in Type 2 diabetes, indicating that insulin is being produced and that diet and/or OHAs with exercise could achieve acceptable control. However, progressive beta cell loss occurs in type 2 diabetes and C-peptide levels fall proportionally.

C-peptide is absent or low in people with type 1 diabetes and can be a useful indicator in slow onset type 1 diabetes (LADA) occurring in adults (Cohen 1996); see Chapter 1. C-peptide is not changed by injecting exogenous insulin. Fasting results are most useful.

Islet cell antibodies (ICA)

ICA are found in most newly diagnosed people with T1DM diabetes, indicating that diabetes is an autoimmune disease. The beta cells of the pancreas are the specific target in diabetes and other pancreatic functions are not affected. In the laboratory, impaired insulin release can be demonstrated when ICA are present but the clinical implication is still unclear.

ICA are present in the prediabetic state before the disease is clinically obvious. They can also be present in close relatives who are at high risk of developing diabetes if they have ICA.

GAD antibodies are also present in 80% of people with T1DM and enable it to be distinguished from T2DM; see Chapter 1.

Creatinine clearance and urea

As indicated, creatinine clearance is used to estimate renal function. It is also used to determine nutritional status in relation to protein especially during TPN and continuous ambulatory peritoneal dialysis (CAPD). An increase in the blood urea nitrogen (BUN) may indicate impaired renal function; however, the BUN can also be increased if the patient is dehydrated, has internal bleeding or is on steroids. Anorexia, a low-protein diet and fasting, can lead to a decrease in urea.

Self-care

The key aspects of self-care are discussed in Chapter 16. Generally assuming responsibility for self-care is an iterative process that falls into three main categories:

(1) Focusing on diabetes after diagnosis to acquire the knowledge and skills, master the self-management tasks, and make life adjustments needed to perform diabetes self-care, which involves individuals and their family/carers. It takes time to accept diabetes and master these significant life changes. Some people take a long time, while others adapt quickly depending on social, environmental, and a range of other factors.
(2) Activating resources, which encompasses being able to identify relevant resources and using them effectively to support their self-care activities. Resources might be family, friends, health professionals, internet, and other media as well as local resources such as libraries, churches, meals on wheels, and transport.
(3) Living with diabetes: people cope with diabetes and successfully integrate it into their lifestyle and grow as individuals (Schulman-Green et al. 2012). This essential stable phase can easily be disrupted by life events and when a complication develops, and the person needs to readapt.

Nurses can ask four simple questions to help make a decision about an individual's diabetes self-care capacity:

(1) Does the individual have the knowledge and skills to manage their diabetes to the best of their ability?
(2) Has the individual access to appropriate resources, equipment, support, and health professional advice?
(3) Is the individual satisfied with their life at present?
(4) Are their cultural issues that need to be considered?

Nurses are in an ideal situation to help determine the barriers to optimal self-care and potential medicine nonadherence (Chapter 5). Barriers might be physical, financial/economic, psychological, cognitive, health literacy/numeracy, social, and environmental (Baumann and Dang 2012). Motivational interviewing, active listening, reflecting, clarifying, being present in the moment (fully focused on the individual and their story), and involving the individual in making management decisions and setting goals and targets are all essential.

The annual review

The annual review/ annual cycle of care describes a comprehensive health assessment undertaken in primary care to do the following:

- Review management goals.
- Assess diabetes complication status.
- Determine whether referral to one of more specialists is warranted.
- Revise the immunisation schedule.
- Undertake other important monitoring process as indicated (Diabetes Australia/Royal Australian college of General Practitioners 2016/18).

Many of the assessments discussed in this chapter are encompassed in the annual review.

Clinical point

Assessments and monitoring are ideal opportunities for interactive discussions between people with diabetes and clinicians to arrive at shared understanding and mutually negotiated care goals and care plans. Some monitoring might occur electronically and some might involve using valid decision aids. As with all aspect of diabetes care, excellent communication and health literacy are key clinician skills.

Summary

The focus should be on the person with diabetes when undertaking assessments and deciding care. Eating a healthy diet, being active, social connection, adequate sleep, and maintaining mental health are important aspects of diabetes self-care.

References

Abraham, M.B., Nicholas, J.A., Smith, G.J. et al. (2018). Reduction in hypoglycemia with the predictive low-glucose management system: a long-term randomized controlled trial in adolescents with type 1 diabetes. *Diabetes Care* 41 (2): 303–310.

American Diabetes Association (2019). Standards of medical care. http://www.diabetes.org/diabetescare.

Australian Diabetes Society (ADS) (2012). Position statement individualization of HbA1c targets for adults with diabetes mellitus. ADS, Canberra. https://diabetessociety.com.au.

Banerjee, S. (2014). HbA1c result, does it depend on testing methods? *Journal of the Association of Physicians of India* 62: 9–12.

Bansal, S., Buning, S., Rifai, N. et al. (2007). Fasting compared with nonfasting triglycerides and risk of cardiovascular events in women. *Journal of the American Medical Association* 18 (298): 309–316.

Baumann, L. and Dang, T. (2012). Helping patients with chronic conditions overcome barriers to care. *Nurse Practitioner* 37 (3): 32–38.

Bergenstal, R., Beck, R., Close, K. et al. (2018). Glucose Management Indicator (GMI) a new term for estimating A1C from continuous glucose monitoring. *Diabetes Care* 41 (11): 2275–2280.

Bloomgarden, Z. (2007). Glucose variability. Comment on sessions presented during the 67th American Diabetes Association, Scientific Sessions (June 22–26), Chicago, Illinois. http://www.medscape.com.viewarticle/560754 (accessed January 2008).

Borch-Johnsen, K., Wenzel, H., Vibert, G., and Mogensen, C. (1993). Is screening and intervention for microalbuminuria worthwhile in patients with IDDM? *British Medical Journal* 306: 1722–1725.

Centers for Disease Control and Prevention (CDC) (2007). Self-monitoring of blood glucose among adults with diabetes – United States, 1997-2006. *Morbidity and Mortality Weekly Report* 56 (43): 1133.

Chadban, S., Briganti, E., and Kerr, P. (2003). Prevalence of kidney disease in Australian adults: the AusDiabe kidney study. *Journal of the American Society of Nephrologists* 14 (7 (Suppl. 2)): S121–S138.

Cohen, M. (1996). *Diabetes: A Handbook of Management*. Melbourne: International Diabetes Institute.

Colman, P., Goodall, I., Garcia-Webb, P. et al. (2008) Glycohaemoglobin: a crucial measurement in modern diabetes management. Progress towards standardization and improved precision of measurement. *EMJA* www.mja.com.au/public/issues/jul21/colan/colman.html (accessed February 2008).

Consensus Committee (2007). Consensus statement on the Worldwide Standardisation of the Haemoglobin A_{1c} measurement. The American Diabetes Association, European Association for the Study of Diabetes, International Federation of Clinical Chemistry and Laboratory Medicine, International Diabetes Federation. *Diabetes Care* 30: 2399–2400.

Cowart, S. and Stachura, M. (1990). Glycosuria, Chapter 138. In: *Clinical Methods: The History, Physical and Laboratory Examinations* (eds. H. Walker, W. Hally and J. Hurst). Boston: Butterworths.

Danne, T., Nimri, R., Battelino, T. et al. (2017). International consensus on continuous glucose monitoring. *Diabetes Care* 40: 1632–1640.

Davis, T. and Bruce, D. (2006). Is self-monitoring of blood glucose appropriate for all type 2 diabetic patients? The Freemantle diabetes study. *Diabetes Care* 29: 1764–1770.

Diabetes Australia (2018). People with type 1 diabetes and do-it-yourself (DIY) technology solutions: Position Statement. diabetesasutralia.com.au.

Diabetes UK (2018). *End of Life Diabetes Care*. London: Diabetes UK.

Dunning, T., Rantzau, C., and Ward, G. (1994). Effect of alcohol swabbing on capillary blood glucose. *Practical Diabetes* 11 (4): 251–254.

Farmer, A. (2007). Self-monitoring of blood glucose does not improve HbA_{1c} levels in patients with non-insulin treated diabetes: The DIGEM study. Presented during the 67th American Diabetes Association, Scientific Sessions (June 22–26), Chicago, Illinois. Also published in the *British Medical Journal Online* June 6, 2007.

Fineberg, S. (2000). Comparison of blood beta-hydroxybutyrate and urine ketones in 4 weeks of home monitoring by insulin-requiring children and adults. American Diabetes Association Scientific Meeting, USA (June 2000).

Franciosi, M., De Berardis, G., Rossi, M.C. et al. (2005). Use of the diabetes risk score for opportunistic screening of undiagnosed diabetes and impaired glucose tolerance: the IGLOO (Impaired Glucose Tolerance and Long-Term Outcomes Observational) study. *Diabetes Care* 28 (5): 1187–1194.

Furler, J., Browne, J., and Speight, J. (2016). Blood glucose: to monitor or not in type 2 diabetes? The practical implications of choosing wisely recommendation. *Diabetes and Primary Care* 1 (2): 55–58.

Grant, R.W., Cagliero, E., Dubey, A.K. et al. (2004). Clinical inertia in the management of Type 2 diabetes metabolic risk factors. *Diabet Med.* 21 (2): 150–155.

HOPE (Outcomes Prevention Evaluation Study Investigators) (2000). Effects of ramipril on cardiovascular and microvascular outcomes in people with diabetes. *Results of HOPE and MICRO-HOPE substudy. Lancet* 355: 253–259.

International Diabetes Federation (IDF) (2007). *Guideline for Management of Postmeal Glucose*. Brussels: IDF.

Jerums, G., Cooper, M., O'srien, R., and Taft, J. (1994). ADS position statement 1993: microalbuminuria and diabetes. *Medical Journal of Australia* 161: 265–268.

Jungheim, K. and Koschinsky, T. (2002). Glucose monitoring at the arm: evaluation of upper dermal blood glucose kinetics during rapid systemic blood glucose changes. *Hormone Metabolism Research* 34: 325–329.

Karter, A.J., Parker, M.M., Moffet, H.H. et al. (2006). Longitudinal study of new and prevalent use of self-monitoring of blood glucose. *Diabetes Care* 29 (8): 1757–1763.

Kessels, R. (2003). Patients' memory for medical information. *Journal Royal Society of Medicine* 96 (5): 219–222.

Kilpatrick, E., Rigby, A., and Atkin, S. (2007). Variability in the relationship between mean plasma glucose and HbA_{1c}: implications for the assessment of glycaemic control. *Clinical Chemistry* 53: 897–901.

Krolewski, A.S., Laffel, L.M., Krolewski, M. et al. (1995). Glycosylated hemoglobin and the risk of microalbuminuria in patients with insulin-dependent diabetes mellitus. *New England Journal of Medicine* 332 (19): 1251–1255.

Nathan, D. (2007). The problem with ADAGE (A1c-derived average glucose equivalent). 67th American Diabetes Association, Scientific Sessions (June 22–26), Chicago, Illinois.

National Kidney Foundation (2017). Glomerular filtration rates. https://medlineplus.gov/ency/article/007305.htm.

O'Kane, M.J., Bunting, B., Copeland, M., and Coates, V.E. (2008). Efficacy of self-monitoring of blood glucose in patients with newly diagnosed type 2 diabetes (ESMON study): randomised controlled trial. *BMJ* 336 (7654): 1174–1177.

O'siordan, M. (2007). Average blood glucose instead of HbA_{1c}? Change appears to be coming for diabetes care. *Heartwire* (July 3). www.medscape.com.viewarticle/559262 (accessed December 2007).

Parchman, M., Pugh, J., Romero, R., and Bowers, K. (2007). Competing demands or clinical inertia: the case of elevated glycosylated hemoglobin. *Annals of Family Medicine* 5 (3): 196–201.

Polonsky, W., Fisher, L., Schikman, C. et al. (2011). Structured self-monitoring of blood glucose significantly reduces A1C levels in poorly controlled non-insulin treated type diabetes: results from the structured testing program study. *Diabetes Care* 34: 262–267.

RACGP/DA (Royal Australian College of General Practitioners & Diabetes Australia) (2016/18). *Diabetes Management in General Practice: Guidelines for Type 2 Diabetes*. Canberra: DA & RACGP.

Rajendran, R. and Rayman, G. (2014). Point-of-care blood glucose testing for diabetes care in hospitalized patients. *Journal Diabetes Science and Technology* 8 (6): 1081–1090.

Rose, M., Fliege, H., Hildebrandt, M. et al. (2002). The network of psychological variables in patients with diabetes and their importance for quality of life and metabolic control. *Diabetes Care* 25: 35–42.

Royal Australian College of General Practitioners/Diabetes Australia (2016-18). General Practice Management of type 2 diabetes. racgp.org.au.

Ruilope, L., Alcazar, J., Hernandez, E., and Rodico, J. (1990). Does an adequate control of blood pressure protect the kidney in essential hypertension? *Journal of Hypertension* 8: 525–531.

San Diego Zoo Global (2018). Koala with diabetes at San Diego Zoo receives help from new technology. https://zoonooz.sandiegozoo.org/2018/06/25/koala-with-diabetes-at-san-diego-zoo-receives-help-from-new-technology/.

Schneider, M., Heinemann, B., Lodwig, L. et al. (2006). The ROSSO study group: self-monitoring of blood glucose in type 2 diabetes and long term outcome: an epidemiological study. *Diabetologia* 49: 271–278.

Schulman-Green, D., Jases, S., and Martin, F. (2012). Self-management in chronic illness. *Journal of Nursing Scholarship* 44: 136–144.

SIGN (Scottish Intercollegiate Guidelines Network) (2010). *Management of Diabetes: A National Guideline*. Edinburgh: SIGN.

Sonksen, P., Fox, C., and Judd, C. (1998). *Diabetes at Your Fingertips*, 105. London: Class Publishing.

Speight, J., Browne, J., and Furler, J. (2015). Challenging evidence and assumptions: is there a role for self-monitoring of blood glucose in people with type 2 diabetes not using insulin. *Diabetes Care* 34: 262–267.

Tobe, S.W., McFarlane, P.A., and Naimark, D.M. (2002). Microalbuminuria in diabetes mellitus. *Cmaj* 167 (5): 499–503.

Treviño, G. (2007). The problem with ADAGE (A1c-derived Average Glucose Equivalent). *Medscape General Medicine* 9 (4): 43.

US Food and Drug Administration (2010). Use of fingerstick devices on more than one person poses risk for transmitting bloodborne pathogens: Initial communication: update 29/11/2010. http://www.fda.gov/medicaldevices/safety/aletsnadnotices/ucm224026/htm.

US Food and Drug Administration (2016). Self-monitoring blood glucose test systems for over-the-counter use. http://www.fda.gov/downloads/medicalDevices/DevicesRegulationsCuidance/GuidanceDocuments/UCM380325.pdf.

Varbo, A., Benn, M., Tybjaerg-Hansen, A. et al. (2007). Nonfasting triglycerides and risk of myocardial infarction, ischemic heart disease, and death in men and women. *Journal of the American Medical Association* 18 (298): 299–308.

Wallace, T., Meston, N., Gardnert, S., and Matthews, D. (2001). The hospital and home use of a 30-second hand-held blood ketone meter: guidelines for clinical practice. *Diabetes Medicine* 18 (8): 640–645.

Wei, N., Wexler, D., Nathan, D., and Grant, R. (2013). Intensification of diabetes medication and risk for 30-day readmission. *Diabetes Medicine* 30 (2): e56–e62.

Young, L.A., Buse, J.B., Weaver, M.A. et al. (2017). Glucose self-monitoring in non–insulin-treated patients with type 2 diabetes in primary care settings: a randomized trial. *JAMA internal medicine* 177 (7): 920–929.

Zuo, L., Ma, Y., and Zhou, Y. (2005). Application of GFR – estimating equations in Chinese patients with chronic kidney disease. *American Journal of Kidney Diseases* 45: 463–472.

Chapter 4

Nutrition and Weight Management

Everybody should eat a healthy balanced diet and undertake regular physical activity – not only people with diabetes and those who are overweight.

Key points

- Dietary advice for people with diabetes is applicable to the whole population. Dietary advice should be personalised to the individual, type of diabetes, life stage and diabetes management.
- Diet and exercise continue to be the cornerstone of diabetes management even when medicines are required.
- Regular dietary assessment is advisable, e.g. change in health status, diabetes management, and annual complication assessments.
- Overweight and obesity are increasing globally and are associated with a range of health risks including type 2 diabetes and gestational diabetes.
- Obesity is associated with more than 30 medical conditions and affects many other conditions. Weight loss can improve some obesity-related conditions including the metabolic syndrome, type 2 diabetes, and hypertension, and can reduce cardiovascular risk.
- The relationship between weight, health outcomes, and life expectancy is complex and is affected by genetic makeup and, significantly, environmental factors, which may play a more dominant role.
- Population-based and targeted screening and prevention programmes are required to address overweight, obesity, and diabetes.

Rationale

Good nutrition is vital to health and well-being and is an essential basis of managing prediabetes/metabolic syndrome and all types of diabetes. Overweight and obesity are significant health issues and a major risk factor for serious disease, including type 2 diabetes. Managing weight is difficult. Regular nutritional assessment is important to maintain the optimal health of people with diabetes as their general health, age, and diabetes-related circumstances change.

The importance of good nutrition

Good nutrition is essential to health. Under- and overnutrition lead to many diseases and affect the health status and response to treatment (Sydney-Smith 2000). Sixty percent of deaths are related to nutrition, for example, diabetes-associated cardiovascular disease (Middleton et al. 2001) and sarrcopenia and frailty (Chapter 12). In particular, micronutrients and protein intake are often inadequate and mineral deficiencies are common, especially in people living in poverty.

Diets low in essential nutrients and vitamins and minerals are also deficient in antioxidants that modulate oxidative tissue damage. Oxidative tissue damage is implicated in the development of long-term diabetes-related complications and is compounded by smoking, excess alcohol intake and chronic inflammatory diseases; see Chapter 8. Vitamins C, E, and A, and some plant chemicals (phytochemicals) are naturally occurring antioxidants present in a well-balanced diet.

A healthy diet rich in fibre and short chain fatty acids also important to the gut microbiome. An increasing body of evidence testifies to a link between the gut microbiome, inflammation and insulin resistance (Chen and Devaraj 2018). The gut microbiome collectively refers to the microbial composition in the gut. Microbiota contains several diverse types of microorganisms such as various types of bacteria, viruses, fungi, and phages (Rajilic-Stojanovic et al. 2014). The five most common types are *Lactobacilli, Proteobacteria, Bacteriodes, Verrucomicrobiota*, and *Abbermansia*. Some studies suggest that some of the beneficial effects of Metformin could be due to alterations in the gut microbiota (Deveraj, Venkatachalam and Chen 2016).

Recent studies of the gut microbiota suggest there is an association between gut microbiota and the brain and schizophrenia (https://newatlas.com/schizophrenia-gut-bacteria-microbiome/58394) and that post prandial blood glucose may be influenced by individual characteristics, including the microbiome and anthropometric variables (Mendes-Soares et al. 2019). A personalised predictive model that encompasses the individual's clinical characteristics, physiological variables, and microbiome in addition to food nutrient content was more predictive of post prandial blood glucose than current methods. This is a new area of research, and more evidence will emerge in the future.

Malnutrition and undernutrition

The focus in diabetes prevention and management is on obesity (overnutrition) but undernutrition and malnutrition are significant problems, especially in older people and those from lower socioeconomic groups and in underdeveloped countries. Malnutrition prevalence ranges are 10–30% in the community, 20–50% in acute care settings, 30–50% in rehabilitation settings, and 40–70% in aged-care facilities in Australia (Dietitians Association of Australia 2009). Malnutrition is associated with increased costs and adverse outcomes and is often underrecognised. Importantly, overweight/obese people can be malnourished.

Dietary management: Diabetes

Diet and exercise are the mainstay and first line of treatment of all types of diabetes to control blood glucose and manage cardiovascular and other health risks. The aim is to achieve an appropriate weight within the healthy weight range for the individual, but focusing on weight might mean that *undernutrition* is not considered, which, as indicated, might confer more health risks than overweight, especially in older people.

Expert dietary advice is essential but the changing role of the nurse and the focus on the preventative aspects of healthcare mean that nurses have a responsibility to develop knowledge about nutrition and its role in preventing disability and disease. A number of basic screening tools can be used to identify dietary intake and nutritional characteristics and can be incorporated into usual nursing assessment and patient care plans and enables useful information to be communicated to the dietitian.

The general dietary principles apply to the whole population as well as all people with diabetes. Precise advice depends on the individual's age, gender, lifestyle, eating habits, cultural preferences and nutritional requirements. It is important that realistic targets are negotiated with the patient, particularly if weight control is necessary. The goal is to achieve gradual progressive weight loss to reduce weight by 5–10%, which is usually achievable and improves the health profile (Pi-Sunyer 2006).

The effect of medications, fasting for procedures, and gastrointestinal (GIT) disturbances such as diarrhoea and vomiting, on food absorption and consequently blood glucose levels is an important consideration especially during illness.

Optimal nutritional care is best achieved by collaboration amongst the individual and their family, nurses, other health professionals and the dietitian to decide the most appropriate management regimen. Nurses have the greatest continuous contact with the patient in hospital; consequently, they have an invaluable role in nutritional management. Nurses are instrumental in these tasks:

(1) Identify patients at high risk of nutritional deficiencies for example poor nutritional intake and/or unintentional weight loss. Approximately 30% of all patients in hospital are undernourished (Kondrup et al. 2003a). People with type 1 diabetes who have repeated admissions to hospital for ketoacidosis (Chapter 7) might have an eating disorder that could be triggered by underlying psychological stress or unrealistic perceptions of obesity. Sensitive discussions with the individual and his or her family and relevant investigations are needed.

(2) Screen patients' nutritional characteristics to identify actual and/or potential problems, for example:

- Inappropriate, erratic, and overeating, and those with eating disorders. Screening processes should be connected to relevant actions. For example, if the person is eating appropriately, arrange for regular screening at specified intervals. If the person is at risk of an eating disorder, an appropriate nutrition plan needs to be determined. If functional, metabolic, or diabetes-related complications are present, standard nutrition plans may not be appropriate and dietitian advice will be needed (Kondrup et al. 2003b). The following factors need to be considered when deciding the level of risk: the current condition, whether the condition is stable (weight loss/gain can be assessed from the health history), the significance of the condition, and whether it is likely to deteriorate or improve, and any disease processes that affect nutritional status such as appetite, diabetes complications, and hyperglycaemia. Managing eating disorders is challenging because people often do not consider their eating behaviour as a problem, or deny they have an eating problem. Repeated episodes of diabetic ketoacidosis (DKA) could indicate an eating disorder and must be investigated. Young people with diabetes often run their blood glucose levels high to lose weight, which puts them at risk of DKA (see Chapters 7 and 13). Cognitive behaviour therapy may be a useful strategy when the eating disorder is mild to moderate. The complex underlying issues need to be ascertained and managed.
- Those with domestic, financial, and/or employment problems are at increased risk.

(3) Provide ongoing patient monitoring on a meal-to-meal basis.

TAKING A DIET HISTORY

Example questions to ask when taking a diet history are shown below. The questions should be asked sensitively as part of a nutritional assessment.

Do you have regular meals?

- It is important to clarify what the individual means by 'regular' and whether they skip meals and if they do when and why. For example, a nurse with diabetes working in the operating theatre might find it difficult to always predict when the operation will finish.

Do you have a good breakfast?

- Poor morning appetite can indicate nocturnal hypoglycaemia and catecholamine production to maintain the falling blood glucose.
- People who do not eat breakfast often snack later in the day on energy-dense foods and can be protein-deficient.
- Missing breakfast interferes with work performance.

How often do you eat takeaway foods?

- Takeaway foods tend to be high in fat, salt and sugar and low in fibre, protein, and essential vitamins and minerals.

Do you eat cream biscuits, chocolates, or lollies (sweets)?

- This question is a way of checking the individual's intake of sugar and fat.

Can you tell me some of the foods you eat that contain carbohydrate?

- Regular carbohydrate intake is important when the individual is using insulin or insulin oral glucose lowering medicines. A minimum of 130 g carbohydrates per day is required to meet the brain demand for glucose (ADA Guidelines).

The information collected from screening, investigations, and questions provides the basis from which nursing staff can quickly and effectively refer patients to the dietitian who can support nursing staff by doing the following:

- Set dietary management goals for the individual consistent with their health status, lifestyle, and healthcare goals.
- Identify possible nutritional problems. Estimating caloric intake is difficult because people generally underestimate their caloric intake by as much as 50% despite trying to keep accurate food records (Fabricatore and Wadden 2004), but three-day food records can be helpful to health professionals and the person with diabetes.
- Identify causes of possible nutritional problems and suggest strategies to overcome them.
- Counsel and educate the patient about how to reduce the risks associated with these problems.
- Support nursing and medical staff on an ongoing basis to ensure most effective nutritional management is achieved and maintained (Dunning and Hoy 1994).

The person with diabetes is in control of what they eat and their activity level and must be actively engaged in planning meals and exercise regimens.

Dietary requirements change with increasing age, activity level, health status, pregnancy, and lactation, and during specific disease processes, for example, renal and cardiac disease.

Method of screening for dietary characteristics and problems

Nutritional status

(1) Identify whether the person is overweight or underweight and whether the person's health is affected by his or her weight status. For example, calculate Body Mass Index (BMI) and/or waist–hip ratio (WHR).

(2) Review any current haematological and biochemical measurements, which reflect the person's nutritional status such as haemoglobin and serum albumin levels, creatinine, folate and cholesterol. Clinical signs such as tiredness, fatigue and obesity can indicate inadequate protein intake and can be confirmed by blood urea nitrogen (BUN) and serum creatinine levels. Low creatinine suggests protein intake is low. Low BUN and creatinine suggests a catabolic state such as hyperglycaemia.

Consider coeliac disease in people with type 1 diabetes; see Chapter 10.

Recent research indicates malnourished patients have a longer length-of-stay, are older and have increased mortality rates compared with well-nourished patients. Most malnourished patients are not identified as being at risk (Middleton et al. 2001). Clues to nutritional deficiency are:

- Weight loss.
- Low lymphocyte count.
- An illness lasting longer than three weeks.
- Serum albumin <3.5 g/dl. Note serum albumin usually falls during acute illness and is not a standalone measure of nutritional deficiency.
- A comprehensive nutrition history and assessment. This includes medicines and possible food-medicine interactions, malabsorption, oral health, anorexia, dysphagia, mental health, and functional ability to identify factors that could contribute to undernutrition, which are likely to be multifactorial.

If a patient is identified as being malnourished, nutritional status should be monitored by weighing the patient regularly, using the same scales and with the person wearing similar clothing, by monitoring nitrogen balance, and using appropriate screening tools such as those listed below. Nutritional supplements may be needed.

Dietary characteristics

The tools and questions described earlier in this chapter can be used to determine:

- The regularity/irregularity of meals and/or snacks
- Whether the person consumes foods and fluids containing refined sugar
- Whether the person omits any of the major food groups

If one or more problems are identified, the person should be referred to the dietitian for further dietary analysis and advice.

Screening tools

Screening tools are used to measure overall risk of malnutrition rather than food consumption and include the following:

- Malnutrition Screening Tool (MST) is widely used in Australia.
- Malnutrition Universal Screening Tool (MUST) is used for adults (Malnutrition Advisory Group [MAG] 2000).
- Simplified Nutritional Assessment Questionnaire (SNAQ).
- Nutritional Risk Screening (NRS-2002) is used in hospital settings.
- Mini Nutritional Assessment (MNA©) is useful for the elderly (Vellas et al. 1999).
- The Healthy Eating Index (HEI) and Modified HEI can be used for children and adolescents (Feskanich et al. 2004).
- Biomarkers identify specific food components in body fluids or tissue, which independently reflect intake of the particular food.

Principles of dietary management for people with diabetes

A number of dietary guidelines have been developed such as the American Diabetes Association, the Diabetes and Nutrition Group of the European Association for the Study of Diabetes, The Canadian Diabetes Association, Diabetes UK, the Indian Council of Medical Research, National Health and Medical Research Council (NHMRC), and Diabetes Australia. The macronutrient content of these guidelines varies despite the fact they are all evidence based and largely draw on the same evidence. Not surprisingly, socioeconomic factors and food availability appear to influence the dietary advice health professionals provide and what people consume, perhaps more than nutrition guidelines (Kapur and Dunning 2007).

Diets such as the traditional Mediterranean, Okinawan, Dietary Approaches to Stop Hypertension (DASH) antihypertensive, anti-inflammatory diet, South Beach diet, Atkins type diet, Omniheart, Onish, and Onish Zone (A to Z) diets all appear to improve metabolic risk factors by reducing lipids and weight to various degrees (Carey et al. 2005; Fung 2007; Gardner et al. 2007; Tay et al. 2008), although they include different combinations of macronutrients. Interestingly, ancestral diets high in acellular carbohydrates could promote an inflammatory microbiota and could be the primary cause of leptin resistance and obesity (Spreadbury 2012). Likewise, consuming high-fat dairy products may reduce obesity risk in Europeans compared to Americans.

The difference could partly be attributed to the different feeding practices adopted in the two countries. Dairy farms are more likely to be highly industrialised in the US where the cows are kept indoors and fed on high protein energy-dense fodder and have little or no exercise. Thus, the milk from US cows has a higher fat content that cows raised on traditional European dairy farms. Ruminant fat consists of more than 400 different fatty acids and is the most complex form of fat in the human diet. These findings are interesting, considering NHMRC and other guideline recommendations to consume low-fat dairy products where possible.

Likewise, vegetarian and vegan diets, which are high in fibre, low in saturated fat and have a low glycaemic index (GI) and lower haem iron, are associated with reduced risk of type 2 diabetes, less weight gain, and better cardiovascular outcomes. However, vegetarian diets may lack essential B group vitamins and iron; thus, supplements might be required. Vegetarian people treated with Metformin are at increased risk of vitamin B_{12} deficiencies because Metformin affects absorption of vitamin B_{12}; see Chapter 5. Although iron is found in vegetables such as spinach and pumpkin, from eggs it is not absorbed as well as haem iron from red meat. Thus, iron supplements might be required (Marsh 2008).

There are various methods of counting carbohydrate, for example, exchanges, portions and carbohydrate counting that help ensure an even distribution of carbohydrate and appropriate ratio of carbohydrate to exercise and glucose lowering medicines doses and administration times when planning meals for individuals. An exchange is equal to 15 g and a portion 10 g of carbohydrate. Exchanges are sometimes used in the United Kingdom whilst Australia often uses GI and glycaemic load (GL).

More recently, portions are making a comeback in programmes such as The German Diabetes Training and Treatment Program (DTTP) and its counterpart the Dose Adjustment for Normal Eating Program (DAFNE). These programmes are being widely adopted and adapted, for example, OzDAFNE in Australia and in group education programmes such as the Royal Derby Hospital in the UK (Shorrock and Hannah 2011).

Using the information they learn in such programmes, people with diabetes estimate their carbohydrate intake based on 10 g portions and calculate their short-acting insulin doses as a ratio to carbohydrate consumption. Basal insulin doses are adjusted to address preprandial and bedtime blood glucose targets, see Chapter 1. HBA1c reductions of ~1% and improved quality of life have been demonstrated without increasing hypoglycaemia or weight (DAFNE Study Group 2002; Muhlhauser and Berger 2002).

In general, people with diabetes should:

- Eat foods high in complex carbohydrate with low GI (50–60% of total intake), high fibre unprocessed foods. Rapidly digested carbohydrates cause a rapid rise in blood glucose and a greater demand on the pancreas to release insulin to maintain the normal blood glucose range. Low GI foods are associated with a lower risk of diabetes and the related complications

(Brand-Miller et al. 2003). GI is a method of ranking foods based on their immediate effect on the blood glucose level. Foods that enter the blood stream quickly have a high GI, for example, sugars. Foods that enter more slowly are known as low GI, for example, cereals. The GI is the area under the glucose response curve measured after ingestion of a test food and multiplied by 100. Foods with a GI <55 are classified as low GI, 56–69 as moderate GI, and >70 are high GI foods. In general, the lower the GI, the smaller the impact on the blood glucose level.

However, many factors affect the rate at which carbohydrate is absorbed including the types of sugar and starch in food, the degree of processing, cooking methods, and the presence of other nutrients such as fat and fibre and the particular combination of foods. Foods high in fat have a low GI because the fat delays their digestion and they are absorbed slowly, but high fat foods are not recommended.

Low GI foods are the preferred basis of a well-balanced diet. They slow food absorption from the gut so the postprandial glucose load is reduced, cause satiety and help control weight, reduce HBA1c, improve insulin sensitivity and help control lipids (Brand-Miller et al. 2003).

People with diabetes are advised to include low GI foods in at least one meal each day. Simple sugars do not have to be excluded using the GI food plan. The move to GI-based diets is not universal and GI can be difficult for some people to understand. Generally, if people are accustomed to working in portions or exchanges and have reasonable metabolic control they should not be expected to change, particularly if they are elderly. Scientists are currently undertaking research to reduce the GI of some foods such as rice by altering their amylopectin structure to improve consumer acceptability (Rahman et al. 2007).

GI is not related to the quantity (portion size) of carbohydrate, which is measured by GL. GI is taken into account when determining GL. That is GI indicates how rapidly the food enters the blood as glucose and the GL indicates how much carbohydrate is in a portion/serving; both are important to understanding the effect of a particular carbohydrate on blood glucose. The type of dietary fibre influences GI, water-soluble fibres such as hemicellulose, mucilages, gums, and pectins have low GI because they slow digestion and absorption of carbohydrate.

Recent advances in blood glucose meter and insulin pump technology and other technological advances include algorithms that calculate insulin doses based on the insulin to carbohydrate ratio, correction factors, and illness and activity levels. Carbohydrate counting is very important when people use insulin pumps.

- Be low in fat (<10% of total energy value), especially saturated fat and trans fatty acids; see Tables 4.1 and 4.2, which depict the main types of dietary fats and their effects on blood lipids, respectively. Some fat is necessary to supply essential fatty acids and fat soluble vitamins A, D, E, and K. Despite an overall reduction in dietary fat, the mean Australian serum cholesterol has not fallen since 1980 (National Heart Foundation 2012). Omega 3 and 6 fatty acids are crucial to healthy brain function, normal growth and development and skin and hair growth, bone health, regulating metabolism, and maintaining reproductive function. Omega 6 fatty acids have an important role in modulating the inflammatory response by generating

Table 4.1 Effect of high carbohydrate, alcohol and fibre on blood fats.

Carbohydrate	Fibre[a]	Alcohol	Non-nutrient components[b]
Increases VLDL and triglycerides	Reduces cholesterol	Increases triglycerides and very-low-density lipo-protein (VLDL) and possibly cholesterol	HMG-CoA-like activity
Lowers HDL		Small increase in HDL	Reduces cholesterol and LDL

[a] Effects depend on the type of fibre. Insoluble fibres only have a small effect on lipoproteins; soluble fibre has a favourable effect.
[b] For example allicin, saponins, isoflavonoids, phyto-oestrogens, and anthocyanins. Individually they only have a small LDL lowering effect but combining several components may produce a cumulative effect.

Table 4.2   Sources of omega-3, -6, and -9 essential fatty acids. And daily intake recommended (RDI) by the National Health and Medical Research Council (2006). A variety of foods high in essential fatty acids should be consumed each day.

Omega-3 (EPA) RDI 50–200 mg/day	Omega-6 RDI 150–1500 mg/day	Omega-9 RDI <50 g/day
Fresh tuna	Safflower	Olive oil
Halibut	Evening primrose	Avocado
Sardines	Sunflower	Almond
Mackerel	Corn and maize	Apricot
Herring	Hempseed	Canola
Trout	Walnut	Peanut
Krill	Pumpkin seed	Butter
Cod liver oil[a]	Borage	Lard
	Blackcurrant	Eggs
	Soya bean	Milk
	Flax and linseed	Coconut

[a] Cod liver oil may be contraindicated in pregnancy without medical advice.

RDI = recommended daily intake. The RDI varies amongst publications. Consider the quantity of EPA and DHA in omega-3 supplements rather than the total quantity of fish oil in the product. Different types of fish contain different quantities of omega-3. Consider the risk of bleeding before recommending supplements if the person is on anticoagulant medicines or has bleeding conditions.

eicosanoids (prostaglandins and leukotrienes) and cytokines (interleukins). For example, gamma-linolenic acid (omega 6) synthesised from linolenic acid reduces inflammation. There is strong evidence that replacing saturated fatty acids with omega 3 and 6 reduces cardiovascular disease in people with diabetes and nondiabetics (Eddy 2008). Dietary sources are not high in gamma-linolenic acid. Some are found in green leafy vegetables and nuts. The richest sources are borage oil, blackcurrant and evening primrose oil, and breast milk. The conversion of linolenic acid into gamma-linolenic acid is inefficient in older age, diabetes, high alcohol consumption, eczema, viral infections, excess fat intake, hypercholestrolaemia, and deficiency of vitamin B_6, zinc, magnesium, calcium, and biotin. Deutsch (2007) suggested *Euphasia superba* (krill) is a better source of omega-3 than plant sources and rapidly reduces C-reactive protein (CRP), a marker of inflammatory disease. However, compared to fish oils, krill oil has less omega-3, so larger doses are needed and krill is more expensive. Sources of omega-3, -6, and -9 are shown in Table 4.3

- Contain adequate protein (15% of total intake).
- Be low in simple sugar, less than 25 g/day.
- Ensure a variety of food is eaten daily from each of the five food groups.
- Ensure that complex carbohydrate is consumed at each meal to reduce the postprandial blood glucose rise and the likelihood of hypoglycaemia in patients on insulin or diabetes medication.
- Limit salt. A typical Western diet contains about ~10 g of salt per day and 75% of salt consumed is added salt. The NHMRC (2003) and The Heart Foundation recommend an upper level of 6 g of salt per day. (The 2003 NHMRC Guidelines have been reviewed and should be available in 2013 but the content is expected to be similar.) High salt diets are leading causes of cardiovascular disease and hypertension (WHO 2002), and reducing salt intake reduces blood pressure.
- Reduce alcohol. Small amounts of alcohol (0.5–1 drink/day) can reduce cardiovascular risk and post prandial blood glucose levels if consumed with the evening meal containing carbohydrate. Greater quantities impair glucose metabolism and contribute to hyperlipidaemia, In Australia, the current recommendation is two standard drinks per day for men and one standard drink per day for women.

Table 4.3 Effects of adipokines and changes that occur in the presence of abdominal obesity, which demonstrates their role in the development of insulin resistance, Type 2 diabetes and cardiovascular disease.

Name of adipokine	Effects in the body	Effect of increasing abdominal obesity on adipokine levels
Tumour necrosis factor-alpha	Disrupts insulin signalling processes in the cell membranes Reduces endothelial vasodilatation by reducing nitric oxide	Higher
Interleukin-6	Stimulates rate of C-reactive protein release from the liver Induces insulin resistance Damages endothelial function	Higher
Plasminogen Activator Inhibitor-1	Enhances prothrombotic state	Higher
Leptin	Regulates: • appetite • energy expenditure • insulin sensitivity Stimulates the sympathetic nervous system Acts as a signalling factor in hypertension	Higher
Adiponectin	Improves tissue sensitivity Anti-inflammatory Reduces atherogenesis	Lower
Angiotensinogen	Contributes to hypertension	Higher

Goals of dietary management

The goals of dietary management are to achieve the following:

- Improve the person's overall health.
- Attain optimal body weight.
- Attain lipid and blood glucose levels as close to normal as practical considering hypoglycaemia risk and its consequences: see Chapter 6.
- Ensure normal growth and development in children.
- Decrease the risk of diabetes- and obesity-related complications and comorbidities.
- Identify nutrition-related disorders that can affect diabetes management and interpreting investigative procedures, such as anaemia.

Overweight and obesity

Obesity is defined as excess body fat and is now recognised as a disease in its own right (Marks 2000; James and Coster 2011). Obesity is emerging as a complex phenomena caused by a number of interrelated factors including high-fat energy-dense diets, inadequate amounts of exercise, and genetic, hormonal, and environmental factors (Brunner and McCarthy 2001; Bouchard et al. 2004; Frayling 2007; Unger and Scherer 2010). The estimated risk of becoming obese using data from the Framlingham Study suggests a normal weight person has a 50% long-term risk of becoming overweight and 25% risk of becoming obese (Reynolds et al. 2005). However, a number of studics suggest underweight might confer greater health risks, especially in older people (Diehr et al. 1998, 2008).

A recent study suggests that normal weight people with type 2 diabetes are more likely to die from any cause than heavier people with type 2 diabetes over 10–30 years after adjusting for demographic factors, smoking and cardiovascular risk (Carnethon et al. 2012). Cardiovascular mortality risk in normal weight individuals was higher by 50% and noncardiovascular risk more than double that of overweight individuals, which is consistent with the *obesity paradox*. Unlike most researchers, Carnethon et al. (2012) measured BMI when diabetes was diagnosed, which helped control for the effect of diabetes duration on complication status. However, lower body weight might be associated with underlying illness or nutritional deficiencies that predisposes individuals to morbidity and mortality risk.

Some medicines such as corticosteroids, antipsychotics, birth control medicines, insulin, sulphonylureas, and thiazolidinediones (TZDs) contribute to weight gain; see Chapter 5. There is increasing evidence that ethnicity, environmental factors, social isolation, being teased about weight, low self-esteem and low global self-worth contribute to obesity in children (Goodman and Whitaker 2002; Eisenberg et al. 2003). Contributing environmental factors include sedentary behaviour including excess television viewing (Wilmot et al. 2012), insufficient physical activity, which might be influenced by living in unsafe areas, and high consumption of fast foods (Burdette and Whitaker 2005).

The prevalence of overweight and obesity are increasing globally but there are differences amongst populations and amongst ethnic groups within populations. Rates of overweight and obesity are also increasing in children and adolescents. A child with one overweight parent has a 40% chance of becoming overweight, and the risk increases to 80% when both parents are overweight. A recent Dutch study showed that more than 75% of severely obese children younger than 18 already has one or more cardiovascular risk factors. Significantly, 62% of severely obese children younger than 12 years have one or more cardiovascular risk factors. Many also have hypertension, low HDL cholesterol, and impaired fasting glucose (Chapter 13).

Obesity prevents people from undertaking many self-care tasks and activities of daily living and increases the burden on joints leading to pain and discomfort that limits exercise capability. In addition, obesity makes it difficult for health professionals to perform some preventative healthcare interventions such as cervical smears and mammograms, and overweight women are more likely to have false-positive results in these tests than nonobese women (Elmore et al. 2004).

Overview of the pathogenesis of obesity

As indicated, environmental factors play an important role in the development of obesity and its related diseases. A simplistic explanation is that increased food intake leads to weight gain and obesity, which lead to insulin resistance and impaired insulin action in muscle, liver, and fat tissue. The pancreas compensates by secreting extra insulin (hyperinsulinaemia). In the long term, the beta cells become exhausted and hyperglycaemia and hypertriglyceridaemia develop (James and Coster 2011). In addition, a novel hypothesis suggests diet-induced obese people homeostatically guard their weight (Spreadbury 2012).

Abdominal fat is not inert. It produces signalling molecules, adipokines, which exacerbate endothelial dysfunction. A number of adipokines are produced; see Table 4.4. In addition, the endocannabinoid neuroregulatory system influences the activity of other neurotransmitter systems, including hormone secretion, and modulates immune and inflammatory responses. Likewise, understanding of the role of leptin-resistance on satiety mediators and white adipose tissue in regulating body metabolism, insulin sensitivity, and food intake has increased rapidly over the past few years (Spreadbury 2012).

The CRB system consists of many endocannabinoids, including CB_1 and CB_2. CB_1 occurs through the body including in the brain, adipose tissue, vascular endothelium, and sympathetic nerve terminals. CB_2 mostly occurs in lymph tissue and macrophages. In addition, a number of endocannabinoid subtypes exist whose function is yet to be determined. Endocannabinoids regulate metabolism in a number of ways. Blocking CB_1 reduces food intake, abdominal fat, triglycerides, low-density lipoprotein (LDL), CRP, and insulin resistance, and it increases high-density lipoprotein (HDL).

Activating CB_1 has the opposite effect. Data from the RIO-Europe Trial showed significant weight reductions and reduction in cardiometabolic risk factors such as waist circumference,

Table 4.4 Dietary fat comes from animal and plant sources and has various effects on blood lipids.[a]

Saturated fatty acids (SFAs)	Monounsaturated fatty acids (MUFAs)	Polyunsaturated fatty acids (PUFAs)	Trans fatty acids (TFAs)
Not essential fatty acids[b]	Not essential fatty acids[b]	Omega-3 Eicosapentaenoic acid (EPA) and Docosahexaenoic acid (DHA) and omega-6 (Gamma-Linolenic acid, GLA) are essential fatty acids (EFA)[c]	Can be MUFAs or PUFAs TFA are formed when hydrogen is added to vegetable oils but small amounts are found in animal fats. Some dietary supplements contain TFA Amounts >0.5 must be listed on the label in the US.
With cholesterol contributes to hypercholesterolaemia	Small beneficial effect on lipoproteins	Has a beneficial effect on cholesterol Increasing omega-3 intake lowers LDL and triglycerides but not as much as reducing dietary SFA. Different omega-3 may have different effects on serum cholesterol. Reduce platelet aggregation and risk of myocardial infarction Retard deposition of atherosclerotic plaque and have anti-inflammatory effects. May help reduce abdominal fat in insulin-resistant people. Improves morning stiffness in rheumatoid arthritis and has additive effects with anti-inflammatory medicines. High doses may increase the risk of bleeding. Omega-9 might reduce cancer risk and reduces abdominal fat but increases HDL but it also increases LDL, cholesterol and triglycerides so it may not be cardio protective (Jepersen 2001)	Increase LDL reduce HDL and lipoprotein[a]

[a] Triglycerides are the most abundant dietary fat. Cholesterol and phospholipid dietary fats have a small but significant impact on serum cholesterol. Provides SFAs, MUFAs, and PUFAs.
[b] Can be obtained from protein and carbohydrate if necessary. Serum cholesterol is more responsive to changes in dietary SFAs than PUFAs or cholesterol. TFAs are found in foods containing hydrogenated vegetable oils and fat from ruminant animals.
[c] Omega-6 is derived from linoleic acid; omega-3 is derived from alpha-linolenic acid. All other longer chain PUFAs can be synthesised in the body from these precursors. Omega-3, -6, and -9 compete for the same desaturase enzymes. The desaturase enzymes show preference for the omega-3, -6, and -9 in that order so that synthesis of some EFAs might only occur when the intake of omega-3 and -6 EFAs is low.

triglyceride levels, and elevated HDL using the CB_1 blocker, Rimonabant, compared to controls (van Gaal, Rissanen and Scheen, 2005). The latter effects occurred independently of weight loss. People taking Rimonabant averaged 4.7 kg weight loss after a year and were more likely to achieve a 10% weight loss than controls.

White adipose tissue has many functions, including acting as a storage depot for triglycerides. It is regarded as an endocrine organ that secretes a range of adipokines, which influence weight, inflammation, coagulation, fibrinolysis, tissue response to insulin, and contributes to the development of metabolic syndrome and Type 2 diabetes. Energy balance is impaired and obesity results if white adipose tissue function is disrupted (Iqbal 2007); see Table 4.4. Ghrelin is produced in the stomach and mediates hunger. Restricting calories and exercising increases Ghrelin levels (Leidy et al. 2007).

Adipose tissue has a major role in hormone metabolism such as synthesising oestrogen in postmenopausal women, which is protective against osteoporosis (Moyad 2004). Likewise, replacing testosterone preserves skeletal muscle and reduces abdominal obesity in nonobese men over 50 years whose testosterone level is <15 nM (Allan 2009). Thus, it contributes to overall well-being.

The Significance of abdominal obesity

People with central or abdominal obesity are at increased risk of obesity-related diseases such as metabolic syndrome, Type 2 diabetes, dyslipidaemia, fatty liver, and therefore, are at significant risk of cardiovascular disease. Obesity is a risk factor for shortened life expectancy in younger but not older people (Heiat et al. 2001) and the importance of overweight and obesity as predictors of health status decline in people >65 years. In fact, some research indicates being overweight is associated with better quality of life and health status in older people (Stevens 2000).

Waist circumference is significantly correlated with triglyceride levels, CRP, cholesterol, and glucose, but not HBA1c in healthy women (Behan and Mbizo 2007). Likewise, the INTERHEART Study Group (Yusuf et al. 2004) demonstrated that a waist circumference is strongly related to myocardial infarction (MI) but the level of risk is unclear. Physical fitness may reduce the inflammation associated with abdominal obesity and reduce cardiovascular risk (Zoeller 2007).

Various cardiovascular risk scores have been developed based on parameters such as age, gender, total cholesterol, LDL, systolic blood pressure, being treated for hypertension and smoking – for example, The Framlingham Risk Score (Expert Panel on Detection, Evaluation, and Treatment of High Blood Cholesterol in Adults 2002) and the Systemic Coronary Risk Evaluation (SCORE) (Third Joint Taskforce of European and Other Societies on Cardiovascular Disease Prevention in Clinical Practice 2003).

However, a 12-year US study of people in their sixties suggests obese people live as long as people of normal weight and are less likely to develop diabetes or lipid abnormalities if they are fit. However, at BMI >30, people experience difficulty performing usual activities of daily living and develop other obesity-related disorders such as musculoskeletal disease that cause pain, lower muscle strength, and reduced cardiovascular fitness (Nantel, Mathieu and Prince, 2011)). Thus, the focus on weight management must also include reducing/managing obesity-related disability.

Other obesity-related diseases include osteoarthritis, rheumatoid arthritis, and other musculoskeletal diseases, some forms of cancer (e.g. breast, oesophagus, colorectal, endometrial and renal cell), sleep apnoea and daytime sleepiness (Chapter 10), gout, urinary stress incontinence, and surgical complications. Significantly, maternal obesity is associated with a higher incidence of birth defects (Chapters 1 and 14).

Nutrition, overweight/obesity and stress

There is a complex association amongst nutrition, stress, and overweight/obesity. Stress affects eating behaviour: most people eat more and gain weight; 30% reduce weight (Stone and Brownell 1994), but the reasons for the increased intake are unclear. Likewise, Groesz et al. 2012 found people are concerned about life stress and 50% eat more calorie-dense food when they are stressed and undertake less activity. A suggested mechanism for the effect of stress on weight is that cortisol levels increase during stress, which stimulates appetite: managing stress reduces stress-related intake. In addition, chronic low level stress reduces insulin sensitivity and contributes to abdominal obesity and the metabolic syndrome.

Significantly, 45% of women and 23% of men think they are overweight and 20% of underweight women think they are overweight and are dieting to lose weight (Better Health Channel, January 2008). People use a range of self-initiated strategies to lose weight, which are often successful initially, but regain half to two-thirds of the weight lost in the first 12 months and nearly all within five years. In contrast, the NHANES 1999–2002 showed 58% of people who lost >5% of their bodyweight maintained the weight loss for up to five years.

Factors associated with weight gain in NAHANES included:

- Mexican-American peoples
- Significant weight loss
- Fewer years since reaching their maximum weight
- Long time spent watching TV: children and adults

- Attempting to control weight
- Sedentary lifestyle
- Frequent attempts to diet were associated with increased risk of developing an eating disorder

Ethnic differences could partly explain the different findings. In addition, people who are supported to lose weight are more likely to stay motivated than those who go it alone. Self-perception and body image influence quality of life and mood and there is a pervasive association amongst perception of being overweight, depression, and disordered body image.

Methods of measuring weight

Measuring obesity is difficult. A number of methods are used. Each has advantages and disadvantages.

Crude weight

Weighing people is the simplest way to estimate obesity using height/weight standards. It does not take into account muscular builds at different heights or that lean body mass weighs more than fat tissue. Mild obesity = 20–40% overweight; moderate obesity = 41–100%, and severe obesity = twice the actual weight for height. Crude weight and BMI are useful to track weight changes over time, but weighing is best undertaken using the same scales at the same time of day wearing the same clothing.

Body mass index

The BMI, sometimes referred to as Quetelet's Index, is a simple method of assessing obesity but, like crude weight, it does not take into account muscular builds at different heights. However, despite the limitations, BMI >30 generally indicates excess adipose tissue. BMI should be interpreted according to growth charts in children. BMI is calculated using the following formula: weight in kilogrammes divided by height in meters squared.

Waist–hip ratio

The WHR is measured with the person standing and specifically measures abdominal obesity. The waist is defined as the largest abdominal circumference midway between the costal margin and the iliac crest. A WHR >90 in men and >80 in women is generally regarded as an accurate predictor of obesity-related disorders, independently of the BMI. WHR can be affected by postprandial status, time of day, and depth of inspiration to an unknown degree. It includes both intra-abdominal fat (the area of interest) and subcutaneous fat, but it is not clear how to adjust the WHR for subcutaneous fat. There are also differences amongst ethnic groups that need to be considered. It is useful to record the WHR on a regular basis.

Other ways of measuring body fat

Dual energy X-ray absorptiometry (DEXA) is often used in research and to determine risk of osteoporosis. Lean body mass, skin fold thickness, densitometry hydrostatic weighing, and bioelectrical impedance analysis are also ways to measure obesity.

Strategies used to measure food consumption

A number of tools are used to estimate food intake over various time periods. These include:

- Food records – the individual keeps a detailed record of their intake for varying periods from three to seven days. Maintaining a food record can be burdensome and requires the person to be literate. In addition, actually recording intake often influences the person to consider what they eat and change their usual eating pattern.

- Food frequency questionnaires (FFQ) retrospectively estimate usual dietary intake over time, usually 6–12 months. Information is collected about specific types of food and the quantities and frequency with which they are consumed. Short (60 foods) and long (100 foods) FFQs are used. FFQs must be culturally relevant, and a number of culturally relevant forms exist. Modified FFQs identify dietary fat, fibre, fruit, and vegetable intake.
- Dietary recall, often over 24 hours, is used to estimate current intake. Accuracy is influenced by the individual's ability to recall the type and quantity of food consumed. Most people underestimate their intake.
- Visual estimation, where trained observers monitor an individual's food choices, classifies foods using a rating scale and estimates serving sizes. This is intimidating and may influence the individual's food selection. Nurses can undertake this type of monitoring process.
- Plate waste methodology has been used extensively in studies of food intake in school children but is not practical in clinical practice.

Managing obesity and diabetes

Obesity and type 2 diabetes are chronic conditions, and long-term management strategies are needed. Usually a combination of strategies is most effective, especially when they are developed in consultation with the individual. In the first instance, energy-dense food intake such as simple carbohydrates and saturated and trans fats should be reduced, exercise increased, and possibly sleep increased (Lamberg 2006). Exercise needs to be enough to increase total energy expenditure to 160–180% of the resting metabolic rate (Erlichman et al. 2002). Increasing exercise with or without a weight loss diet induces a modest weight loss. People with diabetes should have a thorough physical assessment before undertaking exercise and weight loss programmes that need to be individualised for best effect. Along with diet, exercise prescriptions (Elfhag and Rössner 2005) and wearing a pedometer (Richardson et al. 2008) can help the individual achieve weight loss.

Counselling and behavioural strategies that encompass support, exercise, and dietary counselling are effective and in Australia are supported through some health benefit funds. For example, commercial diet-oriented weight loss programmes such as *Step into Life, Lifestyle Integrated Functional Exercise* (LIFE), *Mass Attack Weight Loss Program, Lite n' Easy, ClubOptiSlim*. Some of these programmes deliver nutritionally balanced portion controlled low-fat meals to the individual's home.

Prepared low-energy meals or meal replacements that replace some or all of the individual's diet can be useful as an initial weight-loss strategy or to avoid refeeding syndrome after severe calorie restriction or bariatric surgery. However, they can be expensive in the long term. Avoiding fructose and corn syrup, which are common forms of sugar added to foods and nonalcoholic beverages in the United States.

Self-help programmes often combine lifestyle change, computer-assisted interventions, packaged programmes such as Internet correspondence courses, and take-home weight-loss kits. Self-help programmes are difficult to measure but Latner (2001) claimed 45% of people using such programmes lose weight and keep it off. Knowledgeable clinicians can support individuals likely to benefit from a self-help approach (Tan et al. 2006).

Significantly, public health programmes that involve health providers, legislators, the food industry, and health insurers are needed and must include children and adolescents. Weight-loss strategies may need to include strategies to keep people physically active in the longer term, and recent research suggests it could be important to minimise exercise variation because maintaining exercise at a consistent level moderates age-related weight gain in proportion to the amount of exercise performed (Williams 2008). Even fit people tend to gain weight with increasing age; thus, the amount of exercise may need to be increased to reduce age-related weight gain (Williams 2008).

Significantly, stopping exercise leads to weight gain.

Dietary management: overweight and obesity

Public health strategies are required to have a significant impact on the health, well-being and obesity levels of the population; see Chapter 1. Individual dietary advice should be age-, gender-, and culture-specific and achievable, which means addressing environmental issues such as access to healthy food, safe, accessible areas to exercise, and accurate, understandable food labels.

As well as diet and exercise, a combination of behaviour change strategies tailored to the individual, and support are required. Diets high in fruit, vegetables, whole grains, legumes, and low in fat are generally safe and effective and promote fullness and satiety (Australian Government Department of Health, 2015). However, <20% of people trying to lose weight consume these foods.

As indicated, commercial weight loss programmes such as Weight Watchers, the Slim-Fast plan, Dr Atkin's New Diet, and the Rosemary Conley Program result in significant weight loss and lower WHR after six months compared to controls who gained an average of 0.6 kg. However, the improvements were not sustained after the trial was completed. More sustained benefit was noted in programmes that included a support group (Truby and Baic 2006).

Other popular diets include the following, which all have advantages and disadvantages. People with diabetes should be advised to discuss these diets with a dietitian and/or their doctor before they try them:

- High-protein, low-carbohydrate (ketogenic) diets.
- Meal replacement plans where 1–2 meals per day are replaced with meal supplements.
- Dairy diet. Preliminary data suggest 3 servings/day of calcium-rich food enhances weight loss through a variety of mechanisms, but more research is needed to confirm these preliminary results (Zemel 2003).

Fish oil supplements (3 g fish oil containing 1.8 g polyunsaturated fatty acids) have been shown to reduce adiposity and atherogenic risk factors in a randomised controlled trial of women with Type 2 diabetes (Rizkalla 2007). However, fish oil may affect the INR in patients taking anticoagulants.

If the BMI is >30 or BMI >27 and diabetes or cardiovascular risk factors are present and diet and exercise is ineffective, medicines such as lipase inhibitors (Xenical) or serotonin reuptake inhibitors such as Sibutramine can be used but they only reduce weight by ~10%. Sibutramine can increase blood pressure (Donohoe 2008). Research into future weight loss medicines is likely to focus on the hormones involved in regulating satiety (leptin, ghrelin, and CRBs). Fucoxanthin, an antioxidant obtained from brown seaweed, which is commonly used in Asian cuisine, has been shown to induce weight loss and increase omega-3 fatty acid levels in rats (Miyashita 2006), but its application in humans is unknown.

Bariatric surgery

Gastric bypass surgery (bariatric surgery) is increasingly being recommended for people with type 2 diabetes who have a BMI >35 where lifestyle and medical treatments for obesity and uncontrolled diabetes have not been effective, provided they are fit and over 18 years (Proietto et al. 2012). Bariatric surgery refers to a variety of surgical procedures that induce weight loss by:

- reducing the size of the stomach to restrict the amount of food that can be consumed;
- delaying digestion and absorption of food in the intestines;
- causing a feeling of fullness and satiety due to stimulation of nerves in the stomach or through the hormones that control hunger, or both.

Types of procedures include:

- adjustable gastric banding (the most commonly used procedure);
- partial or sleeve gastrectomy;
- gastric bypass (Roux-en-Y) and bilopancreatic diversion (see Table 4.5).

Table 4.5   Bariatric surgical procedures and the postulated weight loss mechanisms. Complication rates are reported to be low: 1% for gastric banding to between 2 and 10% for the other more complex procedures. Risks increase with increasing age, degree of obesity and concomitant medical conditions.

Bariatric procedure	Outline of the procedure	Postulated weight loss mechanism
Adjustable gastric band	An adjustable gastric band is paced around the upper section of the stomach that creates a small pouch that can only hold a small amount of food.	Restricts the quantity of food consumed
Sleeve gastrectomy	Removal of two thirds of the stomach	Restricts the quantity of food consumed. Affects hunger by stimulating nerves or altering hormones that induce satiety.
Gastric bypass: Roux-en-Y procedure		Restricts the quantity of food consumed Affects hunger by stimulating nerves or altering hormones that induce satiety. Delays digestion and reduces absorption of nutrients.

People most suited to bariatric surgery:

- have type 2 diabetes;
- are obese with a BMI 0.35;
- have tried lifestyle and medical treatments with no success (significant weight loss);
- are over 18 years;
- are fit enough to undergo surgery;
- understand the procedure and the commitment needed for ongoing care and follow-up and to maintain lifestyle changes after surgery;
- are obese adults with a high risk of type 2 diabetes and BMI > 35 and another obesity-related condition or BMI > 40 who meet the other preceding criteria.

The benefits and risks associated with bariatric surgery for people with diabetes have not been established and should be considered on an individual basis.

Bariatric surgery appears to improve blood glucose control through weight loss, reduced insulin resistance, and improved insulin sensitivity (Proietto et al. 2012). Blood glucose normalises in up to 75% of people, especially if they had type 2 diabetes for a short period before undergoing surgery. Procedures such as gastric bypass that involve the small intestine appear to induce hormonal effects apart from weight loss that improves blood glucose control within a few days.

Bariatric surgery effectively reduces weight, improves quality of life, and lowers the risk of comorbidities after two years compared to controls (Adams et al. 2006) and, with 12 months of medical therapy prior to bariatric surgery, achieved glycaemic control in obese people with uncontrolled type 2 diabetes (n = 150) (Schauer et al. 2012).

Schauer et al. did not find significant differences in total and LDL cholesterol levels 12 months post-bariatric surgery or a significant reduction in the number of medicines needed to manage hyperlipidaemia. Adverse events included blood clots requiring surgery, nausea and vomiting, and gastric leak after sleeve gastrectomy. They did not report any deaths, serious hypoglycaemia, malnutrition, or excessive weight loss.

However, some serious adverse events can occur over time and include:

- The gastric band slipping or, less commonly, the band eroding into the stomach wall.
- Vitamin and mineral deficiencies, due to inadequate nutrition or reduced absorption (Encinosa et al. 2006).

Improved mood has been demonstrated using the Beck Depression Inventory (Mitka 2003). Several procedures are used such as Roux-en-Y gastric bypass, stapled gastroplasty, and adjustable gastric banding, all of which reduce the stomach size and control caloric intake. Although the risks are high, people lose weight and blood glucose levels normalise (Encinose et al. 2006). Despite these promising findings, long-term outcomes are not yet available, and it is not clear whether glucose control will be maintained in the long term. Significantly, access to an experienced interdisciplinary team is essential for ongoing follow-up and to minimise complications.

Complementary and alternative weight loss programmes

Many complementary and alternative medicine (CAM) weight loss strategies are similar to conventional programmes, and these are beneficial and effective. However, many CAM medicines have limited evidence of any benefits (Egger 2008) and some are dangerous; for example, weight-loss products that contain ephedra should be avoided and have been banned in some countries. Likewise, creams, soaps, and body wraps are unlikely to lead to weight loss. They may improve body image and self-concept and help the individual mentally. Hypnosis and acupuncture may be useful adjuncts to some other strategies.

People also use topical creams and 'anticellulite' (fat) preparations to improve their body image, and research is continuing into the effectiveness of such medicines. Caruso et al. (2007) reported 11% reduction in waist circumference compared to 5% after 12 weeks in controls with equal reductions in women and men using a 1200-cal balanced diet, a walking programme, and 0.5% topical aminophylline cream applied to the waist The diet and exercise could confound the results. Likewise, the study was not blinded. Thus, there is no compelling evidence to recommend using currently available anticellulite preparations and some that contain aminophylline could affect heart rate and rhythm, which might be undesirable in people with diabetes.

In Australia, weight control products (complementary and conventional) must conform to the Weight Management Industry Code of Practice (http://www.weightcontrol.org/browse.asp?page=349). People should be advised to check whether products conform to this Code before they purchase the product. In addition, websites that show the HonCode logo are likely to contain accurate, unbiased information.

Factors associated with making dietary changes

Kapur et al. (2008) described a number of factors associated with positive dietary changes in India:

- Being older
- A shorter time since being fit and of acceptable weight
- Having strong family support
- Having a less busy work life
- Being conscious of their health
- Having received dietitian advice and frequent visits to a dietitian
- Being interested in overall health not just diabetes

Motivational interviewing in addition to diet and exercise leads to weight loss in African-American in a randomised prospective trial in women. HbA1c was correlated with weight loss at 6 months but was not sustained at 18 months (Smith-West 2007). Galuska et al. (1999) demonstrated cost savings in people being counselled and suggested frequent reminders and support were essential.

These findings suggest important issues for health professionals to consider when developing weight management strategies and delivering dietary advice. They might also indicate that health professionals also need to make some behaviour changes and become better educated about nutrition and how to deliver dietary and weight-loss advice.

Key points

(1) Assess dietary and nutritional characteristics and problems such as poor intake, under- or overweight, and unexplained weight loss/gain and refer to a dietitian as required, for example at a change from tablets to insulin, if there are frequent high or low blood glucose levels, the diagnosis of a complication such as renal disease, if the patient displays inadequate knowledge, or when the person requests a referral.

(2) Observe and, if necessary, record food intake, with particular reference to carbohydrate intake of patients on glucose lowering medication.

(3) Promote general dietary principles to patients in accordance with accepted policies and procedures.

(4) Ensure the meals and carbohydrate content are evenly spaced throughout the day.

(5) Ensure adequate carbohydrate intake for fasting patients and those with diminished intake to avoid hypoglycaemia.

(6) Administer medicines at an appropriate time in relation to food.

(7) Know that the absorption of some medicines can be modified by food, especially antibiotics and their effectiveness may be diminished or increased (see Table 4.6). The pharmacological response to medicines is influenced by the individual's nutritional status. In turn, medicines can affect the nutritional status. The sense of smell and taste play a significant role in adequate dietary intake. Both these senses diminish with age and can be changed by disease processes and some medicines. GIT disorders can lead to malabsorption. pH changes alter the bioavailability of nutrients and medicines, inhibit medicine binding and chelation, and impair the metabolism and excretion of medicines (NHMRC 1999). Interactions can also occur with commonly used dietary supplements; see Chapter 12 and the International Bibliographic Information on Dietary Supplements (National Institute of Health).

(8) Observe for signs and symptoms of hyper- and hypoglycaemia, and correct the blood glucose level by appropriate nutritional management as part of the management plan.

Table 4.6   Medicines whose absorption can be modified by food.

Reduced absorption	Delayed absorption	Increased absorption
Aspirin	Aspirin	Diazepam
Cephalexin	Cefaclor	Dicoumarol
Erythromycin	Cephalexin	Hydrochlorothiazide
Penicillin V and G	Cimetidine	Hydrochlorothiazide
Phenacetin	Digoxin	Metoprolol
Tetracycline	Indoprofen	Nitrofurantoin
Theophylline	Metronidazole	Propranolol

Inadequate nutrition and low protein stores can delay the healing process. Some food-medicine interactions are shown in Table 4.7.

Sugar-free foods

Sugar-free usually refers to the sucrose content of foods. Other sugars are often used to sweeten foods labelled sugar-free (e.g. dextrose, fructose, maltose, lactose, galactose).

Recent evidence suggests that fructose, which is used to sweeten most soft drinks, causes a greater increase in triglycerides and LDL than glucose (American Dietetic Association 2004;

Table 4.7   Some food-medicine interactions.[a]

Food	Medicine	Possible effects
Black liquorice in large doses	Digoxin Diuretics Calcium channel blockers	Irregular heart rhythm Hypertension High serum sodium Muscle pain Weakness
Aged cheese such as brie, parmesan, Roquefort Sauerkraut Over ripe avocadoes Pepperoni	MAO antidepressants	Hypertension
Grapefruit juice	Calcium channel blockers Lipid-lowering medicines Some oral contraceptives Some psychiatric medicines	Modifies medicine metabolism
Orange juice	Aluminium-containing antacids Antibiotics	Increases aluminium
Milk and other dairy products	Tetracycline Digitalis Laxatives containing bisacodyl	Enhanced effects
Oatmeal and high fibre cereals	Many oral medicines including antihypertensive agents	Can affect absorption
Leafy and green vegetables high in vitamin K	Warfarin and other anticlotting medicines	Interferes with blood clotting
Caffeinated foods such as tea, coffee, chocolate	Asthma medications Quinolone antibiotics Some oral contraceptives	Excessive excitability
Alcohol	Medicines containing pseudoephedrine Antidepressant medicines Antipsychotics Muscle relaxants Sedatives Glucose-lowering medicines	Excitability Sedation Hypoglycaemia
High salt foods Iodine-rich food	Steroids Thyroid medicines	Fluid retention Reduced efficacy Might affect blood glucose through its effect on the thyroid

See also Chapter 5.

[a]*Note*: Alcohol interacts with almost all medicines. Some medicines increase the risk of nutritional deficiencies. For example, metformin leads to vitamin B_{12} deficiency; cholestyramine increases excretion of folate and vitamins A, D, E, and K; and antacids interfere with the absorption of many essential minerals. Thus, the person being prescribed medicines should be advised about when to take them in relation to food. People at high risk of a food–medicine interaction are older, taking medicines for chronic diseases such as diabetes, have hypertension, depression hypercholesterolaemia, renal disease, or congestive heart failure.

Havel 2007). The study was undertaken in overweight and obese individuals, but the findings are likely to apply to nonobese people because fructose is more likely to pass into the lipogenic pathway than glucose after being metabolised in the liver. More research is needed to confirm these findings to determine the percentage of total energy consumption at which fructose has an atherogenic effect. These foods may not be appropriate for people with diabetes. Low-calorie and artificially sweetened foods are generally recommended.

Alternative sweeteners

Alternative sweeteners elicit a pleasurable sensation without affecting the blood glucose and are generally safe if used at the recommended doses. They may also play a role in reducing dental caries (American Dietetic Association 2004). They are an acceptable alternative to sugar for people with diabetes. However, a small amount of sugar included in a balanced diet does not adversely affect the blood glucose. There are two types of alternative sweeteners: nonnutritive (or artificial) and nutritive. Nonnutritive sweeteners are kilojoule free, for example:

- Saccharin
- Acesulphame-K
- Aspartame (Equal)
- Cyclamate
- Isomalt
- Neotame
- Sucralose (Splenda)
- Alitame
- Neotame

These products are safe to use. If used in cooking, they are best added after cooking because heat can change the taste. The best choices for pregnant women are Acesulphame-K, Alitame, Aspartame, and Sucralose.

Nutritive sweeteners are usually derived from different types of carbohydrate and products containing these sweeteners are often labelled 'carbohydrate modified'.

Nutritive sweeteners include:

- Sorbitol
- Fructose (Sweetaddin)
- Mannitol
- Xylitol
- Maltilol
- Isomalt
- Polydextrose (Litesse)
- Maltodextrin (hydrolysed corn syrup)
- Thaumatin

Many nutritive sweeteners are sugar alcohols, for example, sorbitol. These sweeteners can cause diarrhoea in high doses. Likewise, 'diet' products containing alternative sweeteners can be high in fat.

Stevia (*Stevia rebaudiana*), an herb much sweeter than sugar, is being promoted as a suitable sugar alternative for people with diabetes and may have glucose-lowering effects, but it has not been extensively evaluated in clinical practice. Only very small quantities are required. Larger doses may cause diarrhoea.

Food additives

Many people are allergic to food additives, which can result in sensitivities or, in severe cases, analphylaxis. Different additives are used for different classes of foods. A list of food additives and their code numbers can be obtained from www.foodstandards.gov.au. Types of additives include acidity regulators, antioxidants, bulking agents, colourings, flavourings, emulsifiers, gelling agents, humectants, preservatives, and thickeners. Some of these additives are also used in some medicines.

It is important to learn to read labels and to get to know the alternative names for foods and additives that commonly cause allergies, such as cow's milk, soy, nuts, and gluten, as well as alternative names for fat and sugar. Key information on a food label people need to look for includes:

- The nutrition claims, e.g. fat free, high fibre, low fat, reduced fat, cholesterol free, low in salt, low in sugar, and sugar free
- How to interpret the list of ingredients

- How to interpret the allergy information
- The country of origin
- Use-by dates and storage recommendations
- The nutrition information
- How to interpret information about recommended daily intake
- Figures and symbols such as the GI symbol, genetically modified foods, and the Heart Foundation logo

These key aspects should be part of routine dietary advice, or the person can be referred to Reid (2007) www.healthyfoodguide.com.au for further information.

Alcohol

Alcohol reduces hepatic glucose output but does not have a direct effect on insulin secretion or glucose disposal (Shai 2007). It is recommended that alcohol consumption be avoided or limited because of its potential to affect blood glucose and contribute to or mask hypoglycaemia (see Chapter 6). Sweet alcoholic drinks can lead to *hyper*glycaemia, whilst the alcohol itself leads to *hypo*glycaemia. The hypoglycaemic effect may depend on the nutritional state and glucose stores. Alcohol should *never* be consumed on an empty stomach.

Alcohol supplies considerable calories and provides little or no nutritional value. In addition, alcohol clouds judgement and can lead to inappropriate decision-making. Drunkenness can resemble hypoglycaemia and treatment of hypoglycaemia may be delayed. Appropriate education about hypoglycaemia risk with alcohol consumption is essential. Alcohol has a range of other physical effects, including liver cirrhosis, malnutrition, and peripheral neuropathy.

Although moderate amounts of alcohol may reduce cardiovascular risk, the current recommended intake still applies: in Australia two standard drinks per day for men and one standard drink per day for women. See also Chapter 10.

Exercise/activity

Exercise has an important role in controlling the blood glucose and increasing overall fitness. It should be combined with a suitable diet. Higher levels of sedentary behaviour are associated with 112% increased risk of developing diabetes, 147% increased risk of developing cardiovascular disease, and 49% risk of all-cause mortality (Wilmot et al. 2012). There is an association between occupational sitting and health outcomes, including diabetes, cardiovascular disease, and mortality (van Uffelen et al. 2010). However, although TV viewing is often cited as a risk factor for diabetes and other diseases, it is a poor measure of overall sedentary behaviour and may underestimate the true effect of overall sitting-related sedentary behaviour (Wilmot et al. 2012). However, people who watch a lot of TV often eat large quantities of energy-dense snacks that increase their risk of obesity and consequently obesity-related diseases. Thus, exercise programmes should include information about how to reduce occupational and TV-related sitting.

People commencing an exercise programme should first have a medical assessment. Structured aerobic and resistance training programmes improve blood glucose levels and lower HBA1c by about 0.6% and reduce cardiovascular risk in type 2 diabetes (Sigal et al., 2007). A 1% reduction was associated with 15–20% reduction in major macrovascular events and 37% reduction in microvascular events. In addition, exercise has mental health benefits, such as improved body image and feelings of self-worth (Goldfield et al. 2007).

Exercise capacity is an independent predictor of nonfatal cardiac events and mortality of patients referred for exercise treadmill testing (ETT) (Peterson et al. 2008). For example, low-exercise capacity is associated with increased risk of MI on ETT, but it is not clear whether limited exercise capacity indicates underlying cardiovascular disease or whether it is a marker of cardiovascular events.

Exercise can result in hypo- or hyperglycaemia. Under normal circumstances exercise stimulates hepatic glucose output and glucose utilisation to maintain glucose in the normal range. However, if exercise occurs in times of metabolic stress, the sympathetic drive can be stimulated, which leads to reduced glucose utilisation (van de Veure et al. 2006).

Before exercising, people should check their blood glucose levels. It is important to make a gradual start to the exercise. Strenuous activity can cause hypoglycaemia; extra carbohydrates may be needed.

Various strategies are suggested to help people begin and maintain an exercise/activity regimen. The beneficial effects of exercise are less evident if exercise is the sole focus of the intervention (Conn et al. 2007). Effective strategies include the following:

- Provide exercise education.
- Set achievable goals and focus on achieving one goal at a time.
- Providing individual supervision is as effective as group programmes and is more acceptable to some people.
- Suggest written 'exercise prescriptions' that take account of the individual's interests, gender, age, and capabilities.
- Wear a pedometer, especially when combined with a step goal diary. Reduction in BMI of $0.38\,kg/m^2$ and reductions in blood pressure by $3.8\,mmHg$ have been described (Bravata et al. 2007). A recent meta-analysis suggests that people lose an average of $0.05\,kg$ representing 2–3% of body weight over 12 months and continues if the individual continues to wear the pedometer (Richardson et al. 2008). People often hope to lose much more weight than this, so it is important that they realise even small weight loss is beneficial and to set reasonable goals. Steps walked increased from ~2000 to ~4000 per day on average in Richardson et al.'s meta-analysis. Pedometers provide feedback on the number of steps a person takes per day, but exercise duration, intensity, and frequency and the long-term benefits are unknown.
- Combine exercise with rehabilitation programmes.
- Tai chi, particularly in older people and those in wheelchairs, has a range of benefits, such as improved muscle strength, flexibility, balance and range of movement, lower risk of falls, improved cardiovascular fitness, and reduced cholesterol and abdominal fat. In addition, people have a younger vital age (ICCMR 2008); see Chapter 12. More recently, combination programmes such as LIFE that teach the principles of balance and lower limb strength training, have been shown to be beneficial, especially for older people (Clemson et al. 2012). Such programmes help reduce falls and improved functional capacity.

References

Adams, T., Walker, J., Litwin, S., and Pendelton, R. (2006). Two-year improvement in morbidity following gastric bypass surgery. NAASO: *The Obesity Society Annual Scientific Meeting*, Dallas, Texas. Abstract 16-0R October.

Allan, C. (2009). Testosterone reduces visceral fat gain in non-obese older men. *Journal of Clinical Endocrinology and Metabolism* 30: 139–146.

American Dietetic Association (ADA) (2004). Guidelines for the use of nutritive and non-nutritive sweeteners. *ADA* 104 (2): 255–275.

Australian Government Department of Health (2015). Australian Dietary Guidelines. https://www.eatforhealth.gov.au/guidelines/about-australian-dietary-guidelines.

Behan, K. and Mbizo, J. (2007). The relationship between waist circumference and biomarkers for disease in healthy non-obese women. *American Society for Clinical Pathology* 38 (7): 422–427.

Better Health Channel (2008). Better Health Channel Fact Sheet: Weight Loss – Common Myths. http://www.betterhealth.vic.gov.au/bhcv2/bhcarticles.nsf/pages/Weight_loss_common (accessed January 2008).

Bouchard, L., Drapeau, V., Provencher, V., and Lemieux, S. (2004). Neuromedin beta: a strong candidate gene linking eating behaviours and susceptibility to obesity. *American Journal of Clinical Nutrition* 80 (6): 1478–1486.

Brand-Miller, J., Hayne, S., petocz, P., and Coalgiuri, S. (2003). Low glycaemic index diet in the management of diabetes: a meta-analysis of randomized controlled trial. *Diabetes Care* 26 (8): 2261–2267.

Bravata, D., Smith-Sprangler, C., and Sundaram, V. (2007). Using pedometers to increase physical activity and health. A systematic review. *Journal of the American Medical Association* 298: 2296–2304.

Burdette, H. and Whitaker, R. (2005). A national study of neighbourhood safety, outdoor play, television viewing, and obesity in preschool children. *Pediatrics* **116** (3): 657–662.

Brunner, E. and McCarthy, N. (2001). Adult obesity depends on genes and environment. *BMJ* **323**: 52.

Carey, V., Bishop, L., and Charleston, J. (2005). Rationale and design of the optimal macronutrient intake heart (Omni-Heart) trial. *Clinical Trials* **2** (6): 529–537.

Carnethon, M., de Chaves, P., Biggs, M. et al. (2012). Association of weight status with mortality in adults with incident diabetes. *Journal of the American Medical Association* **308** (6): 581–590.

Caruso, M., Pekarovic, S., Raum, W., and Greenway, F. (2007). Topical treatments for fat reduction do they work? A best evidence review. *Diabetes Obesity and Metabolism* **9**: 300–303.

Chen, X. and Devaraj, S. (2018). Gut Microbiome in Obesity, Metabolic Syndrome, and Diabetes. *Current Diabetes Reports* **18**: 129. https://doi.org/10.1007/s11892-018-1104-3.

Clemson, L., Fiatarone, S.M., Bundy, A. et al. (2012). Integration of balance and strength training into daily life activity to reduce falls in older people (the LIFE study): randomized parallel trial. *British Medical Journal*: 345.

Conn, V.S., Hafdahl, A.R., Mehr, D.R. et al. (2007). Metabolic effects of interventions to increase exercise in adults with type 2 diabetes. *Diabetologia* **50** (5): 913–921. https://doi.org/10.1007/s00125-007-0625-0.

DAFNE Study Group (2002). Training in flexible, intensive insulin management to enable dietary freedom in people with Type 1 diabetes: dose adjustment for normal eating (DAFNE) randomized controlled trial. *British Medical Journal* **325**: 746.

Deutsch, L. (2007). Evaluation of the effect of Neptune krill oil on chronic inflammation and arthritis symptoms. *Journal of American College of Nutrition* **26** (1): 39–48.

Devaraj, S., Venkatachalam, A., and Chen, X. (2016). Metformin and the gut microbiome in diabetes. *Clinical Chemistry* **62**: 1554–1555.

Diehr, P., Bild, D., and Harris, T. (1998). Body mass index and mortality in non-smoking older adults. The cardio-vascular effects. *Journal of Public Health* **88**: 623–629.

Diehr, P., O'seara, E., Fitzpatrick, A., and Newman, A. (2008). Weight, mortality, years of healthy life and active life expectancy. *Journal American Geriatric Society* **56** (1): 76–83.

Dietitians Association of Australia (2009). Evidence based practice guidelines for the nutritional management of malnutrition in adult patients across the care continuum. *Nutrition and Dietetics* **66** (Supp): S4–S10.

Donohoe, M. (2008). Weighty matters: Public health aspects of the obesity epidemic. *Medscape Obstetrics and Gynaecology and Women's Health* (April 10). https://www.medscape.com/viewarticle/571139 (accessed September 2019).

Dunning, T. and Hoy, S. (1994). *What To Do Till the Dietitian Gets There*. Melbourne: Servier Australia.

Eddy, S. (2008). Omega-6 and 9 fatty acids. *Journal of Complementary Medicine* **7** (2): 34–39.

Egger, G. (2008). Helping patients lose weight: what works? [online]. *Australian Family Physician* **37** (1-2): 20–23.

Eisenberg, M.E., Neumark-Sztainer, D., and Story, M. (2003). Associations of weight-based teasing and emotional well-being among adolescents. *JAMA Pediatrics* **157** (8): 733–738. https://doi.org/10.1001/archpedi.157.8.733.

Elfhag, K. and Rössner, S. (2005). Who succeeds in maintaining weight loss? A conceptual review of factors associated with weight loss maintenance and weight regain. *Obesity Reviews* **6** (1): 67–85. https://doi.org/10.1111/j.1467-789X.2005.00170.x.

Elmore, J., Carney, P., and Abraham, L. (2004). The association between obesity and screening mammography accuracy. *Archives of Internal Medicine* **164**: 1140–1147.

Erlichman, J., Kerbey, A., and James, W. (2002). Physical activity and its impact on health outcomes. Paper 2: prevention of unhealthy weight gain and obesity by physical activity: An analysis of the evidence. *Obesity Review* **3**: 273–287.

Fabricatore, A.N. and Wadden, T.A. (2004). Psychological aspects of obesity. *Clinics in Dermatology* **22** (4): 332–337.

Feskanich, D., Rockett, H., and Colditz, G. (2004). Modifying the healthy eating index to assess diet quality in children and adolescents. *Journal of the American Dietetic Association* **104** (9): 1375–1383.

Frayling, T., Timpson, N., Weedon, M. et al. (2007). A common variant in the FTO gene is associated with Body Mass Index and predisposes to childhood and adult obesity. *Science* **316**: 889–894.

Fung, T. (2007). DASH-style diet may reduce risk of CHD and stroke. *American Heart Association Scientific Sessions*, Abstract 2369 (5 November).

Galuska, D., Will, J., Serdula, M., and Ford, E. (1999). Are health care professionals advising obese patients to lose weight? *Journal of the American Medical Association* **282**: 1576–1578.

Gardner, C., Kiazand, A., and Alhassan, S. (2007). Comparison of the Atkins, Zone, Ornish and LEARN diets for change in weight and related risk factors among overweight premenopausal women: the A to Z weight loss study: a randomized trial. *Journal of the American Medical Association* **297**: 969–977.

Goldfield, G., Mallory, R., Parker, T. et al. (2007). Effects of modifying physical activity and sedentary behaviour on psychosocial adjustment in overweight/obese children. *Journal of Pediatric Psychology* **32** (7): 783–793.

Goodman, E. and Whitaker, R. (2002). A prospective study of the role of depression in the development and persistence of adolescent obesity. *Pediatrics* **110**: 497–504.

Groesz, L.M., McCoy, S., Carl, J. et al. (2012). What is eating you? Stress and the drive to eat. *Appetite* **58** (2): 717–721.

Havel, P. (2007). Fructose but not glucose consumption linked to atherogenic lipid profile. *American Diabetes Association 67th Scientific Sessions*, Abstract 0062-0R (June).

Heiat, A., Vaccarino, V., and Krumholz, H.M. (2001). An evidence-based assessment of federal guidelines for overweight and obesity as they apply to elderly persons. *JAMA Internal Medicine* **161** (9): 1194–1203.

ICCMR (2008). International Council Complementary Medicine Research (29–31 March), Sydney.

Iqbal, O. (2007). Endocannabinoid system and pathophysiology of adipogenesis: Current management of obesity. *Personalised Medicine* **4** (3): 307–319.

James, D. and Coster, A. (2011). Identifying the enemy in the battle against diabetes and obesity. *Diabetes Management Journal* **37**: 68.

Jespersen, I. (2001). The effect of dietary oils on blood lipids and the risk of ischemic heart disease with special emphasis on olive oil. A literature review. *Ugeskr Laeger* **163** (35): 4736–4740.

Kapur, K. and Dunning, T. (2007). Global nutritional recommendations: a combination of evidence and food availability. *Practical Diabetes International* **24** (9): 1–8.

Kapur, K., Kupur, A., Ramachandran, S. et al. (2008). Barriers to changing dietary behaviour. *Journal of the Association of Physicians in India* **56**: 27–32.

Kondrup, J., Rasmussen, H., and Hamberg, O. (2003b). Nutritional risk screening (NRS 2002): a new method based on an analysis of controlled clinical trials. *Clinical Nutrition* **22**: 321–336.

Kondrup, S., Allison, S., Elia, M. et al. (2003a). EPSEN guidelines for nutrition screening 2002. *Clinical Nutrition* **22** (4): 415–421.

Lamberg, L. (2006). R$_x$ for obesity: eat less, exercise more, and – maybe get more sleep. *Journal of the American Medical Association* **295** (20): 2341–2344. http://www.medscape.com/viewarticle/566056 (

Latner, J. (2001). Staff help in the treatment of obesity. *Obesity Review* **2**: 87–97.

Malnutrition Advisory Group (MAG) (2000). *MAG – Guidelines for Detection and Management of Malnutrition*. Redditch, UK: British Association for Parenteral and Enteral Nutrition.

Marks, S. (2000). Obesity management. *Current Therapeutics* **41**: 6.

Marsh, K. (2008). Vegetarian diets and diabetes. *Diabetes Management Journal* **26**: 14–15.

Mendes-Soares, H., Raveh-Sadka, T., Azulay, P. et al. (2019). Assessment of a personalized approach to predicting post prandial glycaemic responses to food among individuals without diabetes. *JAMA Network Open* **2** (2): e188102. https://doi.org/10.1001/jamanetworkopen.2018.8102.

Middleton, M., Nazarenko, G., Nivison-Smith, I., and Smerdely, P. (2001). Prevalence of malnutrition and 12-month incidence of mortality in two Sydney teaching hospitals. *Medical Journal of Australia* **31**: 455–461.

Mitka, M. (2003). Surgery for obesity: demand soars amid scientific, ethical questions. *Journal of the American Medical Association* **289**: 1761–1762.

Miyashita, K. (2006). Brown seaweed may burn away brown fat. American Chemical Society. 232nd National Meeting and Exposition, San Francisco (10–14 September).

Moyad, M. (2004). Fad diets and obesity-Part 1: measuring weight in a clinical setting. *Urology Nurse* **24** (2): 114–119.

Muhlhauser, I. and Berger, M. (2002). Patient education – evaluation of a complex intervention. *Diabetologia* **45**: 1723–1733.

Nantel, J., Mathieu, M.E., and Prince, F. (2011). Physical activity and obesity: biomechanical and physiological key concepts. *Journal of Obesity* https://doi.org/10.1155/2011/650230.

National Health and Medical Research Council (NHMRC) (1999). *Diet for Older Australians*. Canberra: Commonwealth of Australia.

National Health and Medical Research Council (NHMRC) (2003). *Dietary Guidelines for Australian Adults*. NHMRC Ref. No. N29-N34.

National Health and Medical Research Council (NHMRC) (2006). Healthy eating Club Fact Sheets: fat & cholesterol. http://www.healthyeatingclub.org/info/articles/fats-chol/index.htm (accessed January 2008).

National Heart Foundation of Australia and the Cardiac Society of Australia and New Zealand (2012). *Reducing risk in heart disease: an expert guide to clinical practice for secondary prevention of coronary heart disease*. Melbourne: National Heart Foundation of Australia.

Peterson, P.N., Magid, D.J., and Ross, C. (2008). Association of exercise capacity on treadmill with future cardiac events in patients referred for exercise testing. *Archives of Internal Medicine* **168**: 174–179.

Pi-Sunyer, F. (2006). Use of lifestyle changes, treatment plans and drug therapy in controlling cardiovascular disease and obesity. *Obesity* **14** (Suppl. 3): 135S–142S.

Proietto, J., Aly, A., Barton, M. et al. (2012). Diabetes Australia position statement on bariatric surgery. *Diabetes Management Journal* **39**: 26–30.

Rahman, S., Morell, M., Topping, D. et al. (2007). Low glycaemic response cereals for enhanced human health. *International Diabetes Monitor* **19** (3): 21–25.

Rajilić-Stojanović, M. and de Vos, W.M. (2014). The first 1000 cultured species of the human gastrointestinal microbiota. *FEMS Microbiology Reviews* **38**: 996–1047. https://doi.org/10.1111/1574-6976.12075.

Reid, C. (2007). www.healthyfoodguide.com.au.

Reynolds, S., Yasuhukio, S., and Crimmins, E. (2005). The impact of obesity on active life expectancy in older Americans. *Gerontologist* **45**: 438–444.

Richardson, C., Newton, T., Abraham, J. et al. (2008). A meta-analysis of pedometerbased walking interventions and weight. *Annals of Family Medicine* **6** (1): 69–77.

Rizkalla, S. (2007). Fish oil supplements cut adiposity in Type 2 diabetes. *American Journal of Clinical Nutrition* **86**: 1670–1679.

Schauer, P., Kashyap, S., Wolski, K. et al. (2012). Bariatric surgery versus intensive medical treatment in obese patients with Type 2 diabetes. *New England Journal of Medicine* https://doi.org/10.1056/NEJMoa1200225.

Shorrock, I. and Hannah, J. (2011). Carbohydrate counting and insulin dose adjustment – group education for people with Type 2 diabetes. *Journal of Diabetes Nursing* **15** (6): 239.

Sigal, R.J., Kenny, G.P., Boulé, N.G. et al. (2007). Effects of aerobic training, resistance training, or both on glycemic control in type 2 diabetes: a randomized trial effects of aerobic and resistance training on glycemic control in type 2 diabetes. *Annals of Internal Medicine* **147** (6): 357–369. https://doi.org/10.7326/0003-4819-147-6-200709180-00005.

Smith-West, D. (2007). Motivational interviewing improves weight loss in women with Type 1 diabetes. *Diabetes Care* **30**: 1018–1087.

Spreadbury, I. (2012). Comparison with ancestral diets suggest dense acellular carbohydrates promote an inflammatory microbiota, and may be the primary dietary cause of leptin resistance and obesity. *Diabetes, Metabolic Syndrome and Obesity* **2012** (5): 175–189.

Stevens, J. (2000). Impact of age on associations between weight and mortality. *Nutrition Review* **58**: 129–137.

Stone, A. and Brownell, K. (1994). The stress eating paradox: multiple daily measurements in adult males and females. *Psychological Health* **9**: 425–436.

Sydney-Smith, M. (2000). Nutritional assessment in general practice. *Current Therapeutics* **41** (9): 13–24.

Tan, J.O., Hope, T., Stewart, A., and Fitzpatrick, R. (2006). Competence to make treatment decisions in anorexia nervosa: thinking processes and values. *Philosophy, Psychiatry, & Psychology* **13** (4): 267–282.

Tay, J., Brinkworth, G., and Noakes, M. (2008). Metabolic effects of weight loss on a very-low-carbohydrate diet compared with an isocaloric high-carbohydrate diet in abdominally obese subjects. *American Journal of Cardiology* **51**: 59–67.

Third Joint Taskforce of European and Other Societies on Cardiovascular Disease Prevention in Clinical Practice (2003). European guidelines on cardiovascular disease prevention in clinical practice. *European Journal of Cardiovascular Prevention Rehabilitation* **10** (Suppl. 1): S1–S78.

Truby, H. and Baic, S. (2006). Randomised controlled trial of four weight loss programmes in the UK: initial findings from the BBC "diet trials". *British Medical Journal* **332**: 1309–1314.

Unger, R. and Scherer, P. (2010). Gluttony, sloth and the metabolic syndrome: a roadmap to lipotoxicity. *Trends in Endocrinology and Metabolism* **216**: 345–352.

van de Veure, N., de Winter, O., Gir, M. et al. (2006). Fasting blood glucose levels are related to exercise capacity in patients with coronary artery disease. *American Heart Journal* **152** (3): 486–492.

van Gaal, L., Rissanen, A., and Scheen, A. (2005). RIO-Europe Study group. Effects of the cannabinoid-1 receptor blocker rimonabant on weight reduction and cardiovascular risk factors in overweight patients: 1-year experience from the RIO-Europe Study. *Lancet* **365**: 1389–1397.

van Uffelen, J., Wong, J., and Chau, J. (2010). Occupational sitting and health risks: a systematic review. *American Journal of Preventative Medicine* **39**: 379–388.

Vellas, B., Guigoz, Y., and Garry, P. (1999). The Mini Nutritional Assessment (MNA) and its use in grading nutritional state of elderly patients. *Nutrition* **15**: 116–122.

Williams, P. (2008). Asymmetric weight gain and loss from increasing and decreasing exercise. *Medicine Society for Sports Exercise* **40** (2): 296–302.

Wilmot, E., Edwardson, C., Achana, F. et al. (2012). Sedentary time in adults and the association with diabetes, cardiovascular disease and death: a systematic review and meta-analysis. *Diabetologia* https://doi.org/10.1007/s00125-012-2677-z.

World Health Organisation (WHO) (2002). *Reducing Risks, Promoting Healthy Life: World Health Report*. Geneva, Switzerland: WHO.

Yusuf, S., Hawken, S., Ôunpuu, S. et al. (2004). Effect of potentially modifiable risk factors associated with myocardial infarction in 52 countries (the INTERHEART study): case-control study. *The Lancet* **364** (9438): 937–952.

Zemel, M. (2003). Role of dietary calcium and diary products in modulating adiposity. *Lipids* **38**: 139–146.

Zoeller, R.F. (2007). Physical activity and obesity: Their interaction and implications for disease risk and the role of physical activity in healthy weight management. *American Journal of Lifestyle Medicine* **1** (6): 437–446. https://doi.org/10.1177/1559827607306889.

Further reading

Australian Government (1991). *Australian Dietary Guidelines*. Canberra: Australian Government Publications.

Barclay, A. (2012). Fructose. *Diabetes Management Journal* **39**: 1213.

Block, G. (1982). A review of validations of dietary assessment methods. *American Journal of Epidemiology* **115**: 492–505.

British Diabetic Association (1992). Dietary recommendations for people with diabetes. *Diabetic Medicine* **9**: 189–202.

Encinosa, W., Bernard, D., Steiner, C., and Chen, C. (2006). Healthcare utilization and outcomes after bariatric surgery. *Medical Care* **44**: 706–712.

Grontved, A. and Hu, F.B. (2011). Television viewing and risk of Type 2 diabetes, cardiovascular disease and all-cause mortality: a meta-analysis. *Journal of the American Medical Association* **305**: 2448–2455.

Jespersen, I. (2001). The effect of dietary oils on blood lipids and the risk of ischemic heart disease with special emphasis on olive oil. A literature review. *Ugeskr Laeger* **163** (35): 4736–4740.

Katan, W. (1990). Biochemical indicators of dietary intake. *European Journal of Clinical Nutrition* **52**: S5.

Keleman, L., Jacobs, D., and Cerham, J. (2005). Association of dietary protein with disease and mortality in a prospective study of postmenopausal women. *American Journal of Epidemiology* **161** (3): 239–249.

National Cholesterol Education Program (NCEP) Expert Panel on Detection, Evaluation and Treatment of High Blood Cholesterol in Adults (2002). (Adult Treatment Panel 111) Final Report. *Circulation* **106** (25): 3143–3421.

National Institutes of Health (NIH) Office of Dietary Supplements IBIDS database. http://grande.nal.usda.gov/index.php (accessed January 2008).

Tsai, A. and Wadden, T. (2005). Systematic review: an evaluation of major commercial weight loss programmes in the United States. *Annals of Internal Medicine* **142**: 56–66.

Weiss, E. (2007). Certain factors associated with weight regain after weight loss. American Journal of Preventative Medicine Online (5 June 2007). http://healthaffairs.org/blog/author/anneweiss (accessed December 2012).

Chapter 5

Medicine Management

All things are poison and nothing is without poison. Only the dose distinguishes the killer from the cure.

(Paracelsus circa 1493–1541)

Paracelsus' statement is still true. For example, insulin is a high-risk medicine. It is also an essential lifesaving medicine but it is associated with significant adverse effects, including death. Balancing the risk/benefit ratio is an essential aspect of prescribing and monitoring any medicine.

Key points

- Medicines should be managed within the principles of the quality use of medicines (QUM) and pharmacovigilance.
- Understanding the pharmacology of the different glucose-lowering medicines (GLM) and other medicines enables meals, activity, medicine administration times and the blood glucose monitoring regimen to be planned appropriately to suit the individual.
- Medicines are the cause of many preventable adverse events including death in people in hospital.
- Medicine-related outcomes need to be proactively monitored according to management target ranges, the indications for their use and the benefits and risks to the individual.
- Type 2 diabetes is a progressive disease of beta cell decline, and insulin will eventually be needed by >50% of people with type 2 diabetes.
- Polypharmacy is common in diabetes, especially type 2 and older people, and could be considered best practice, but it increases the risk of adverse events, including medicine interactions and the medicine self-care burden.
- Medicine-related nonadherence is common, complex, and multifactorial. It has its basis in patient and health professional-related issues as well as environmental and system-related issues.
- People with diabetes frequently use complementary medicines/therapies (CM), which needs to be considered when selecting diabetes management options. Some CM are safe, appropriate nonmedicine options.

Introduction

The main types of 'diabetes medicines' discussed in this chapter are listed below. Other medicines are described in the relevant chapters: likewise, the management target ranges for blood glucose, HbA1c, lipids, blood pressure, and weight are described in Chapter 1 and other relevant chapters.

(1) Oral glucose-lowering medicines (GLM)
(2) Insulin
(3) Other injectable GLMs
(4) Lipid lowering agents
(5) Cardiovascular agents
(6) Antiplatelet agents.

The authors prefer to use the term *medicines* rather than *drugs*, which is used to describe illegal drugs in this book. Medicines should be managed within a quality use of medicine framework (QUM), which is an holistic risk management approach that encompasses all types of medicines and recommends using non-medicine options first. The other key principle is pharmacovigilance to reduce the risk of adverse events and monitor medicine use appropriately to achieve optimal outcomes. People with diabetes also frequently use complementary medicines (CM), and these are discussed throughout the book but principally in Chapter 18. Medicines are also mentioned in other chapters throughout the book where relevant.

QUM

The information in this section was adapted from *The Quality Use of Medicines in Diabetes* (QUM) (2005), a paper developed by the Pharmaceutical Health and Rational use of Medicines (PHARM) Committee, a Committee of the Australian Commonwealth Department of Health and Ageing (DoHA). Figure 5.1 is reproduced with DoHA's permission. The Australian medicines system has been reviewed and revised since 2005 and PHARM no longer exists, but QUM is still central to medicines use and policies in Australia and many other countries. QUM also encompasses CM (Dunning 2005); see Chapter 18.

QUM aims to help health professionals and consumers make the best possible use of medicines if/when they are needed to improve their health outcomes. QUM recognises the central role of the consumer in medicines use and that many people maintain their health without using medicines, while for others medicines are important, even essential, to their health and well-being. It also recognises that medicines may be needed for prevention as well as treatment. QUM means:

- 'Selecting management options wisely;
- Choosing suitable medicines if a medicine is considered necessary;
- Using medicines safely and effectively', which includes monitoring the outcomes, dose adjustments, undertaking structured medicine reviews and de-prescribing when indicated (DoHA 2002).

Thus, QUM highlights health professionals' responsibility for safe, effective medicines use in addition to the need to consider patient adherence, which is influenced by health professionals' knowledge, attitudes, behaviours, and communication and teaching skills. People with diabetes' and health professionals' medicine-related beliefs and attitudes individually and collectively influence medicine use and outcomes.

QUM and diabetes

Medicines are central to effective diabetes management to control metabolic abnormalities and manage the complications of diabetes and other concomitant conditions. However, even when medicines are required, lifestyle factors, diet, exercise, and smoking cessation, are necessary to

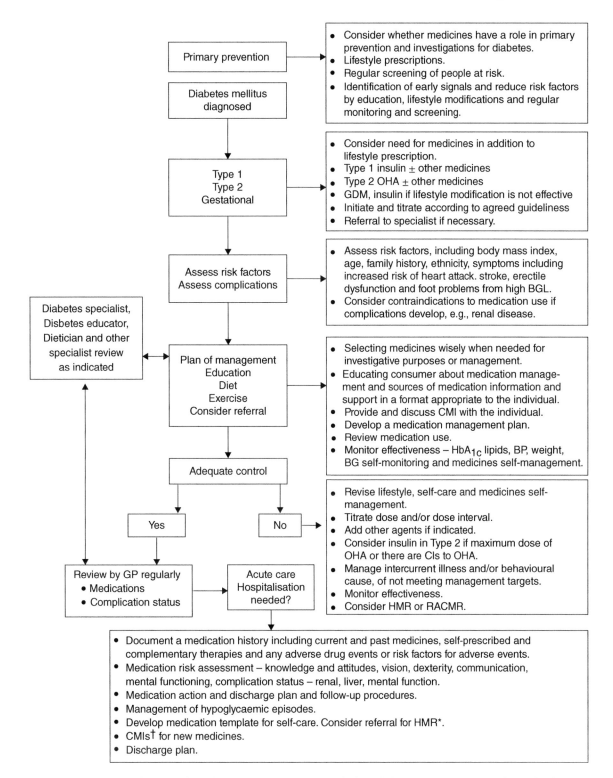

Figure 5.1 The Quality Use of Medicines (QUM) process applied to diabetes care reproduced from the QUM in Diabetes Pharmaceutical Health And Rational use of Medicines (PHARM) Committee, Commonwealth Department of Health and Ageing (2005). The medication regimen should be reviewed each time a new medicine is required, if an adverse event occurs, and at least annually as part of routine diabetes complication procedures (included with permission). *HMR = home medicines reviews, †CMI = consumer medicines information.

achieve optimal outcomes. Prevention programmes have a central, primary, and ongoing role (DoHA 2016-2020).

Medicines are used in four main areas in diabetes:

(1) *Primary prevention* focuses on lifestyle factors to prevent or delay the need for medicines in those at risk of diabetes and its complications. However, medicines may be needed for prevention, for example, lipid-lowering and antihypertensive medicines, and flu vaccine to prevent intercurrent illness in at-risk individuals.

(2) *Secondary prevention* where medicines are usually necessary to reduce the risk of diabetes complications, such as renal disease, atherosclerosis, and retinopathy.

(3) *Clinical care*, which involves using medicines to achieve optimal metabolic, psychological, and quality-of-life targets by appropriately selecting management options, including choosing suitable medicines if they are required, obtaining informed consent, enhancing informed decision-making by ensuring people have the information and skills needed to actively participate in medicine self-management, and monitoring the outcomes to ensure medicines are used safely and effectively. Educating the individual with diabetes and their carers and supporting them to manage their diabetes generally, and medicines in particular, are key aspects of QUM. Medicines prescribed for other conditions, self-initiated nonprescription medicines, and complementary and alternative medicine (CAM) use need to be considered as part of a holistic assessment and care plan. Significantly, polypharmacy is usually necessary to achieve optimal outcomes for/with people with diabetes and may be considered best practice. However, polypharmacy increases the complexity, risks, and costs of the management regimen. Therefore, as few medicines as possible should be used. Insulin and sometimes other medicines are needed at diagnosis in type 1 diabetes and for many people with type 2 and Latent Autoimmune Diabetes of Adults (LADA). Type 2 diabetes is a progressive disease and, consequently the medication regimen becomes progressively complex with increasing duration of the diabetes.

(4) *Clinical trials* commonly investigate new medicines and other interventions before they are licensed for use to ensure they are safe and efficacious, and to determine cost–benefit. Information from trials is also used to develop clinical practice guidelines, medicine prescribing algorithms, and consumer and health professional information. Health professionals are often asked to help recruit participants for clinical trials. The fact that an individual is participating in a clinical trial should be clearly documented in the person's medical record.

QUM is a useful framework for reducing polypharmacy and duplicate prescribing and for de-prescribing because it encompasses prevention using nonmedicine options, regular medication reviews, and effective communication among health professionals and with people with diabetes (National Prescribing Service (NPS) 2001).

Medicines are selected taking into account:

• The individual's social, physical, and mental health status.
• Whether suitable nonmedicine option/s are available.
• The risks and benefits of using medicines for the individual, including health literacy, functional and cognitive ability, and support available.
• Dosage, dose interval, and duration of treatment.
• Other medicines, CM, and therapies that the individual might be using or considering.
• The process required to monitor the outcomes of medicine use, including adverse events, medication self-management and other relevant self-care such as blood glucose monitoring, processes for communicating the medication plan among the relevant health professionals when the individual makes transitions among health providers and services, and strategies for regularly reviewing the continued benefits and risks of the medication regimen and the individual's self-care capacity.
• The costs to the individual, the community, and the health system. A process for integrating QUM into existing care is shown in Figure 5.1.

GLM

Different GLMs target the various underlying abnormalities of glucose homeostasis in T2DM (Chapter 1). People with T1DM require insulin. T2DM is a progressive disease of beta cell decline; thus, the medication regimen needs to be constantly monitored and adjusted and medicines included or de-prescribed as necessary. The United Kingdom Prospective Diabetes Study (UKPDS) study (Turner et al. 1999) showed monotherapy was ineffective in 75% of people with T2DM. Importantly, appropriate diet and activity/exercise regimen are essential, even when medicines are required.

Sulphonylureas were the first GLMs to become available in the 1940s. The Biguanides followed in the 1950s. The value of these medicines has been established, and they have been consistently improved over time with new generations of the original medicines. In addition, new classes of GLMs have been introduced, some of which might extend the life of the remaining beta cells and delay the need for insulin in T2DM (Dornhorst 2001) Some, such as the SGLT-2 inhibitors, also have additional cardiovascular and other benefits (Abe et al. 2018).

GLMs target the different underlying abnormalities of glucose homeostasis associated with T2DM. These GLMs are:

- Biguanides, which reduce hepatic glucose production and might improve peripheral glucose disposal and promote weight loss. It activates the energy regulating enzyme AMP-kinase in liver and muscle. Metformin is the medicine of first choice in overweight people with type 2 diabetes (United Kingdom Prospective Diabetes Study (UKPDS 33) 1998). Biguanides are insulin sensitisers.
- Sulphonylureas and Glitinides are insulin secretagogues that stimulate insulin release from the beta cells. Therefore, the beta cells must be capable of responding by producing insulin. First-generation sulphonylureas such as chlorpropramide and tolbutamide are now rarely used in many countries and have been removed from the market in others. Secretagogues might be first-line treatment in people who are not overweight or who have contraindications to metformin.
- Meglitinides, which act on the same beta cell receptor as the sulphonylureas but are chemically different.
- Thiazolidinediones (TZD), which increase whole-body sensitivity to insulins by activation of nuclear receptors and prompting esterifiation and storage of free fatty acids in subcutaneous fat tissue. They reduce daytime preprandial hyperglycaemia, and have some effect on the fasting blood glucose. The two main TZDs are Rosiglitazone and Pioglitazone. The latter can be added to metformin and sulphonylureas or substituted for these medicines if the individual is intolerant of them.
- Alpha-glucosidase inhibitors, which slow carbohydrate digestion and glucose absorption from the gut by inhibiting alpha-glucosidases in the brush border of the small intestine. Alpha-glucosidases are essential to the release of glucose from complex carbohydrates. Alpha-glucosidases reduce postprandial glucose levels.
- Dipeptidyl peptidase-4 inhibitors (DPP-4), which inhibit the activity of DPP-4, an enzyme that prolongs the activity of endogenous glucagon like peptide 1 (GLP-1).
- GLP-1 agonists; GLP-1 is an incretin hormone secreted in the gut in response to food. GLP-1 amplifies insulin secretion from the beta cells and inhibits inappropriate glucagon secretion. GLP-1 also slows gastric emptying, which slows postprandial food absorption and helps control postprandial blood glucose, reducing appetite. GLP-1 agonists mimic the activity of endogenous GLP-1 but are more resistant to being broken down by DDP-4, which prolongs their action.
- Sodium-glucose cotransporter-2 inhibitors (SGLT-2) act independently of insulin secretion or action and target glucose reabsorption in the kidney and induce glycosuria (Whaley et al. 2012). They reduce blood glucose proportional to the ambient blood glucose and glomerular filtration of glucose from the blood. Glucose lowering is greater in people with 'poor' blood glucose control than those with 'good control (Abe et al. 2018; Hwang et al. 2019). SGLT-2

are less effective in people with eGFR <60 ml/min/1.73m² and not significant <30 ml/min/1.73m² (Cherney et al. 2018). They often induce weight loss but can contribute to urinary incontinence in people with or at risk of incontinence. Various insulin preparations are available. Insulin can be used alone or in combination with metformin and some other GLMs. Metformin and sometimes sulphonylureas are continued when insulin is initiated in people with type 2 diabetes, but the risk of hypoglycaemia must be considered when insulin and suphonylureas are combined (NICE 2017; Davies et al. 2018); American Diabetes Association 2019).

The commonly available GLM are described in Table 5.1.

Blood glucose and HbA1c monitoring are essential to assess whether, when, and which GLM should be commenced, decide doses and the dose frequency and when insulin is required. When GLMs are commenced it is necessary to monitor the blood glucose in order to appropriately adjust the dose and dose interval. However, the other factors that affect blood glucose and HbA1c must be considered. Normal endogenous insulin secretion consists of two components:

(1) Basal secretion, a constant low secretion rate to suppress hepatic glucose production between meals and overnight (fasting).
(2) Bolus secretion, which occurs in response to increasing glucose levels after meals (postprandial). These insulin bolus doses also consist of two phases. The first phase is an initial high spike, which is lost early in the development of T2DM. The second is a lower, more prolonged phase. Insulin release is influenced by the incretins DPP-4 and GLP-1.

The different classes of GLMs, including insulin, target the different components of glucose homeostasis. Monitoring blood glucose is a key to determining medicine effectiveness. HbA1c only provides an overall average blood glucose level and does not account for glucose variability, which influences complication risk (see Chapters 3 and 8). Thus, both measures provide important information as part of the total situation. Key blood glucose testing times are:

(1) Before breakfast to assess the fasting blood glucose, an indicator of overnight hepatic glucose output. High blood glucose can indicate nocturnal hypoglycaemia OR inadequate insulin doses the previous evening.
(2) Postprandial, usually two hours after food, to assess glucose disposal. Postprandial hyperglycaemia is common in T2DM because of the loss of first-phase insulin response early in the course of the disease. It is also associated with increased risk of cardiovascular disease.

Sometimes monitoring pre- and postprandial blood glucose is required and sometimes overnight (2–3 a.m.) is used to detect nocturnal hypoglycaemia; see Chapter 6.

Biguanides

Biguanides are still the medicine of first choice for overweight people with type 2 diabetics when the HbA1c is >7%. Metformin effectively lowers all-cause mortality and diabetes complications among overweight people with diabetes (UKPDS 1998). It is also used to manage insulin resistance associated with PCOS, where it may delay the progression to type 2. Metformin is the most commonly used biguanide. It acts by:

- impairing the absorption of glucose from the gut;
- inhibiting hepatic glucose output;
- increasing glucose uptake in peripheral tissues (muscle and fat);
- increasing the effects of insulin at receptor sites;
- suppressing the appetite (mild effect) (Minamii et al. 2018).

Table 5.1 Glucose lowering medicine classes, dose range and dose frequency, possible side effects, the duration of action and main site of metabolism.

Medicine	Usual daily dose	Frequency	Possible side effects	Duration of action (DA)	Site of metabolism
Sulphonylureas: these are sulphonamides, urea derivatives that close K ATP channels on beta cell plasma membranes and increase insulin secretion.	Depends on the specific medicine. Often used with other GLMs that address other changes in glucose homeostasis.		Hypoglycaemia is the most significant side effect. Doses need to be adjusted for renal disease. Some blunt myocardial ischaemic preconditioning. Weight gain.		Increase insulin secretion
Reduce HbA1c by 1–2% when used as monotherapy.					
Glibenclamide					
Daonil 5 mg	2.5–20 mg	Up to 10 mg as a single dose	Side effects rarely encountered include: Nausea, anorexia, skin rashes. Severe hypoglycaemia, especially in elderly and those with renal dysfunction.	DA: 6–12 h Peak: 6–8 h	Liver
Euglucon 5 mg Glimel 5 mg		>10 mg in divided doses Taken with, or immediately before food			
Glipizide					
Minidiab 5 mg	2.6–40 mg	Up to 15 mg as a single dose >15 mg in a twice daily dosage Taken immediately before meals	GIT disturbances Skin reactions Hypoglycaemia (rare).	DA: Up to 24 h Peak: 1–3 h	Liver
Gliclazide					
Diamicron MR (a sustained release preparation)	30–120 mg Dose increments should be two weeks apart. Should not be crushed.	Daily	Hypoglycaemia	Released over 24 hours	Liver
Glimepiride (Amaryl)					

(Continued)

Table 5.1 (Continued)

Medicine	Usual daily dose	Frequency	Possible side effects	Duration of action (DA)	Site of metabolism
(2) *Biguanides activate Amp-kinase and reduce hepatic glucose production.* Reduce HbA1c by 1–2% when used as monotherapy.	1–4 mg	2–3 per day	Gastrointestinal disturbances, especially when first commenced. Long-term use contributes to vitamin B_{12} deficiency. Dose adjustments are required in stage 3 renal disease: eGFR 30-44 ml/min $(1.73 m)^2$.	DA: 5–8h	Liver
Metformin Diaformin 500 mg Diabex 500 mg Glucophage 500 mg	0.5–1.5 g May be increased to 3–0 g	1–3 times/day Taken with or immediately after food	GIT disturbances Lactic acidosis Hypoglycaemia with other GLMs	DA: 5–6h	Suppresses gluconeogenesis in the liver and affects glucose handling in the colon. It inhibits mitochondrial respiratory complex 1, which increases cellular AMP, which activates ATP and ultimately has various effects on energy metabolism. Including down regulating glyconeogenic genes. Secreted unchanged in urine.
Combination sulphonylurea and biguanide Glucovance (G): Metformin (M) and Glibenclamide (G): M 250 mg G 1.25 mg M 500 mg, G 2.5 mg M 500 mg G 5 mg Combination Metformin and Rosiglitazone (TZD) e.g. Avandamet in various dose combinations. Combination Metformin and Sitagliptin (DPP-4) e.g. Janumet in various dose combinations.			Hypoglycaemia, especially in older people. Side effects associated with each medicine.		Liver
(3) *Meglitinides close K-ATP channels on beta cell plasma membranes and increase insulin secretion.* Repaglinide Nataglitinide	0.5–16 mg	2–3 per day	Hypoglycaemia with other OHAs Weight gain GIT disturbance		Liver

	Dose	Frequency	Side effects		
(4) *Thiazolidinediones activate the nuclear transcription factor peroxisome-proliferator-activated receptor (PPAR-γ) and increase insulin sensitivity* Reduce HbA1c by 0.5–1.4% Rosiglitazone: 4, 8 mg Pioglitazone: 15, 30, 45 mg.	4–8 mg	Daily	Oedema, weight gain, congestive heart failure Raised liver enzymes, Bone loss and osteoporotic hip and non-vertebral fractures Rosiglitazone increases LDL-C Pioglitazone has been linked to bladder cancer. Might contribute to macularoedema. Rosiglitazone: pregnancy risk in women with polycystic ovarian disease, increased LDL-C and MI risk Pioglitazone: might increase bladder cancer risk	DA: 24 h	Liver
(5) *Alpha-glucosidase inhibitors* Acarbose: 50, 100 mg Reduce HbA1c by 0.5–0.8%	50–100 mg Reduce post prandial blood glucose	TDS with food	GIT problems, for example, flatulence, diarrhoea Hypoglycaemia Dose adjustment in renal disease		Faeces and urine
(6) *DPP-4 inhibitors increase postprandial GLP concentration, which increases insulin secretion and reduces glucagon secretion.* Reduce HbA1c 0.5–0.8% Sitagliptin Vildagliptin Saxagliptin Linagliptin Alogliptin	100 mg per day in BD regimen in combination with other GLMs when indicated. Moderate renal failure 50 mg Saxagliptin has been associated with heart failure and hospital admissions. Severe renal disease 25 mg	With or without food	Low risk of hypoglycaemia – reduce dose of sulphonylurea if used as dual therapy to reduce hypoglycaemia risk associated with sulphonylureas Dose adjustment for renal disease deepening on the particular medicine.		Most can be used in people with renal disease, except saxagliptin, which is not recommended in end-stage renal disease. Secreted unchanged in urine.
DPP-4 combination medicines Janumet and metformin	Daily dose				

(Continued)

Table 5.1 (Continued)

Medicine	Usual daily dose	Frequency	Possible side effects	Duration of action (DA)	Site of metabolism
(7) GLP-1 receptor agonists Reduce HbA1c by 0.5–1% Short acting: Exenatide, Lixisenatide Longer acting Liraglutide Dulaglutide Semaglutide Byetta Glucose-dependent insulin secretion, reduce glucagon and enhance satiety. Short acting medicines slow gastric emptying and reduce postprandial glucose rise.	Once to three times per day depending on the medicine: Lixisenatide is administered daily Exanatide extended release can be administered one/ week.		Flatulence and abdominal bloating. Dose adjustments required in renal disease. May cause gall bladder disease. May increase heart rate. Rare acute pancreatitis.		
Sodium-glucose cotransporter-2 inhibitors (SGLT-2) Reduce HbA1c by 0.6–0.9% Dapagliflozin Canagliflozin Empagliflozin	Reduces weight and blood pressure.		Increased incidence of urinary tract and genital infections, including vaginal candidiasis. Possibility of polyuria in volume sensitive people and volume depletion. Increase LDL-C. Canagliflozin has been associated with amputations, fracture risk and DKA (euglycaemic DKA). Dose adjustment required for renal disease.		Enhance urinary glucose excretion in the kidney. Some also have antihypertensive effects and cardiovascular benefits. Stop three days prior to surgery; may need to stop during acute illness because of the risk of euglycaemic DKA.
SGLT_2 combination medicines Saxagliptin 10 mg and Metformin 500 mg (Xigduo) XR, Saxagliptin 5 mg and metformin (Kombiglyze) XR metformin dose can be 500, 1000, or 2000 mgs.					

Note: Only some of the many trade named formulations are listed. Formulations in each class have similar actions, although there are minor differences among them. The table is a guide only. Specific prescribing information for each medicine should be consulted as well as relevant regulatory authority licensing and approvals. Combination medicines such as Glucovance (Metformin and Glibenclamide) may be useful in reducing the medicine burden (overall number of medicines an individual needs to take).

Note: Information is based on pharmaceutical company prescribing information as well as the Nice (2017), Australian Medicines Handbook (2018), Therapeutic Guidelines: Diabetes (2019) and Joint Formulary Committee (2018), ADA (2019). There are many brand names for the main classes of glucose-lowering medicines (GLMs) and their availability and the brand names differ among countries not all the GLM brands or generic GLMs are shown in the table. Insulin is described separately.

Practice points

(1) Biguanides do not stimulate the production or release of insulin, and therefore are unlikely to cause hypoglycaemia.
(2) They have favourable effects on the lipid profile and slow glucose absorption from the intestine.
(3) They do not stimulate the appetite and are unlikely to cause weight gain.
(4) They have similar effects on HbA1c as sulphonylureas (Table 5.1).
(5) The gut microbiome may play a role in enhancing or inhibiting medicine effectiveness. Many orally administered medicines are processed by intestinal microbial enzymes before they are absorbed into the blood stream. They also metabolise nondigestible fibre and play a role in metabolism. Thus, the gut microbiome influences medicine metabolism (Wang et al. 2018).

Possible side effects

(1) Nausea and/or diarrhoea occur in 10–15% of patients. Most patients tolerate biguanides if they are started at a low dose, the tablets are taken with or immediately after food, and the dosage is increased gradually.
  • Lactic acidosis is the most significant side effect, but it is rare and could be prevented by appropriate assessment, monitoring, and prescribing; see Chapter 7. It occurs in at-risk people during acute infections, acute kidney injury, and decompensated heart failure, which are independently associated with lactic acidosis (Iedema and Russell 2011). Although lactic acidosis is rare, 48 cases were reported to the Australian Adverse Drug Reactions Advisory Committee (ADRAC) between 1985 and 2001. Of these, known risk factors were present in 35 of the 48 cases (Jerrall 2002). Salpeter et al. (2006) found no cases of lactic acidosis in a systematic review of comparative trials and cohort studies ($n = 59\,320$ patient years of metformin use). Salpeter et al. estimated the upper limit of true incidence of lactic acidosis per 100 000 patient years was 5.1 in people using metformin, and there was no difference in lactate levels for metformin compared with non-metformin therapies. However, the true clinical incidence is unknown and could be higher because not all adverse events are reported. Nisbet et al. (2004) identified 13 cases of lactic acidosis possibly related to metformin since 2000. Of these, two died, three required dialysis for renal failure, and one had severe neuro-logical deficits and required nursing home care. The average age was 67 and average serum creatinine was 0.31 mmol/l (normal 0.05–0.11 women; 0.06–0.12 men mmol/l). Nisbet et al.'s study highlighted the importance of appropriate clinical assessment before prescribing or represcribing medicines, especially in older people. The risk of lactic acidosis is increased in people with diseases likely to cause hypoxia, such as alcohol abuse and liver, renal, and cardiac disease. However, Ekstrom et al. (2012) found a reduced risk of all-cause mortality in an observational study of people on metformin monotherapy with eGFR 45–60 ml/min/1.73 squared and no increased risk of all-cause mortality, acidosis, serious infection, or cardiovascular disease in people with eGFR 30–45 ml/min/1.73 squared ($n = 51\,675$). The authors concluded the benefits of metformin outweigh the risks. Early signs of lactic acidosis include:
    ○ Anorexia
    ○ Nausea and vomiting
    ○ Abdominal pain
    ○ Cramps
    ○ Weight loss
    ○ Lethargy
    ○ Respiratory distress

(2) Biguanides should not be prescribed under these conditions:
- Pregnancy
- Chronic renal failure
- Type 1 diabetes
- Any disease likely to cause hypoxia, such as severe respiratory diseases and hepatic or cardiovascular disease

There is some evidence that at higher doses and longer duration of use, metformin inhibits absorption of vitamin B_{12}. The metformin dose is the strongest predictor of vitamin B_{12} deficiency (Ting et al. 2006). However, Ting and colleagues did not assess calcium intake or measure vitamin B_{12} metabolites (homocysteine and methylmalonic acid), which could have affected the results. Nevertheless, vitamin B_{12} deficiency should be considered in people at high risk of malnourishment, such as older people and those with eating disorders, people who have been on metformin for long periods of time especially at high doses, and those with malabsorption syndromes such as coeliac disease.

Biguanides should be ceased for two days before intravenous pyelogram (IVP), computerized axial tomography (CAT) scans and investigations that require IV-iodinated contrast media to be used (Calabrese et al. 2002).

Sulphonylureas

Sulphonylureas can be used alone or combined with metformin. They can be used as first-line therapy in nonobese people who are intolerant of, or have contraindications to, metformin (Scottish Intercollegiate Guideline Network (SIGN) 2010). They are usually well tolerated, but there is a tendency for people to gain weight, especially with older sulphonylureas, although these are rarely used nowadays. Weight gain occurs to a less extent with newer sulphonylureas (Inzucchi 2002). They generally have a rapid onset of action except for long-acting formulations. Hypoglycaemia is a risk, especially in older people on long-acting agents, although these are rarely used and are no longer available in some countries. However, glibenclamide is available in combination with metformin (Glucovance). People with renal impairment and those who are malnourished are also at risk of hypoglycaemia.

Sulphonylureas act in the following ways:

- Stimulate insulin secretion from the pancreatic beta cells.
- Increase the effects of insulin at its receptor sites.
- Sensitise hepatic glucose production to inhibition by insulin.

Possible Side Effects
(1) Hypoglycaemia may result due to oversecretion of insulin if the dose of the medicine is increased, food is delayed, meals are missed, or activity is increased; see Chapter 6.
(2) Liver dysfunction.
(3) Nausea, vomiting.
(4) Various skin rashes.
(5) Increased appetite.
(6) Rarely, agranulocytosis and red cell aplasia can occur.

Note: Points 2–6 are very uncommon. Sulphonylureas are contraindicated in pregnancy, although they are used during pregnancy in some countries. They are mostly metabolised in the liver so severe liver disease is a contraindication to their use. Caution should be taken in people who are allergic to sulphur medicines because the sulphonylureas have a similar chemical makeup.

Meglitinides

These medicines increase insulin secretion at mealtimes and they should only be taken with meals, usually two to three times per day. They have the same effect on the beta cell receptor but a different chemical structure. They are short acting and have a low hypoglycaemic risk, but hypoglycaemia is possible. They have not been assessed for beneficial effects on reducing micro- and macrovascular disease and are generally more expensive than other GLMs (SIGN 2010).

Meglitinides target early phase insulin secretion, which is essential for postprandial glucose and control the postprandial glucose load (Dornhorst 2001). In this way, they initiate an insulin response pattern close to normal. They can be used in combination with biguanides and possibly TZD. The two main formulations are repaglinide and nataglinide. These medicines are rarely used in Australia because they are not listed on the Pharmaceutical Benefits Scheme (PBS). However, because of their short duration of action and the requirement to take them with meals, they could be very useful in older people at high risk of hypoglycaemia.

Thiazolidinediones (TZD)

The TZD are also known as peroxisome-proliferator-activated receptor (PPAR-γ). TZDs lower fasting and postprandial blood glucose by increasing insulin sensitivity in muscle, fat, and liver cells. Some improve lipid profiles, enhance insulin sensitivity and may restore the beta cell mass. They are given as a daily dose. It takes several days before they show an effect.

There are two forms: pioglitazone and rosiglitazone. Pioglitazone can be used as dual therapy in combination with metformin OR a sulphonylurea in type 2 diabetes when the HbA1c is >7% when combining metformin and a sulphonylurea is contraindicated. Pioglitazone can be combined with insulin in type 2 diabetes if the HbA1c is >7% despite treatment with OHAs and insulin, OR insulin alone OR if metformin is contraindicated. Rosiglitazone can be combined with metformin AND a sulphonylurea in type 2 diabetes when the HbA1c is >7% despite maximum tolerated doses of these medicines.

TZDs reduce HbA1c by ~1–2% (Ko et al. 2006) with similar improvements to adding insulin. If adding a TZD does not adequately reduce HbA1c to <8 5% in three months, insulin should be commenced (Nathan and Buse 2006). It is usual to start at a low dose and monitor the person closely for signs of heart failure, especially those with preexisting cardiovascular disease. Significant cardiovascular disease is a contraindication to TZDs.

Rosiglitazone might prevent or delay the transition to type 2 diabetes in at-risk individuals (DREAM (Diabetes Reduction Assessment with Ramipril and Rosiglitazone Medication Investigators) 2006). However, subsequent modelling of the Diabetes Reduction Assessment with Ramipril and Rosiglitazone Medication (DREAM) data suggests that people taking rosiglitazone to prevent diabetes would end up taking more medicines than those who start medicines after diabetes is diagnosed and are at risk of TZD side effects (Montori and Isley 2007). SIGN (2010) stated that there is no convincing evidence that rosiglitazone as monotherapy has benefits over metformin and sulphonylureas.

Pioglitazone is associated with the risk of bladder cancer in people who use the medicine for over 12 months (Lewis et al. 2011). The risk is greater in people with bladder cancer or a history of bladder cancer. People should be advised of the risk when discussing their medicine options. Pharmaceutical companies have revised their product information to reflect the risk.

Possible side effects
- Localised oedema, which can be significant and may occur to a greater extent in people treated with TZD and insulin (SIGN 2010).
- Congestive cardiac failure and heart failure. People with diabetes are 2.5 times more likely to develop heart failure than nondiabetics (Nichols et al. 2001) and TZDs increase the risk of heart failure. Rosiglitazone doubles the risk among those with preexisting cardiovascular disease (Home et al. 2009). Both TZDs are contraindicated in people with New York Heart Association

Class III or IV heart failure. The person should be closely monitored for signs of heart failure such as oedema and rapid weight gain, and importantly, informed about these risks.

- Myocardial infarction and death associated with rosiglitazone (Nissen and Wolski 2007). This report caused significant debate among diabetes experts and stress for patients prescribed Rosiglitazone. The risk appears to be small (DREAM 2006). The information should be used in the context of individual risk. For example, rosiglitazone might increase the risk of MI in people with ischaemic heart disease, those on insulin or nitrates, those with an atherogenic lipid profile, and those at high risk of MI (ADRAC 2007). Pioglitazone does not appear to carry the same risk because it has fewer adverse effects on lipids (Dormandy et al. 2005). The RECORD study Home et al. 2005, 2009) suggested that there is a possible increase in cardiovascular events with rosiglitazone in people with existing heart disease, but the association was not statistically significant. The European Medicines Agency (EMA) (2005, 2010) reviewed all medicines containing rosiglitazone and concluded the risks of rosiglitazone outweigh the benefits and recommended marketing authorisation for all products containing rosiglitazone be suspended across the European Union (http://bit.ly/ Rosi 2011; Blind et al. 2011). Likewise, the US Federal Drug Administration (FDA) added information about the cardiovascular risks of rosiglitizone to the physician labelling and medication guide (FDA (US Federal Drug Administration) 2011).
- Reduced red and white cell count.
- Weight gain, especially deposition of subcutaneous fat, while visceral obesity is reduced. Weight gain appears to continue as long as TZDs are continued. Gains between 2 and 5 kg are reported (Dormandy et al. 2005). However, insulin also causes weight gain (~3 kg), as do sulphonylureas (~4 kg). Weight gain is lower when patients are taking metformin before a TZD is added (Strowig et al. 2004).
- Hypercholesterolaemia, especially LDL-C (rosiglitazone).
- Liver damage, although it is uncommon. TZDs are contraindicated if liver disease is present or serum transiminase is >2.5 times the upper limit of the normal. Liver function tests should be performed before starting a TZD and then monitored regularly while the patient remains on TZDs. Signs of liver toxicity include nausea, vomiting, jaundice, dark urine, and right upper abdominal discomfort.
- Macular oedema (European Medicines Agency, 2010). Macular oedema is a known complication of diabetes, and there some reports the condition worsens with TZD.
- Fractures occurring in the arms and lower leg, usually in women (Meier et al. 2008); however, the risk is small. Fracture risk may be significant in older women at risk of osteoporosis and increase the risk of falls if the fractures occur in the feet or legs. People prescribed TZD, especially women, should be informed about the risk.
- Women with polycystic ovarian disease should be counselled about contraception because TZDs may improve fertility in these women.
- They are contraindicated in pregnancy and during breast feeding.
- Care should be taken in lactose intolerant people because TZDs contain a small amount of lactose.
- Hypoglycaemia is possible because TZDs reduce insulin resistance and enhance the effectiveness of endogenous insulin.

These data suggest a thorough assessment, including a medication review, is warranted before commencing TZDs. Health professionals and people with diabetes should be alert to the possibility of silent MI.

Alpha-glucosidase inhibitors

These medicines are usually taken in a TDS regimen.

They act by slowing glucose uptake of many carbohydrates by inhibiting alpha-glucosidase, which slows the metabolism of complex and simple carbohydrates in the brush border of the proximal small intestine so glucose absorption is spread over a longer time frame. Alpha-glucosidase inhibitors reduce fasting and postprandial glucose (Rosak and Mertes 2012).

Their major side effects are due to the arrival of undigested carbohydrate in the lower bowel – bloating, flatulence, and diarrhoea. These symptoms can be distressing and embarrassing, and people often stop their medications because of these side effects. Taking the medicines with meals, starting with a low dose and increasing slowly to tolerance levels, and careful explanation to the patient can reduce these problems.

Hypoglycaemia is possible if alpha-glucosidase inhibitors are combined with other GLMs. They may be contraindicated or need to be used with caution in people with gastrointestinal disease such as gastroparesis, coeliac disease, and irritable bowel syndrome.

Practice point

Oral glucose may not be an effective treatment for hypoglycaemia occurring in people on alpha-glucosidase inhibitors because absorption from the gut can be delayed. IM Glucagon is an alternative.

The incretin hormones

The incretins enhance glucose-mediated insulin secretion by the beta cells. Approximately 60% of insulin secreted in response to food is due to the activity of incretins. The incretin effect is due to peptide hormones released by K and L cells in the intestine directly into the blood stream. The incretins include:

(1) Glucose-dependent insulinotropic peptide (GIP) secreted by the K-intestinal cells. Postprandially, GIP levels are about 10 times higher than GLP-1 and have similar insulinotrophic actions when the glucose level is >6 mmol/l, but its effects are limited at blood glucose levels >7.8 mmol/l. GIP does not inhibit glucagon secretion.

(2) Glucagon-like peptide (GLP-1) is secreted by the L-cells in the intestine. It primarily regulates postprandial glucose by slowing gastric emptying and reducing glucagon. It reduces appetite and may induce weight loss (SIGN 2010), and it may stimulate beta cell proliferation (Abraham et al. 2002). GLP-1 binds to its specific receptor but has a very short half-life (60–90 seconds) because it is rapidly broken down by DPP-4. Exanetide, liragulitide, and lixisenatide are GLP-1 receptor agonist analogues and may improve metabolic control in people with BMI >30 kg/m squared with type 2 diabetes. Lixisenatide is administered daily. GLP-1 agonists may not be beneficial in people with inadequate glycaemic control for >10 years: insulin may be the medicine of choice in these people (SIGN 2010). Bydureon (Exanetide) can be given using a disposable pen weekly.

(3) DPP-4 inhibitor analogues are oral GLMs such as sitagliptin, vildagliptin, and saxagliptin that inhibit the action of DDP-4 and consequently increase postprandial GLP concentration, which increases insulin secretion, reduces glucose-dependent glucagon secretion and reduces HbA1c 0.5–0.8% (Nathan and Buse 2006; Richter et al. 2008; Inzucchi et al. 2012; Vashisht et al. 2018). DPP-4 are listed in most countries as add-on therapy with metformin or a sulphonylurea where a combination of the latter two medicines is contraindicated and particular prescribing recommendations may apply in particular countries (NICE 2008; NPS 2012; SIGN 2019). Recently, The European Commission approved the combination of metformin and linagliptin, a DPP-4 inhibitor.

Possible side effects
- Side effects include nasopharyngitis and upper respiratory tract infections and hypersensitivity reactions.
- Pancreatitis has been reported with Sitagliptin and Vildagliptin (DeVries and Rosenstock 2017).
- Vildagliptin and saxagliptin should be avoided in people with renal impairment, creatinine clearance <50 ml/mim.

- Vildagliptin is not recommended in people with liver disease. Sitagliptin should be used cautiously in people with liver disease.
- Sitagliptin has been associated with anaphalyxis, angioedema, rashes, urticaria, and exfoliative skin conditions, but these side effects are rare (NPS 2012).
- Weight gain can occur when the gliptins are used with a sulphonylurea.
- Hypoglycaemia can occur when the gliptins are used with a sulphonylurea.
- Gastrointestinal side effects.

SGLT2 Inhibitors

SGLT2 inhibitors target renal glucose reabsorption and induce glucose excretion in the urine independently of insulin secretion or action and are used in type 2 diabetes (Whaley et al. 2012; Thomas 2018). SGLT2 medicines reduce hyperglycaemia, fasting and postprandial blood glucose and HbA1c, hypertension, and weight. They have a low hypoglycaemia risk and may be able to be combined with insulin and other GLMs (Whaley et al. 2012; Abe et al. 2018; Cherney et al. 2018). Empagliflozin and canagliflozin significantly reduce occurrence of nonfatal myocardial infarction, nonfatal stroke and cardiovascular, independently of the glucose lowering effect (Zinman et al. 2015). SGLT-2 reduce total mortality by 32–38%, depending on the particular medicine (Zinman et al. 2015).

The glucose-lowering effects of SGLT-2 are negligible in people with renal impairment; however, some studies suggest some SGLT-2 might reduce rates of albuminuria, renal failure and the need for dialysis (Wanner et al. 2016).

Possible side effects
Reported side effects include:

- Increased incidence of urinary tract infections, which could put individuals with autonomic neuropathy affecting the bladder at particular risk and can contribute to incontinence.
- Increased incidence of genital fungal infections.
- Polyuria in volume-sensitive people, which could predispose them to dehydration, e.g. older people.
- Euglycaemic ketoacidosis (euDKA) in people with type 2 diabetes can occur and lead to severe acidosis requiring hospital admission (Peacock and Lovshin, 2018). euDKA is more likely to occur when people are fasting/starving, during surgery, active infection, excess alcohol intake and dehydration (Peters et al. 2016; Fralick et al. 2017). Consequently, a number of diabetes organisations released position statements/recommendations that encompass preoperative assessment, routine blood ketone monitoring, and referral to an endocrinologist. SGLT_2 should be stopped three days prior to surgery and recommenced when the individual is on full oral intake (American Association of Clinical Endocrinologists (AACE) 2011).
- The glycosuria effects of SGLT-2 might affect calcium, phosphate, and vitamin D homeostasis. Canagliflozin is associated with reduced bone mineral density, which could represent a fracture risk. Recent research suggests the fracture risk (pelvis, hip, radius, humerus, ulna, carpal, metacarpal, and ankle) is low in middle-aged people with type 2 diabetes: 22 events/1000 person years compared to 2.3 event/100 person years in people commencing GLP-1 ($n = 79\,964$ matched with $79\,964$ on GLP-1) (Fralick et al. 2017).

Canaglifozin increases LDL cholesterol but it also increases HDL.

Practice point

- Individual medicines within a class can have different effects and side effects. These differences must be considered when prescribing, monitoring effectiveness and when deprescribing GLMs.
- GLM medicine names and GLM availability can differ among countries.

A range of algorithms is available to help health professionals prescribe individual GLMs, combine GLMs, and initiate insulin. These are regularly revised as new medicines are introduced and include: ADA (2019); Australian Diabetes Society (2007); Gunton et al. 2016; Diabetes Australia/Royal Australian College of General Practitioners (2016/2018); NICE (2017).

Medicine interactions

Some possible interactions between GLMs and other commonly prescribed medicines are shown in Table 5.2. Some medicines interact with GLM and can cause hypo- or hyperglycaemia. A number of mechanisms for the interactions are known:

- Displace the medicine from binding sites.
- Inhibit or decrease hepatic metabolism.
- Delay excretion.
- Reduce insulin release.
- Antagonise insulin action.

Potential medicine and herb or herb/herb interactions and food/medicine interactions should also be considered when introducing a new medicine or reviewing the medicine regimen; see Chapter 19 (Hui et al. 2009). For example, over 95 medicines administered by mouth can interact with grapefruit, including antihypertensive agents, some antibiotics, cancer and cardiovascular medicines (Bailey et al. 2013), and interactions can occur even if grapefruit is taken several hours before taking the medicine. In addition, other citrus fruits may also interact but have not been widely studied to date. Interactions can also lead to micronutrient deficiency (Braun and Rosenfeldt 2012).

Table 5.2 Potential medicine interactions between glucose-lowering medicines (GLM) and other medicines.

Medicine	Possible mechanism
Medicines that increase blood glucose	
Clonidine	Adrenergic response
Clozapine	Impaired insulin secretion
Corticosteroids	Oppose insulin action
Diuretics, especially thiazides	Oppose insulin action
Nicotinic acid	Unknown
Nifedipine	Delays insulin action
Oral contraceptives	Unknown
Phenytoin	Impairs insulin secretion
Glucocorticoids	Cause insulin resistance and weight gain
Antipsychotics, especially atypical antipsychotics	
Sugar-containing medicines, for example, cough syrup	Increase blood glucose
Medicines that lower blood glucose	
ACE inhibitors	Enhance insulin action
Alcohol	Reduce hepatic glucose production
Fibrates such as gemfibrosil	Unknown
MOA inhibitors	Unknown
Salicylates in high doses (some herbal medicines contain salicylic compounds)	Unknown

Note: See Shenfield (2001). It is important to consider interactions with glucose lowering complementary medicines (CM) (Honxiang et al. 2009; Hunter et al. 2017).

Potential interactions have not yet fully emerged for TZIs and the incretins (gliptins) and SGLT-2. Medicines that alter hepatic enzymes have the potential to cause interactions with these GLMs because they are metabolised in the liver. Medicines that interfere with access to the gut by alpha-glucosidase inhibitors can inhibit their action, such as charcoal, digestive enzymes, Cholestyramine, Neomycin, and some CAM medicines such as slippery elm.

Practice points

(1) The clinical relevance of some postulated medicine interactions is uncertain.
(2) Other miscellaneous interactions that should also be considered are:
   - Beta blockers can mask tachycardia and other signs of hypoglycaemia resulting in delayed recognition and treatment increasing the risk of hypoglycaemic coma.
   - Chronic alcohol consumption can stimulate the metabolism of sulphonylureas and delay their effectiveness, cause hypoglycaemia, mask signs of hypoglycaemia, and with metformin, predispose the individual to lactic acidosis. It may also increase the bioavailability of ACE-1.

Combining GLMs and insulin

Any combination of currently available GLM only lowers HbA1c by ~3% (American Association of Clinical Endocrinologists (AACE) 2011, thus people with HbA1c > 10% are unlikely to achieve management targets using GLM alone. Therefore, insulin is assuming an increasingly important role in type 2 diabetes. As indicated, most people with type 2 diabetes have progressive beta cell dysfunction and a decline in beta cell mass. Proposed mechanisms for these defects include the interplay among a range of factors that reduce beta cell mass and secretory function such as hyperglycaemia, elevated free fatty acids, and inflammatory processes associated with adipocyte-derived cytokines. Apoptosis appears to be a key underlying mechanism (Leiter 2006). In addition, lifestyle factors, concomitant diseases, and often medicines compound the metabolic abnormalities. In some cases, medication nonadherence may be a factor and should be assessed in a nonjudgmental manner.

Goudswaard et al. (2004) showed continuing metformin when insulin is commenced is associated with lower HbA1c (by up to 0.6%) and less weight gain without increasing hypoglycaemia risk. Continuing sulphonylurea when initiating a daily insulin dose was associated with a greater HbA1c reduction than monotherapy. Likewise, continuing metformin, sulphonylurea, or both when insulin is commenced results in lower insulin requirements compared with monotherapy.

As indicated, various algorithms are available for initiating insulin and continuing one or more GLM. The medicines selected and the dose and dose regimen must be tailored to the individual's needs. Generally, bedtime neutral protamine hagedorn (NPH) or a basal insulin analogue should be used when adding insulin to metformin and/or a sulphonylurea, depending on the hypoglycaemia risk.

Practice points

- GLMs, including insulin, are not substitutes for healthy eating, weight management, and regular activity/exercise.
- Medication administration times should be planned so that GLMs that cause hypoglycaemia are administered with or before meals to reduce the risk of hypoglycaemia.

When should insulin be initiated in Type 2 diabetes?

Commencing insulin should be a planned, proactive decision and should not be delayed. Some experts refer to 'tablet failure' as a reason for initiating insulin. The choice of language/words should be considered carefully when conveying the need for insulin to a person with diabetes: they may interpret 'tablet failure' to mean *they* have failed (Diabetes Australia (DA) and Royal Australian College General Practitioners (RACGP) 2011/2012).

Clinical observations

- The challenge for health professionals is to balance the optimal time to initiate insulin with the time the individual is ready to accept insulin.
- Culture, literacy, beliefs, experience, and social situation are some of the factors that affect people's readiness to accept insulin.
- Interestingly, doctors, and probably other health professionals frequently do not follow recommended guidelines, including initiating insulin, for various reasons such as resource and time constraints, because they are 'slow adopters', or because they use complex individual decision-making heuristics (Choudhry and Fletcher 2005; Tung 2011).

The time of day to administer insulin in type 2 diabetes depends on the individual's blood glucose pattern, HbA1c, adherence to medicines, and complication status, especially cardiovascular and renal status, and willingness to use insulin. Often, a basal insulin is initiated at bedtime and the dose adjusted according to the fasting (prebreakfast) blood glucose (Kuritzky, 2006).

Prandial insulin before one or more meals is added if HbA1c and blood glucose targets are not achieved. A general guide to deciding insulin requirements when initiating insulin follows: individual needs, the blood glucose pattern, and frequency of hypo- and hyperglycaemia must be considered.

Indications for insulin include:

- Women with type 2 diabetes who become pregnant and sometimes women with gestational diabetes; see Chapter 14.
- When the person actually has LADA (see Chapter 1).
- As rescue therapy in diabetic ketoacidosis (DKA), hyperosmolar hyperglycaemic states (HHS), during other acute illnesses, and surgical procedures; see Chapters 7 and 9.
- Persisting hyperglycaemia indicated by elevated fasting blood glucose and/or elevated postprandial blood glucose and HbA1c above the individual's target (e.g. HbA1c > 7%).
- Symptoms, especially polyuria, polydipsia, and weight loss.
- GLM intolerance or contraindication, for example, metformin if creatinine is high.
- People on two GLMs and not achieving target ranges where insulin may be preferable to adding a third GLM, given that most people with type 2 diabetes eventually need insulin, especially if the GLMs are at maximal doses. However, there is no consensus about whether the second agent added to Metformin should be another GLM or insulin. Insulin might be preferable if the HbA1c is >8.5% or the person is very symptomatic (Nathan and Buse 2006) or when there is a high tablet burden (polypharmacy). In such presentations, LADA should be considered, especially if the individual is thin. The National Prescribing Service (NPS) advised health professionals to be '… more aggressive in their management of people with type 2 diabetes' (NPS media release, 26 March 2008), a sentiment echoed by other experts. However, the benefits of 'insulin aggression' need to be balanced against the risks such as hypoglycaemia and its consequences (falls in older people, MI, effects on cognition).
- Recent research suggests insulin has anti-inflammatory properties in addition to its other actions (Dandona et al. 2008; Sun et al. 2014). It attenuates the anti-inflammatory effects of hyperglycemia through metabolic regulation, directly modulates inflammatory mediators, and acts on immune cells to enhance immunocompetence (Sun et al. 2014).

The goals are to achieve optimal control without causing hypoglycaemia or excessive weight gain and with minimal impact on lifestyle. Thus, understanding the individual's perspective is essential.

For some people, commencing insulin and ceasing GLMs may represent a simpler, more manageable medication regimen; for others, it represents 'the end of the line' or 'the last resort'.

Insulin is often added to the GLM regimen at bedtime to reduce fasting glucose levels (Riddle et al. 2003; Janka et al. 2005). The dose is adjusted according to the fasting blood glucose pattern, including self-adjustment by the person with diabetes to achieve targets with minimal hypoglycaemia according to a simple algorithm (Yki-Jarvinen et al. 2007). Yki-Jarvinen et al. showed insulin could be successfully initiated in groups and achieve glycaemic targets. In addition, group insulin initiation was acceptable to patients.

The specific initiation process depends on the policies and guidelines of individual health services. Over recent years, research has demonstrated the efficacy of several processes for initiating and titrating insulin in type 2 diabetes using various insulins and usually starting with small doses. They all used a stepwise approach and include:

- The Treat-to-Target study used basal Glargine at bedtime and titrated the dose weekly in 10 weeks (Riddle et al. 2003). This regimen is suitable for older people because it is associated with fewer hypoglycaemic events and is well tolerated (Janka et al. 2005). Isophane insulin can also be used as the basal insulin but has a higher risk of hypoglycaemia.
- The 1-2-3 study, which used daily bedtime doses of NovoMix 30 initially and subsequently added doses pre-breakfast then pre-lunch if necessary to achieve targets (Raskin et al. 2005).
- The INITIATE study that used BD doses of NovoMix 30 (Gabbay et al. 2005; Jain et al. 2005).

The stepwise approach is also used with insulin analogues such as long-acting basal lantus, Detemir and Degludec, an ultralong acting preparation currently in phase three clinical trials, and rapid-acting prandial insulins such as Novorapid.

The advantage of using basal bolus insulin dose regimens is that they usually achieve better postprandial control, but eating after injecting the insulin is important. BD lispro/isophane mix and metformin also improve pre- and postprandial blood glucose with few episodes of nocturnal hypoglycaemia (Malone et al. 2005).

Many researchers have compared different brands of insulin and dose regimens. Overall, the findings suggest the pharmacokinetic differences among insulin brands may not be clinically relevant and there are likely to be variations in individual patient's response to the different formulations Evans et al. 2011. The ultralong acting basal insulin in phase three testing, Degludec, appears to cause less nocturnal hypoglycaemia in type 1 and type 2 diabetes and to reduce fasting glucose (Wang et al. 2012). In reality, the choice of insulin may actually be made according to prescriber preference and local availability. Despite the similarities, indiscriminate switching between different insulin brands or using different brands together is not generally recommended.

Outpatient or community-based insulin initiation is preferable, except in specific circumstances. A proforma initiation process is outlined in this chapter that can be adapted as necessary and a simple algorithm for commencing insulin in type 2 diabetes is shown in Table 5.3 and Figure 5.2. Often, GLMs are continued with basal insulin regimens if there are no contraindications to their use. When bolus insulin doses are added, insulin secretagogue doses usually need to be reduced or the medicines discontinued.

The proforma is based on the premise that the individual undertakes blood glucose monitoring, relevant monitoring and assessments are undertaken, relevant education is provided, and the response to therapy is monitored at each step. Consider LADA if the person is not overweight, loses weight, has significant hyperglycaemia, and is very symptomatic, because insulin should not be delayed in these people; see Chapter 1.

Table 5.3   Issues to consider when deciding insulin doses and dose regimen when commencing insulin.

Issues to consider	HbA1c %	Insulin doses and administration times
Consider current diabetes management and glycaemic status and whether it is safe to continue existing GLM.		Insulin in units/kg depends on preinsulin treatment and weight.
Decide on a safe blood glucose target range for the individual.	<7	Refer to guidelines and consider risk of hypoglycaemia.
Decide whether to administer insulin as a daily basal dose and/or bolus doses and when the insulin will be administered on the basis of the amount of insulin required per day and whether oral GLMs will be continued.	>7	Diet and activity 0.3 GLMs 0.4
Morning blood glucose high and evening blood glucose is acceptable.		Pre-bed basal insulin
Morning blood glucose is acceptable and evening blood glucose high.		Morning basal insulin
Morning blood glucose is high and evening blood glucose high.		Basal bolus regimen could be with a long-acting analogue before bed or before breakfast and TDS rapid-acting insulin OR BD premixed insulin OR morning Isophane insulin and TDS rapid-acting insulin. Choose insulin type/s, doses, and dose regimens to minimize the hypoglycaemia risk. Note insulin might be a lower risk than insulin secretagagues.

Note: See NICE 2008; DA and RACGP 2011/2012; ADA 2019. However, guidelines and protocols in use should be followed. Insulin doses are adjusted by 2–4 units according to the blood glucose pattern every 3–4 days to reach the target blood glucose range and avoid hypoglycaemia.

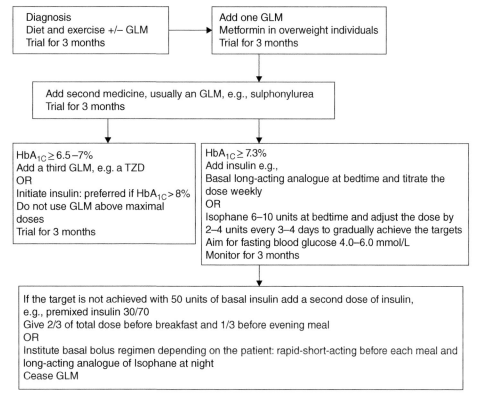

Figure 5.2   Algorithm for achieving blood glucose targets in Type 2 diabetes that encompasses a Quality Use of Medicines approach and adopts a proactive stepwise approach to initiating insulin.

Management aims:

(1) Proactively initiate insulin. Insulin should not be delayed.
(2) Control fasting and postprandial hyperglycaemia without causing serious hyperglycaemia.
(3) Achieve HbA1c target relevant to the age hypoglycaemia risk and health status of the individual, generally <7% but may be higher in older people.
(4) Normalise lipids to reduce cardiovascular risk.
(5) Control symptoms.

A range of prescribing algorithms is available and the algorithms are updated regularly to accommodate emerging evidence about GLM safety and benefit and include new GLMs. It is important to consider any limitations to prescribing second- and third-line GLMs from an individual perspective as well as regulatory requirements and the medicine burden for the individual. Increasingly, cardiovascular and other risks are considered when selecting GLMs. Thus, many algorithms include SGLT-2 inhibitors and DPP-4 inhibitors as second-line choices.

Pharmacovigilance is essential (Dunning and Sinclair 2014). GLM prescribing algorithms include:

- Algorithm for blood glucose lowering therapy in adults with type 2 diabetes (NICE guideline NG28 2017).
- A new blood glucose management algorithm for type 2 diabetes: a position statement of The Australian Diabetes Society (Gunton et al. 2016).
- American Diabetes Association and European Association for the Study of Diabetes (Davies et al. 2018). Management of hyperglycaemia in type 2 diabetes: a consensus report. diabetologia-journal.org/wp-content/uploads/2018/09/EASD-ADA.pdf.
- ADA Standards of Medical care: diabetes (2019).
- How to commence insulin: Guiding you through that first prescription (Soldatus and Pease 2018).
- Second steps in managing type 2 diabetes. (Petersen/Australian Prescriber 2018).

Challenges to initiating insulin therapy

There are many barriers to initiating insulin therapy in type 2 diabetes: most relate to the individual with diabetes and some to health professional factors (Dunning and Martin 1997). Although patients often view insulin negatively, early explanations about the nature of type 2 diabetes (from diagnosis), and with support and encouragement, most people usually accept they need insulin. However, their fears and concerns must be acknowledged, respected, and explored. People often regard insulin as 'the last resort', and fear hypoglycaemia and weight gain (Dunning and Martin 1999). The DAWN study (Rutherford et al. 2004) showed that people on insulin worried about hypoglycaemia more than noninsulin users, and insulin was associated with worse quality of life in people with type 2 diabetes. This finding continues to emerge in other studies (e.g. MILES; see Speight et al. 2011).

Type 2 diabetes is a silent disease with few symptoms; thus, it is often difficult for people to accept they have a serious, progressive disease. Many worry about weight gain associated with insulin use. They are often reluctant to test their blood glucose frequently and feel blood glucose monitoring and insulin interferes with their lifestyle. For some people, the stigma associated with needles is an issue.

Many doctors are reluctant to use insulin in type 2 diabetes and often compound the patient's concerns, albeit usually unintentionally, by delaying insulin initiation. Such health professional behaviour has been referred to as 'clinical inertia' (Shah et al. 2005), and, like non-adherence, is a complex multifactorial issue (Tung 2011). Other health professional-related barriers include inadequate knowledge, lack of time, support and resources, worry about causing hypoglycaemia, and complicating the management regimen. For example, UK practice nurses felt commencing insulin in primary care was beneficial for patients but lack of time, support, and confidence, and concerns about medico-legal implications and personal accountability made it difficult to achieve (Greaves et al. 2003).

Some strategies to overcome the barriers

The therapeutic relationship between the patient and the health professional has a significant effect on health outcomes and patient behaviours including adherence to medicines and improved safety (Worthington 2003). Thus, a first step is to establish a non-judgmental, trusting relationship. Specific approaches depend on the individual and the circumstances in which insulin is required. Health professionals need to acknowledge that:

- People's previous experience of insulin and beliefs about insulin.
- Listen to their story and clarify relevant issues.
- Managing insulin is a complex process and is only one self-care and life task the person is expected to fulfill.
- 'Things might get worse before they get better'. For example vision often deteriorates temporarily.
- The ability to self-care changes over time due to physical and mental functional changes: normal age-related changes and changes associated with diabetes complications.
- Insulin side effects especially hypoglycaemia.
- There are usually added costs involved.

The transformational model of change can be a useful framework for addressing the need to commence insulin, especially if it is integrated with aspects of the health belief model, QUM and holistic care, where insulin is discussed as one aspect to be addressed, not an isolated event in a person's life. Research suggests timing is important when trying to initiate change. That is, it needs to be linked to an individual's stage in the change process (Prochaska and Velicer 1997) and significant life transitions, which are often also accompanied by changes in identity and behaviour (George 1993; Dunning 2017; Rasmussen 2018).

Providing personalised and customised advice and written information is most useful when it is delivered in a caring relationship where the individual's concerns are acknowledged and they are invited to suggest ways they could address the issues they identify. Thus, listening, clarifying, and following up by asking about progress are essential. However, despite the focus on patient-centred care, the patient's views are often not sought and they are inadvertently placed in a passive rather than an active role particularly when communication barriers such as language, religion, culture, health literacy and numeracy, hearing impairment or other disabilities are present.

Identifying and discussing the person's concerns is essential. For example, 'needle phobia', weight gain, and hypoglycaemia. Demonstrating the various insulin delivery devices often helps reduce some concerns about needles. People on insulin gain more weight than those on diet for over 10 years (Mayfield and White 2004), partly due to better glycaemic control and losing less glucose in the urine, the fact that insulin is an anabolic hormone, lower metabolic rate and people may eat more to prevent hypoglycaemia (Birkeland et al. 1994). Levemir appears to cause less weight gain in both type 1 and type 2 diabetes (Dornhorst et al. 2007), whereas Glargine is associated with a modest weight increase and hypoglycaemia (ORIGIN 2012).

Strategies to avoid weight gain include selecting insulin formulations and other medicines least likely to contribute to weight gain if possible, regular exercise perhaps using a pedometer, and individualised nutrition advice. Once symptoms are controlled people often feel more active and exercise helps control weight and blood glucose.

Understanding and exploring the person's concerns about hypoglycaemia and helping them identify strategies to reduce hypoglycaemic episodes. Although the UKPD showed the frequency and severity of severe hypoglycaemia was lower in people with type 2 diabetes than type 1 diabetes (UKPDS 1998), more recent research suggests hypoglycaemia is a significant risk in both types of diabetes (Chapter 6). The risk increases when the HbA1c is <7.4% and with insulin and oral insulin secretagogues. Carefully identifying hypoglycaemia risk factors with the individual and helping them develop strategies to minimise their individual risk, is important.

Vision can deteriorate when insulin is commenced. Sight is not usually threatened, but it is very distressing for the person with diabetes and they need a careful explanation and reassurance to help them understand. Activities of daily living such as reading and driving can be affected. Visual changes occur because the lens absorbs excess glucose in much the same way as sponge soaks up water. Changes in the amount of glucose in the lens can lead to blurred vision and can occur with high and low blood glucose levels. This phenomenon is quite different from diabetic retinopathy, which can threaten the sight.

The starting dose may not be the 'right' dose and the 'right' dose changes according to specific circumstances and individual need.

Insulin therapy

Insulin is a high-risk medicine (Dooley et al. 2011) and is associated with significant adverse events, including in hospitals and aged-care facilities. For example, 30% of unplanned hospital admissions for older people are associated with medicine-related adverse events (Australian Commission on Safety and Quality in Health Care 2012).

High-risk medicines are likely to cause significant harm or death when given incorrectly. Even when used correctly, insulin can cause significant harm. Over one third of medical errors that result in death involve insulin use within 48 hours of the death (Roughhead et al. 2013). Thus, when considering insulin, the individual's risk of harm must be considered and preventative strategies used when possible.

Overview of insulin action

Insulin is a hormone secreted by the beta cells of the pancreas. Normal requirements are between 0.5 and 1.0 units/kg/day. Insulin synthesis and secretion are stimulated by an increase in the blood glucose level after meals. Insulin attaches to insulin receptors on cell membranes to facilitate the passage of glucose into the cell for utilisation as fuel or storage, and reduces hepatic glucose production. Insulin also stimulates the storage of fatty acids and amino acids, facilitates glycogen formation, and storage in the liver and skeletal muscle, and limits lipolysis and proteolysis. Therefore, insulin deficiency results in altered protein, fat, and carbohydrate metabolism (also refer to Chapter 1). As indicated earlier in this chapter, it also has anti-inflammatory properties.

Insulin is vital to survival for people with type 1 diabetes, and 90% of people with type 2 diabetes eventually require insulin (Thomas 2018).

Objectives of insulin therapy

(1) Achieve blood glucose, HbA1c and lipid levels within a safe, acceptable individual range by replacing absent insulin secretion in type 1 and supplementing insulin production in type 2 diabetes (see previous section).
(2) Approximate physiological insulin secretion and action.
(3) Avoid the consequences of too much insulin (hypoglycaemia) or too little insulin (hyperglycaemia).
(4) Improve quality of life and reduce the risk of long-term diabetes complications.

Types of insulin available

Insulin cannot be given orally at this stage. It is a polypeptide. Polypeptides are digested by gastric enzymes and do not reach the circulation. Research is currently underway to coat insulin in a substance that can withstand gastric juices and enable it to pass unchanged into the intestine before breaking down. Recently, a formulation that delivers the insulin into the mouth as a metered-dose spray, which enables it to be rapidly absorbed (Kennedy and Oliver 2017). Oral-Lyn was launched in Ecuador in 2005 and is available in other countries such as United Arab Emirates and India.

Inhaled insulin is also the subject of research where it is absorbed via the alveoli in the lungs. Approximately 60% of inhaled insulin is absorbed from the lungs and 40% is swallowed and enters to gastrointestinal tract (Cefalu et al. 2001; Skyler et al. 2001).

Exubera was withdrawn within 12 months of being launched, largely on the basis of cost, restrictive labelling, and confusing dose equivalence and side effects such as persistent cough and increased risk of lung cancer. Afrezza, a rapidly acting prandial insulin, is associated with bronchospasm, and two cases of lung cancer were reported in clinical trials compared with no cases in the control group. Two additional cases of lung cancer in nonsmokers were reported in the treatment group after the trial ended (Kennedy and Oliver 2017). Active marketing of Afrezza has stopped and it is rarely prescribe.

In addition, glucose-responsive insulins or smart insulins and BioChaperoned peptide insulins are under development. They are designed to release insulin into the blood stream when needed, Smart insulins use glycosylated insulins in combination with glucose-binding lectins, but they are in the early stages of development. BioChaparoned Lisoro is an ultrarapid formulation that showed promising results; trials have been suspended at present.

A number of different brands of insulins are available, for example, Novo Nordisk, Eli Lilly, and SanofiAventis. As indicated, the insulins are all effective and safe.

Animal insulins (bovine and porcine) are almost never used nowadays but are still available in some countries, often under special access schemes. 'Human' insulin (HM) is manufactured by recombinant DNA technology. The amino acid sequence of HM insulin is the same as that of insulin secreted by the beta cells of the human pancreas. Rapid-acting insulin analogues (prandial insulins) have been developed that give a more physiologic response after injection and improve the blood glucose profile, for example, lispro, aspart, and apidra. The advantages of these insulins are reduced postprandial hyperglycaemia and reduced risk of hypoglycaemia.

Long-acting analogues are glargine (brand names Lantus, Basaglar, Toujeo), Levemir, and degludec. Glargine has a slower onset than isophane insulins and a smooth peakless action profile for up to 24 hours (Buse 2001). Levimir may be shorter acting than glargine and has its maximal effect between 3 and 14 hours. Recently an ultra-long-acting insulin, degludec, was introduced. It appears to have longer duration of action and low hypoglycaemia risk profile. These insulins enable greater management flexibility and lower risk of hypoglycaemia.

Insulin doses can be estimated based on the person's weight and doses range from 0.4–1.0 units/kg/day. Higher doses are require in special circumstances, e.g. puberty, pregnancy, acute illnesses, and significant insulin resistance (ADA 2019).

Rapid-acting insulin

Rapid-acting insulin should be clear and colourless. Examples are:

- Lispro (Humalog)
- Aspart (Novorapid)
- Apidra (Glulisine)

They have a rapid onset of action, within 10–15 minutes, peak at 60 minutes, and act for 2–4 hours.

They need to be given *immediately* before meals and are used in basal bolus regimes, in combination with intermediate acting insulin and long-acting analogues, or used in combination with oral hypoglycemic agents (OHAs) or in insulin pumps.

Combining rapid-acting insulin with alpha-glucosidase inhibitors, which reduce glucose absorption from the gut, can increase the risk of hypoglycaemia the first hour after injection and two to three hours after exercise are other peak times for hypoglycaemia.

Short-acting insulin

This should be clear and colourless. Examples are:

- Actrapid
- Humulin R

They begin to take effect in 20–30 minutes after injection and act between 4 and 8 hours. Rapid- and short-acting insulins can be used:

- Alone two to four times per day
- In combination with intermediate- or long-acting insulins
- For correction doses
- As IV insulin infusions
- In continuous subcutaneous insulin infusions (CSII) via insulin pumps

Intermediate-acting insulin

Intermediate-acting insulins must be mixed gently before use and should be milky after mixing. Examples are:

- Protophane
- Humulin NPH
- Hypurin (isophane)

They begin to act in 2–3 hours. The duration of action is between 12 and 18 hours. They can be used:

- In combination with short-acting insulin – this is the usual method.
- Alone for patients who are sensitive to short-acting insulin, or in combination with oral hypoglycaemic agents.

Long-acting basal insulin

- Glargine (Lantus) acts for about 20 hours.
- Detemir (Levemir) as described in the preceding section.
- Insulin degludec (Tresiba) has a long-acting flat action profile and is less likely to cause hypoglycaemia. It is injected with the largest meal of the day and not necessarily the same time each day.

Recent research comparing glargine 300 units/ml with degludec 100 units/ml showed similar improvements in glycaemic control and comparable hypoglycaemia rates but lower in favour of glargine (Rosenstock et al. 2018).

Biphasic insulins

Biphasic insulins are often prescribed for people with type 2 diabetes.

These contain both short- or rapid- and intermediate-acting or long insulins in various combinations. Most must be mixed before using. They do not enable independent adjustment of the short or intermediate/long acting components. Examples of mixed fast and intermediate acting insulins are:

- NovoMix 30 (30% Aspart /70% protamine)
- Humalog Mix 25 (Lispro 25%/Lispro protamine 75%)

- Humalog Mix 50 (Lispro 40%/ Lispro protamine 50%)
- Humalin 30/70 (Humulin 30%/Isopahane 70%)
- Mixtard 50/70 (Actrapid 50%/Isopahne 50%)

Mixed fast- and long-acting insulin

- Aspart 30% Degludec 70%

Many insulins are available in prefilled disposable insulin devices. Each insulin administration device has advantages and disadvantages, and patient preference should be considered. The diabetes educator can help individuals decide which device (and therefore, to some extent which insulin) suits them best. Generally, the insulin device should be used with the insulin designed by the same manufacturer. Insulin syringes still have a role, and some people with diabetes prefer to use syringes.

A number of insulins are no longer protect under patent. Thus, biosimilar insulins (copies) are appearing. They are not an exact copy of the original and can have different action profiles. Regulatory authorities in Europe and the United States have published guidelines on medicine biosimilars, including insulin. Abasaglar, a glargine biosimilar, is in phase 3 clinical trials (Kapitza et al. 2017). Thus, clinicians can expect to see biosimilar insulins in use in the future.

Storing insulin

The temperature at which insulin is stored is important to maintaining its efficacy. Insulin should be stored according to the manufacturer's directions. Unopened vials should be stored in the refrigerator at 2–8 °C. Insulin vials in use can be stored out of the refrigerator, for example, in the patient's medication drawer, provided they are not stored near a source of heat or light (Campbell et al. 1993; see individual product prescribing information). People with diabetes need to be educated about correct storage and handling of insulin, as well as sharps disposal, as part of their education about insulin therapy.

Exposure to heat and light accelerates the formation of insulin transformation products (ITP) and denatures insulin. Insulin undergoes a chemical transformation in solution and ITP are formed. The main ITPs are deanimated insulin, covalent dimers, and oligomers (Pryce 2009).

Clinical observation

Hyperglycaemia can occur when using incorrectly stored insulin and insulin that has passed the expiry date.

Practice points

(1) Long-acting analogues cannot be mixed with other insulins. Nor can they be injected in the same site.
(2) They are clear, and great care must be taken to ensure they are not mistaken for rapid- or short-acting insulins. Look-alike medicine alert policies should be initiated. For example, consider storing them in a different part of the refrigerator and clearly flagging them with a 'look-alike' medication alert label.
(3) Carefully check the dose to be administered of NovoMix 30 and Humalog Mix 25 or 50 and do not mistake the numbers in the name of the insulin for the insulin dose, which has occurred and led to serious adverse medicine events.

Injection sites and administration

Administer at the appropriate time before the meal. The abdomen is the preferred site; but upper arms, thighs, and buttocks can also be used. Injection sites must be rotated to avoid lipoatrophy and lipodystrophy. Injection sites and technique should be checked on a regular basis, e.g. annual complication assessment and periods of unexplained glucose variability. Injection sites should also be rotated when people use insulin pumps. These recommendations also apply to insulin pump infusion sites. Insulin infusion cannula need to be changes every 48–72 hours, depending on the manufacture's recommendations.

How to inject

The insulin injection technique can influence insulin absorption and, therefore, its action. Insulin should be administered subcutaneously. IM injections lead to unstable blood glucose levels (Vaag et al. 1990; Frid et al. 2016).

- Choose and appropriate needle size and length: 4 mm (ADEA 2017; Frid et al. 2016).
- Pinch up a fold of skin if children use 5 mm needle or inject on a 45° angle.
- Prime insulin pens before use and use according to the manufacturer's directions.
- Needles should be removed from the pen and disposed into a sharps container immediately after use.
- Remove the needle, and apply gentle pressure to the site.
- Document dose and time of the injection.
- Injection sites should be regularly checked for swelling, lumps, pain, or leakage of insulin.

Practice points

(1) A range of needle sizes is available. Needle size is important to people with diabetes. Most modern guidelines recommend using 4 mm gauge needles to reduce the likelihood of intramuscular injection.

(2) Injection with fine-gauge needles is relatively painless.

(3) Giving the first injection is often very difficult for people with diabetes. Support and encouragement and allowing them to take their time and inject at their own pace is important.

(4) Insulin leakage from injection sites is rare when a skinfold is not pinched using modern short needles. However, the loss of even small amounts of insulin can result in unpredictable increases in the blood glucose and inappropriate dose adjustment especially in lean people and children. Careful observation and estimation of the amount of insulin lost is necessary to make appropriate adjustments to the individual's injection technique – this applies to both patients and clinicians.

(5) The larger the volume of insulin to be injected, the greater the likelihood of some insulin leaking back along the needle track. Likewise, leakage can occur if the injection is too shallow or given intradermally.

(6) To minimise the risk of insulin loss during injection, inject slowly and leave the needle in place for three to six seconds after the insulin is delivered.

(7) Long-acting and premixed insulins dispensed in insulin pens must be mixed gently before administration.

Instructions for teaching people how to draw up and administer insulin using a syringe appear in Chapter 16. Refer also to the manufacturer's instructions and patient information material.

Practice points

(1) Insulin syringes and pen needles are approved for single use only.
(2) Pen needles should be removed after administering an insulin dose and a new needle used for the next dose especially with premixed insulins, which can block the needle.
(3) Most insulin administration devices, except syringes, were designed to enable patients to administer their own insulin. In hospital, patients should remove the needle and place it in the sharps container after injecting to avoid needle stick injury to staff.
(4) In hospital, aged-care and community settings staff should NOT recap needles.
(5) If the patient cannot remove the needle from the pen, a removal device should be used, or the insulin administered using a syringe until the patient is well enough to self-inject again.

Mixing short/rapid acting- and intermediate-acting insulins

General points

There is less need to mix insulins now, due to the range of modern premixed insulin combinations and insulin analogues. However, it is still necessary in some settings and in some countries. Mixing short- and intermediate-acting insulins before injecting may diminish the effect of the short-acting peak, which is more marked when there is substantially more long-acting insulin in the mixture (as is usually the case), especially if the insulin is left to stand for a long time before being injected.

The clinical significance of these changes is unknown. It is more likely to apply to in home situations where home-care/domiciliary nurses or relatives draw up doses for several days in advance for people to self-administer; see Chapter 18. This practice may not be ideal, but it does enable people to retain a measure of independence where syringes are still the device of choice.

The long-acting insulin analogues cannot be mixed with other insulin or injected into the same site.

Commonly used insulin regimens

Daily injection

A combination of:

- Rapid- or short- and long-acting insulin combinations, which are usually given before breakfast. Biphasic premixed insulins such as Mixtard 30/70 are sometimes used.
- Long- or intermediate-acting insulin is often given at bedtime when it is combined with GLMs for type 2 diabetes. Daily regimes are commonly used for:
  ○ Older people
  ○ Those not willing to have more than one injection per day
  ○ Some situations where people require assistance to inject, are living in aged-care facilities, or depend on home nursing care when staff are not available to inject more than once per day
- Daily regimens are not recommended for people with type 1 diabetes

It can be difficult to attain good control using biphasic insulin because the dose of the individual insulins in the mix cannot be altered, which can increase the risk of hypoglycaemia if eating is erratic, the carbohydrate intake is low, or after vigorous exercise. However, premixed insulins can reduce the medicine burden on individuals.

BD regimens

A combination of rapid- or short- and intermediate or long-acting insulin is usually given before breakfast and before the evening meal. Biphasic insulins are commonly used but do not allow a great deal of flexibility in adjusting doses. The evening dose may effectively control overnight

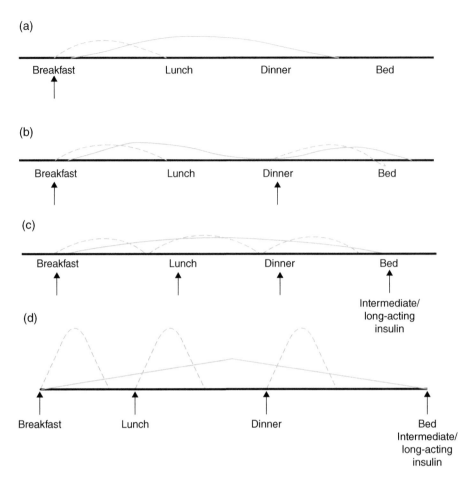

Figure 5.3 Diagrammatic representation of insulin action showing different regimens: (a) daily, (b) twice a day, (c) basal bolus using short-acting insulins and (d) basal bolus using rapid-acting insulins. *Note:* The broken line depicts short-acting insulin, the unbroken line intermediate/long-acting insulin. The arrows indicate the time of injection. Note that the action profile depends on the specific insulin and many individual factors.

hyperglycaemia. There is a risk of nocturnal hypoglycaemia; see Chapter 6. Usually two-thirds of the total dose is given in the morning and one-third in the evening.

Figure 5.3 depicts the action profiles of the various insulins. Understanding the action profile enables hypoglycaemia risk times to be identified so that meals, activity, and medication administration times can be planned accordingly. They also help decide which insulin to adjust when considered in conjunction with the blood glucose profile. Consideration should always be given to other factors that affect blood glucose levels; see Chapter 3.

Practice point

Rapid-acting insulins act very quickly. They should be given immediately before a meal, or within 15 minutes after the meal to reduce the risk of hypoglycaemia.

Basal bolus regimen

Basal bolus regimens simulate the normal pattern of insulin secretion, that is, a small amount of circulating insulin is present in the blood and restrains gluconeogenesis and glycogenolysis; this is the basal insulin. A bolus amount of insulin is stimulated by the blood glucose rise after a meal. Bolus injections of rapid- or short-acting insulin are given before each meal. The longer-acting insulin, often an analogue, is often given before bed to supply the basal insulin requirement and restrain hepatic glucose output overnight and control the pre-breakfast blood glucose (fasting) level.

Basal bolus regimens offer more flexibility to adjust insulin doses and mealtimes, and therefore lifestyle is not affected as much. The amount of insulin given at each dose is usually small; therefore, the likelihood of hypoglycaemia is reduced. Basal bolus regimens are commonly used for young people with type 1 diabetes and increasingly for type 2. Despite the number of injections per day, basal bolus therapy using analogues may be safer for older people, with a lower risk of hypoglycaemia and falls. Nocturnal hypoglycaemia is less frequent when long-acting analogues are used.

Interpreting morning hyperglycaemia

There are three main reasons for fasting hyperglycaemia:

(1) Insufficient basal insulin to restrain overnight hepatic glucose output. It is a common finding with daily insulin regimens when the insulin is given in the morning. A larger dose of insulin may be needed or a second dose of insulin introduced at lunch or bedtime, or if the person is on GLM and a basal analogue insulin, the insulin could be given at night.
(2) The Somogyi effect, which is due to the counter-regulatory response to nocturnal hypoglycaemia. The cause needs to be sought (see Chapter 6) but the basal insulin dose may need to be reduced.
(3) *Dawn phenomenon* reflects insufficient insulin and insulin resistance. There is a normal physiological increase in many hormones early in the morning. However, elevated fasting blood glucose may indicate general hyperglycaemia. A thorough assessment is needed and the medication regimen adjusted.

CSII

Insulin pumps continuously deliver subcutaneous insulin, usually a rapid-acting analogue, at a pre-programmed steady basal rate or rates through a needle inserted subcutaneously, which stays in place for about three days. Bolus doses are delivered before meals or as corrective doses for hyperglycaemia. Bolus doses can be preprogrammed or delivered manually when needed. Insulin pumps enable a more physiological insulin profile to be attained and greater flexibility in meeting individual insulin requirements and lifestyle. Insulin pumps use rapid- or short-acting insulin only; therefore, if they malfunction or are removed (e.g. during surgery), the patient must be given insulin via another method to avoid hyperglycaemia (e.g. subcutaneously or via an IV insulin infusion, depending on the circumstances).

Modern insulin pumps are generally reliable and have an inbuilt alarm system that identifies a number of faults such as kinks/blockages in the tubing, tubing disconnections from the pump and low batteries, so that malfunctions can be identified early and appropriate steps taken to avoid hyperglycaemia. Some do not sound an alarm if the tubing disconnects from the insertion site. If this occurs, insulin is not delivered and can go unnoticed until the blood glucose is tested. In people with T1DM, hyperglycaemia can occur quickly and increase the risk of DKA. Reported rates vary between 2.7 and 9 episodes per 100 patient years.

Pumps are expensive and require a great deal of commitment on the part of the person with diabetes to use them safely and effectively. Readily available support and advice from insulin pump expert clinicians are vital. People need time to adjust to the pump regimen and become accustomed to not having intermediate-acting insulin. Pumps offer a great deal of flexibility and can have significant psychological benefits. However, pumps do not suit everybody and some people dislike the thought of being constantly connected to a device.

People need to learn to count carbohydrates when they commence using an insulin pump. Structured education programmes such as Dose Adjustment for Normal Eating (DAFNE, 2002) and OzDAFNE are often used to help individuals learn how much insulin is required per meal (~0.5 units/10 g of carbohydrate). DAFNE is based on 10 g of carbohydrate. Recently, a blood glucose meter and smart phone apps have appeared on the market and can be useful decision aids for people with diabetes. Combining continuous blood glucose monitoring with an insulin pump is becoming a reality and will be welcomed by people with diabetes (Chapter 1).

Practice points

(1) Insulin pumps are not a cure for inadequate metabolic control, but they can help some people achieve better control.
(2) They enable the insulin regimen and food intake to be matched to individual requirements and greater flexibility.
(3) Hypoglycaemia unawareness may be reversed and hypoglycaemia frequency and severity may be reduced.
(4) Insulin injections are not required, except if the pump malfunctions.
(5) Blood glucose monitoring at least four-hourly is necessary unless the person uses continuous blood glucose monitoring.
(6) Training and readily available support and advice from skilled pump experts are essential.
(7) People with existing psychological problems do worse on pumps than on other insulin regimes (DCCT (Diabetes Control and Complications Trial Research Group) 1993).
(8) Pumps are expensive to purchase and the ongoing cost of consumables is high. In Australia some health insurance funds subsidise the initial outlay for the pump according to specified guidelines. The cost of consumables is subsidised by the Commonwealth government under the National Diabetes Supply Scheme but subsidies for diabetes products is currently under review and could change in the future (Australia Government Department of Health 2019).

Currently there is no national Australian guideline for selecting which patients could benefit from using a pump, but most diabetes centres offering pump therapy have guidelines for selecting patients and initiating pump therapy. In 2016 the Australian Government introduced subsidies for CGM under the National Diabetes Supplies Scheme, but only for people younger than 21. NICE (2003) recommended that pumps be funded for people with T1DM who suffer recurrent severe hypoglycaemia. Thus, although CGMs provides very useful information about ambient blood glucose and glucose variability, it is not used as widely as it could be, largely because of cost. Commonly used CGM systems include Dexcom, MiniMed 640G and Guardian Connect.

Continuous blood glucose sensors

Continuous glucose monitoring is a step towards a closed-loop system that links continuous blood glucose measurements to a computer-driven insulin infusion system to approximate normal glucose homeostasis. Modern sensors consist of a disposable sensor probe, which is inserted into subcutaneous tissue using an insertion device and connected to a battery-powered transmitter. The transmitter sends a signal to a receiver, which displays the blood glucose reading. The sensors last for approximately three to five days.

After the sensor is attached to the transmitter, warm-up periods between 2 and 10 hours are required and capillary blood glucose testing is required to calibrate the system. There are at least three sensors on the market and each manufacturer recommends ongoing calibration. In addition, abnormal sensor readings need to be confirmed with a capillary test before corrective

Table 5.4   Some commonly encountered factors that affect insulin absorption.

Accelerated	Delayed
Type of insulin	Type of insulin
Exercise	Low body temperature
High body temperature	Condition of injection sites
Condition of injection sites	Poor circulation, hypertrophy, and hyperlipodystrophy from constantly injecting into the same area
Massage round injection site	Smoking
Depth of injection	Long-acting insulins

action is taken. Thus, the current sensors are adjuncts to, rather than replacements for, capillary blood glucose testing but they enable people to have several days break from finger pricking. The cost is prohibitive for many people.

The choice of regimen and insulin delivery system depends on personal preference, management targets and the willingness and ability of the patient to monitor their blood glucose. Many factors can influence insulin absorption and consequently blood glucose; some of these factors are shown in Table 5.4.

Subcutaneous insulin sliding scales and top-up regimens

A sliding insulin scale refers to subcutaneous insulin doses administered to reduce hyperglycemia detected on routine blood glucose monitoring. Supplemental insulin is administered at mealtimes added to the usual insulin dose based on the blood glucose level and pattern according to an algorithm or programs such as DAFNE and Diabetes Education and Self-Management for Ongoing and Newly Diagnosed (DESMOND).

However, many insulin sliding scales (top-up doses) are reactive and may not treat the underlying cause of the hyperglycaemia (Hirsch et al. 1995). Sliding scale/top up doses are not recommended, especially for older people (American Geriatrics Society [AGS] Beers Criteria 2019).

Using subcutaneous sliding scales in day-to-day management can lead to disassociation between the insulin regimen and the other parameters that affect the blood glucose such as the timing of meals, effects of illness, and medications, for example, corticosteroids and the counter-regulatory response to hypoglycaemia.

Using sliding scales to stabilise blood glucose for newly diagnosed, unstable or brittle diabetes is *not* generally recommended (Katz 1991). It is preferable to monitor the blood glucose over 24–48 hours and adjust the insulin regimen according to the emerging pattern considering the action profile of the various insulins and other factors that affect the blood glucose level. Top-up doses can predispose the individual to hypoglycaemia- and hypoglycaemia-related adverse events (Queale et al. 1997, AGS (American Geriatrics Society) 2018).

Top-up or stat doses of insulin

Sliding scale top-up insulin doses continue to be used, especially in aged care facilities despite there being no evidence of any benefit and long term evidence of harm. In fact, diabetes experts have been advocating for a proactive prospective approach to managing hyperglycaemia in hospital and in aged care facilities rather than using sliding scale/top-up since 1981 (Queale et al. 1997; AGS 2018).

Top-up or stat doses of insulin refer to temporary supplementary doses of insulin, usually rapid- or short-acting, given to correct hyperglycaemia found on routine blood glucose monitoring. Such doses are often given independently of meals and of any possible underlying cause. Top-up dosing commonly occurs in aged-care homes, is reactionary, and does not address the underlying causes of hyperglycaemia. Top-up doses to correct isolated hyperglycaemia are not recommended in older people (AGS 2018). See Chapter 12. When necessary, extra supplementary insulin (correction dose) is best added to the next due dose of insulin rather than being given in isolation.

Adopting a proactive problem-solving approach, considering the management regimen, and nursing/medical actions occurring at the time will provide important insight into the cause/s of the hyperglycaemia, which can be appropriately treated. For example, hyperglycaemia might be a consequence of pain or fear, in which case the most effective strategy would be to manage the pain/fear. In addition, non-medicine options might be effective. Often, top-up doses continue for days before the overall blood glucose profile and medicine requirements or the underlying causes are considered and have serious adverse consequences such as DKA, HHS, and death.

Practice points

(1) There are no documented benefits of insulin sliding scales or top-up doses in people in hospital (Gearhart et al. 1994; Queale et al. 1997; AGS 2018).
(2) Insulin sliding scales are associated with a threefold higher risk of hyperglycaemia, especially when basal insulin is not used (Queale et al. 1997).
(3) Sliding scales are not recommended for older people (AGS 2018).
(4) Sliding scales could help maintain acceptable blood glucose levels in hospital if they are used proactively according to a logical algorithm based on the action profiles of the relevant insulin regimen and delivered in relation to meals.
(5) IV insulin infusions require a sliding insulin scale and are an example of proactive hyperglycaemia management.

Intravenous insulin infusions

The IV route is preferred for very ill patients because the absorption of insulin is rapid and more reliable than from poorly perfused muscle and fat tissue. Absorption may be erratic in these patients, especially if they are hypotensive. The aims of the insulin infusion are to:

- Prevent the liver converting glycogen and fatty acids into glucose and therefore avoid hyperglycaemia, that is, restrain hepatic glucose output.
- Prevent utilisation of fatty acids and therefore limit ketone formation.
- Reduce protein catabolism and therefore limit production of glucose substrates.
- Enhance wound healing by limiting protein catabolism and normalising neutrophil function.
- Reduce peripheral resistance to insulin.
- If hyperglycaemia is present, gradually lower the blood glucose concentration to ~10 mmol/l without subjecting the patient to hypoglycaemia.

Intravenous insulin infusions are associated with lower morbidity and mortality in surgical settings (see Chapter 9), during acute illness such as MI (see Chapter 8), in patients requiring parenteral nutrition (Cheung et al. 2005), and in intensive care settings (Quinn et al. 2006). In fact, van den Berghe et al. (2001) demonstrated improved outcomes using insulin infusions in acutely ill nondiabetics as well as people with diabetes.

However, a recent systematic review was inconclusive about the benefits of IV insulin infusions for people with diabetes in hospital who are not critically ill (Colunga-Lozano et al. 2018). The authors suggested basal bolus insulin regimens result in better short-term glycaemic control, but could increase the risk of severe hypoglycaemia.

Two main insulin delivery methods are used:

(1) Insulin given via an infusion pump, and fluid administered separately.
(2) Glucose, insulin, potassium, and fluids are combined (GIK), which is efficient and safe. The glucose component is usually 5% or 10% dextrose, depending on the calories required (Dagogo-Jack and Alberti 2002).

The medication order for the infusion must be clearly and legibly written on the treatment sheet. Insulin doses for IV insulin infusions are usually 0.1 unit/kg/hour. Sometimes an initial bolus of 5–10 units is given. In general, a low-dose infusion such as this has been shown to reduce the blood glucose and prevent ketosis and acidosis as effectively as high-dose regimens, without the added risk of hypoglycaemia. The rate at which the insulin is to be administered should be written in ml/hour and units to be delivered. Several protocols exist; the following is one example only. People with insulin-treated type 2 diabetes may require one to two units/hour if they are overweight and insulin resistant.

The infusion rate is adjusted according to the patient's blood glucose results (tested one to two-hourly). For example:

Blood glucose (mmol/l)	Insulin (units/hour)
0–5.9	0
6–11.1	1
12–15.1	2
16–19	3
>19.1	4
>24	Notify doctor

The insulin order and blood glucose results should be reviewed regularly. The duration of the infusion depends on the clinical status of the patient.

Preparing the Insulin Solution to be Infused

Two people should check and make up the solution according to the medication order and hospital protocols. In many cases, it is prepared and labelled in the pharmacy.

Practice points

(1) Only clear rapid- or short-acting insulin is used for insulin infusions. Great care should be taken not to use clear long-acting insulin analogues in insulin infusions.
(2) Insulin is known to bind to plastic. Flushing the first 50 ml through the giving set tubing prevents this nonspecific absorption into the infusion equipment.

Uses of insulin infusions

General use (during surgical procedures)

Insulin is added to 4% dextrose in one-fifth normal saline or 5% dextrose. The infusion is often given via burette or more commonly an infusion pump at 120 ml/hour (i.e. eight-hourly rate; see previous example scale). Monitor blood glucose one to two-hourly and review with medical staff *regularly*.

Special needs

- Myocardial infarction. In many areas an IV insulin infusion is commenced when the patient presents to the emergency department and continues for ~24 hours, after which time subcutaneous insulin is commenced (Malmberg 1997); see Chapter 8.
- Open heart and other surgery.
- Ketoacidosis.
- Hyperosmolar states.
- Severe septicaemia or other infections.
- Intensive care unit (ICU) situations.

These situations always require the use of a controlled-rate infusion pumps to ensure accurate insulin dosing. It is often necessary to limit the amount of fluid administered to avoid cerebral oedema in these situations, especially in young children and the elderly. Standard regimens include:

(1) Haemaccel 100 ml + 100 units rapid or fast-acting insulin = 1 unit/1 ml, used in ICU and administered via an infusion pump.
(2) Haemaccel 500 ml + 100 units rapid or short-acting insulin = 1 unit/5 ml via an infusion pump.

People who are insulin-resistant, such as those who:

• Have liver disease
• Are on corticosteroid therapy
• Are obese
• Have a serious infection
• May require more insulin, that is, a high-dose infusion (more units per hour)

Practice points

  • Subcutaneous insulin must be given before removing the infusion and the patient must be eating and drinking normally to avoid hyperglycaemia because of the short half-life of insulin given IV.
  • Ceasing the infusion before a meal enables a smooth transition to subcutaneous insulin.

Risks associated with insulin infusions

• Hypoglycaemia
• Cardiac arrhythmias
• Sepsis at the IV site
• Fluid overload and cerebral oedema especially in children, which is associated with high morbidity and mortality rates

Factors affecting insulin delivery via IV infusions:

• Accuracy of the system, including blood glucose testing
• Stability of the solution
• Circulatory insufficiency

Mistakes associated with insulin infusions

(1) Where a burette is used and if insulin is added to the burette rather than the bag of IV fluid, refilling the burette from the bag results in no insulin being administered and hyperglycaemia results.
(2) An incorrect amount of insulin added to the bag/burette can be a result of inadequate checking, not using an insulin syringe to draw up the insulin or failing to check illegible medical orders, especially where insulin doses are written as 'U/s' instead of 'units' and the dose is misinterpreted.
(3) Problems can arise if the insulin infusion is run at the same time through the same site as other intravenous fluids, for example, 4% dextrose in 1/5 normal saline. The most common method is to infuse the different fluids through the one IV cannula using a three-way adaptor (octopus): see Figure 5.4.

Usually, the dextrose or saline is running at a faster rate than the insulin infusion. Problems can arise if there is a complete or partial blockage of the cannula. The force of gravity pushing the fluid towards the vein can actually cause the dextrose/saline to flow back up the slower-flowing insulin

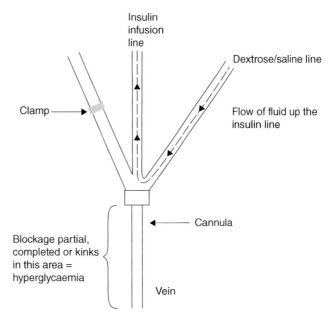

Figure 5.4 Possible results of a blockage in the IV cannula and three-way adaptor during the concurrent administration of insulin and dextrose/saline.

line resulting in high blood glucose levels. Figure 5.4 depicts the result of a blockage in the IV cannula and three-way adaptor during the concurrent administration of insulin and dextrose/saline.

If hyperglycaemia occurs during an insulin infusion check the following:

- The tubing and adaptors are patent.
- Insulin has been added to the burette/bag.
- The amount of insulin added is correct.
- Determine possible sources of infection, for example, UTI, the feet.

Insulin allergy

Insulin allergies are rare with modern, highly purified insulins but they do occasionally occur.

Two types of reaction have been reported:

(1) Localised weal and flare with itching due to antihistamine reactions
(2) Generalised anaphylaxis, which is rare

Clinical observation

Indicating insulin doses by writing 'U/s' still occurs despite the known association with adverse events and incorrect, in some cases fatal, insulin doses being administered. Incorrect, usually excess, insulin has been administered and can result in serious hypoglycaemia. For example, in Australia, in an aged-care facility, a patient died and a court case ensued. Both the nurse who administered the insulin and the doctor who wrote the prescription were found to have contributed to the person's death. There were other issues involved with the particular patient, but the case highlights the importance of accurate documentation and the nurse's responsibility to check.

Insulin doses should always be indicated by writing or typing 'units' after the amount to be given.

Allergic reactions are most likely to occur where people have been on insulin previously, for example, during gestational diabetes mellitus (GDM), surgery or acute illness in people with type 2 diabetes where insulin is used intermittently, for example, during surgery and with corticosteroid medications, and when injection sites are not rotated. The reaction may be due to the preservatives and other incipients in insulin rather than insulin itself.

To diagnose insulin allergy a careful case history is required. The person should be given insulin and observed where resuscitation equipment is available. Any reaction should be carefully documented. Blood test for IgG and other immune response factors can be helpful. If insulin allergy is present, a desensitisation programme may be required. Local reactions can be managed by using a different insulin and antihistamine creams (Williams 1993; Dunning et al. 1998).

Pancreas transplants

Pancreas transplants of either the whole pancreas or islet cells or the pancreas and kidneys is available to some people with diabetes (e.g. those with autonomic neuropathy causing life-threatening hypoglycaemic unawareness and end-stage renal failure). Immunosuppressive therapy is required, and if rejection does not occur, the response is good. The transplanted pancreas/beta cells secrete insulin and HbA1c normalises in approximately three months.

Obtaining pancreases for transplantation or to harvest islet cells is difficult, as is actually separating the islet cells from pancreatic tissue. Other options are under study, such as beta cell engineering and stem cell cloning. Islet cell transplants have been undertaken successfully in Canada, Australia, the United States, and in the United Kingdom and an international islet cell consortium has been established to try to reproduce positive results.

Stabilising diabetes

Rationale

Optimal blood glucose control can prevent or delay the onset of long-term complications. Insulin is frequently required by people with type 2 diabetes to achieve optimal control, as indicated.

Stabilising diabetes refers to the process of achieving an optimal blood glucose range, helping the person acquire appropriate diabetes knowledge and managing diabetic complications, either acute or chronic, but the term usually specifically refers to commencing insulin. Stabilisation may occur at initial diagnosis of diabetes, when a change of treatment is indicated, for example, transfer from GLM to combination therapy or insulin, and for antenatal care in GDM.

Some people need to be admitted to hospital to stabilise their diabetes, for example, complex issues that cannot be identified in outpatient/primary care settings, where clinical observation is necessary, or where the person is admitted with a concurrent illness or is diagnosed during an admission and commences insulin while in hospital.

Stabilising diabetes in hospital

People admitted to hospital to improve their metabolic control (stabilisation) are not generally ill and should be encouraged to:

(1) Keep active.
(2) Wear clothes instead of pyjamas.
(3) Perform diabetes self-care tasks such as blood glucose monitoring and insulin administration.

They will require support, encouragement, and consistent advice. The time spent in hospital should be kept to a minimum.

Nursing responsibilities

(1) Inform the appropriate staff about the person's admission, especially the diabetes nurse specialist/diabetes educator, specialist team, and dietitian soon after they are admitted.

(2) Assess the patient carefully (refer to Chapter 2).

(3) Monitor blood glucose according to the individual's need or usual protocols; for example, 7 A.M., 11 A.M., 4 P.M., and 9 P.M. In some cases, postprandial levels are also performed (see Chapter 3).

(4) Assess the patient's ability to monitor his or her own blood glucose and/or administer insulin, or teach these skills if the person is newly diagnosed.

(5) Ensure diabetes knowledge is assessed and updated regularly, refer to a diabetes educator.

(6) Refer to a dietitian to decide an appropriate food and exercise plan with the individual. New learning may include insulin techniques, sharps disposal, hypoglycaemia and home management during illness.

(7) Check temperature, pulse and respiration (TPR) daily, or every second day, if indicated.

(8) Check blood pressure (BP), lying and standing, daily if indicated.

(9) Ensure all blood samples, urine collections, and special tests are performed accurately. The opportunity is often taken to perform a comprehensive complication screen and education assessment while the person is in hospital, especially if they often miss appointments with health professionals or it has not been performed for some time. Inspection of injection sites and assessment of the person's psychological status should be included. These tests include electrocardiogram (ECG), eye referral, spot urine collection for creatinine, and microalbumin and blood tests such as lipids, HbA1c, and kidney function.

(10) Ensure the person has supplies, such as test strips, lancets, insulin device, before discharge and that the appropriate follow-up appointments are made.

(11) Ensure the individual has a contact telephone number in case they need advice.

Community and outpatient insulin stabilisation

The types of outpatient service provided for people with diabetes include:

- Diabetes education
- Commencement on diabetes medication (GLM, insulin)
- Complication screening and assessment
- Blood glucose testing
- Consultations with dietitian, diabetes nurse specialist/diabetes educator or diabetes specialist
- Clinical assessment
- Education is a key factor in a person's understanding and acceptance of diabetes. Diabetes educators often know the person well from the outpatient service and can assist ward nurses to plan appropriate nursing care and understand the person's needs.

Practice point

The specific protocol and policy of the relevant healthcare setting should be followed and all contacts including telephone advice documented. An example protocol for insulin stabilisation in the community or on an outpatient basis is shown on pages 166 and 167.

Objectives of stabilisation onto insulin

Short-Term Objectives

(1) Reassure the individual and their family and allay the fear that everything about diabetes must be learned at once.

(2) Lifestyle should be modified as little as possible.
(3) Establish trust between the patient and the diabetes team.
(4) Gradually normalise blood glucose and lipids.
(5) Teach the 'survival skills' necessary for the person to be safe at home:
- How to draw/dial up and administer insulin
- Blood glucose monitoring
- Recognising and treating hypoglycaemia
- Sick day management
- How and when to obtain advice, e.g. provide contact telephone number

Long-Term Objectives
The aim in the long term is for the individual to:

(1) Develop appropriate coping and problem-solving skills and resilience to manage their diabetes and life in general.
(2) Accept diabetes as part of their life and recognise their role and responsibility in the successful management of the diabetes.
(3) Be able to make appropriate changes in insulin doses, carbohydrate intake and activity to maintain acceptable blood glucose levels.
(4) Be able to maintain an acceptable range of blood glucose, HbA1c, and lipids.
(5) Be able to maintain a healthy weight range.
(6) Modify risk factors to prevent or delay the onset of the long-term complications of diabetes and therefore the need for hospital admissions.
(7) Attend regular medical/education appointments.
(8) Receive ongoing support and encouragement from the diabetes team.
(9) Maintain psychological well-being and quality of life.

Clinical observations

- People are often overwhelmed, unsure what to do and confused by conflicting or inaccurate advice from health professionals, family and friends, and the media, or obtained on the internet.
- These issues frequently need to be addressed and clarified before commencing the insulin stabilisation process.
- The therapeutic relationship and trust between health professional and the person with diabetes is a vital aspect of their adjustment to having diabetes and changes in their diabetic management or status. Therapeutic relationships should be cultivated nurtured and treasured.

Rationale for choosing community/outpatient stabilisation

Community/outpatient stabilisation onto insulin is preferred for the following reasons:

(1) It can avoid the 'sick role', which is often associated with a hospital admission.
(2) It is cost effective; that is, does not require a hospital bed.
(3) It involves less time away from work and usual activity for the patient, who can therefore be stabilised according to their usual routine, rather than hospital routines and food.
(4) To encourage self-reliance and confidence.

The person must be:

- Able to attend the service for the required period, which depends on the individual service. In some cases twice a day visits may be necessary. Telephone contact should be maintained as long as necessary.

- Physically and mentally capable of performing blood glucose monitoring and insulin administration, or have assistance to do so.

In addition, some social/family support is helpful initially for older people and is required for children.

The process of stabilisation

(1) The process should involve members of the diabetes team and relatives/carers as appropriate.
(2) Communication, especially among the doctor, practice nurses, diabetes nurse specialist/diabetes educator, dietitian, and patient, is essential.
(3) People should be assessed on an individual basis so that appropriate education goals and blood glucose ranges can be determined. The insulin regimen and insulin delivery system depends on individual requirements; follow-up advice and early reassessment must be available.
(4) Formal teaching times should take account of the individual's commitments as far as is practicable.
(5) Adequate charting and documentation of progress should be recorded after each session: blood glucose results, ability to manage insulin technique, goals of management.
(6) Effective education strategies should be used. Stabilisation can be undertaken in groups (see Chapter 16).

A sample protocol for outpatient stabilisation is shown at the end of this chapter. It is included here to give nurses an overview of the kind of information required and the complex issues people with diabetes have to deal with, often when they feel vulnerable. Other protocols also exist.

Practice points

(1) People of all ages can be overwhelmed and unable to manage emergencies.
(2) Clinicians and well-meaning family and friends often give inaccurate advice that either confuses the person with diabetes or causes them to ignore all advice.
(3) People with T1DM are at risk of ketoacidosis but often do not have ketone testing equipment at home, or if they do, it can be out of date (Sumner et al. 2000; Tay et al. 2001).
(4) Constant, diplomatic reminders are important. An episode in hospital represents an opportunity to remind people about diabetes self-management and care during intercurrent illness; see Chapter 7.

Traditionally, initiation of insulin occurred on an individual basis. Recent reports suggest that group education programmes for commencing insulin can be effective and achieve reductions in HbA1c and competent insulin self-care by individuals (Almond et al. 2001; Yki-Jarvinen et al. 2007). Such programmes could be a cost-effective way to manage the increasing numbers of people being commenced on insulin as a result of the DCCT and UKPDS trials, provided competent facilitation is available.

Lipid-lowering agents

Normalising the lipid profile is an essential component of diabetes management guidelines. People with diabetes, especially T2DM, are at significant risk of cardiovascular disease, which is often present at diagnosis, unless the blood glucose and lipids can be kept within normal limits. Generally, the aim is to reduce cholesterol, especially LDL-c and triglycerides, and increase HDL-c. HDL helps remove LDL cholesterol but it might also have anti-inflammatory and antithrombotic properties. HDL-c is inversely related to triglycerides in that high triglyceride levels are associated with the removal of cholesterol from HDL-c to more atherogenic lipopro-teins and lipoprotein precursors. HDL-c is often low in T2DM, partly because of the increased production of triglyceride-rich lipoproteins. LDL-c may not be elevated because of the increased level of cholesterol LDL, which suggests relying on LDL-c levels may underestimate the cardio-vascular risk in people with type 2 diabetes (Sullivan 2008).

High triglycerides >1.7 mmol/l (>150 mg/dl) significantly increases the risk of myocardial infarction, but other risk factors such as obesity and inflammatory processes are important and are often exacerbated by low levels of HDL <immol/l (40 mg/dl in men and < 1.3 (50 mg/dl) in women (Colquhoun 2002; ADA 2019). The cholesterol content of HDL, HDL-c, could be protective in that it reflects removal of cholesterol from atherosclerotic plaque. Low HDL-c is an independent risk factor for cardiovascular disease (Lee et al. 2017).

Weight loss, reducing saturated fat in the diet, exercise, and stopping smoking all effectively raise HDL-c. Alcohol increases HDL-c but excess consumption is associated with significant health risks because it causes weight gain, especially around the abdomen, liver damage, contrib-utes to malnutrition, and reduces LDL-c and triglycerides, and increases the risk of breast cancer in women. Controlling blood glucose is integral to controlling lipids (Lipid Study Group 1998; RACGP study 2016-2018; see Gunston et al. 2016; ADA 2019). Current lipid targets aim for total cholesterol <4 and triglyceride and LDL-C < 2 and HDL-C > 1 generally and especially in people with existing heart disease (National Heart Foundation of Australia 2001).

The ADA (2019) recommended using statins to prevent cardiovascular disease in all people with T2DM, particularly reducing LDL-c 100 mg/dl, and initiating statins in people with diabetes over 40 years without cardiovascular disease to reach the LDL-c target. Likewise, the Collaborative Atorvastatin Diabetes Study (CARDS) suggested that statins are indicated in most people with type 2 diabetes (Colhoun et al. 2004), whereas the atorvastatin study for the preven-tion of coronary heart disease endpoints in non-insulin dependent diabetes mellitus (ASPEN) (Knopp et al. 2006) suggested people at low risk of cardiovascular disease might receive less benefit from statin therapy. Not all people with diabetes have the same 10-year risk of cardio-vascular disease; thus, lipid-lowering therapy needs to be commenced according to individual level of risk (Grundy et al. 2004). However, lipid-lowering agents, including statins, must be used with an appropriate diet and exercise regimen (Ridker 2012). Major cardiovascular prevention trials include:

- Antihypertensive and Lipid-Lowering Treatment to Prevent Heart Attack Trial (ALLHAT), which was one of the first trials to assess the efficacy of statins (Pravostatin) in people with and without diabetes. It failed to show a significant reduction in mortality but there was a trend towards a higher mortality risk in people with LDL-c > 130 mg/dl. The findings were similar for those with and without diabetes.
- Heart Protection Study, which also included people with and without diabetes. The all-cause mortality and major cardiovascular event rate were significantly lower in the Simvastatin group. The outcomes were similar for those with and without diabetes in the Simvastatin group, but people with diabetes in the placebo group had more vascular events than nondia-betics, and the risk was additive. The researchers suggested people with diabetes have a risk equivalent to those with preexisting cardiovascular disease and that statin therapy is beneficial for people with diabetes without cardiovascular disease and LDL-C close to the target.
- Anglo-Scandinavian Cardiac Outcomes Trial-Blood Pressure Lowering Arm (ASCOTBPLA) compared two antihypertensive regimens in people with at least three cardiovascular risk fac-tors. A substudy (ASCOT-LLA), compared Atorvastatin to placebo. ASCOT was stopped after an average of 3.3 years because there was no significant difference in the primary endpoints. There was an overall benefit from using Atorvastatin but it was not significant in people with diabetes. However, the researchers recommended statin therapy should be considered in peo-ple with type 2 diabetes and hypertension.
- CARDS included people with type 2 diabetes, LDL-c, no history of cardiovascular disease, and one additional cardiovascular risk factor and used 10 mg of Atorvastatin. There was a trend that failed to reach significance, towards lower all-cause mortality and LDL-c was lower (<100 mg/dl)

in the Atorvastatin group than in the placebo group. CARDS researchers suggested that there was no specific LDL-c threshold at which statins should be initiated in people with type 2 diabetes. The American Diabetes Association Standards of Medical Care in Diabetes, developed in 2007 (American Diabetes Association 2007), recommendation that people with diabetes > age 40 and no cardiovascular diseases should be commenced on a statin regardless of their LDL-c level. The Canadian Diabetes Association (CDA) (Lau et al. 2007) recommended the LDL-c target for people with diabetes be lowered to 2 mmol/l from 2.5 mmol/l and placed less emphasis on the LDL/HDL ratio as a primary endpoint of treatment. The triglyceride level at which treatment should be commenced was also revised to >10 mmol/l from 4.5 mmol/l. The CDA suggested fenofibrate be commenced to reduce the risk of pancreatitis and a second lipid-lowering agent be added if targets were not achieved after four to six months.

- ASPEN included people with type 2 diabetes and a history of cardiovascular disease and compared 10 mg Atorvastatin with placebo. The protocol was amended to include people with no history of cardiovascular disease following changes in the cardiovascular management guidelines. The results were not statistically significant, but there was a trend towards clinical improvements. The researchers concluded that the level of risk (presence of multiple risk factors) affects the degree to which statins reduce the cardiovascular risk in type 2 diabetes without cardiovascular disease.
- Veterans Affairs High-Density Lipoprotein Cholesterol Intervention Trial (VA-HIT) indicated low HDL-c is a treatable risk factor in people with and without diabetes. VA-HIT results indicate fibrates reduce cardiovascular risk by lowering LDL-c but only had a small effect on increasing HDL-c.
- FIELD study, which used fenofibrate, showed reductions in the rates of macular oedema and proliferative retinopathy but did not show a significant increase in HDL-c. It lowered LDL-c and there was a reduction in major cardiovascular events in the intervention group (Keech et al. 2005). Statins were added in the placebo group, which may have influenced the results.
- The Framingham Study indicated that low HDL-c is an independent risk factor for cardiovascular disease in people with diabetes and nondiabetics and developed a cardiovascular disease risk calculator (Anderson et al. 1991).
- PROSPER, which studied the effects of pravastatin on all-cause mortality in people aged 70–82 years with cardiovascular risk factors or cardiovascular disease, but failed to show a reduction in all-cause mortality. However, a later meta-analysis that included the 4S, cholesterol and recurrent events (CARE), long-term intervention with pravastatin in ischaemic disease (LIPID), heart protection study (HPS) trials, and unpublished data from PROSPER showed a reduction in all-cause mortality by 22%, as well as cardiovascular mortality by 30%, nonfatal MI by 26% and the need for revascularisation by 30% and stroke by 25% (Afilalo et al. 2008). Afilalo et al. also suggested that older people do not have higher rates of serious adverse events than younger people but they did experience higher rates of myalgia in the statin and placebo groups. Masoudi (2007) showed ruvastatin reduced LDL-c and C-reactive protein but did not significantly reduce the combined risk of cardiovascular disease in older people (mean age 73 years), and there were fewer admissions to hospital than in the placebo group.
- Other studies such as the West Scotland Coronary Prevention Study (WESTCOPS), Air Force/Texas Coronary Athersclerosis Prevention Study (AFCAPS/TexCAPS), also showed cardiovascular benefits (Ridker 2012).

Management strategies should be based on the absolute risk rather than the lipid level alone. Individual risk assessment should include cardiovascular status, age, gender, the presence of hypertension, smoking, and family history of hyperlipidaemia, hypertension, and cardiac disease (Chapter 8). Management strategies consist of:

- Dietary modification, including reducing salt, alcohol, and saturated fat in the diet and increasing omega-3 fatty acids (see Chapter 4).
- Low-dose aspirin to reduce platelet aggregation.
- ACE inhibitors (ACEI) to control blood pressure and other antihypertensive agents as indicated.

- Stopping smoking; see Chapter 10.
- Lipid-lowering agents are recommended when the absolute cardiovascular risk is >15% in the next 5 years or when the risk is >10–15% in people with a family history of premature heart disease or who have metabolic syndrome (National Heart Foundation of Australia and Cardiac Society of Australia and New Zealand 2005). Most people will be commenced on a statin unless they are contraindicated. Diet and exercise therapy must continue, even when lipid-lowering medicines are indicated. Metformin and TZDs might have some small effect on increasing HDL-c and Rimonabant is associated with significant improvements in HDL-c, possibly because of the associated weight loss.
  - Statins reduce LDL-c and have some effect on HDL. They reduce the risk of future cardiovascular disease by about 30%. However, long-term adherence to statins is poor and many older people are not commenced on these agents despite the improved cardiovascular outcomes (Diamond and Kaul 2008).
  - Nicotinic acid very effectively increases HDL-c, but is associated with side effects and non-adherence is significant. In addition, it increases blood glucose. Although the increase is not significant, it contributes to overall increased cardiovascular risk.
  - Ezetimibe can be administered with a statin but it only has a modest effect on HDL-c.
  - Fibrates.
  - A new class of lipid-lowering agents, Cholesterol Ester Transfer Protein (CEPT), which block the transfer of cholesterol from HDL-c to more atherosclerotic lipoproteins, is under trial. The first agent, Torcetrapib, significantly raised HDL-c but did not prevent the progression to atherosclerosis. The trial (ILLUMINATE) was stopped early due to the rate of cardiovascular events in the treatment group (Nissen et al. 2007). The adverse results triggered debate about the advisability of using medicines to treat HDL. Other lipid-lowering agents under trial include Liver-X-receptor agonists, which promote cholesterol transport and reduce atherosclerosis in animal models, endothelial lipase inhibitors, which raise HDL-c and apolipoprotein A-1 mimetic peptides that improve HDL function in animal models (Zadelaar et al. 2007).
  - Coaching.

Table 5.5 depicts the major classes of lipid-lowering agents (Colquhoun 2000, 2002; Australian Medicines Handbook 2019; ADA 2019).

Side effects

The side effects of lipid-lowering agents often contribute to nonadherence to these medicines:
- Statins: tendonitis and myositis occurs in ~2% of people (Marie et al. 2008). Regular assessment to detect these side effects should occur, especially during the first year. Poor sleep quality has been associated with simvastatin but not pravastatin (Golomb 2007). Taking simvastatin earlier in the day may reduce these effects. Simons (2002) suggested measuring creatine kinase (CK) before commencing statins and then six-monthly when lipids are checked could help interpret minor changes in muscle enzymes, especially in people at risk of muscle effects such as in women, and those with a small body frame, multisystem disease, polypharmacy, perioperative, interactions with medicines such as cyclosporin, azole antifungals, macrolide antibiotics, some antidepressants, large amounts of grapefruit juice, and alcohol. The American College of Cardiology, American Heart Association, and National Heart Lung and Blood Institute (Pasternak et al. 2002) recommended:
  - Advising people with no symptoms and raised CK to immediately report generalised muscle aches and pains.
  - Monitoring the individual if the CK is normal and the muscle effects are mild or change to another statin or another lipid-lowering agent.
  - Referring people with very high CK to a lipid specialist but continue statin therapy until the individual is assessed.
  - Carefully monitoring muscle enzymes in people with raised CK and muscle aches. Discontinue statin therapy if clinically indicated, for example, severe symptoms such as fatigue, significant pain, or an interaction with statin occurs.
  - Stop statins if CK is ≥10 (upper limit of normal).

Table 5.5 Lipid-lowering agents.

Lipid-lowering agent and main action	Management considerations
HMG-CoA reductase inhibitors (statins): reduce LDL-c and have a modest effect on triglycerides and HDL, may increase bone mineral density, for example: Atorvastatin Simvastatin Fluvastatin Rouvastatin	Test liver function on commencing and six months after commencing. Use caution if liver disease is present. Reduce the dose if the patient commences cyclosporine. Monitor creatinine kinase (CK) and effects on muscles and tendons. Generally not recommended during pregnancy[a].
Ezetimebe reduces LDL-c by ~18% and by up to 20% if combined with a statin Ezetimebe combined with simvastatin	Prescribing authority is required in Australia and specific criteria need to be met.
Fibrates: Reduce cholesterol and triglycerides and increase HDL-c, for example: Fenofibrate Gemfibrosil	Can be combined with HMG-CoA after a trial on monotherapy but the risk of muscle toxicity is increased if used with statins or other fibrates. Monitor CK and liver function six weeks after starting and again in six months.
Bile acid sequestrants (resins) enhance LDL-c lowering effects of HMG-CoA agents – reduce triglyceride and HDL-c, for example: Cholestyramine Cholestyramine hydrochloride	It allows lower doses of the resins to be used. It slows absorption of oral hypoglycaemic agents. Hypoglycaemia risk increases when used with these agents. Administer 1.5 hours apart. They can impair the absorption of other medicines such as statins, fat-soluble vitamins, and thyroxine. Can be used with a statin.
Low-dose nicotinic acid	Can be given with HMG-CoA agents.

Note: The main classes of lipid-lowering medicines are depicted. Relevant prescribing information should be consulted. Combinations of statins and antihypertensive agents are also available, for example, amlopipine bensylate with Atorvastatin in eight dose combinations, which are indicated for people with hypertension and/or angina who meet the prescribing criteria for lipid-lowering agents. Educating and supporting the person to maintain a healthy lifestyle and enhance their medication self-management and improve medication adherence is essential.
[a]Karamermer and Roos-Hesselink (2007).

- GIT (glucose impaired tolerance) disturbances (clofibrate).

Many people discontinue taking their lipid-lowering agents because they are unconvinced about the need, perceive that they have poor efficacy, or dislike the associated side effects. Nurses can play a key role in encouraging people to adhere to their medications by explaining the reason they need them and suggesting ways to limit minor side effects. For example, tai chi might help reduce the muscle effects of statins.

Monitoring lipid medicines

Current lipid and other management guidelines recommend that blood lipids should be tested at diagnosis and then at least yearly. People using lipid-lowering agents should have their lipid levels measured more frequently. Lipid targets were discussed in Chapter 3. Not achieving targets is not necessarily a failure: any reduction in lipid levels has a beneficial effect.

Blood glucose should also be monitored and GLMs adjusted as needed to reach blood glucose targets. Persistent hyperglycaemia can cause hypertriglyceridaemia, which usually falls along with cholesterol if blood glucose and weight improve. Mixed hyperlipidaemia is best treated with a statin or a fibrate initially depending on the underlying lipid abnormality. Doses are usually adjusted at four-week intervals. For example, more than 80% of the lipid-lowering effect of statins is achieved at 50% of the maximal dose (Jackowski 2008a).

Liver function tests and CK should be tested before commencing lipid-lowering therapy, then in approximately four to eight weeks and subsequently when doses are adjusted or if clinically indicated. For example, renal impairment, older people, severe muscle weakness. Statins may need to be temporarily ceased if the person requires macrolide antibiotics. Stopping statins is associated with an increased risk of a cardiac event, especially in the first weeks (Rossi 2007).

If the triglycerides are <4.0 mmol/l or between 2 and 4 mmol/l and HDL is <1 mmol/l, gemfibrozil may be the medicine of choice. Consider whether vitamin A, D, E, and K (the fat-soluble vitamins) supplements are needed if bile acid resins are used in high doses for long periods of time.

Omega-3 fish oils 2–5 mg/day effectively lower triglycerides (Rossi 2007) and may be a beneficial addition to other agents for hypertriglyceridaemia or mixed hyperlipidaemia. However, several products are available on the market and doses are not the same in all products or brands. It is important that people read labels and seek professional advice when using these medicines. In addition, they can interact with other medicines.

Antihypertensive agents

Hypertension is a significant risk factor for cardiovascular disease. Thus, achieving and maintaining normotension is a major therapeutic goal. There are many medicines that reduce blood pressure. Therefore the particular antihypertensive agent used depends on the underlying cardiovascular abnormality/ies and specific benefits and risks to the individual. Diabetes is associated with several cardiovascular abnormalities; thus several agents are often required. Generally, beta blockers are started at a low dose and the dose gradually increased, depending on the agent used to improve left ventricular function and reduce the risk of death in patients with heart failure (Jackowski 2008b). Side effects of beta blockers include:

- Fluid retention, which might be exacerbated by concomitant use of TZDs, nonsteroidal anti-inflammatory drugs (NSAIDs), and COX-2 selective agents.
- Hypotension, which might increase the risk of falls and may be the result of an interaction with another antihypertensive agent or tricyclic antidepressants.
- Bradycardia.
- Severe fatigue; other causes should be considered such as depression, hypothyroidism, and hyperglycaemia.
- Bronchospasm can occur with beta blockers in patients with asthma and chronic obstructive pulmonary disease (COPD).
- Weight gain with some beta blockers such as atenolol, which was still apparent at the 20-year follow-up of the UKPDS (Standl et al. 2012). Atenolol was also associated with a slight increase in tryglycerides and a mean HbA1c increase of 0.6% that required an increase in GLM doses in the UKPDS.

ACEI are considered first-line therapy in diabetes because they have renoprotective, cardioprotective and probably retinoprotective properties as well as reducing blood pressure. In addition, they might improve insulin sensitivity. ACEI and metabolites are predominantly excreted via the kidney and doses may need to be adjusted or another antihypertensive agent used if renal function is impaired. *Post hoc* data analysis suggests ACEI and angiotensin-11 receptor blockers reduce the risk of progression to type 2 diabetes; however, there may be different effects in different racial groups. For example, Wright et al. (2006) reported lower risk of progression to diabetes in African-Americans receiving ramipril compared to amlodipine and metoprolol. However, in the

DREAM trial, ramipril did not reduce the incidence of diabetes in non-African Americans with impaired fasting glucose or glucose tolerance, although it did increase the regression to normoalbuminuira (Bosch et al. 2006).

The ACCOMPLISH trial (2008) to determine the effects of the ACE inhibitor benazepril and a calcium channel blocker, amlodipine on morbidity and mortality was stopped early because the combination treatment was more effective than an ACE inhibitor and a diuretic (Jamerson 2008). Cardiovascular morbidity and mortality was reduced by 20%.

The main side effects of ACEI are:

- The 'ACEI cough' is a well-known side effect that is benign but often irritating to the individual and family/friends. It is less common with some of the newer agents.
- Diabetes is often associated with hyporeninaemic hypoaldosteronism syndromes, particularly if renal impairment is present. The syndrome presents with unexplained hyperkalaemia, which can be exacerbated by concomitant ACEI use.
- Using an ACEI in the presence of renal artery stenosis (RAS) may critically reduce glomerular filtration. Prevalence of RAS does not appear to be higher in people with diabetes but it may be associated with, though not a cause of, hypertension. Risk factors include male gender, smoking, and peripheral vascular and coronary artery disease. Ensuring absence of RAS is important in such patients before commencing ACEI. Plasma potassium and creatinine should be regularly monitored in all patients on ACEI prior to and within one week commencing therapy (Gilbert et al. 1998).

Long-term use of antihypertensive agents is associated with zinc loss, which may be clinically relevant if people are already at risk of low zinc (e.g. people with type 2 diabetes, alcoholism, renal insufficiency and malabsorption syndromes) (Braun and Rosenfeldt 2012). Antihypertensive medicines associated with zinc loss are thiasizide diuretics, ACE inhibitors angiotension-2 receptor antagonists, and is especially noticeable with captopril.

Zinc deficiency is associated with anorexia, poor appetite, compromised immune function and changes in smell and taste and can complicate neurological diseases and age–related degenerative diseases. Improving the diet to include foods that contain zinc and supplements might be indicated and could be tested and evaluated and continued if benefits were demonstrated.

The main types of antihypertensive medicines are shown in Table 5.6.

Antiplatelet agents

Antiplatelet agents are indicated to reduce cardiovascular risk. Commonly used antiplatelet agents are:

- Aspirin (Salicylate). Salicylates were traditionally used to reduce inflammation, fever, and pain. They are also commonly used as antiplatelet agents to reduce the risk of cardiovascular disease, particularly in people at high risk, such as those who have had an MI, smoke, have hypertension, and/or high cholesterol. Aspirin may be contraindicated if the individual has a bleeding disorder and sometimes asthma. Aspirin occasionally causes indigestion and a tendency to bleed freely (e.g. from blood glucose testing, nosebleeds, and bruises).
- Clopidogrel hydrochloride sulphate is used if aspirin poses a significant risk of bleeding and is usually used to prevent recurrent stroke, transient ischaemic attack (TIA), or ischaemic event.
- Dipyridamole can be used alone or with low-dose aspirin or where aspirin represents a bleeding risk. A combination formulation is available – Dipyridamole with aspirin. These agents are used to prevent recurrent stroke, TIA, or ischaemic event.
- Warfarin and heparin. These agents are rarely combined with antiplatelet agents except when the individual is at high risk.

Table 5.6   Antihypertensive medications.

Class of medicine	Generic name
Diuretics used for hypertension	
Thiazide diuretics	Hydrochlorothiazide
Sulphonamide diuretics	Chlorthalidone
	Indapamide hemihydrate
Diuretics used for heart failure	
High ceiling diuretics	Frusemide
Aryloxyacetic acid derivatives	Ethacrynic acid usually used if the person is sensitive to other oral diuretics
Potassium sparing agents:	Eplerernone
Aldosterone antagonists	Amiloride hydrochloride
Amiloride hydrochloride	
Combination potassium sparing agents and low ceiling diuretics	Hydrochlorothiazide with amiloride hydrochloride
	Hydrochlorothiazide with triamterene
Nonselective beta blockers used for hypertension	Oxyprenolol hydrochloride
	Pindolol
	Propranolol hydrochloride
Selective beta blockers used for hypertension	Atenolol
	Metoprolol tartarate
Alpha beta-blocking agents	Labetalol hydrochloride
Beta blocking agents used in heart failure	
Alpha and beta-blocking agents	Carvedilol
Selective beta-blocking agents	Bisoprolol fumarate
	Metropolol succinate
Beta-blocking agents used as antiarhythmics	Sotalol hydrochloride
Calcium channel blockers[a]	
Selective calcium channel blockers with predominantly vascular effects – Dihydropyridine derivatives	Amlodipine bensylate
	Felodipine
	Lercanidipine hydrochloride
	Nifedipine
Selective calcium channel blockers with direct cardiac effects – phenylalkylamine derivatives	Verapamil hydrochloride
Calcium channel blockers with cardiac and vascular effects	Diltiazem hydrochloride
Agents acting on the renin–angiotensin system (ACE inhibitors (ACEI))[a]	
Plain ACEI	Captopril
	Enalapril maleate
	Fosinopril sodium
	Lisinopril
	Perindopril
	Quinapril hydrochloride
	Ramipril
	Tandolapril
ACEI and diuretic combinations	Enalapril maleate with hydrocholorothiazide
	Fosinopril sodium with hydrocholorothiazide
	Perindopril erbumine with indapamide hemihydrate
	Quinapril hydrochloride with hydrocholorothiazide

Table 5.6 (Continued)

Class of medicine	Generic name
Angiotensin-11 antagonists	Candesartan cilexetil
	Eprosartan mersylate
	Irbesartan
	Telmisartan
Angiotensin-11 antagonist combinations	Candesartan cilexetil with hydrocholorothiazide
	Eprosartam mesylate with hydrocholorothiazide
	Irbesartan with hydrocholorothiazide
	Telmisartan with hydrocholorothiazide
Centrally acting antiadrenergic agents	Methyldopa
Imidazoline receptor antagonists	Clonidine
	Moxonidine
Peripherally acting antiadrenergic agents	Prazosin hydrochloride
Hydrazinophthalazine derivatives	Hydralazine hydrochloride
Pyramidine derivatives	Minoxidil

Note: Often more than one antihypertensive agent will be required in diabetes to manage the underlying cardiovascular abnormalities. Prescribing information should be followed.
[a] May be contraindicated in pregnancy.

A recent study suggests aspirin is associated with increased risk of macular degeneration (MD) in a prospective 15-year study involving 2389 participants (Liew et al. 2013). In the study, 275 were on aspirin, 63 of whom developed MD. Adjusting for age and other confounders suggest the cumulative risk of MD is 9.3% in aspirin users versus 3.7% risk in nonusers, and this is a dose–response effect. The risk of stopping aspirin must be weighed against the cardiovascular benefits and should be carefully discussed when aspirin is commenced. Caution may be required in people at risk of MD but no such warnings have been issued at the time of writing.

It is important for people to understand how their medicines work and the potential interactions with CM such as St John's wort and glucosamine, which might potentiate the action of warfarin and lead to bleeding. Regular INR monitoring is essential and frequent dose adjustment may be required. Home INR monitoring systems are available but regular medical review is essential.

Medication safety, adherence, and medication self-management

Factors that affect medication safety and contribute to harm are complex and can be patient-related, system/environment-related, product-related and health-professional related, therefore risks in all these categories must be considered and managed. Strategies for reducing health professional-related medicine-related errors include the following:

- Identify individuals at risk.
- Use QUM as a decision-making framework.
- Consider safety standards, guidelines, and advisories such as NICE, US Institute of Safe Medicine Practice, prescribing information, and the Beers Criteria (AGS 2019).
- Use computerised prescribing, ALERTs, and reminders.
- Implement automated ALERT systems, e.g. to allergies, high risk medicine alerts.
- Educate health professionals. Education is more effective if it is interactive and clinically based.
- Implement ward-based pharmacies, which enhance interprofessional communication.
- Undertake regular comprehensive medicine reviews, including home-based reviews.

- Use structured medicine validation processes in hospital.
- Ensure that practice environments are supportive. Supportive practice environments enhance nurses' ability to intercept medicine errors before they occur (Flynn et al. 2012).
- Improve communication among professionals, especially when the individual is discharged and during transitions among care facilities (Dooley et al. 2011; Dunning 2013a).
- Conduct team briefings (e.g. concerning medicine alerts, high-risk patients, and new medicines).

Medication self-management is an essential aspect of diabetes self-care. It becomes increasingly complex as more medicines are added to the regimen, often, as the individual grows older. Medicine nonadherence is widely documented. For example, two out of three people with diabetes adhere to <80% of their insulin doses (Donnelly et al. 2007). The preceding information indicates that polypharmacy is common and is probably best practice diabetes care. Polypharmacy is variously defined as using 2–10 medicines, depending on the source sometimes including prescribed, over-the-counter and CAM medicines.

Polypharmacy contributes to:

- Difficulty remembering the medicine regimen, which affects medicine adherence, medication reviews and complicates prescribing.
- Increased risk of medicine interactions.
- Increased risk of nonadherence. Approximately half the medicines prescribed for people with chronic conditions are not taken. Krapek et al. (2004) reported people with high scores on the Morisky Medication Adherence Scale had lower HbA1c levels. Nonadherence results in high HbA1c and related health risks (Grant et al. 2007). Nonadherence to cardiovascular medications is high: 10–25% discontinue medicines within six months of starting, increasing to 21–47% by 24 months (Senes and Penm 2007). Significantly, people who do not have their prescriptions filled after discharge from hospital post-MI are more likely to die within a year than those who have their prescriptions filled (Jackevicius et al. 2008). Nonadherence to lipid-lowering agents is also high, often because people are not sure they have any benefits or feel health professionals are not interested in the individual's input into their management plan, and the associated side effects (McGinnis et al. 2007). These findings suggest actually prescribing and monitoring medicines in the spirit of the newer term, *concordance*, which denotes shared decision-making and agreement might be more effective than current strategies.
- Increased likelihood of presenting to emergency or being admitted to hospital with a medication-related event. Budnitz and Knight (2007) reported one third of all presentations to emergency in the US involved older people with adverse medication events.
- Increased risk of a medication-related error in hospital. As already stated, insulin, warfarin, and digoxin are the top three high-risk medicines, all of which are frequently prescribed in diabetes. Adverse medicine-related events occurred in 28 500 hospital admissions in 2004–2005 predominantly in people >65 years and is probably an underestimation (AIHW 2007).
- High medicine costs.
- Increased risk of falls.
- Increased risk of driving accidents.
- Relying on medicines rather than continuing mandatory healthy lifestyle.
- Reduced quality of life and well-being.
- Health professionals not prescribing needed medicines on the basis of inadequate patient self-care (Grant et al. 2007) or because they do not want to complicate the regimen or for other individual decision heuristics (Tung 2011).

Other factors that contribute to patient nonadherence include:

- Low health literacy and health numeracy (Chapter 16).
- Sensory deficits such as vision and hearing loss.
- Reluctance to take medicines and a desire to minimise medicine intake (Pound et al. 2005).
- Cultural and other beliefs and attitudes about medicines.

- Inadequate or unclear medicines education, especially when the education is not personalised for the individual and for each medicine (Dunning 2013a).
- Misinterpreting medicine labels and medicine information, which is common even when labelling requires minimal reading skills (Davis et al. 2008). For example instructions to take medicine twice daily (which is imprecise because 'daily' means once per day) or every 12 hours means people have to make addition decisions about what the words actually mean. 'Take medicines as directed' is even more difficult to interpret (Dunning 2013b). People are more likely to understand specified medicine administration times such as 8 A.M., 6 P.M. but using time periods might suit some people better (Davis et al. 2008). Complex medicine regimens independently predict the likelihood people will misinterpret medicine instructions, advice, or education.
- Variations in medicine colour and appearance, e.g. when generic medicines are substituted for the individual's usual medicine (Kesselhiem et al. 2012). Kesslheim et al.'s study concerned antiepileptic medicines but the concept is likely to apply to all medicines. Earlier studies show many people identify their medicines by the colour, size, and shape.
- Medicine costs.

Medicine nonadherence is higher among people who do not attend appointments and is associated with increased rates of all-cause mortality (Currie et al. 2012). Currie's study concerned insulin adherence, but most of the findings are likely to apply to other medicines. In addition, medicine nonadherence was common in a web-based survey of community pharmacy patients in the United States ($n = 2000$) (Shrank et al. 2011). Caregivers were more likely to report they did not adhere to their medicine regimens than noncaregivers, 38% of Shrank's et al.'s sample described themselves as caregivers and most were women. The finding suggest health professionals may need to consider caregiver behaviours and the potential effect on their medicine adherence (and possible the adherence of the person they care for).

Enhancing medication self-care

Adherence is a complex mixture of acceptance, adherence, and persistence – not merely taking a medicine. In addition, each component is itself complex. For example, acceptance involves informed decision-making that can be affected by the health professional's assessment, diagnostic, prescribing, and communication skills. Significantly, agreement of all people involved in medicine adherence is essential to optimal compliance.

Barriers to appropriate medication self-care include the complexity of the regimen, the number of medicines prescribed, the dose frequency, not understanding the regimen or when or how to take the medicines, poor communication, inadequate information or information in a format the individual does not understand, beliefs and attitudes to medicines. Adherence to beneficial medicines reduces morbidity and mortality, which suggests adherence is a surrogate marker of healthy behaviour (Johnson and Shalansky 2007). Several meta-analyses have been undertaken but few show a benefit of any one strategy, which is not surprising given the complex and changing nature of managing diabetes medicines and more importantly, the fact that most strategies focus on changing patient's behaviour rather than also considering health professional's contribution to nonadherence. A truly concordant strategy would/should also address health professional- and systems-related factors that affect medicine adherence.

Nevertheless, a number of strategies for measuring and promoting patient-related medication adherence have been proposed. Some show short-term benefits, but long-term benefits are unclear. Strategies include:

- The Assessment, Individualization, Documentation, Education, and Supervision (AIDES) method based on a meta-analysis of 53 studies, which suggested no single strategy is more effective than any other but that strategies that combine cognitive, behavioural, and affective interventions are more likely to be effective (Roter et al. 1998). However, the AIDES method appears complicated and there is still limited evidence to support its benefit.

- Federal Study of Adherence to Medications in the Elderly (FAME) (Lee et al. 2006), which specifically addressed people >65 years and encompasses education, regular follow up, and customised blister packs. The strategy was based on a review of 12 interventions and was associated with improved adherence over six months from 61% at baseline to >96% and significant reductions in systolic blood pressure and LDL-c.
- Education materials such as those developed by the Australian National Prescribing Service, Consumer Medicines Information (CMI), which are available for all PBS-listed medicines in Australia, Internet sites such as familydoctor.org, and the International Alliance of Patient Organisations, however, these are largely passive and their effect on medicines use is unclear. Part of medicines education is helping people understand risks and benefits and putting these into their individual context. Woloshin and Schwartz (2007) developed a booklet designed to help people understand risks using colon cancer and medical investigations as examples. It was said to be user-friendly and used eighth-grade literacy level. The booklet was tested in a high socioeconomic group and the investigators reported 'significant improvements in participants' ability to interpret risk'. It is not clear whether the information would be applicable to lower socioeconomic groups or whether behaviour changed as a consequence of enhanced ability to interpret risk.
- Education programmes for health professionals such as improving adherence to cardiovascular medicine (National Heart Foundation of Australia 2011).

From these strategies, relevant meta-analysis and the author's clinical experience using a QUM approach, the following strategies are useful. They can be used alone or in combination, depending on the individual's need and agreement. That is, patient-centred medication self-management:

- Understand the health professionals' impact on patient adherence.
- Understand the individual's beliefs and attitudes towards medicines, their capabilities, and their life goals.
- Understand their usual lifestyle and daily activities.
- Assess their physical and mental capability to manage medicines, whether help is available, and whether they will accept it if it is.
- Identify triggers to nonadherence, for example, on more than five medicines, complex dosing regimen, sound-alike medicine names, look-alike medicines, low literacy, cognitive deficits, and being a carer.
- Develop strategies to address specific issues. These should be developed in consultation with the individual, such as, 'How do you think you could remember to take your insulin?' Some useful strategies include personal cues, reminders, and medicine boxes such as blister packs.
- Provide medicine information in a relevant format and language level using appropriate words suitable for the individual. Work through the information with the individual and ask them to repeat back what they learned. Explain the benefits and risks but apply them to the individual's context, that is, personalise the information. Information could include:
  - Why the medicines were prescribed, which will include stressing the importance of maintaining a healthy lifestyle.
  - The name of the medicine, the difference between generic and other medicines, and what brand names mean.
  - What the medicine is expected to do (outcomes) and how the person will know if it is effective.
  - How soon an effect will show.
  - The dose and dose frequency.
  - Special instructions such as when to take the medicine in relation to meals.
  - What to do if they forget a dose.
  - When to stop taking the medicine, if relevant.
  - Where and when to seek medicine advice, for example, fasting for a procedure or investigation.

- Common side effects, how to recognise them and what to do about minimising or reporting them.
  - Storing and disposing of unused medicines or medicines that have passed their use-by date.
- How to use other self-care information to interpret the effects of medicines adherence and nonadherence on relevant outcomes; for example, their blood glucose pattern.
- How to keep their medication list up-to-date and ensure it includes over-the-counter and CAM medicines.
- Help them formulate questions to ask their doctor at the next appointment if necessary.
- Follow-up medicines self-management regularly.

Clinical observation

From the list of strategies it is clear that person-centred, individualised medicine education is complex, time consuming, and probably not accomplished in the majority of people with diabetes. Reflect on how you and/or your team could improve the way you provide medicine education.

Strategies that can be used to monitor medicine adherence

In research settings, MEMs medicine containers are used. MEMs containers have microprocessors in the lid that record the date and time the container was opened. Opening the container is a proxy measure of medicines' actual use. MEMs also acts as a behavioural intervention; people are more likely to adhere if they think they are being watched. However, MEMs is impractical in clinical settings. Other strategies involve:

- Provide appropriate education with behavioural support.
- Use case management and effective interprofessional communication.
- Use systems approaches to reduce the cost of medicines.
- Discuss medicine use using open communication, blood glucose, and other self-monitoring and laboratory results in a nonjudgemental way.
- Know the 'right' questions to ask.
- Use open, neutral language and choose words and sentences carefully and avoid passive language and ambiguity to enhance memory and understanding.
- Use questionnaires such as the:
  - Brief Medication Questionnaire (BMQ) that measures current and potential nonadherence and can be self-completed by the individual.
  - The Morisky Scale, which measures attitudinal and behavioural factors that affect adherence. However, the language is judgemental (e.g. Are you careless at times about taking your medicine? It has low internal reliability).
  - Medication Adherence report (MARS), which views medicine use on a continuum.
  - Beliefs about Medication Questionnaire (BaMQ).
  - Revised Illness Perception Questionnaire (IPQ-R).

Reflecting on their own medicine-related behaviours might help them understand people with diabetes medicine-related behaviours. After all, health professionals fall into the category of carers: caring is a known risk factor for nonadherence.

Based on the preceding information about adherence, one could ask:

(1) Is adherence a patient problem?
(2) Is adherence a health professional problem?
(3) Is adherence an interrelated responsibility of the individual, the health professional, service providers, and funders?
(4) Should we be promoting rights and responsibilities rather than merely adherence?

Example protocol for outpatient stabilisation onto insulin

Suggested protocol

These are guidelines only and should be modified to suit individual needs.

The information can be delivered individually or in groups and over various time frames and include other information relevant to individuals:

(1) Introduce the diabetes team and area facilities.
(2) Test blood glucose; individuals should test their own blood glucose if possible.
(3) Insulin dose/frequency is determined in consultation with the doctor.
(4) The educator demonstrates insulin technique and explains the procedure to the patient and encourages the patient to practice them.
(5) It is important to encourage patients to discuss their feelings about diabetes and to assess current diabetes knowledge, learning capacity, style, psychological status, and social situation.

Education goals
(1) To give a basic explanation of what diabetes is and what an acceptable blood glucose range is.
(2) To explain the reason for instituting insulin therapy.
(3) To explain the effects of insulin on blood glucose levels, i.e. insulin action and the role of long- and short-acting insulin in control of blood glucose levels.
(4) To explain insulin technique:
   • Preparing the dose depending on the insulin delivery system chosen
   • Sites for injection
   • Expiry dates of insulin bottles/cartridges
   • Care and storage
   • Appropriate sharps disposal
(5) To explain why insulin must be given by injection and allow patient to handle insulin device or bottles and practice preparing the insulin dose.
(6) To explain hypoglycaemia:
   • Recognising symptoms of low blood glucose levels.
   • Causes and prevention.
   • Effective management.
   • Patient should carry carbohydrates for emergencies.
(7) Blood glucose monitoring should be encouraged, to provide feedback to the patient and enable them to telephone in the afternoon with a result if necessary. The role of monitoring should be explained as well as the timing of testing and how to record results.
(8) Basic introduction to a food plan: role of carbohydrate in blood glucose control and the need to reduce fat and the need for regular meals.
(9) Explain and enrol the patient in the National Diabetes Supply Scheme (in Australia).
(10) Explain responsibilities with respect to self-care, medicine management, complication screening, and driving.
(11) Ensure patient has the equipment to administer insulin and monitor blood glucose and knows how and where to obtain future supplies and knows who to contact for advice.

Other important self-care issues
(1) Discuss how to manage illness at home, in relation to:
   a. Who to contact
   b. Effects of illness on blood glucose
   c. Emergency diet
   d. Monitoring and recording of blood glucose and urine or blood ketones
   e. Adjusting/continuing insulin
   f. Need to rest

(2) Discuss precautions to be taken relating to driving, work, etc.

(3) Discuss the role of exercise/activity in controlling blood glucose levels.

(4) Encourage patient to wear some form of identification.

(5) Ensure that patient has a contact telephone number and knows who to contact for advice.

(6) Provide appropriate follow-up appointments for doctor, nurse specialist/educator according to patient needs.

(7) Provide ongoing individual teaching as required.

(8) Ensure patient knows about other services available for people with diabetes, for example, diabetes associations and relevant support groups.

(9) Arrange for consultation with family if necessary.

References

Abe, T., Matsubayashi, Y., Yoshida, A. et al. (2018). Predictors of the response of HbA1c and body weight after SGLT2 initiation. *Diabetes & Metabolism* **44**: 172–174. https://doi.org/10.1016/j.diabet.2017.10.003.

Abraham, E., Leech, C., Lin, J. et al. (2002). Insulinotrophic hormone glucagonslike peptide-I differentiation of human pancreatic islet-derived progenitor cell into insulin producing cells. *Endocrinology* **143**: 3152–3161.

Afilalo, J., Duque, G., and Steele, R. (2008). Statins for secondary prevention in elderly patients. *Journal of the American College of Physicians* **51**: 37–45.

AGS (American Geriatrics Society) (2018). Identifying medicines that older adults should avoid or use with caution: the updated AGS Beers criteria). https://www.americangeriatrics.org/.../2018%20AGS%20Beers%20Criteria%20-%20F.

Almond, J., Cox, D., Nugent, M. et al. (2001). Experience of group sessions for converting to insulin. *Journal of Diabetes Nursing* **5** (4): 102–105.

American Association of Clinical Endocrinologists (AACE) (2011). Guidelines for clinical practice for developing a diabetes mellitus comprehensive care plan. *Endocrine Practice* **17** (2 Suppl 2): 1–53.

American Diabetes Association (2007). Standards of Medical Care in Diabetes—2007. *Diabetes Care* **30**: S4–S41.

American Diabetes Association (2019). Pharmacologic approaches to glycemic treatment: *Standards of Medical Care in Diabetes*—2018, Figure 8.2. *Diabetes Care* **41** (Suppl. 1): S73–S85.

American Geriatrics Society Beers Criteria® Update Expert Panel (2019). American Geriatrics Society 2019 Updated AGS Beers Criteria® for Potentially Inappropriate Medication Use in Older Adults. *Journal of the American Geriatrics Society* **67**: 674–694.

Australian Adverse Drug Reactions Advisory Council (ADRAC) Bulletin (2007). *Emerging cardiovascular concerns with rosiglitazone* **26**: 6. http://www.tga.gov.au/hp/aadrb-0712.htm (accessed August 2019).

Australian Commission on Safety and Qualtiy in Health Care (2012). *Safety and Quality Improvement Guide Standards 4: Mediation Safety*. Sydney: ACSQHC.

Australian Diabetes Educators Association (2017). Clinical Guiding Principles for Subcutaneous Injection https://www.adea.com.au/wp.../10/Injection-Technique-FINAL_170815.docx-1.pdf.

Australian Diabetes Society (ADS) (2007). *ADS Position Statement on Rosiglitzone* (AVANDIA®) May 28th, 2007. Canberra: ADS.

Australia Government Department of Health (2019). National Medicines Policy. https://www1.health.gov.au/internet/main/publishing.nsf/Content/National+Medicines+Policy-1 (accessed September 2019).

Australian Medicines Handbook (2019). Adelaide: Australian Medicines Handbook Pty Ltd; 2019. https://amhonline.amh.net.au/.

Bailey, D.G., Dresser, G., and Arnold, J. (2013). Grapefruit–medication interactions: Forbidden fruit or avoidable consequences? *Canadian Medical Association Journal* **185**: 309–316.

Birkeland, K., Torjesen, P., Eriksson, J. et al. (1994). Hyperproinsulinemia of type II diabetes is not present before the development of hyperglycemia. *Diabetes Care* **17** (11): 1307–1310.

Blind, E., Dunder, K., De Graeff, P.A., and Abadie, E. (2011). Rosiglitazone: a European regulatory perspective. *Diabetologia* **54** (2): 213–218.

Braun, L. and Rosenfeldt, F. (2012). Pharmoco-nutrient interactions – a systematic review of zinc and antihypertensive therapy. *International Journal of Clinical Practice* https://doi.org/10.1111/ijcp.12040.

Budnitz, D. and Knight, S. (2007). Common drugs trigger most ER visits by seniors. www.medicinenet.com/script/main/art.asp?articlekey=85633.

Buse, J. (2001). Insulin analogues. *Current Opinion in Endocrinology* **8** (2): 95–100.

Calabrese, A., Coley, K., Da Pos, S. et al. (2002). Evaluation of prescribing practice: risk of lactic acidosis with metformin. *Archives of Internal Medicine* **162**: 434–437.

Campbell, M., Anderson, D., Holcombe, J., and Massey, E. (1993). Storage of insulin: a manufacturer's view. *Practical Diabetes* **10** (6): 218–220.

Cefalu, W., Skyler, J., Kourides, I. et al. (2001). Inhaled insulin treatment in patients with type 2 diabetes. *Annals of Internal Medicine* **134**: 242–244.

Cherney, D., Cooper, M., Tikkanen, L. et al. (2018). Pooled analysis of phase 111 trials indicate contrasting influences of renal function on blood pressure, bodyweight and HbA1c reductions aith empagliflozin. *Kidney International* **93** (1): 231–244. https://doi.org/10.1016/j.kint.2017.06.071.

Cheung, N., Napier, B., Zaccaria, C., and Fletcher, J. (2005). Hyperglycaemia is associated with adverse outcomes in patients receiving total parenteral nutrition. *Diabetes Care* **28**: 2367–2371.

Choudhry, N. and Fletcher, R. (2005). Systematic review:the relationship between clinical experience and quality of health care. *Annals of Internal Medicine* **114**: 260–273.

Colquhoun, D. (2000). Unstable angina – a definitive role for statins in secondary prevention. *International Journal of Clinical Practice* **54**: 383–389.

Colquhoun, D. (2002). Lipid lowering agents. *Australian Family Physician* **31** (1): 25–30.

Colhoun, H.M., Betteridge, D.J., Durrington, P.N. et al. (2004). Primary prevention of cardiovascular disease with atorvastatin in type 2 diabetes in the Collaborative Atorvastatin Diabetes Study (CARDS): multicentre randomised placebo-controlled trial. *The Lancet* **364** (9435): 685–696.

Colunga-Lozano, L., Gonzalez Torres, F., Delgado-Figueroa, N. et al. (2018) Sliding scale insulin for non-critically ill hospitalized adults with diabetes mellitus. Cochrane Library. https://www.cochranelibrary.com/cdsr/doi/10.1002/14651858.CDO11296.pub2/full.

Currie, C.J., Peyrot, M., Morgan, C.L. et al. (2012). The impact of treatment noncompliance on mortality in people with type 2 diabetes. *Diabetes Care* **35**: 1279–1284.

DAFNE Study Group (2002). Training in flexible, intensive insulin management to enable dietary freedom in people with type 1 diabetes: Dose Adjustment of Normal Eating (DAFNE) randomized controlled trial. *British Medical Journal* **325**: 746.

Dagogo-Jack, S. and Alberti, G. (2002). Management of diabetes mellitus in surgical patients. *Diabetes Spectrum* **15**: 44–48.

Dandona, P., Topiwala, S., Chaudhuri, A., and Ghanim, S. (2008). Insulin is an antiatherogenic hormone. *International Diabetes Monitor* **20** (1): 9–16.

Davies, M.J., D'Alessio, D.A., Fradkin, J. et al. (2018). Management of hyperglycaemia in type 2 diabetes, 2018. A consensus report by the American Diabetes Association (ADA) and the European Association for the Study of Diabetes (EASD). *Diabetologia* **61** (12): 2461–2498.

Davis, T., Federmann, A., Bass, P. et al. (2008). Improving patient understanding of prescription drug label instructions. *Journal of General Internal Medicine* **24** (1): 57–62.

DCCT (Diabetes Control and Complications Trial Research Group) (1993). Effects of intensive insulin therapy on the development and progression of long-term complications in IDDM. *New England Journal of Medicine* **329**: 977–986.

DeVries, J.H. and Rosenstock, J. (2017). DPP-4 Inhibitor–Related Pancreatitis: Rare but Real! *Diabetes Care* **40**: 161–163.

Diabetes Australia/ Royal Australian College of General Practitioners is Diabetes Australia/The Royal Australian College of General Practitioners (2016). General practice management of type 2 diabetes: 2016–18. East Melbourne, Vic: RACGP (2016). https://www.racgp.org.au/FSDEDEV/media/documents/Clinical%20Resources/Guidelines/Diabetes/General-practice-management-of-type-2-diabetes_1.pdf.

Diamond, G.A. and Kaul, S. (2008). The disconnect between practice guidelines and clinical practice—stressed out. *Journal of the American Medical Association* **300**: 1817–1819.

DoHA (Australian Government Department of Health and Ageing) (2016) National Diabetes Strategy (2016-2020). https://www1.health.gov.au/internet/main/publishing.nsf/Content/nds-2016-2020.

DoHA (Australian Government Department of Health and Ageing) (2002). The National Strategy for Quality Use of Medicines. https://www1.health.gov.au/internet/main/publishing.nsf/Content/EEA5B39AA0A63F18CA257BF0001DAE08/$File/National-Strategy-for-Quality-Use-of-Medicines.pdf.

Donnelly, L., Morris, A., Evans, J., and DARTS/MEMO Collaboration (2007). Adherence to insulin and its association with glycaemic control in patients with type 2 diabetes. *Quality Journal of Medicine* **100**: 345–350.

Dooley, M., Wiseman, M., McRae, A. et al. (2011). Reducing potentially fatal errors associated with high doses of insulin: A successful multifaceted multidisciplinary prevention strategy. *British Medical Journal Quality and Safety* https://doi.org/10.1136/bmjqs.200.049668.

Dormandy, J., Charbonnel, B., and Eckland, D. (2005). Secondary prevention of macrovascular events in patients with type 2 diabetes in the PRO active Study (PROspective pioglitAzone Clinical Trial in Macrovascular Events): a randomised controlled trial. *Lancet* **366**: 1279–1289.

Dornhorst, T. (2001). Insulinotropic meglitinide analogues. *Lancet* **17** (358): 1709–1716.

Dornhorst, A., Luddeke, H.J., Sreenan, S. et al. (2007). Safety and efficacy of insulin determined in clinical practice: 14-week follow-up data from type 1 and type 2 diabetes patients in the PREDICTIVE™ European Cohort. *Clinical Practice* **61** (3): 52–58.

DREAM (Diabetes Reduction Assessment with Ramipril and Rosiglitazone Medication Investigators) (2006). Effect of Rosiglitazone on the frequency of diabetes in patients with impaired glucose tolerance or impaired fasting glucose: a randomized controlled trial. *Lancet* **355**: 2427–2443. (correction in Lancet (2006) 368, 1770).

Dunning, T. (2005). Applying a quality use of medicines framework to using essential oils in nursing practice. *Complementary Therapies in Clinical Practice* **11**: 172–181.

Dunning, T. (2013a). Medicine self-management: More than just taking pills. In: *Diabetes Education: Art, Science and Evidence* (ed. T. Dunning), 177–197. Chichester, UK: Wiley Blackwell.

Dunning, T. (2013b). Turning points and transitions. In: *Diabetes Education: Art, Science and Evidence* (ed. T. Dunning), 117–131. Chichester, UK: Wiley Blackwell.

Dunning, T. (2017). Turning points and transitions: crises and opportunities, Chapter 8. In: *Diabetes Education: Art, Science and Evidence* (ed. T. Dunning), 117–132. Oxford: Wiley Blackwell.

Dunning, T. and Martin, M. (1997). Using a focus group to explore perceptions of diabetes severity. *Practical Diabetes International* **14** (7): 185–188.

Dunning, T. and Martin, M. (1999). Health professionals' perceptions of the seriousness of diabetes. *Practical Diabetes International* **16** (3): 73–77.

Dunning, T., Rosen, S., and Alford, F. (1998). Insulin allergy: a diagnostic dilemma. *Journal of Diabetes Nursing* **2** (6): 188–190.

Dunning, T. and Sinclair, A. (2014). Glucose lowering medicines and older people: the importance of comprehensive assessments and pharmacovigilance. *The Journal of Nursing Care* **3**: 1–4.

Ekstrom, N., Schioler, L., Svensson, A.M. et al. (2012). Effectiveness and safety of metformin in 51 675 patients with type 2 diabetes and different levels of renal function: a cohort study from the Swedish National Diabetes Register. *British Medical Journal Open* **2**: e001076. https://doi.org/10.1136/bmjopen-2012-001076.

Evans, M., Schumm-Draeger, P.M., Vora, J. et al. (2011). A review of modern insulin analogue pharmacokinetic and pharmacodynamic profiles in type 2 diabetes: improvements and limitations. *Diabetes Obesity & Metabolism* **13**: 677–684.

European Medicines Agency (2010). Questions and answers on the suspension of rosiglitazone-containing medicines (Avandia, Avandamet, and Avaglim). Outcome of a procedure under Article 20 of Regulation (EC) No724/2004.https://www.ema.europa.eu/en/documents/medicine-qa/questions-answers-suspension-rosiglitazone-containing-medicines-avandia-avandamet-avaglim_en.pdf.

FDA (US Federal Drug Administration) (2011). Avandia (rosiglitazone): REMS – Risk of Cardiovascular Events: includes Avandia, Avandamet, and Avandaryl. www.fda.gov/Drugs/DrugSafety/ucm241411.htm (accessed November 2012).

Flynn, L., Liang, Y., Dickson, G., and Xie, M. (2012). Nurses' practice environments, error interception practices, and inpatient medication errors. *Journal of Nursing Scholarship* **44** (2): 180–186.

Fralick, M., Schneeweiss, S., and Patorno, E. (2017). Risk of Diabetic Ketoacidosis after Initiation of an SGLT2 Inhibitor. *New England Journal of Medicine* **376**: 2300–2302.

Frid, A., Kreugel, G., Grassi, G. et al. (2016). New insulin delivery recommendations. *Mayo Clinic Proceedings* **91** (9): 1231–1255. http://dc.doi.org.10.1016/j.mayocp.2016.06.010.

Gabbay, R., Hu, P., Bode, B., and Garber, A. (2005). The INITIATE Study group: Initiating insulin therapy in type 2 diabetes: a comparison of biphasic insulin analogs. *Diabetes Care* **28**: 254–259.

Gearhart, J.G., Replogle, W.H., Forbes, R.C., and Walley, E.J. (1994). Efficacy of sliding-scale insulin therapy: a comparison with prospective regimens. *Family Practice Research Journal* **14** (4): 313–322.

George, L. (1993). Sociological perspectives on life transitions. *Annual Review of Sociology* **19**: 353–373.

Gilbert, R., Cooper, M., and Krum, H. (1998). Drug administration in patients with diabetes mellitus. *Drug Safety* **1** (6): 441–456.

Golomb, B. (2007). Simvastatin but not pravastatin, may reduce sleep quality. American Heart Association Scientific Sessions. Abstract 3725 (November), Orlando.

Goudswaard, A., Furlong, N., Valk, G. et al. (2004). Insulin monotherapy versus combinations of insulin with oral hypoglycaemic agents in patients with type 2 diabetes mellitus. *Cochrane Database of Systematic Reviews* **4** The Cochrane Library, London.

Grant, R., Adams, A., Trinacty, C. et al. (2007). Relationship between patient medication adherence and subsequent clinical inertia in type 2 diabetes glycemic management. *Diabetes Care* **30**: 807–812.

Greaves, C., Brown, P., Terry, R. et al. (2003). Converting to insulin in primary care: an exploration of the needs of practice nurses. *Journal of Advanced Nursing* **42** (5): 487–496.

Grundy, S., Cleeman, J., Merz, C. et al. (2004). Implications of recent clinical trials for the National Cholesterol Education Treatment Panel 111 guidelines. *Circulation* **110**: 227–239.

Gunton, J., Cheung, N., Davis, T. et al. (2016). A new blood glucose management algorithm for type 2 diabetes: A position statement of the Australian Diabetes Society. https://diabetessociety.com.au/documents/ADS_POSITIONSTATEMENT_v2.4.pdf.

Hirsch, I., Paaun, D., and Brunzell, J. (1995). Inpatient management of adults with diabetes. *Diabetes Care* **18** (6): 870–877.

Home, P., Pocock, S., Beck-Neilsen, H. et al. (2009). Rosiglitazone evaluated for cardiovascular outcomes in oral agent combination therapy for type 2 diabetes (RECORD): a multicentre, randomized open-label trial. *Lancet* **373** (681): 2125–2135.

Home, P., Pocock, S., and Beck-Nielsen, H. (2005). Rosaglitazone evaluated for cardiac outcomes and regulation of glycaemia in diabetes (RECORD): study design and protocol. *Diabetologia* **48**: 1726–1735.

Hui, H., Tang, G., and Go, V. (2009). Hypoglycaemic herbs and their action mechanisms. *Chinese Medicine* **4**: 11. https://doi.org/10.1186/1749-8546-4-11.

Hunter, J., Arentz, S., and Deed, G. (2017). Protocol for a rapid evidence review of traditional and complementary medicine for people with diabetes receiving palliative or end-of-life care. *Hospital Palliative Medicine International Journal* (7). https://doi.org/10.15406/hpmij.2017.01.00039.

Hwang, Y.C., Kim, J.H., Lee, B.W., and Lee, W.J. (2019). A lower baseline urinary glucose excretion predicts a better response to the sodium glucose cotransporter 2 inhibitor. *Diabetes & Metabolism Journal* **43**: e36. https://doi.org/10.4093/dmj.2018.0257.

Iedema, J. and Russell, A. (2011). Optimising metformin benefits in type 2 diabetes. *Diabetes Management Journal* **34**: 22–24.

Inzucchi, S. (2002). Oral antihyperglycemic therapy for type 2 diabetes: scientific review. *Journal of the American Medical Association* **287**: 360–372.

Inzucchi, S., Bergenstal, R., Buse, J. et al. (2012). Management of hyperglycaemia in type 2 diabetes: a patient-centred approach. *Diabetes Care* **35** (6): 1364–1379. care.diabetesjournals.org/content/35/6/1364.long (accessed May 2012).

Jackevicius, C., Li, P., and Tu, J. (2008). Prevalence, predictors, and outcomes of primary non-adherence after acute myocardial infarction. *Circulation*. https://doi.org/10.1161/CIRCULATIONAHA.107.706820.

Jackowski, L. (2008a). Lipid lowering therapy. *Australian Family Physician* **37** (1/2): 39–41.

Jackowski, L. (2008b). Beta blockers in systolic heart failure. *Australian Family Physician* **37** (3): 137–139.

Jain, R., Allen, E., and Wahl, I. (2005). Premixed insulin analogues for the treatment of diabetes. *Diabetes* **54** (Suppl. A69).

Jamerson, K. (for the ACCOMPLISH investigators) (2008). Avoiding cardiovascular events in combination therapy in patients living with systolic hypertension. American College of Cardiology Scientific Sessions, Chicago (March). www.sbm.org/meetings/2012/rapid-communication-abstracts.

Janka, H., Plewe, G., Riddle, M. et al. (2005). Comparison of basal insulin added to oral agents versus twice daily premixed insulin as initial therapy for type 2 diabetes. *Diabetes Care* **28**: 254–259.

Jerrall, M. (2002). Warning over metformin use. *Archives of Internal Medicine* **162**: 434–437.

Johnson, G. and Shalansky, S. (2007). Predictors of refill non-adherence in patients with heart failure. *British Journal of Clinical Pharmacology* **63** (4): 488–493.

Joint Formulary Committee (2018). British National Formulary. http://www.medicinescomplete.com (accessed:August 2018).

Kapitza, C., Nowotny, I., Lehman, A. et al. (2017). Similar pharmacokinetics and pharmacodynamics of rapid-acting insulin lispro products SAR342434 and US- and EU-approved Humalog in subjects with type 1 diabetes. *Diabetes, Obesity and Metabolism* **19** (5): 622–627.

Karamermer, Y. and Roos-Hesselink, J. (2007). Coronary heart disease and pregnancy. *Future of Cardiology* **3** (5): 559–567.

Katz, C. (1991). How efficient is sliding scale insulin therapy? Problem with a 'cookbook' approach in hospital patients. *Postgraduate Medicine* **5** (5): 46–48.

Keech, A., Simes, R., and Barter, P. (2005). Effects of long term fenofibrate therapy on cardiovascular events in diabetes mellitus (the FIELD study): randomized controlled trial. *Lancet* **366**: 1649–1861.

Kennedy, E. and Oliver, N. (2017). Emerging technologies for diabetes. *Practical Diabetes* **34** https://www.practicaldiabetes.com/article/emerging-technologies-diabetes/.

Kesselhiem, A., Misono, A., Shrank, W. et al. (2012). Variations in pill acceptance of antileptic drugs and the risk of nonadherence. *Archives of Internal Medicine* **173** (3): 1–7.

Knopp, R., d'Emden, M., and Smilde, J. (2006). Efficacy and safety of Atorvastatin in the prevention of cardiovascular disease in people with type 2 diabetes: the Atorvastatin study for the prevention of coronary heart disease endpoints in non-insulin dependent diabetes mellitus (ASPEN). *Diabetes Care* **29**: 1478–1485.

Ko, G.T.C., Tsang, P.C.C., Wai, H.P.S. et al. (2006). Rosiglitazone versus bedtime insulin in the treatment of patients with conventional oral antidiabetic drug failure: a 1-year randomized clinical trial. *Advances in Therapy* **23** (5): 799–808.

Krapek, K., King, K., Warren, S. et al. (2004). Medication adherence and associated hemoglobin A1c in type 2 diabetes. *The Annals of Pharmacotherapy* **38** (9): 1357–1362.

Kuritzky, L. (2006). Addition of basal insulin to oral antidiabetic agents: a goal directed approach to type 2 diabetes therapy. *Medscape General Medicine* **8** (4): 34–47.

Lau, D.C., Douketis, J.D., Morrison, K.M. et al. (2007). 2006 Canadian clinical practice guidelines on the management and prevention of obesity in adults and children [summary]. *Canadian Medical Association Journal* **176**: S1–S13.

Lee, J.S., Chang, P.-Y., Zhang, Y. et al. (2017). Triglyceride and HDL-C dyslipidemia and risks of coronary heart disease and ischemic stroke by glycemic dysregulation status: The strong heart study. *Diabetes Care* **40**: 529–537.

Lee, J., Grace, K., and Taylor, A. (2006). Effect of a pharmacy care program on medication adherence and persistence, blood pressure, and low density lipoprotein cholesterol. *Journal of the American Medical Association*. https://doi.org/10.1001/jama.296.21.joc60162.

Leiter, L. (2006). Can thiazolidinediones delay disease progression in type 2 diabetes? *Current Medical Research and Opinion* **22** (6): 1193–1201.

Lewis, J., Ferrara, A., Peng, T. et al. (2011). Risk of bladder cancer among diabetic patients treated with pioglitazone: interim report of a longitudinal cohort study. *Diabetes Care* **34**: 916–922.

Liew, G., Mitchell, P., Wong, F.Y. et al. (2013). Aspirin association with wet macula oedema. *Journal of Internal Medicine* **213** (3): 1–7.

Lipid Study Group (1998). The long-term intervention with pravastatin in ischaemic disease. Prevention of cardiovascular events and death with pravastatin in patients with coronary heart disease and a broad range of initial cholesterol levels. *New England Journal of Medicine* **339**: 1349–1357.

Malmberg, K. (1997). Prospective randomised study of intensive insulin treatment on long-term survival after acute myocardial infarction. *British Medical Journal* **314**: 1512–1515.

Malone, J., Campaigne, B., Reviriego, J., and Augendre-Ferrrante, B. (2005). Twice daily pre-mixed insulin rather than basal insulin therapy alone results in better overall glycaemic control in patients with type 2 diabetes. *Diabetic Medicine* **22**: 374–381.

Marie, I., Delafenêtre, H., Massy, N. et al. (2008). Tendinous disorders attributed to statins: A study on ninety-six spontaneous reports in the period 1990–2005 and review of the literature. *Arthritis Care & Research* **59**: 367–372.

Masoudi, F. (2007). Can statins benefit elderly patients with ischaemic heart disease. *Journal Watch Cardiology* **6** (11): 10–16.

Mayfield, J. and White, R. (2004). Insulin therapy for type 2 diabetes: rescue, augmentation, and replacement of beta-call function. *American Family Physician* **70** (3): 100–115.

McGinnis, B., Olson, K., Magid, D. et al. (2007). Factors related to adherence in statin therapy. *Annals of Pharmacotherapy* **41** (11): 1805–1811.

Meier, C., Kraenzlin, M., Bodmer, M. et al. (2008). Use of thiazolidinediones and fracture risk. *Archives of Internal Medicine* **168**: 820–825.

Minamii, T., Nogami, M., Ogawa, W. et al. (2018). Mechanisms of metformin action: in and out of the gut. *Journal Diabetes Investigation*. http://onlinelibrary.wiley.com/journal/jdi https://doi.org/10.1111/jdi.12864.

Montori, V. and Isley, W. (2007). Waking up from the DREAM of preventing diabetes with drugs. *British Medical Journal* **334**: 882–884.

Nathan, D. and Buse, J. (2006). Management of hypertension in type 2 diabetes: a consensus algorithm for the initiation and adjustment of therapy. A consensus statement from the American Diabetes Association and the Diabetes Association for the Study of Diabetes. *Diabetologia* **49**: 1711–1721.

National Heart Foundation of Australia (2001). *Lipid Management Guidelines*. Melbourne: National Heart Foundation.

National Heart Foundation of Australia (2011). *Improving Adherence in Cardiovascular Care*. Melbourne: National Heart Foundation.

National Heart Foundation of Australia and Cardiac Society of Australia and New Zealand (2005). Position statement on lipid management. *Heart, Lung & Circulation* **14**: 275–291.

National Institute for Clinical Excellence (NICE) (2003). Guidance on the use of continuous subcutaneous insulin infusion for diabetes. *Technology Appraisal Guidance. NICE* **57**: 1–23.

National Institute for Health and Clinical Excellence (NICE) (2008). *Type 2 diabetes: The Management of type 2 Diabetes*. London: National Health Service.

National Institute for Health and Clinical Excellence (2017). Algorithm for blood glucose lowering therapy in adults with type 2 diatebes. https://www.nice.org.uk/guidance/ng28.

National Prescribing Service (NPS) (2001). *Improving Treatment of Systolic Heart Failure*. Canberra: NPS.

National Prescribing Service (NPS) (2008). *Managing Hyperglycaemia in Type 2 Diabetes. NPS News*. Canberra: NPS.

National Prescribing Service (NPS) (2012). Type 2 diabetes drug table. www.nps.org.au (accessed November 2012).

NICE (2017). Algorithm for blood glucose lowering therapy in adults with type 2. https://www.nice.org.uk/.../algorithm-for-blood-glucose-lowering-therapy-in-adults-w.

Nichols, G., Hillier, T., and Erbey, J. (2001). Congestive heart failure in type 2 diabetes: prevalence, incidence, and risk factors. *Diabetes Care* **24**: 1614–1619.

Nisbet, J., Sturtevant, J., and Prons, J. (2004). Metformin and serious adverse events. *Medical Journal of Australia* **180** (2): 53–54.

Nissen, S., Tardif, J., and Nicholls, S. (2007). Effect of Torcetrapib on the progression of coronary atherosclerosis. *New England Journal of Medicine* **356**: 1304–1316.

Nissen, S. and Wolski, K. (2007). Effect of rosiglitazone on the risk of myocardial infarction and death from cardiovascular causes. *New England Journal of Medicine*. https://doi.org/10.1056/NEJMoa072761.

ORIGIN (2012). Basal insulin and cardiovascular and other outcomes in dysglycaemia. *New England Journal of Medicine* **367**: 319–328.

Pasternak, R.C., Smith, S.C. Jr., Bairey-Merz, C.N. et al. (2002). ACC/AHA/NHLBI Advisory on the Use and Safety of Statins. *Journal of American College of Cardiology* **40**: 568–573.

Peacock, S. and Lovshin, J. (2018). Risk of diabetic ketoacidosis after initiation of an SGLT2 inhibitor sodium-glucose cotransporter-2 inhibitors (SGLT-2i) in the perioperative setting. *Canadian Journal Anaesthesiology* **65**: 143–147.

Peters, A., Henry, R., Thakkar, P. et al. (2016). Diabeteic ketoacidosis with canagliflozin, a sodium-glucose cotransporter 2 inhibitor in patients with type 1 diabetes. *Diabetes Care* **39** (4): 532–538.

Petersen, C. (2018). Second steps in managing type 2 diabetes. *Australian Prescriber* **41141**: 4. https://doi.org/10.18773/austprescr.2018.043.

Pound, P., Britten, N., Morgan, M. et al. (2005). Resisting medicines: a syntheses of qualitative studies of medicine taking. *Social Science and Medicine* **61**: 133–155.

Prochaska, J. and Velicer, W. (1997). The transtheoretical model of health behaviour change. *American Journal of Health Promotion* **12**: 38–48.

Pryce, R. (2009). Diabetic ketoacidosis caused by exposure of insulin pump to heat and sunlight. *British Medical Journal* **338**: 1077–1078.

Queale, W., Seidler, A., and Brancati, F. (1997). Glycaemic control and sliding scale insulin use in medical inpatients with diabetes mellitus. *Archives of Internal Medicine* **157**: 545–552.

Quinn, J., Snyder, S., Berghoff, J. et al. (2006). A practical approach to hyperglycaemia management in the intensive care unit: evaluation of an intensive insulin infusion protocol. *Pharmacotherapy* **26** (10): 1410–1420.

Raskin, P., Allen, E., Hollander, P. et al. (2005). The INITIATE study group: initiating insulin therapy in type 2 diabetes: a comparison of biphasic and basal insulin analogues. *Diabetes Care* **28**: 260–265.

Rasmussen, B. (2018). Older people with diabetes and life transitions, Chapter7. In: *The Art and science of Personalising Care with Older People with Diabetes* (ed. T. Dunning), 121–135. Switzerland: Springer.

Richter, B., Bandeira-Echtler, E., Bergerhoff, K., and Lerch, C. (2008). Dipeptidyl peptidase-4 (DDP-4) inhibitors for type 2 diabetes mellitus. *Cochrane Database of Systematic Review* www.ncbi.nlm.nih.gov/pubmedhealth/PMH0014112/, Cochrane Library, London.

Riddle, M., Rosenstock, J., and Gerich, J. (2003). The insulin Glargine 2004 study investigators; The treat-to-target trial: randomized addition of glargine to human NPH insulin to oral therapy in type diabetes patients. *Diabetes Care* **26**: 3080–3086.

Ridker, P. (2012). What works and in whom? A simple, easily applied, evidence-based approach to guidelines for statin therapy. *Circulation. Cardiovascular Quality and Outcomes* **5**: 592–593.

Rosak, C. and Mertes, G. (2012). Critical evaluation of the role of Acarbose in the treatment of diabetes: Patient considerations. *Diabetes Metabolic Syndrome Obesity: Targets and Therapy* **3**: 357–367.

Rosenstock, J., Cheung, A., Ritzel, R. et al. (2018). More similarities than differences testing insulin glargine 300 unit/mL versus insulin degludec 100 units/mL in insulin-naïve type 2 diabetes: the randomized head-to-head BRIGHT trial. *Diabetes Care* **41** (10): 2147–2154. https://doi.org/10.2337/dc18-0559.

Rossi, S. (ed.) (2007). *Australian Medicines Handbook*. Adelaide: Australian Medicines Handbook Pty Ltd.

Roughhead, L., Semple, S., and Rosenfeld, E. (2013). *Literature Review: Medication Safety in Australia*. Sydney: ACSQHC. https://www.safetyandquality.gov.au/sites/default/files/migrated/lit-review.pdf.

Roter, D., Hall, J., Mersica, R. et al. (1998). Effectiveness of interventions to improve patient compliance: a meta-analysis. *Medical Care* **36**: 1138–1161.

Rutherford, E., Wright, E., Hussain, Z. et al. (2004). *DAWN: Diabetes Attitudes, Wishes and Needs*. NovoNordisk Australasia, Sydney: The Australian Experience.

Salpeter, S., Greyber, E., Pasternak, G., and Salpeter, E. (2006). Risk of fatal and non-fatal lactic acidosis with metformin use in type 2 diabetes mellitus. *Cochrane Database of Systematic Reviews* **Jan 25** (1). www.ncbi.nlm.nih.gov/pubmed/16437448 Cochrane Library, London.

Scottish Intercollegiate Guideline Network (SIGN) (2010). *Management of Type 2 Diabetes: A National Guideline*. Edinburgh: SIGN.

Scottish Intercollegiate Guideline Network (SIGN) (2019). *Management of Type 2 Diabetes: A National Guideline*. Edinburgh: SIGN. https://www.guidelines.co.uk/diabetes/sign-type-2-diabetes-guideline/453869.article.

Senes, S. and Penm, E. (2007). *Medicines for Cardiovascular Health: Are They Used Appropriately?* Canberra: Australian Institute of Health and Welfare (AIHW). http://citeseerx.ist.psu.edu/viewdoc/download?doi=10.1.1.541.1766&rep=rep1&type=pdf.

Shah, B., Hux, J., Laupacis, A. et al. (2005). Clinical inertia in response to inadequate glycemic control. *Diabetes Care* **28** (3): 600–606.

Shenfield, G. (2001). Drug interactions with oral hypoglycaemic agents. *Australian Prescriber* **24** (4): 83–84.

Shrank, W., Libeman, J., Fischer, M. et al. (2011). Are caregivers adherent to their own medicines. *Journal of the American Pharmacists Association* **51** (41): 492–498.

Simons, L. (2002). Test CK before starting on statins. *Medical Observer* (30 August), p. 5.

Skyler, J., Cefalu, W., Kourides, I. et al. (2001). Efficacy of inhaled human insulin in type 1 diabetes mellitus. *Lancet* **357**: 331–335.

Soldatus, G. and Pease, A. (2018). How to commence insulin: guiding you through that first prescription. *Diabetes Management Journal* **2018**: 10–14.

Speight, J., Browne, J.L., Holmes-Truscott, E. et al. (2011). *Diabetes MILES – Australia 2011 Survey Report.* Melbourne: Diabetes Australia – Vic.

Standl, E., Erbach, M., and Schnell, O. (2012). What should be the antihypertensive drug of choice in diabetic patients and should we avoid drugs that increase glucose levels? Pros and cons. *Diabetes/Metabolism Research and Reviews* **28** (Suppl 2): 50–66.

Strowig, S., Aviles-Santa, L., and Raskin, P. (2004). Improved glycaemic control without weight gain using triple therapy in type 2 diabetes. *Diabetes Care* **27**: 1577–1583.

Sullivan, D. (2008). Raising HDL cholesterol in diabetes. *Diabetes Management Journal* **22**: 16.

Sumner, J., Barber, C., and Williams, V. (2000). What do people with type 1 diabetes know about hypoglycaemia? *Practical Diabetes International* **17** (6): 187–190.

Sun, Q., Li, J., and Gao, F. (2014). New insights into insulin: The anti-inflammatory effect and its clinical relevance. *World Journal of Diabetes* **5** (2): 89.

Tay, M., Messersmith, R., and Lange, D. (2001). What do people on insulin therapy remember about safety advice. *Journal of Diabetes Nursing* **5** (6): 188–191.

Therapeutic Guidelines (2019). *eTG Complete*. West Melbourne, Australia: Therapeutic Guidelines. https://tgldcdp.tg.org.au/etgcomplete.

Thomas, M. (2018). Combining SGLLT2 and DPP-4 inhibition in type 2 diabetes. *Healthed Expert Monograph* www.healthed.com.au.

Ting, R.Z.-W., Szeto, C.C., Chan, M.H.-M. et al. (2006). Risk factors of vitamin B(12) deficiency in patients receiving metformin. *Archives of Internal Medicine* **166** (18): 1975–1979.

Tung, A. (2011). The mystery of guideline non-compliance: why don't doctors do the right thing? *Anaesthesiology* **503**: 3–10.

Turner, R., Cull, C., Frighi, V., and Holman, R. (1999). Control with diet, sulphonylurea, metformin, or insulin in patients with type 2 diabetes mellitus: Progressive requirement for multiple therapies (UKPDS 49). *Journal of the American Medical Association* **281**: 2005–2012.

United Kingdom Prospective Diabetes Study (UKPDS 33) (1998). Intensive blood glucose control with sulphonylureas or insulin compared with conventional treatment and risk of complications in patients with type 2 diabetes. *Lancet* **352**: 837–853. (correction in *Lancet* (1999) 354, 602).

Vaag, A., Handberg, A., Lauritzen, M. et al. (1990). Variation in insulin absorption of NPH insulin due to intramuscular injection. *Diabetes Care* **13** (1): 74–76.

van den Berghe, G., Wouters, P., Weekers, F. et al. (2001). Intensive Insulin Therapy in Critically Ill Patients. *New England Journal of Medicine* **345**: 1359–1367.

Vashisht, R., Jung, K., Schuler, A. et al. (2018). Association of hemoglobin A1c levels with use of sulfonylureas, dipeptidyl peptidase 4 inhibitors, and thiazolidinediones in patients with type 2 diabetes treated with metformin: analysis from the observational health data sciences and informatics initiative. *JAMA Network Open* **1** (4): e181755–e181755.

Wang, A., Nagpal, R., and Yaday, H. (2018). Bi-directional drug microbiome interactions of anti-diabetics. *eBioMedicine*. https://doi.org/10.1016/ebiom.2018.11.o46.

Wang, F., Surh, J., and Kaur, M. (2012). Insulin degludec as an ultralong-acting basal insulin one a day: a systematic review. *Diabetes Metabolism and Obesity Targets and Therapy* **5**: 191–204.

Wanner, C., Inzucchi, S.E., Lachin, J.M. et al. (2016). Empagliflozin and Progression of Kidney Disease in Type 2 Diabetes. *New England Journal of Medicine* **375**: 323–334.

Whaley, J., Reilly, T., Poucher, S. et al. (2012). Targeting the kidney and glucose excretion with Dopagliflozin: Preclinical and clinical evidence for SGLT2 inhibition as a new option for treatment of type 2 diabetes mellitus. *Diabetes Metabolic Syndrome and Obesity: Targets and Therapy* **5**: 135–138.

Williams, P. (1993). Adverse effects of exogenous insulin: Clinical features, management and prevention.

Woloshin, S. and Schwartz, L. (2007). The effectiveness of a primer to help people understand risk. *Annals of Internal Medicine* **146**: 256–265.

Worthington, B. (2003). The nurses' role in patient-centred medicines management. *Professional Nurse* **19** (3): 142–144.

Wright, J., Randall, O., Miller, E. et al. (2006). Differing effects of antihypertensive drugs on the incidence of diabetes mellitus among patients with hypertensive kidney disease. *Archives of Internal Medicine* **166**: 797–805.

Yki-Jarvinen, H., Juurinen, L., Alvarsson, M. et al. (2007). Initiate insulin by aggressive titration and educate (INITIATE). *Diabetes Care* **30**: 1364–1369.

Zadelaar, S., Kleemann, R., Verschuren, L. et al. (2007). Mouse models for atherosclerosis and pharmaceutical modifiers. *Arteriosclerosis, Thrombosis, and Vascular Biology.* http://www.atvbaha.org. https://doi.org/10.1161/ATVBAHA.107.142570.

Zinman, B., Wanner, C., Lachin, J.M. et al. (2015). Empagliflozin, Cardiovascular Outcomes, and Mortality in Type 2 Diabetes. *New England Journal of Medicine* **373**: 2117–2128.

Chapter 6

Hypoglycaemia

Key points

- Hypoglycaemia is one of the most common short-term complications of diabetes treatment with insulin and sulphonylurea medicines.
- The brain depends on a constant supply of glucose because it is mainly depend on glucose as a source of metabolic energy and does not synthesise or store glucose.
- Severe hypoglycaemia is associated with cognitive changes that affect the person's ability to self-manage the hypoglycaemic episode and function normally during hypoglycaemia. It has longer-term effects on various aspects of cognition.
- Hypoglycaemia symptoms are often atypical, especially in older people, who usually present with predominantly neurogenic symptoms.
- Glucagon and the other counter-regulatory hormone response to hypoglycaemia diminishes with longer duration of both type 1 and type 2 diabetes and can be lost early in the course of type 1 diabetes.
- Hypoglycaemia is associated with clinically significant effects on wellbeing and quality of life.
- Hypoglycaemia is the most feared side effect of insulin, especially in the presence of hypoglycaemic unawareness (HU).

Rationale

Hypoglycaemia can be prevented by proactive self-care, including regular blood glucose monitoring, appropriate nursing care, and recognising impending hypoglycaemia and managing it appropriately. The prevalence of hypoglycaemia is increasing due to the focus on achieving blood glucose levels as close to normal as possible and initiating insulin early in people with type 2 diabetes. Hypoglycaemia can be a barrier to optimal control and is an independent cause of excess morbidity, mortality, and increased costs (Brod et al. 2012; Leonard et al. 2016; Davis et al. 2018). People who have hypoglycaemia appear to be more affected by diabetes than people who do not have hypoglycaemia and often report lower general health (Lundkvist et al. 2005).

Care of People with Diabetes: A Manual for Healthcare Practice, Fifth Edition. Trisha Dunning and Alan Sinclair.
© 2020 John Wiley & Sons Ltd. Published 2020 by John Wiley & Sons Ltd.

The US National Plan for Adverse Drug Prevention (2014) listed hypoglycaemia as one of three high-priority adverse medicine event prevention targets.

Introduction

Hypoglycaemia mainly occurs in people with diabetes treated with insulin and sulphonylureas (Leonard et al. 2016) but it can also occur in people without diabetes receiving palliative care, commonly due to multiorgan dysfunction or failure (Kok and Lee 2016). It can also occur in critical illness due to increased metabolic stress, which increases glucose utilisation in the tissues (Kok and Lee 2016). It can also be due to endocrine disorders such as insulinoma. The focus of this chapter is people with diabetes rather than nondiabeteic-related causes of hypoglycaemia.

Hypoglycaemia is the most common and the most serious adverse event associated with insulin use. The prevalence of hypoglycaemia has increased since the results of the Diabetes Control and Complications Trial (DCCT) in people with type 1 diabetes (DCCT Trial Group 1997; DCCT/EDICT 2003) and the United Kingdom Prospective Diabetes Study (UKPDS) (UKPDS 1998) in type 2 diabetes demonstrated that keeping blood glucose in the normal range reduced the risk of long-term diabetes complications. The blood glucose target range and HbA1c indicators of 'good glycaemiac' control are now as close as possible to the normal ranges, which increases the risk and frequency of, hypoglycaemia.

Severe hypoglycaemia occurred three times more frequently in the intensive insulin treatment group compared to conventional treatment in the DCCT (61 events per 100 people). Hypoglycaemia was more common in men than women and in adolescents than adults. The risk of severe hypoglycaemia was 1 in 3 and the risk of coma 1 in 10 (DCCT 1991). Concern about hypoglycaemia was thought to contribute to the difficulty achieving glycaemic targets. Likewise, Pramming et al. (1991) reported mild hypoglycaemia was 1.8 episodes per patient per week, and 1.4 episodes of severe hypoglycaemia per patient per year.

The increased rate of hypoglycaemia is largely due to the focus on achieving normoglycaemia by intensifying management in people with type 1 and type 2 diabetes and to initiating insulin earlier in people with type 2 diabetes, since the results of these studies were released. In early reports from the UKPDS, major hypoglycaemia occurred between 0.4 and 2.3% of insulin-treated patients per year compared with 0.4% of those treated with diet or sulphonylureas (UKPDS 1998). Later studies also show the frequency and severity of hypoglycaemia in people with type 2 diabetes is lower than type 1 (Yki-Jarvinen et al. 1999).

Wright et al. (2006) recorded self-reported hypoglycaemia rates and graded severity as: (i) transient; (ii) temporarily incapacitated; (iii) requiring assistance; (iv) requiring medical attention in various treatment groups who remained on their prescribed therapy for six years from diagnosis as part of the UKPDS. Grades 1 and 2 occurred in 0.8% in the diet and 1.7% in the Metformin groups per year and 0.1% and 0.3%, respectively, for grades 2–4 per year. Rates for those on sulphonylureas were 7.9% and 1.2%, 21.2% and 3.65 on basal insulin, and 32% and 5.5% on basal and premeal insulin.

Younger people (<45 years), women, those with HbA1c <7%, and islet autoantibody-positive people were twice as likely to report hypoglycaemia. Wright *et al.* claimed the low rates of hypoglycaemia in type 2 diabetes were unlikely to have a major negative impact on people's ability to achieve glycaemic targets. Approximately 30% of people initially recruited were lost from the study, possibly due to intensifying treatment to achieve optimal glycaemic control; thus, the numbers of people in each treatment group was small, and the overall hypoglycaemia rate was low.

Not surprisingly, hypoglycaemia risk was greater in people on insulin with poorer control but lower doses of insulin were associated with a 35% lower rate of hypoglycaemia. Older people (>65) were not included in the study; thus, their risk and ability to recognise hypoglycaemia is unclear from the study, but subsequent research suggests they are at high risk and often unable to recognise or treat hypoglycaemia (Seaquist et al. 2013) (Chapter 12).

A number of researchers suggest the rate of mild and severe hypoglycaemia is lower in insulin-treated type 2 diabetes than in type 1. However, hypoglycaemia risk increases once insulin is commenced and with increasing duration of diabetes (Henderson et al. 2003) and the loss of counter-regulatory hormone function in type 2 diabetes of longer duration parallels progressive beta cell loss and increases the risk of hypoglycaemia (Rajan 2002; Amiel et al. 2008; Unger 2012). Significantly, insulin is classified as a high-risk/high-alert medicine because it has a narrow therapeutic index and a high likelihood of causing harm or death, even when it is used appropriately.

Hypoglycaemic unawareness (HU) is uncommon in type 2 diabetes, but when present, it is associated with a higher incidence of severe hypoglycaemia. HU in adolescents with type 1 diabetes is influenced by duration of diabetes, but can occur early after the diagnosis (Johnston et al. 2012).

The DARTS study in Scotland suggests the hypoglycaemia rate in people with type 2 diabetes on insulin is the same as those with type 1 (Leese et al. 2003) and that insulin treatment is a predictor of hypoglycaemia in people with type 2 diabetes (Donnelly et al. 2005) and people treated with insulin for long periods of time are particularly at risk (Unger 2012). Significantly, hypoglycaemia is likely to become more prevalent in people with type 2 diabetes given the increasing prevalence of type 2 diabetes and the trend towards early initiation of insulin in people with type 2 diabetes.

The cost of treating hypoglycaemia is higher for people with type 2 than type 1 diabetes (Farmer et al. 2012). Farmer collected retrospective data over 12 months (2009–2010) from the South Central Ambulance Service National Health Service Trust in the UK to estimate the incidence of severe hypoglycaemia requiring ambulance assistance. Farmer et al.'s findings suggest ambulance services manage a high prevalence of hypoglycaemia in younger than older age groups: 2.1% over age 15; and 7.5% in the 15–35-year age group. The prevalence was 1.9% in people over 65 years.

The researchers concluded that, despite the higher hypoglycaemia rates in young adults the absolute number of incidents was higher in older people. The authors acknowledged that ambulance services may not attend all cases of severe hypoglycaemia, thus, the study may underestimate the incidence of severe hypoglycaemia. Field et al. (2018) also reported a high level of self-reported ambulance service use by people with type 1 diabetes for severe hypoglycaemia. Interestingly, they also reported low levels of specialist follow-up and therapy change.

The rate of severe hypoglycaemia is higher in young children: 0.49 in children <6 years compared to 0.16 in children >6 (Davis et al. 1997). Daneman et al. (1989) reported 31% of children (n = 311); mean age 11.6 and mean duration of diabetes 4.6 years, had at least one coma or convulsion since diagnosis. Other researchers report rates ranging from 6.8 to 12%. In contrast, Nordfeldt and Ludvigsson (1997) stated that the incidence of hypoglycaemic coma did not increase when HbA1c improved from 8.1 to 6.9%, but episodes of severe hypoglycaemia increased from 1.01 to 1.26 per patient per year. Early recognition and treatment of hypoglycaemia in young children is essential because their brains are vulnerable to hypoglycaemia, which may cause permanent cognitive deficits (Tattersall 1999).

Leonard et al. (2017) indicated the standard ranking of severe hypoglycaemia occurrence due to noninsulin-glucose lowering medicines was: Glyburide, Glimepiride, Glipizide Repaglinide, Nateglinide, Rosiglitazone, Pioglitazone, and Metformin at higher than average daily doses. Hypoglycaemia occurred within 180 days of commencing the medicines. These are interesting findings, given many people with type 2 diabetes require more than one glucose lowering medicine (American Diabetes Association 2019).

Wiegers et al. (2016) reported people with type 1 diabetes experience an average of two hypoglycaemic episodes per week and one severe event per year. More recently, Misra-Herbert et al. (2018) noted episodes of hypoglycaemia increased between 2006 (0.12%) and 2015 (0.31%) in people with type 2 diabetes in the Cleveland Clinic (n = 50 439). Significantly, people with severe hypoglycaemia had previous mild hypoglycaemic events.

Practice point

People's perceptions of and beliefs about hypoglycaemia differ significantly from clinical definitions and those of health professionals. People with diabetes use different language and explanatory models to explain hypogylycaemia and its severity. It is essential to understand people's perceptions of hypoglycaemia to help them develop personalised hypoglycaemia prevention/management strategies based on their hypoglycaemia risk.

The counter-regulatory response

Normal glucose homeostasis was discussed in Chapter 1. Counter-regulatory hormones, especially glucagon, the catecholamines, growth hormone, and cortisol are released when the blood glucose falls below the normal range to maintain the blood glucose level and ensure a constant supply of energy to the brain. Glucagon and the catecholamines stimulate gluconeogenesis and reduce glucose utilisation. The severity and duration of hypoglycaemia determines the magnitude of the counter-regulatory response and begins as the blood glucose falls to about 3.5–3.7 mmol/l before cognitive function is impaired around 3.0 mmol/l (Heller and Macdonald 1996).

The counter-regulatory hormones are largely responsible for the autonomic signs and symptoms of hypoglycaemia through activating the autonomic nervous system. Several researchers have compiled lists of hypoglycaemic symptoms, and most diabetes-related textbooks and chapters list the signs and symptoms of diabetes. Recognising the signs and symptoms enables early treatment to be initiated. Significantly, symptoms are often specific to the individual and individuals interpret them differently from health professionals. For example, people report symptoms differently if they are asked to indicate the relevance of each symptom to themselves (Tattersall 1999, p. 57; Unger 2012).

In the author's experience, some people think 'a hypo means you go into a coma' and do not associate mild symptoms with hypoglycaemia. Other people and their relatives associate trembling, vagueness, and aggressive behaviour as 'having a fit', which suggests some information included in hypoglycaemia education programmes may not be appropriate to everybody, and that hypoglycaemia education must be individualised, taking account of the person's hypoglycaemia risk profile. Worryingly, a US national survey (n = 2530) found many people reported they are not informed about hypoglycaemia risk factors and often experience hypoglycaemia in their daily lives while they are working and driving (Moghissi 2011), which puts them at significant risk of adverse events.

When the blood glucose is <3.0 mmol/l, fine motor coordination, mental speed and concentration, and some memory functions become impaired. Reaction times are slower, especially when the individual needs to make decisions, do mental arithmetic, and short-term verbal memory and working memory are impaired (Sommerfield et al. 2003). McAuley et al. (2001) also demonstrated significant impairment of attentional ability during hypoglycaemia but found fluid intelligence (problem-solving ability) was not impaired. Thus, many everyday tasks appear to be impaired during hypoglycaemic events, including the individual's ability to manage the hypoglycaemic episode.

Factors associated with increased cognitive deficits include male gender, HU, type1 diabetes, and high IQ. These findings have implications for effective hypoglycaemia self-management and safety. For example, people drive slowly, swerve more, steer inappropriately, spend more time driving off the road and position the car badly on the road when the blood glucose is <2.6 mmol/l (Chapter 10). The counter-regulatory response to recurrent hypoglycaemia may be blunted in subsequent hypoglycaemia and the individual may not recognise hypoglycaemia signs and symptoms. Often, people do not recall severe hypoglycaemic episodes.

Results from continuous glucose monitoring systems (CSII) suggest people taking four insulin injections per day have at least one blood glucose level <2.8 mmol/l of varying duration per day, which may not cause symptoms. The hypoglycaemia frequency and severity is affected by a number of factors, including the number of injections per day, the type of insulin, and variations in food absorption within individuals and among injection sites.

Emotions are also affected and mood changes in the three basic mood types: energetic arousal (feel active), tense arousal (feel anxious), and hedonic state (feel happy) occur during or in anticipation of hypoglycaemia. Many people with diabetes fear hypoglycaemia, which can lead them to inappropriately lower their insulin doses to reduce the risk of hypoglycaemia; see Chapter 15. Thus, the effects of hypoglycaemia are complex and multifactorial.

Education and strategies to prevent/manage hypoglycaemia should be individualised and accompany changes in medication management and include family and significant others. The education and care plan should be informed by the person's hypoglycaemia risk profile. The risk assessment should be a collaborative decision-making endeavor *with* the individual and family and other carers, when relevant. Figure 6.1 outlines the main hypoglycaemia risk factors (Dunning et al. 2019). People are either at risk (one or more risk factors present) or not at risk (no risk factors present).

Definition of hypoglycaemia

Hypoglycaemia is defined in various ways using different parameters by various organisations and many differ in the low threshold set for hypoglycaemia, which ranges from <3.9 to <3 mmol/l. The American Diabetes Association (ADA 2019) *Standards of Medical Care in Diabetes* defined hypoglycaemia as:

Hypoglycaemia alert: 3.9 mmol/l
Clinically significant: 3.0 mmol/l

Severe hypoglycaemia: no specific threshold; has significant cognitive impairment and people are unable to self-manage the episode.

However, hypoglycaemia is no longer only defined biochemically as blood glucose below a specific level. It is also defined according to severity as:

- Mild: symptomatic where the individual is able to self-treat. The symptoms are often vague and may not be related to the actual blood glucose level. The most commonly reported initial symptoms that closely reflect the actual blood glucose level are trembling, sweating, tiredness, difficulty concentrating and hunger.
- Severe: symptoms associated with neuroglycopaenia where help is required to treat the episode. People do not always remember a severe hypoglycaemic episode because of retrograde amnesia or denial. Severe hypoglycaemia can occur without coma.
- Profound: associated with coma and sometimes convulsions (Tattersall 1999, pp. 55–87).

In addition, a grading system is sometimes used, especially in research, as follows:

- Grade 1 – mild: the person recognises and self-treats.
- Grade 2 – moderate: the person requires assistance but oral treatment normalises the blood glucose.
- Grade 3 – severe: the person is semiconscious and requires assistance, and glucagon or IV glucose may be needed.

None of the definitions appear to state the important fact that most hypoglycaemia occurs in people with diabetes treated with insulin or oral glucose-lowering medicines (GLMs), especially supphonyulureas. As indicated, hypoglycaemia can occur as a consequence of terminal disease,

Why complete the tool?

To determine the person's risk of hypoglycaemia use the outcome of the risk assesment to proactively manage the risk.

How to complete

- Complete with the person/family where possible and consult the medical record.
- Place a cross in all the boxes that apply to the person.
- At risk–one or more risk factors identied. plan care to reduce/manage the risk
- If no boxes were crossed complete the risk assessment at regular intervals.

When to complete

- Complete when the person first presents for care as part of a comprehensive assessment.
- Review risk at any change in health status, before commencing or changing medicines and following a hypoglycaemic episode.

Hypoglycaemia unawareness

☐ The person does not recognise hypoglycaemia signs or symptoms (hypoglycaemic unawareness). Ask the person whether he/she knows when they are having a hypoglycaemic episode.

☐ The person has dementia/cognitive impairment.

Individual factors

☐ Long duration of diabetes.

☐ Consistently low HbA1c (≤ 7%, 53 mmol/mol).

☐ Recent hypoglycaemia episode.

☐ Incorrect insulin and other injectable GLM injection technique or oral GLM management.

☐ Fasting ketones before breakfast can indicate nocturnal hypoglycaemia.

☐ Pacing/wandering behaviour.

☐ Fasting for a procedure or religious customs.

☐ Alchohol use.

Medicine-related factors

☐ On insulin.

☐ On sulphonylureas (SU)such as gliclazide, glibenclamide, glimepiride, glipizide.

☐ On SGLT-2 inhibitor with insulin or SU.

☐ On insulin and sulphonylureas.

☐ On sedative medicines.

☐ CM such as **Panax gingseng, Mormordica charantia.**

Comorbidities

☐ Renal disease.

☐ Liver disease.

☐ Cardiovascular disease.

☐ Gastrointestional problems e.g. malabsorption conditions such as coeliac disease, gastrointestinal autonomic neuropathy.

☐ Frailty.

☐ Cahexia related to cancer.

☐ Depression.

Food-related factors

☐ Eating disorder.

☐ Low carbohydrate content in meals.

☐ Swallowing difficulties.

☐ Diarrhoea, vomiting or nausea.

☐ Erratic appetite.

Clinician-related factors

☐ Meal times do not match the action profile of the GLMs prescribed.

☐ Inappropriate prescribing: e.g. medicine choice, dose, dose frequency.

☐ Incorrect insulin injection technique.

☐ BGM regimens in hospital and RACF that do not reflect the action profile of prescribed GLMs.

☐ Over correcting hyperglycaemic episodes using stat/top-up insulin doses, often used in aged care facilities.

Abbreviations:

GLM – Glucose lowering medicine

CM – Complementary medicine

RACF – Residential aged care facility

BGM – Blood glucose monitoring

SU – Sulphonylureas

Figure 6.1   Primary hypoglycaemic risk factors.

in acute illness, and rare endocrine conditions such as insulinoma. Concomitant insulinoma and diabetes is very rare. Significantly, part of the diagnostic process for suspected insulinoma includes screening for surreptitious insulin or other GLM use.

Practice points

(1) People with diabetes managed on diet do not usually have hypoglycaemia and do not require treatment of low blood glucose levels.
(2) People treated with insulin and/or sulphonylureas are at the greatest risk of hypoglycaemia.
(3) Hypoglycaemia is the most significant side effect of insulin, including the newer insulin analogues. However, hypoglycaemia risk is lower with insulin analogues, particularly nocturnal hypoglycaemia.

In addition to insulin and/or GLM treatment, age, gender, and associated medical conditions such as liver disease, cerebrovascular disease, autonomic neuropathy, and the rate at which the blood glucose falls, influences the development and recognition of hypoglycaemic symptoms. In general, a rapid fall in blood glucose results in the development of the classic symptoms of hypoglycaemia described in Table 6.1. The classic presentation is more likely to occur in people treated with insulin.

The onset of hypoglycaemia is usually slower with sulphonylureas especially in older people and hypoglycaemia can be prolonged and recur for >24 hours, despite treatment. Mortality rates of 4–10% are reported and permanent neurological damage is present in 5% of those who

Table 6.1   Signs and symptoms of hypoglycaemia (Edinburgh Hypoglycaemia Scale Deary 1993)[a].

Sympathetic or adrenergic[b]	*Neuroglycopaenic*[c]
Weakness	Headache
Pale skin	Tiredness
Sweating	Hypothermia
Tachycardia	Visual disturbances
Palpitations	Difficulty concentrating
Shaking	Difficulty speaking
Tremor	Confusion
Nervousness or feeling anxious	Amnesia
Irritability	Seizures
Tingling of the mouth and fingers	Coma
Hunger	Inappropriate behaviour

[a] Symptoms can be different in young children, adults and older people and may vary between episodes in the same individual. Some people may not experience any of the symptoms listed; therefore it is important for people to learn to recognise *their own* hypoglycaemia cues.
[b] Caused by increased activity of the autonomic nervous system triggered by a rapid fall in blood glucose. Also referred to as sympathetic and sympathomedullary.
[c] Caused by decreased activity of the central nervous system because of very low blood glucose. Psychomotor function deteriorates. Some people appear withdrawn, others become restless and irritable. They may refuse treatment. Recovery can be slow, or rarely the person may die if they do not have help. Nausea and vomiting may occur but are unusual.

survive (Salas and Caro 2002). Long-acting sulphonylureas increase the risk because of their long duration of action, active metabolites, and the reduced ability to mount a counter-regulatory response that occurs with increasing duration of diabetes and increasing age.

Presenting symptoms may be neuroglycopaenic, often confusion, dizziness, and altered behaviour, rather than sympathetic, and the hypoglycaemia can be mistaken for stroke, transient ischaemia, or early dementia and lead to unnecessary investigations and delayed treatment (Dunning 2005; Sinclair 2006; Seaquist et al. 2013; Hope et al. 2017). Risk factors for hypoglycaemia are shown in Figure 6.1.

Most recent management guidelines recommend personalising diabetes management, including blood glucose and HbA1c targets, to suit individual needs and to enhance patient safety (Del Prato et al. 2010; IDF 2013; Dunning et al. 2014; ADA 2018).

Recognising hypoglycaemia

Some, or all, of the signs and symptoms listed in Table 6.1 can be present. A number of factors affect the individual's ability to recognise hypoglycaemia, as indicated. In addition, some commonly consumed substances such as caffeine, which can increase the intensity of the symptoms, and alcohol, which clouds judgement, can make it difficult for people to recognise hypoglycaemia.

Symptoms are more varied in children than adults and between hypoglycaemic episodes in the same child, and they have more difficulty recognising the symptoms. Young children may become naughty, aggressive, complain of abdominal pain, feeling 'awful', yawning, daydreaming, and warm to the touch (Ross et al. 1998). As indicated, older people with type 2 diabetes commonly present with neurological symptoms. Many emergency departments now have a policy of testing the blood glucose in all unconscious patients to detect hypoglycamia.

A number of factors affect the individual's ability to detect and treat hypoglycaemia, including:

- Their blood glucose level.
- Usual metabolic control.
- Recent hypoglycaemia.
- Chronic hypoglycaemia, which can occur 'acutely' in older people as a result of repeated unrecognised hypoglycaemia or as a result of HU; see Chapter 8.
- Counter-regulatory response and amount of adrenaline secreted. The ability to mount counter-regulatory response diminishes over time.
- Medications such as beta blockers can mask the sympathetic warning signs, and caffeine can cause trembling and sweating that can be mistaken for hypoglycaemia. Smoking confers a 2.6 times greater risk of severe hypoglycaemia in type 1 diabetes (Klein 2007) as well as contributing to the long-term complications of diabetes and other diseases.
- Distractions such as concentrating on work, when anxious and stressed, which also activates the autonomic nervous system ('fight or flight' response).
- Knowledge such as not recognising the symptoms.
- HU or impaired mental function, which inhibits appropriate management.
- Cognitive impairment.

Other research shows older people, especially those living alone, young children who depend on their parents, adolescents, those determined to achieve strict glycaemic control, lower socio-economic status, and pregnant women with type 1 diabetes, experience more hypoglycaemia. For example, 45% of pregnant women with type 1 diabetes experience severe hypoglycaemia during pregnancy, particularly in the first trimester and 3–5 mild hypoglycaemic events per patient-week especially in the presence of previous severe hypoglycaemia and impaired or hypoglycaemia unawareness (Ringholm and Nielsen 2008).

The brain and glucose homeostasis

Glucose homeostasis is described in Chapter 1. The brain requires 120–140 g glucose per day to function normally and has limited capacity to manufacture its own glucose. Therefore, it depends on adequate levels of circulating blood glucose. A major function of glucose homeostasis is to ensure the brain receives sufficient glucose, which is its main source of energy. Glucose homeostasis depends on tight regulation of glucose use by liver, muscle, white and brown fat, and glucose production, and release into the bloodstream by the liver (Thorens 2011).

In addition to the hormones described in Table 6.2, glucose homeostasis is controlled by the autonomic nervous system through glucose-excited neurons (activated) or glucose-inhibited neurons (inhibited). Most of these neurons are located in the brainstem and hypothalamus. They are activated by hyper- and hypoglycaemia. The loss of glucose sensing by these neurons as well as diminished beta cell responses are a feature of type 2 diabetes. The effects on the counter-regulatory response could be due to initial defects in these glucose sensing neurons (Thorens 2011).

Causes of hypoglycaemia

Although hypoglycaemia is associated with insulin and GLM use, the relationship among these agents and food intake, exercise, and a range of other contributory factors is not straightforward. Some episodes can be explained by altered awareness or mismatch between food intake and/or food absorption and insulin. It should be noted that serum insulin levels and glucose clearance following insulin injections varies in the same individual even when the same dose is injected at the same time, dose, and approximate site each day (Galloway and Chance 1994), even with modern purified insulins (Del Prato et al. 2010) and insulin analogues.

Exercise is also a contributing factor in many cases but the effect of exercise is also difficult to predict and depends on exercise intensity and duration, planned or spontaneous, time of the day, previous food intake, when it occurred in relation to insulin/GLM dose, and the insulin injection site. For example, absorption is enhanced if exercise commences immediately after injecting insulin but not if exercise commences >35 minutes after injecting.

As indicated, sulphonylureas cause hypoglycaemia but less often than insulin; however, when sulphonylurea-induced hypoglycaemia does occur, it causes significant morbidity and mortality, may be prolonged, and may accompany or precipitate a stroke or myocardial infarction. Interactions with other medicines, including complementary medicines, should be considered especially in the setting of compromised renal function; see Chapters 8 and 18. Alcohol may be a contributing factor. Frequent hypoglycaemia might indicate changing renal function and insulin doses may need to be reduced. GLMs may be contraindicated. Lowered appetite and nausea accompanying renal disease may contribute to hypoglycaemia risk.

Table 6.2 The counter-regulatory hormonal response to hypoglycaemia. The response is reduced by 50% by antecedent hypoglycaemia.

Hormone	Action
Glucagon	Increases glucose output from liver and muscle (glycogenolysis)
Adrenaline and noradrenaline	Becomes the main defense when the glucagon response is lost, but is also impaired over time. Enhances glycogenolysis in liver and muscle. Enhances gluconeogenesis. Reduces insulin secretion. Causes many of the signs and symptoms of hypoglycaemia (autonomic response, see Table 6.1)
Cortisol	Mobilises the substrates for gluconeogenesis
Growth hormone	Acts with cortisol and adrenaline to inhibit peripheral glucose utilisation

If no reasonable common contributing factor can be identified, less common causes such as endocrine disorders, gastroparesis, and coeliac disease should be considered; see Chapter 10. Psychological factors also need to be considered; see Chapter 15. However, a specific reason for the episode cannot always be found, which makes prevention difficult: the cause for 19–38% of hypoglycaemic events cannot be identified.

Various authors attribute hypoglycaemia to 'patient noncompliance' such as manipulating insulin doses, reducing intake, or omitting meals. While these behaviours do occur, especially in adolescents (Chapter 13), health professionals need to understand the reason for the behaviour and the very significant burden (workload) involved in self-managing diabetes and medicines, rather than attaching a label to the individual. They need to appreciate the complexity of achieving diabetes balance and the frustration it causes many people with diabetes and the fear associated with hypoglycaemia (Jones 2011; Bernard et al. 2012). Blood glucose balance is sometimes viewed as an equation:

$$\text{Insulin/glms} + \text{Appropriate diet} + \text{Appropriate exercise} = \text{Target glucose levels}$$

However, this is simplistic. It ignores significant individual factors not included in the equation. Likewise, many older people with diabetes are overtreated (Tucker et al. 2018) and sliding-scale insulin use in hospital and aged-care facilities persists despite the risks and recommendation that it is not used (Pandaya et al. 2008; ADA 2019).

Preventing and managing hypoglycaemia

Preventing hypoglycaemia is challenging and may be impossible to achieve. It is possible to help people recognise their unique hypoglycaemia symptoms, signs, and personal hypoglycaemic risk factors and plan care to limit the severity and frequency of hypoglycaemia. Key management strategies include the following:

- Undertake a personalised hypoglycaemia risk assessment (Figure 6.1), especially with vulnerable older people, children, those with recurrent severe hypoglycaemia, HU, cognitive impairment, renal and liver disease, and people who consume excess alcohol. The assessment should include helping people identify situations that increase their risk of hypoglycaemia. In hospital settings, people at high risk of hypoglycaemia, include those fasting for procedures and people on insulin infusions. In-hospital hypoglycaemia is associated longer length of stay, increased morbidity and mortality, and costs (Hulkower et al. 2014). HU is common in people with diabetes in hospital. The prevalence varies and can be as high as 45% when people receive intensive treatment (Boucai et al. 2011).
- Use the information to develop a personalized hypoglycaemia management plan with the individual and/or their family.
- Use the information to determine safe blood glucose and HbA1c target ranges for the individual. The joint British Diabetes Society and Diabetes UK suggested 'making 4 (mmol/l) the floor' (Umpierrez et al. 2012).
- Appreciate the emotional and psychological components of hypoglycaemia and the associated fear and impacts on self-care. These aspects should be part of an individualised, comprehensive assessment when people commence insulin and at regular intervals, especially when the person experiences an hypoglycaemic event.
- Appropriate prescribing and medicine reviews and dose adjustment.
- Include medicine reviews in annual complication screening programmes.
- Educate the person about insulin action, hypoglycaemia symptoms, and food intake and exercise in relation to insulin action, and managing hypoglycaemic episodes. The education might include adjusting insulin doses, insulin types, and the dose regimen using programmes such as DAFNE and DESMOND and structured blood glucose monitoring programmes, especially for people using insulin pumps and those on basal bolus regimens. Regular education revision is advisable.

- Educate the person about the risks associated with driving any type of motorised vehicle and operating machinery when blood glucose is low.
- Regular blood glucose-self-monitoring is essential; the information can be used to tailor food, exercise, and medicine doses.
- The individual must wear appropriate identification and carrying hypogycaemic treatment at all times.
- Use new technologies such as blood glucose meters and algorithms embedded in insulin pumps and glucose sensor systems that can be programmed to identify high and low blood glucose. Systems are available that suspend insulin for two hours when hypoglycaemia is detected. Continuous glucose monitoring can be used as part of a risk assessment and a range of mobile phone apps are available to help people manage their diabetes.
- Have back-up and support systems in place if the individual is unable to manage the hypoglycaemic episode themselves.
- Help people with hypoglycaemia unawreness recognise changed body signs of hypoglycaemia, including structured programmes such as blood glucose awareness training (BGAT) (Cox et al. 2001).

In addition, organisations such as hospital and aged-care homes must have relevant policies and procedures in place and ensure staff are competent to recognise and manage hypoglycaemic episodes.

Hypoglycaemic unawareness

The ability to recognise hypogycaemia warning signs is essential to prevention of severe hypoglycaemia and associated risk of injury, falls and coma. People's experience of hypoglycaemia varies considerably from each other and between hypoglycaemic episodes (Speight 2011). HU is defined as the onset of neuroglycopenia before the appearance of autonomic warning signs (Martin-Timón and del Cañizo-Gomez 2015). The underlying causes are multifactorial; it manifests as the inability to recognize impending hypoglycemia signs and symptoms. HU increased the risk of severe hypoglycaemia sixfold in people with type 1 diabetes and 17-fold in those with type 2 diabetes (Schopman et al. 2010).

HU also affects glucose uptake in the brain. People with type 1 diabetes have more profound cognitive dysfunction during acute hypoglycaemia, which persists for longer following recovery. In type 2 diabetes. HU is associated with cardiovascular complications that increase the risk of myocardial infarction that remains for up to six months. They are also at risk of neurologic complications.

HU means people no longer recognise the early autonomic hypoglycaemic signs and do not recognise hypoglycaemia; thus, they do not treat it and are at risk of severe hypoglycaemia and coma.

Recurrent episodes of hypoglycaemia reduce the counter-regulatory response, associated symptoms and cognitive responses, which affects the individual's ability to recognise and treat the episode. People with type 1 and type 2 diabetes have compromised counter-regulatory responses over time, and a cycle of recurrent hypoglycaemia where each episode becomes increasingly severe may develop. If counter-regulation is compromised endogenous insulin secretion is not inhibited.

Significantly, glucagon release in response to hypoglycaemia is impaired soon after diagnosis of diabetes and becomes progressively defective in people with diabetes. Adrenaline release is also reduced, which ultimately contributes to HU (DCCT Research Trial Group 1991; Unger 2012).

HU can develop when the usual blood glucose is in the low/normal range and people may begin to recognise the symptoms again if the blood glucose targets are raised. Chronic HU develops with long duration of diabetes usually as a result of autonomic neuropathy and diminished counter-regulatory response. Both acute and chronic HU can be aggravated by medicines such as beta blockers, alcohol, and stimulants such as caffeine. HU increases the risk of severe and profound hypoglycaemia and is one criterion for islet cell transplants.

Prevalence of HU

Determining the prevalence of HU is difficult because experts use different definitions and assessment methods. An estimated 19.5–25% of adults with type1 diabetes have HU and are older than people who recognise hypoglycaemic symptoms (Geddes et al. 2008). Rates for people with type2 diabetes are more difficult to determine because fewer data are available, but increasing age and duration of diabetes contribute to HU, which may be present in 8% of people with type2 diabetes (Speight 2011). However, HU in people with type2 diabetes could be under-recognised and underreported.

Indicators that chronic hypoglycaemia might be present in older people, especially those on GLMs, include confusion, changes in cognition, personality changes, and disordered behaviour and must be distinguished from other less easily reversible causes of these signs. Accurately monitoring the blood glucose levels is important to detect chronic hypoglycaemia, and continuous glucose monitors (CGMs) can be useful. Management consists of revising the care plan and checking:

- That carbohydrate intake is adequate and evenly distributed.
- The individual is able to accurately prepare and administer their insulin.
- Whether any new medications or complementary therapies (CM) were commenced and reviewing the individual's medication self-management practices.
- Teeth/dentures to ensure there is no infection or mouth ulcers and that false teeth fit and are worn.
- Presence of diabetic complications or comorbidities that can affect self-care ability.

Knowledge might mean relatives and friends need information about managing hypoglycaemia, including how and when to use. People may benefit from education programmes such as BGATT (see Chapter 16) and some regain the ability to recognise hypoglycaemia or their new body cues after a period free from hypoglycaemia.

Clinical observations

Clinicians need to learn to recognise 'hypo clues' during diabetes consultations, especially people at high risk of hypoglycaemia (Hope et al. 2017).

Several methods are used to assess HU and include careful questioning when HU is suspected, for example changed hypoglycaemic symptoms over time, combined with appropriate use of the individuals blood glucose monitoring pattern and serial HbA1c levels, frequent presentations to emergency for hypoglycaemia, and continuous blood glucose monitoring (CGM). Clinical trial methods include the following:

- Clarke method assesses people's threshold for and symptomatic response to hypoglycaemia but is limited by outdated definition of severe hypoglycaemia and lack of consensus about the glycaemic thresholds for hypoglycaemic severity.
- Gold method is a single item measure of HU and is the most frequently used method, but it is limited by the difficulty of interpreting scores between 1 (awareness) and 4 (unawareness).
- Pederson-Bjergaad method could overestimate the prevalence of HU.
- Functional neuroimaging to measure regional brain metabolism, which is a proxy measure of neuronal activation, during hypoglycaemic episodes (Dunn et al. 2007).

- Hypoglycaemicia Awareness Questionnaire (HYPOA-Q) is a new tool that consists of 18 items that assess a range of issues related to HU. In the future, the HYPOA-Q could enable earlier diagnosis and evaluation of HU and proactive management and might be the most clinically relevant measure.

Nocturnal hypoglycaemia

Nocturnal hypogycaemia is defined as blood glucose, 3.3 mmol/l occurring during the night and mainly occurs in type1 diabetes, usually as a consequence of relative insulin excess and impaired glucose production overnight. Increased insulin sensitivity overnight plays a role. More than 80% of people treated with insulin experience nocturnal hypoglycaemia; 40% of these episodes are severe and are associated with significant morbidity and, rarely, death. CGSM suggests the prevalence of nocturnal hypoglycaemia is 10–56%, lasts for ~6 hours, the time of the lowest level (nadir) depends on the insulin type and regimen (Raju et al. 2006). Raju et al. (2006) did not find differences in mean nocturnal blood glucose or mean nadir using CGSM to compare four insulin regimens in people with type1 diabetes with HbA1c <7.1%, but detected high rates of under- and overestimation of the glucose level.

Pramming et al. (1985) tried to identify predictors of early-morning hypoglycaemia. They suggested if the blood glucose was <6 mmol/l at 11 p.m. there was an 80% chance of nocturnal hypoglycaemia compared to 12% risk if the blood glucose was >5 mmol/l. Other researchers report similar predictive blood glucose levels, but the likelihood of nocturnal hypoglycaemia increases if multiple injections are used compared to CSII (Whincup and Milner 1987; Bendtson et al. 1988). Vervoort et al. (1996) found the bedtime blood glucose level predicted hypoglycaemia in the early part of the night but not hypoglycaemia occurring in the early morning and that a fasting blood glucose (before breakfast) <5.5 mmol/l indicated early morning hypoglycaemia.

However, the only risk factor Cooperberg et al. (2008) identified in a study to determine the amount of glucose needed to prevent exercise-induced hypoglycaemia, was frequent exercise. In Young et al.'s study, nocturnal hypoglycaemia occurred on both exercise and sedentary nights. Blood glucose 7.2 mmol/l at 9 p.m. predicted overnight hypoglycaemia on sedentary days. Exercise has multiple effects on fuel utilisation and mobilisation. Initially, in the first 5–10 minutes muscle glycogen is the primary fuel source, followed by circulating glucose and then fuel derived from gluconeogenesis and fatty acid oxidation (Silverstein 2008). When the counter-regulatory response is abnormal, people are unable to effectively mobilise glucose stores for gluconeogenesis.

In many cases, the individual does not recognise the signs of nocturnal hypoglycaemia and does not wake up. Repeated episodes of nocturnal hypoglycaemia reduce the counter-regulatory response to hypoglycaemia. Undetected autonomic dysfunction and nocturnal hypoglycaemia can increase the risk of fatal cardiac ventricular dysrrhythmias ('dead in bed' syndrome).

Indicators of nocturnal hypoglycaemia

- Night sweats
- Nightmares or vivid dreams
- Unaccustomed snoring
- Morning lethargy or chronic fatigue
- Headaches or 'hung over' feeling
- Mood change, particularly depression
- High blood glucose before breakfast (Somogyi effect)
- Morning ketouria
- Relatives notice unusual behavior such as snoring or 'sleep walking'

Factors that contribute to nocturnal hypoglycaemia include preceding physical activity that may have occurred many hours previously, insufficient carbohydrate in meals, excess insulin as a result of these factors, enhanced sensitivity to insulin, and/or inappropriate insulin dose and alcohol consumption.

The Somogyi effect refers to pre-breakfast hyperglycaemia following an overnight hypoglycaemic episode. If any of the above symptoms occur, the blood glucose should be measured at 2–3 a.m. over several nights to establish whether nocturnal hypoglycaemia is occurring. The insulin is then adjusted accordingly by decreasing the morning long-acting dose for those on a daily insulin, the afternoon long-acting dose for those on BD insulin or the pre-evening meal or bedtime dose for basal bolus regimes.

Clinical observations

(1) Sometimes the evening short-acting insulin, rather than the intermediate or long-acting insulin, causes nocturnal hypoglycaemia, depending on the time the insulin was administered.
(2) Rapid-acting insulins have a shorter duration of action and are less likely to cause nocturnal hypoglycaemia.
(3) Stress and illness are usually associated with hyperglycaemia; however, they can induce hypoglycaemia in some people with type 1 diabetes.

Practice point

The Somogyi effect should be distinguished from another condition that results in morning hyperglycaemia, the *dawn phenomenon*. The dawn phenomenon refers to a situation where insulin requirements and blood glucose concentration increase between 5 a.m. and 8 a.m., which occurs in up to 75% of people with diabetes. Treatment consists of *increasing* the insulin dose.

Many other hormones have a normal physiological rise in the early morning (e.g. testosterone, which causes early-morning erections).

Managing nocturnal hypoglycaemia

Not surprisingly, people with diabetes and their relatives are very fearful of hypoglycaemia at any time, but particularly at night, and careful explanations about the possible causes and suggestions of ways to prevent nocturnal hypoglycaemia are essential. Families/significant others need to know how to manage the hypoglycaemia by maintaining the person's airway and calling an ambulance. If they have glucagon at home, they should give the injection.

Various methods have been used to prevent nocturnal hypoglycaemia. These include providing carbohydrate snacks at bedtime, although there is no real evidence to support the practice (Allen and Frier 2003) or demonstrate efficacy (Raju et al. 2006), and adjusting the insulin regimen. The long-acting insulin analogues, with their more predictable action profile, are associated with significantly lower rates of nocturnal hypoglycaemia. Helping the individual and their family/carers recognise cues to hypoglycaemia through hypoglycaemia training programmes, such as HYATT and BGATT, may be effective (Cox et al. 2004). CGSM may provide important clues to assist in such training.

More recently, antihypoglycaemic agents such as ß₂-adrenergic agonists (Terbutaline) were trialled and a significant reduction in the frequency and severity of nocturnal hypoglycaemia was demonstrated (Raju et al. 2006). The morning blood glucose was significantly higher after Terbutaline and the pulse rate was elevated. Acarbose with a carbohydrate bedtime snack also reduced the mean blood glucose nadir but did not prevent nocturnal hypoglycaemia.

Relative hypoglycaemia

People who are accustomed to high blood glucose levels for long periods of time may experience the symptoms of hypoglycaemia when blood glucose control improves and blood glucose levels normalise. In general, it is not necessary to treat the symptoms once the blood glucose is recorded, but reassurance, support, and education are necessary until the person adapts to the new blood glucose range.

Medicine interactions

Some commonly prescribed medicines can interact with sulphonylureas and increase the possibility of hypoglycaemia (see Table 6.3).

Practice points

- Consider whether the person is using complementary medicines such as herbs, supplements, and other CM such as massage and relaxation therapies. These therapies can exert hypoglycaemic effects themselves, interact with conventional medicines or cause liver or renal damage that alters the pharmacokinetics and pharmacodynamics of medicines and predisposes the person to hypoglycaemia, or indirectly affect the blood glucose by reducing stress (see Chapter 18).
- People with diabetes are high CAM users.

Table 6.3 Commonly prescribed medicines that can increase the hypoglycaemic effect of sulphonylurea medicines.

Medicines	Means of potentiation if known
Sulphonamides	Displaces sulphonylureas from protein binding sites
Salicylates	
Warfarin	
Clofibrate	
Phenylbutazone	
Coumarin derivatives	Inhibits/decreases hepatic metabolism of the sulphonylurea
Chloramphenicol	
Phenylbutazone	
Probenecid	Delays urinary excretion of the sulphonylurea
Salicylates	
Tuberculostatics	
Tetracyclines	
MAO inhibitors	Increases action by an unknown mechanism

Objectives of care

In hospital settings, staff must be alert to the possibility of hypoglycaemia in all people on insulin or GLMs, and should hypoglycaemia occur, staff must take the following steps:

(1) Supply quick-acting carbohydrate to immediately raise blood glucose levels if the person is conscious and able to eat.
(2) Maintain blood glucose levels within the acceptable range of 4–8 mmol/l most of the time for most people, but the range may vary in specific situations such as surgical procedures.
(3) Ascertain the cause of the hypoglycaemic episode.
(4) Limit further episodes of hypoglycaemia.
(5) Allay fear and anxiety including that of relatives.
(6) Prevent trauma occurring as a result of hypoglycaemia; for example, falls.
(7) Assess the individual's knowledge about managing hypoglycaemia and educate or refer to a diabetes educator if necessary. In particular, people should be assisted to recognise their personal risk of hypoglycaemia and learn to recognise their individual *hypo symptoms* rather than being provided with a list of textbook signs and symptoms.
(8) Consider including an alert in the individual's medical record if they are at high risk of hypoglycaemia.
(9) Consider safety issues related to hypoglycaemia, such as falls and associated fractures in older people, and plan care and organise the environment to reduce such risks. One Australian hospital lists severe hypoglycaemia as a reason for a Medical Evaluation Team (MET) call.

Johnston et al. (2012) examined hypoglycaemic events and fall-related fractures in people with type2 diabetes over 65 years over two consecutive 12-month periods. They also collected data about the presence of other falls risk factors such as vascular disease, medicines including thiazolidinediones (TZDs). Johnston et al. found hypoglycaemia was independently associated with increased risk of falls-related fractures. Common fractures include hip, spine, pelvis, leg, and upper arm. The findings suggest that hypoglycaemia should be included on falls risk assessment tools when the individual has GLM-treated diabetes (Dunning 2005).

Treatment

Rapid treatment is important to prevent mild hypoglycaemia progressing to severe hypoglycaemia and limit the potential adverse risks associated with severe episodes. The following management refers to people in hospital but can be applied in other settings (Green 2016).

Mild hypoglycaemia

Test and record the blood glucose level.

Provide 15–20g of carbohydrate as quick-acting glucose or other high glycaemic index carbohydrate to raise the blood glucose immediately, for example:

Three level teaspoons sugar in 50ml (1/2 cup) water

or 150ml (1/2 can) regular sugary/soft drink (*not low calorie* [joule])

or proprietary glucose preparation, such as glucose gels/tablets or person's usual hypoglycaemia treatment (e.g. seven jellybeans).

Traditional treatment advice is to follow the initial glucose treatment with long-acting carbohydrate to maintain blood glucose until the next meal. However, the extra carbohydrate may not always be necessary if the hypoglycaemia is due to rapid-acting insulin with short duration of action. The person's experience and clinical judgement are important determinants of the need for extra carbohydrate, but remember, many people overtreat hypoglycaemia. If follow-up carbohydrate is required, provide:

1/2 sandwich or 1 slice of bread
or 2–4 dry biscuits (unsweetened)
or 1 piece of fruit.

Check blood glucose in one hour and then as necessary. The next dose of insulin or GLM is not usually withheld following a mild hypoglycaemic episode. However, if hypoglycaemia occurs frequently, the management regimen might need to be adjusted, for example, extra carbohydrate in the diet, reduced medication dose.

Severe hypoglycaemia with impaired conscious state

Note: Do not give anything by mouth if the person is unconscious. Confused patients often spit fluids out or refuse to swallow. Gels are preferable and can be smeared onto the buccal mucosa but do little to raise the blood glucose.

(1) Place the person on their side.
(2) Clear airway.
(3) Notify the doctor in hospital settings or call an ambulance.
(4) Test the blood glucose level and confirm with the laboratory (i.e. urgent glucose).
(5) Give IM glucagon. Instructions for glucagon administration are shown at the end of the chapter. Prepare an IV tray containing 50% dextrose. Fifty percent glucose should be given into an antecubital vein because injection into hand veins often results in extravasation and thrombophlebitis. Ten percent glucose is recommended for children to reduce the risk of hyperosmolality. Dose: adult 20–30 ml 50% glucose; child 2–5 ml/kg bolus 10% glucose then 0.1 ml/kg/min until the child regains consciousness. Consciousness usually returns within five minutes (Therapeutic Guidelines (TG) 2004).
(6) Monitor blood glucose every one to two hours until blood glucose level is stable above 5 mmol/l and then revert to the usual testing regimen.
(7) Give complex carbohydrate low glycaemic index food to maintain the blood glucose level when consciousness returns. The patient may still be confused and may need to be reminded to chew and swallow.

The patient should be monitored for at least 36 hours. Ascertain the time and dose for the next insulin injection/OHA dose. Provide education, counselling, and support to the individual and their family/carers.

Prolonged hypoglycaemia

Recovery from hypoglycaemia can be prolonged if the episode is severe, prolonged, and/or associated with coma and/or seizures. Other causes of impaired consciousness should be considered such as stroke and insulin overdose. Insulin overdose should be excluded when high doses of IV glucose are needed to maintain the blood glucose >5 mmol/l.

Hypoglycaemia related to long-acting sulphonylureas is a medical emergency, and the person should be managed in hospital. Prolonged infusion of 10% IV and one to two hourly blood glucose monitoring is often necessary. Some experts recommend using 50 mg of subcutaneous octreotide eight hours for three doses (TG 2004). In some cases, a brain scan will be indicated, and if cerebral oedema is present, IV mannitol is administered. Shorr et al. (1996) suggested the crude rate of prolonged hypoglycaemia associated with long-acting sulphonylureas is 16.6% per 1000 person years compared to 1.9% in second-generation agents. However, long-acting sulphonylureas are no longer used in most countries. Significantly, recent discharge from hospital is a significant predictor of serious medicine-associated hypoglycaemia in older people (days 1–30), especially the very old, frail, those on more than five medicines (Shorr et al. 1997).

Recovery should be rapid. If recovery does not occur in 10–15 minutes, exclude other causes of unconsciousness.

(1) Record episode and blood glucose level on the appropriate chart/s and in patient's medical record. Consider whether an alert sticker should be included in their medical record.
(2) Monitor progress/recovery from the episode.
(3) Look for the cause of hypoglycaemia, such as meal delayed or missed, inadequate intake of carbohydrate, unaccustomed activity, excessive medication, medication/medication, medication/herb, or herb/herb interactions.
(4) Reassure the patient and relatives.
(5) Ensure patient has an understanding of causes and management of hypoglycaemia (refer to diabetes nurse specialist/diabetes educator, and/or geriatric assessment).
(6) See Chapter 12 for information about managing hypoglycaemia in older people.

Patients most at risk of hypoglycaemia

A number of factors significantly increase the risk of hypoglycaemia. These include:

- Those taking insulin or GLM, especially long-acting formulations and intensive insulin therapy; see Chapter 12. However, the long-acting insulin analogues have lower hypoglycaemia risk than the other long-acting and biphasic insulins.
- Medicine doses not adjusted for changes such as weight loss, increased activity, following acute illness, and when reducing oral corticosteroid doses.
- Beginning an exercise/diet regimen or prolonged aerobic exercise. Hypoglycaemia can occur many hours after exercise, often during the night. Unaccustomed activity such as rehabilitation programmes should be considered 'exercise'.
- People on insulin achieving blood glucose within the normal range.
- History of hypoglycaemia.
- People with an irregular lifestyle and irregular meal and exercise patterns and when carbohydrate content of the meal is low.
- Eating disorders.
- Young children. It is difficult to predict their activity levels and food intake, and the presenting signs may be difficult to distinguish from other causes such as tiredness and misbehaving. It is important to support and educate the family.
- Adolescents, possibly because of their erratic eating patterns and experimentation with alcohol and striving for 'good control'.
- Older people, especially those who live alone.
- Insulin-treated pregnant women and newborn babies of women with GDM or on insulin.
- Those with renal or hepatic disease. Severe hypoglycaemia is independently associated with microalbuminuria in people with type 2 diabetes (Yun et al. 2013).
- Those with long-standing diabetes who may have autonomic neuropathy are at risk of HU, and effects on the gastrointestinal tract may delay gastric emptying and food absorption.
- People with brittle diabetes (Chapter 10).
- People fasting for a procedure/surgery or religious reasons (e.g. Ramadan and Buddhist Lent).
- People with diarrhoea and vomiting where food absorption is impaired. Hypoglycaemia may impair gastric emptying (Russo et al. 2005).
- Those with an impaired conscious state.
- Those sedated or on narcotic infusions.

- Endocrine diseases such as insulinoma, hypothyroidism, and hypoadrenalism.
- Alcohol may also cause hypoglycaemia, particularly if food is not eaten at the same time. The hypoglycaemia can occur hours after consuming alcohol.
- People taking a lot of medications and/or complementary medicines, especially those that lower blood glucose.
- Social class where people may not be able to afford appropriate food or hypoglycaemia treatment and prevention.

Practice points

(1) The signs of alcohol intoxication can make hypoglycaemia difficult to recognise. Alcohol impairs cognitive function and reduces the ability to recognise and effectively treat hypoglycaemia. Self-care and diet are often inadequate. In addition, chronic alcohol abuse leads to malnutrition and limited glucose stores to mount an effective counter-regulatory response.
(2) People with chronic alcohol addiction are very difficult to manage because OHAs are often contraindicated and insulin puts them at high risk of hypoglycaemia.

Psychological effects of hypoglycaemia

Hypoglycaemia is feared and hated by many people with diabetes, and the effects are often underrated by health professionals. The importance of recognising and accepting these concerns cannot be overemphasised. Hypoglycaemia has profound effects on people's quality of life, social activities such as driving and work, and they fear brain damage and death from hypoglycaemia. It is not unusual for people to deliberately run their blood glucose levels high to avoid hypoglycaemia (Dunning 1994) (see Chapter 15). They can then be termed noncompliant and be placed in a conflict situation. Commonly expressed concerns about hypoglycaemia are:

- Loss of control of the situation
- Reminder that they have diabetes
- Losing face and making a fool of themselves
- Blood glucose rising too high after treatment
- Sustaining brain damage; however, the DCCT and EDIC studies did not show a relationship between hypoglycaemia and declining cognitive function (DCCT Trial Group/EDICT 1993). The DCCT is not relevant to older people. Hershey et al. (2005) found impaired spatial long-term memory performance and repeated episodes of severe hypoglycaemia, particularly when the hypoglycaemia commenced before five years of age. Severe, repeated hypoglycaemia has also been associated with a lower volume of grey matter in the left superior temporal region of the brain, which is associated with episodic memory, in young people with type 1 diabetes (Perantie et al. 2007).
- recovery can take days following serious hypoglycaemia and the person may experience residual headache and tiredness;
- death.

Hypoglycaemia can affect the individual's confidence in their ability to cope. Support and understanding, and exploring all of the issues, physical, mental, and social that affect coping are important parts of management.

Clinical observation

Pet dogs sometimes recognise their owner's hypoglycaemia and alert them in time for them to be able to treat the hypoglycaemia or rouse another family member.

There are a number of physical sequels to hypoglycaemia in addition to the psychological consequences that include:

- *Neurological impairment.* Two main areas of the brain function are affected: cognitive ability, most commonly hippocampal functions such as memory, and affective ability, which affects mood and anxiety level. Blood glucose <1 mmol/l is referred to as neurogycopaenia and usually results in coma, loss of consciousness, seizures, and death or permanent brain damage (McNay and Cotero 2010). Less-profound hypoglycaemia, blood glucose <2 mmol/l, can interfere with the individual's ability to perform usual activities and lead to irritability, drowsiness, vision changes, difficulty speaking, and confusion (Unger and Parkin 2011). These neurological changes are particularly dangerous in older people and contribute to or accelerate dementia. Zhang et al. (2010) suggested that the risk of dementia attributable to hypoglycaemia is 2.9% per year. However, the longer-term neurological effects are controversial. Interestingly, Dunn et al. (2007) suggested that although hypoglycaemia is distressing, it might also be weakly rewarding because the brain regional networks serving hedonic responses are relatively unaffected in hypoglycaemic people. Amiel, one of the coauthors, used the term *hypo junkies* in a presentation in Melbourne to refer to a very small group of people who derived pleasure from hypoglycaemia.
- *Cardiovascular outcomes.* Symptomatic mild and severe hypoglycaemia is associated with increased cardiovascular events, hospital admissions from all causes, and mortality from all causes (Pai-Feng et al. 2012; Davis et al. 2018; Misra-Herbert et al. 2018). Likewise, Zoungas (2010) found a significant increase in risk of major macrovascular events (hazard ratio (HR) 2.88; 95% confidence interval (CI)), microvascular events (HR1.81, 95% CI 1.19–2.74), death from macrovascular events (HR 2.68 95% CI 1.72–4.19), and death from any cause (HR 2.69, 95% CI 1.97–3.67) (p all < 0.001) associated with severe hypoglycaemia. The presence of macroalbuminuria predicts severe hypoglycaemia (Jae-Seung et al. 2013).
- *Nonvascular outcomes* are also affected (Zoungas 2010). There are associations between severe hypoglycaemia and outcomes such as respiratory, digestive, and skin conditions.
- Falls and fall-related fractures (Johnston et al. 2012) compromise self-care and mobility, increase anxiety, and could mean admission to an aged-care facility.
- Accidents when driving and/or operating equipment.

Guidelines for administering glucagon

Glucagon is a hormone produced by the alpha cells of the pancreas. Glucagon stimulates glycogenolysis and hepatic glucose output. Glucagon is available in a single-dose pack containing one vial of glucagon hydrochloride powder (1 mg) and a glass syringe prefilled with sterile water (for injection).

Indication

Glucagon is used to treat severe hypoglycaemia in people with diabetes treated with insulin or GLMs, primarily people who are unable to take glucose orally, for whom oral glucose is ineffective, who are unconscious or uncooperative, or who are having a seizure. Glucagon can be administered by relatives.

Instructions for use

(1) Individual patients must be assessed to determine the appropriate dose and route of administration. Glucagon is given according to body weight and muscle bulk (intramuscularly or subcutaneously). The buttock is the ideal injection site.
(2) The intravenous route may be the preferred route in hospital in profound hypoglycaemia to ensure rapid absorption and reversal of the hypoglycaemia. DCCT data suggest unconscious patients recover within approximately 6 minutes of the glucagon injection. Glucagon may be ineffective in people with low glycogen stores, such as thin, frail older people and those with liver disease, including alcoholics.
(3) Check the expiry date. Do not reconstitute the glucagon until just before it is administered (prepare and administer). Glucagon should be used soon after reconstitution. Do not use if reconstituted solution is not clear and colourless.
(4) Follow the instructions in the package to prepare the injection and the medical order for the dose.
(5) Record the time and route of administration, the dose, and the patient's response.

Dosage

- Adults and children of weight >25 kg: full dose (1 mg).
- Children of weight <25 kg: half dose (0.5 mg).

Practice points

(1) A second dose of glucagon can be given; however, repeated injections can cause nausea, making subsequent food intake difficult, thus, repeat dosing is not recommended.
(2) If recovery does not occur within 10–15 minutes, IV glucose might be required. Slow recovery could indicate limited glucose stores, but other causes of unconsciousness should be considered.
(3) Glucagon may be contraindicated where glycogen stores are low, for example, in fasting states, chronic hypoglycaemia, chronic adrenal insufficiency, and malnutrition where the individual is unable to mount an effective counter-regulatory response.

Adverse reactions

Adverse reactions are rare. Occasionally, transient nausea occurs that can make it difficult to consume sufficient oral carbohydrates, which is necessary to avoid the blood glucose dropping again. Vomiting occurs occasionally, usually only after a second dose.

Glucagon is a peptide, so theoretically hypersensitivity is possible and is more likely in atopic patients. In reality, hypersensitivity is rare.

Clinical observations

- Hypothermia can prolong recovery from hypoglycaemia, especially in the elderly in winter. Management of the hypothermia as well as the hypoglycaemia is usually required.
- Hypothermia represents a poor prognosis.

References

Allen, K. and Frier, B. (2003). Nocturnal hypoglycaemia: clinical manifestations and therapeutic strategies towards prevention. *Endocrine Practice* **9**: 530–543.

American Diabetes Association (2018). Classification and Diagnosis of Diabetes: Standards of Medical Care in Diabetes—2018. *Diabetes Care* **41** (Supplement 1): S13–S27.

American Diabetes Association (2019). Glycemic Targets: Standards of Medical Care in Diabetes—2019. *Diabetes Care* **42** (Supplement 1): S61–S70.

Amiel, S., Dixon, T., Mann, R., and Jameson, K. (2008). Hypogycaemia in type2 diabetes. *Diabetic Medicine* **25** (3): 245–254.

Bernard, K., Cavan, D., Ziegler, R. et al. (2012). The ticking time bomb: Fear of hypoglycaemia and its impact on diabetes control: Baseline results from ABACUS. Poster presented at the European Association for the Study of Diabetes, Berlin.

Brod, M., Rana, A., and Barnett, A.H. (2012). Impact of self-treated hypoglycaemia in type 2 diabetes: a multinational survey in patients and physicians. *Current Medical Research Opinion* **28** (12): 1947–1958.

Boucai, L., Southern, W.N., and Zonszein, J. (2011). Hypoglycemia-associated mortality is not drug-associated but linked to comorbidities. *The American Journal of Medicine* **124** (11): 1028–1035.

Cooperberg, B., Breckenridge, S., Arbelaez, A. et al. (2008). Terbutaline and the prevention of nocturnal hypoglycemia in type 1 diabetes. *Diabetes Care* **31**: 2271–2272.

Cox, D.J., Gonder-Frederick, L.A., Kovatchev, B.P., and Clarke, W.L. (2001). Self-treatment of hypoglycemia while driving. *Diabetes Research and Clinical Practice* **54** (1): 17–26.

Cox, D., Kovatchev, B., and Koev, D. (2004). Hypoglycaemia anticipation, awareness training (HYATT) reduces occurrences of severe hypoglycaemia among adults with type1 diabetes. *International Journal Behavioural Medicine* **11**: 212–218.

Daneman, T., Frank, M., Perlman, K. et al. (1989). Severe hypoglycaemia in children with insulin dependent diabetes: frequency and predisposing factors. *Journal of Paediatrics* **115**: 681–685.

Davis, E., Keating, B., Byrne, G. et al. (1997). Hypoglycaemic incidence and clinical predictors in a large population based sample of children and adolescents with IDDM. *Diabetes Care* **20**: 22–25.

Davis, S., Duckworth, W., Emanuele, N. et al. (2018). Effects of severe hypoglycaemia on cardiovascular outcomes and death in the Veterans Affairs Diabetes Trial. *Diabetes Care*. https://doi.org/10.2337/dc18-1144.

DCCT (Diabetes Control and Complication Trial Research Group) (1991). Epidemiology of severe hypoglycaemia in the Diabetes Control and Complications Trial. *American Journal of Medicine* **90**: 450–459.

DCCT (Diabetes Control and Complication Trial Research Group) (1997). Hypoglycaemia in the Diabetes Control and Complications Trial. *Diabetes* **46**: 271–286.

Deary, I. (1993). Effects of hypoglycaemia on cognitive function. In: *Hypoglycaemia and Diabetes: Clinical and Pyysiological Aspects* (eds. B. Frier and B. Fisher), 80–92. London: Edward Arnold.

Del Prato, S., LaSalle, J., Mattheai, S., and Bailey, C. (2010). Tailoring treatment to the individual in type2 diabetes practical guidance from the Global Partnership for Effective Diabetes Management. *International Journal of Clinical Practice* **64** (3): 295–304.

Diabetes Control and ComplicationsTrial (DCCT)/Epidemiology of Diabetes Interventions and Complications Research Group (2003). Intensive diabetes therapy and carotid intima-media thickness in type 1 diabetes mellitus. *New England Journal Medicine* **348**: 2294–2903.

Diabetes Control and ComplicationsTrial (DCCT)/Epidemiology of Diabetes Interventions and Complications Research Group (DCCT) (1993). The effect of intensivetreatment of diabetes on the development and progression of long-term complications in insulin dependent diabetes mellitus. *New England Journal Medicine* **329**: 977–986.

Donnelly, L., Morris, A., and Frier, D. (2005). Frequency and predictors of hypoglycaemia in type1 diabetes and insulin treated Type 2 diabetes: a population based study. *Diabetic Medicine* **22** (6): 749–755.

Dunn, J., Cranston, I., Marsden, P. et al. (2007). Attenuation of amydgala and frontal cortical responses to low blood glucose concentration in asymptomatic hypoglycaemia in type1 diabetes: a new player in hypoglycaemic unawareness. *Diabetes* **36**: 2706–2773.

Dunning, P. (1994). Having diabetes: young adult perspectives. *The Diabetes Educator* **21** (1): 58–65.

Dunning, T. (2005). *Managing Diabetes in Older People*. Chichester: Wiley Blackwell.

Dunning, T., Sinclair, A., and Colagiuri, S. (2014). New IDF Guideline for managing type 2 diabetes in older people. *Diabetes Research and Clinical Practice* **103** (3): 538–540.

Farmer, A., Brockbank, K., Keech, M. et al. (2012). Incidence and costs of severe hypoglycaemia requiring attendance by the emergency medical services in South Central England. *Diabetic Medicine* Mar 21. https://doi.org/10.1111/j.1464-5491.2012.03657.x.

Field, B., Nayar, R., Kilvert, A. et al. (2018). A retrospective observational study of peole with tyoe 1 diabetes with self-reported severe hypoglycaemia reveals high level of ambulance attendance but low levels of therapy change and specialist intervention. *Diabetic Medicine*. https://doi.org/10.1111/dme.13670.

Galloway, J. and Chance, R. (1994). Improving insulin therapy: achievements and challenges. *Hormone and Metabolic Research* **26**: 591–598.

Geddes, J., Schopman, J., Zammitt, M., and Frier, B. (2008). Prevalence of impaired awareness of hypoglycaemia in adults with Type 1 diabetes. *Diabetic Medicine* 24 (4): 501–504.

Heller, S. and Macdonald, I. (1996). *Diabetic Medicine* 13 (7): 607–615.

Henderson, J., Allen, K., Deary, I., and Frie, H. (2003). Hypoglycaemia in insulin-treated type2 diabetes: Frequency, symptoms and impaired awareness. *Diabetic Medicine* 20 (12): 1016–1021. The measurement of cognitive function during acute hypoglycaemia: experimental limitations and their effect on the study of hypoglycaemia unawareness.

Hershey, T., Perantie, D., and Warren, S. (2005). Frequency and timing of severe hypoglycaemia affects spatial memory in children with type1 diabetes. *Diabetes Care* 28: 2372–2377.

Hope, S., Taylor, P., Shields, B. et al. (2017). Are we missing hypoglycaemia? Elderly patients with insulin treated diabetes present to primary care frequently with non-specific symptoms associated with hypoglycaemia. *Primary Care Diabetes* http://www.elsevier.com/locate/pcd.

Hulkower, R., Pollack, R., and Zomszein, J. (2014). Understanding hypoglycaemia in hospitalized patients. *Diabetes Management* 4 (2): 165–176.

Jae-Seung, Y. and Sun-Hye, K. (2013). Presence of macroalbuminuria predicts severe hypoglycemia in patients with Type 2 Diabetes Mellitus: a 10-year follow-up study. *Diabetes Care* December 17, 2012. https://doi.org/10.2337/dc12-1408.

Johnston, S., Conner, C., Aagren, M. et al. (2012). Association between hypoglycaemic events and fall-related fractures in Medicare-covered patients with type2 diabetes. *Diabetes, Obesity and Metabolism* 14: 634–643.

Jones, T. (2011). Strategies for preventing hypoglycaemia in intensively managed type1 diabetes patients. *Diabetes Management* 37: 30–34.

Klein, R. (2007). Smoking is linked to hypoglycaemia in type1 diabetes. *Diabetes Care* 30: 1437–1441.

Kok, V. and Lee, P.-H. (2016). Management of hypoglycaemia in non-diabetic palliative care patients: a prognosis-based approach. *Palliative Care Research and Treatment* 10: 1–5. https://doi.org/10.4137/PCRT.S38956.

Leese, G., Wang, J., and Broomhall, J. (2003). Frequency of severe hypoglycaemia requiring emergency treatment in type1 and type2 diabetes: a population based study of health service resource use. *Diabetes Care* 26 (4): 1176–1180.

Leonard, C.E., Bilker, W.B., Brensinger, C.M. et al. (2016). Severe hypoglycemia in users of sulfonylurea antidiabetic agents and antihyperlipidemics. *Clinical Pharmacology & Therapeutics* 99 (5): 538–547.

Leonard, C., Han, X., Brensinger, C. et al. (2017). Comparative risk of hypoglycemia with oral antidiabetic monotherapy: a retrospective cohort study. *Pharmaceutical Drug Safety*. https://doi.org/10.1002/pds.4337.

Lundkvist, J., Bolinder, C., and Johnson, L. (2005). The economic and quality of life impact of hypoglycaemia. *European Journal of Health Economics* 6: 197–202.

Martín-Timón, L. and del Cañfizo-Gomez, F. (2015). Mechanisms of hypoglycaemia unawareness and implications in diabetic patients. *World Journal of Diabetes* 6 (7): 912–926.

McAuley, V., Deary, I., Ferguson, S., and Frier, B. (2001). Acute hypoglycaemia in humans causes attentional dysfunction while nonverbal intelligence is preserved. *Diabetes Care* 24: 1745–1750.

McNay, E. and Cotero, V. (2010). Mini-review: Impact of recurrent hypoglycaemia on cognitive and brain function. *Physiology Behaviour* 100 (3): 234–238.

Misra-Herbert, A., Pantalone, K., Ji, X. et al. (2018). Patient characteristics associated with severe hypoglycaemia in a type 2 diabetes cohort in a large, integrated health care system from 2006 to 2015. *Diabetes Care*. https://doi.org/10.2337/dc17-1834.

Moghissi E. (2011). Patients with diabetes lack knowledge about hypoglycaemia. Presented at the 20th Annual Meeting and Clinical Congress of the American Association of Clinical Endocrinologists. San Diego, California.

Nordfeldt, S. and Ludvigsson, J. (1997). Severe hypoglycaemia in children with IDDM. A prospective study, 1992–1994. *Diabetes Care* 20: 497–503.

Pai-Feng, H., Shih-Hsien, S., Hao-Min, C. et al. (2012). Association of clinical symptomatic hypoglycaemia with cardiovascular events and total mortality in type2 diabetes mellitus: A nationwide population-based study. *Diabetes Care*. https://doi.org/10.2337/dc12-0916.

Pandaya, N., Thompson, S., and Sambamoothi, L. (2008). The prevalence and persistence of sliding scale insulin use among newly admitted elderly nursing home residents with diabetes mellitus. *Journal American Dir Association* 9 (9): 663–669.

Perantie, D., Wu, J., and Koller, J. (2007). Regional brain volume differences associated with hyperglycaemia and severe hypoglycaemia in youth with type1 diabetes. *Diabetes Care* 30: 2331–2337.

Pramming, S., Thorsteinsson, B., Bendtson, I., and Binder, C. (1991). Symptomatic hypoglycaemia in 411 type1 diabetic patients. *Diabetic Medicine* 8: 217–222.

Pramming, S., Thorsteinsson, B., Ronn, B., and Binder, C. (1985). Nocturnal hypoglycaemia in patients receiving conventional treatment with insulin. *British Medical Journal* 291: 376–379.

Rajan, A. (2002). Mechanisms of hypoglycaemia counterregulation. *Medscape Diabetes and Endocrinology*. http://www.medscape.org/viewarticle/438362_print.

Raju, B., Arbelaez, A., Breckenridge, S., and Cryer, P. (2006). Nocturnal hypoglycaemia in type1 diabetes: an assessment of preventative bedtime treatments. *Journal Clinical Endocrinology and Metabolism* 91: 2087–2092.

Ringholm, N. and Nielsen, L. (2008). Hypoglycaemia most common in early pregnancy in women with type1 diabetes. *Diabetes Care* **31**: 9–14.

Ross, L., McCrimmon, R., Frier, B. et al. (1998). Hypoglycaemic symptoms reported by children with type1 diabetes mellitus and by their parents. *Diabetic Medicine* **15**: 836–843.

Russo, A., Stevens, J., Chen, R. et al. (2005). Insulin-induced hypoglycaemia accelerates gastric emptying of solids and liquids in long standing type1 diabetes. *Journal of Clinical Endocrinology and Metabolism* **90**: 4489–4495.

Salas, M. and Caro, J. (2002). Are hypoglycaemia and other adverse effects similar among sulphonylureas? *Adverse Drug Reactions Toxicology Review* **21**: 205–217.

Seaquist, E., Anderson, J., Childs, B. et al. (2013). Hypoglycaemia and diabetes: a report of a working group of the American Diabetes Association and the Endocrine Society. *Diabetes Care* https://doi.org/10.2337/dc12-2480.

Shorr, R., Daugherty, W., and Griffin, M. (1996). Individual sulfonylureas and serious hypoglycaemia in older people. *Journal of the American Geriatric Society* **44** (7): 751–755.

Shorr, R., Ray, W., Daugherty, J., and Griffin, M. (1997). Incidence and risk factors for serious hypoglycaemia in older persons using insulin or sulphonylureas. *Archives of Internal Medicine* **157** (15): 1681–1686.

Silverstein, J. (2008). The lows of exercise: another piece of the puzzle. *International Diabetes Monitor* **20** (1): 44–46.

Sinclair, A. (2006). Special considerations in older adults with diabetes: meeting the challenge. *Diabetes Spectrum* **19**: 229–233.

Sommerfield, A., Deary, I., McAuley, V., and Frier, B. (2003). Short-term delayed, and working memory are impaired during hypoglycaemia in individuals with type1 diabetes. *Diabetes Care* **26**: 390–396.

Speight, J. (2011). Assessing impaired awareness of hypoglycaemia. *Diabetes Management* **34**: 36–37.

Tattersall, R. (1999). Frequency, causes, and treatment of hypoglycemia. In: *Hypoglycemia in Clinical Diabetes* (eds. B. Frier and B. Fisher), 55–87. Chichester, UK: Wiley.

Therapeutic Guidelines (TG) (2004). *Hypoglycaemia*. http://www.tg.com.au/etg_demo/tcg/edg/1473.htm (accessed December 2007).

Thorens, B. (2011). Brain sensing and neural regulation of insulin and glucagon secretion. *Diabetes Obesity and Metabolism* **13** (sup 1): 82–88.

Tucker, J.L., Zoberi, K.A., Hooks-Anderson, D.R. et al. (2018). Race in Older but Not Younger Patients Associated with Greater Glycemic Burden in Primary Care Patients. *The Diabetes Educator* **44** (6): 549–557.

UKPDS (1998). Intensive blood glucose control with sulphonylureas or insulin compared with conventional treatment and risk of complications in patients with type2 diabetes (UKPDS 33). *Lancet* **352**: 837–853. (correction *Lancet* (1999) **354**, 602).

Umpierrez, G.E., Hellman, R., Korytkowski, M.T. et al. (2012). Management of hyperglycemia in hospitalized patients in non-critical care setting: an endocrine society clinical practice guideline. *The Journal of Clinical Endocrinology & Metabolism* **97** (1): 16–38.

Unger, J. (2012). Uncovering undetected hypoglycaemic events. *Diabetes Metabolic Syndrome and Obesity* **5**: 57–74.

Unger, J. and Parkin, C. (2011). Hypoglycaemia in insulin-treated diabetes: a case for increased vigilance. *Postgraduate Medical Journal* **123** (4): 81–91.

US Department of Health and Human Services, Office of Disease Prevention and Health Promotion (2014). *National Action Plan for Adverse Drug Event Prevention*. Washington, DC: Author.

Vervoort, G., Goldschmidt, H., and van Doorn, L. (1996). Nocturnal blood glucose profiles in patients with type1 diabetes on multiple (>4) daily insulin injection regimens. *Diabetic Medicine* **13**: 794–799.

Whincup, G. and Milner, R. (1987). Prediction and management of nocturnal hypoglycaemia in diabetes. *Archives of Diseases in Childhood* **62** (4): 333–337.

Wiegers, E., Becker, K., Rooijackers, H. et al. (2016). Cerebral blood flow response to hypoglycaemia is altered in patients with type 1 diabetes and impaired awareness of hypoglycaemia. *Journal od Cerebral Blood Flow and Metabolism*. https://doi.org/10.1177/0271678X16658914.

Wright, A., Cull, C., Macleod, K., and Holman, R. (2006). Hypoglycaemia in type2 diabetic patients randomized to and maintained on monotherapy with diet, sulphonylurea, Metformin, or insulin for six years from diagnosis. UKPDS 73. *Journal of Diabetes Complications* **20**: 395–401.

Yki-Jarvinen, H., Ryysy, L., Nikkila, K. et al. (1999). Comparison of bedtime insulin regimens in patients with type2 diabetes mellitus. A randomised, controlled trial. *Archives of Internal Medicine* **130**: 399–396.

Yun, J.S., Ko, S.H., Ko, S.H. et al. (2013). Presence of macroalbuminuria predicts severe hypoglycemia in patients with type 2 diabetes: a 10-year follow-up study. *Diabetes Care* **36** (5): 1283–1289.

Zhang, Y., Wieffer, H., Modha, R. et al. (2010). The burden of hypoglycaemia in type2 diabetes: a systematic review of patient and economic perspectives. *Journal of Clinical Outcomes Management* **17** (12): 547–557.

Zoungas, S. (2010). Severe hypoglycaemia and risks of vascular events and death. *Results in Diabetes* **3** (1): 3.

Chapter 7

Hyperglycaemia, Acute Illness, Diabetic Ketoacidosis (DKA), Hyperosmolar Hyperglycaemic States (HHS), and Lactic Acidosis

---

Key points

- Acute illness most commonly causes hyperglycaemia and less commonly hypoglycaemia.
- Untreated hyperglycaemia can precipitate ketoacidosis and/or hyperosmolar states, which are serious short-term complications of diabetes, even when they are managed competently.
- Meticulous attention to detail and proactive insulin use reduces morbidity and mortality.
- Monitor hydration status closely, especially in children and older people.
- *Gradually* lower the blood glucose level to avoid hypoglycaemia.
- Monitor ketone clearance in blood.
- Consider whether infection could be an underlying cause, but note the white cell count is often elevated in hyperglycaemic states and may not indicate infection.
- Hyperglycaemia-related abnormalities lead to thrombosis, inflammatory changes and impair ischaemic preconditioning, which is a protective mechanism and predisposes the individual to cardiac events, and the formation of superoxide anion (oxidative stress) that cause tissue damage.
- Hyperglycaemia is associated with cerebral neuronal damage possibly due to elevated tissue acidosis and lactate levels that occur in hyperglycaemia.
- Insulin is the most effective way to manage hyperglycaemia-induced abnormalities and reduce the associated complications.
- Educate the person with diabetes and their family about how to manage future intercurrent illnesses and develop a personalised sick-day-care plan with them.
- Consider psychological and social issues, especially if there are repeated admissions for diabetic ketoacidosis (DKA).

Care of People with Diabetes: A Manual for Healthcare Practice, Fifth Edition. Trisha Dunning and Alan Sinclair.
© 2020 John Wiley & Sons Ltd. Published 2020 by John Wiley & Sons Ltd.

Rationale

This chapter primarily concerns managing hyperglycaemia associated with illnesses in hospital settings, but preventative self-care is also discussed. Hyperglycaemia, DKA, and hyperosmolar hyperglycaemic states (HHS) are preventable short-term complications of diabetes. When hyperglycaemia does occur, effective proactive management can reduce the progression to DKA or HHS and limit the attendant metabolic derangements should these conditions occur. Hyperglycaemia induces a range of metabolic abnormalities that predispose the individual to cardiovascular, cerebrovascular and cognitive complications and other adverse events.

People with well-controlled diabetes do not usually experience higher rates of intercurrent illness than those without diabetes. However, people with persistent hyperglycaemia may have lower immunity, delayed wound healing, and are at increased risk of infections, including infections caused by organisms that are not normally pathogenic such as tuberculosis, and have a poorer response to antibiotics (Australasian Paediatric Endocrine Group [APEG] 2005; Australian Diabetes Society [ADS] 2012). Infection is the most common cause of DKA and HHS. Thus, optimal blood glucose target ranges, and the most appropriate method to achieve the target range for people in hospital need to be decided. Maintaining the blood glucose range between 5 and 10 mmol/l is appropriate for most patients (ADS 2012), including those on corticosteroid medicines (Chapter 10) (Clement et al. 2004).

However, a number of factors affect clinical decisions, and where possible decisions should be made with the individual concerned and their relatives and carers, or according to their advanced care plan (ACP) (Chapter 18). Key factors that affect clinical decisions are:

- Previous hyperglycaemic events and the outcomes
- Duration and acuity of the presenting problem
- Risks associated with hyperglycaemia and/or ketosis
- Duration of diabetes: longstanding diabetes or new diagnosis
- Presence of existing diabetes complications and/or other comorbidities
- Nutritional status
- Medicine regimen and risk of hypoglycaemia and consequent adverse events (Chapter 6)
- Life expectancy
- Available resources and expertise (ismail-beigi et al. 2011)

Prevention: proactively managing intercurrent illness

Prevention strategies consist of educating the person with diabetes and their family about how to prevent intercurrent illness or proactively manage intercurrent illnesses to limit the metabolic consequences. Illness prevention/management strategies should be individualised and based on a thorough physical, psychological, and social assessment using a risk management and quality use of medicines (QUM) approach (Chapter 5). General healthcare should be considered as well as diabetes-related issues and encompass risk screening for periodontal problems, breast and other forms of cancer such as bowel and prostate disease, and preventative vaccinations in children, adults and older people.

Illness prevention education should encompass the following:

- Engage in proactive healthcare such as identifying key illness risk times, for example, colds and flu during winter, having an individualised documented plan for managing illness, and a kit containing essential equipment and information such as in-date ketone test strips and relative's and health professional's telephone numbers.
- Recognise and manage the signs and symptoms of DKA and HHS, which includes the importance of monitoring blood glucose and ketones and using the information to adjust glucose-lowering medicine (GLM) doses or to seek medical advice, what to tell the doctor and how to maintain fluid intake.

- Know how to adjust insulin/GLMs and dietary intake to manage blood glucose levels.
- Know when to seek assistance.
- Evaluate the performance of the sick day care plan when the episode resolves and revising it, if necessary.

In addition, clinicians should regularly reassess the individual's illness self-care capability:

- Determine knowledge, according to the factors outlined in the preceding list.
- Assess physical ability to manage such as mobility, sight, manual dexterity, cognitive changes associated with hyperglycaemia, and other activities of daily living, bearing in mind that these may all be compromised by hyperglycaemia. Assessing these factors is an important aspect of long-term complication-screening programmes. Groups likely to need assistance are children, pregnant women, frail older people who live alone, people with disabilities, those who are acutely ill, and those who are depressed. The most effective management strategy for these people may be to seek health professional advice quickly.
- Evaluate psychosocial factors such as mental health and coping skills, cognitive function, and available support from family or other carers, considering the carer's state of health and coping ability, especially older people.
- Review preventative healthcare strategies such as vaccinations, mammograms, prostate checks, bowel screening, usual metabolic control, and their sick-day management plan and kit. Annual influenza and pneumococcal vaccinations are recommended for people with diabetes, COPD and cardiovascular disease, including children with these conditions (National Asthma Council 2005). Mortality increases by 5–15% in people with diabetes during influenza epidemics, especially those with cardiovascular and renal complications (Smith and Poland 2004). The increased risk may be due to older age, cardiovascular disease, or to the diabetes itself due to the impaired immune function because of DKA/HHS (Diepersloot et al. 1990). Kornum (2007) suggested that type 2 diabetes predicts mortality associated with pneumonia and further, hyperglycaemia on admission, >11 mmol/l in people with diabetes and >6 mmol/l in people without diabetes, predicts pneumonia-related mortality.
- Observational data suggest that influenza vaccination prior to and during an influenza epidemic reduces the associated hospital admissions and mortality in people with diabetes (Wang et al. 2004). Thus, all people with diabetes aged six months and older should receive annual influenza vaccination unless contraindicated. Contraindications include allergy/anaphylactic reaction to eggs and/or the vaccine, intercurrent illness with fever >38 °C.
- Regularly review medication, including asking about complementary and over-the-counter medicines. In particular, assess the continued need for diabetogenic medicines such as atypical antipsychotic medications, glucocorticoids, and thiazide diuretics. If these medicines are necessary and there are no alternatives, the lowest effective dose should be used for the shortest possible time.

Early recognition of new presentations of diabetes is important. Diabetes can be diagnosed during a hospital admission: ~7% of people admitted via the emergency department have blood glucose levels that meet diagnostic criteria (>11.1 mmol/l). These people must be followed up after discharge and a definitive diagnose made or excluded:

- Ensure that they have good access to competent medical and nursing care and ongoing education. Both the person with diabetes and the health professionals caring for them should have good knowledge of the individual's care.
- Ensure good communication/therapeutic relationship between the person with diabetes and their health professionals; see Chapter 2.
- Incorporate psychological screening into routine complication assessment programmes (Ciechanowski et al. 2000; Dunning 2001; ADA 2017).

Self-care during illness

People with type 1 diabetes are at greatest risk of DKA, but DKA can occur in seriously ill people with type 2 diabetes. HHS most commonly occurs in people with type 2 diabetes and is associated with significant morbidity and mortality. A suggested plan for monitoring blood glucose and ketones is shown in Table 7.1 (American Diabetes Association 2002; Laffel et al. 2005; Australian Diabetes Educators Association [ADEA] 2006; Kitabchi et al. 2006). In the early stages of the illness, people may be able to be managed at home if they are capable of performing self-care, have support, and can contact their doctor/diabetes educator at least every one to two hours and these clinicians can respond when contacted. Admission to hospital is advised in the following situations:

- Children, especially younger than two years
- Persistent vomiting and/or bile-stained vomitus
- Persistent diarrhoea
- Blood glucose persistently ≤4 mmol/l or >15 mmol/l and ketones present
- Severe localised abdominal pain
- Hyperventilation (Kussmaul's respirations), a late sign
- Dehydration
- Coexisting serious illness
- Impaired conscious state
- The individual, parent or care providers are unable to cope

Hyperglycaemia

Hyperglycaemia refers to an elevated blood glucose level (>10 mmol/l) due to a relative or absolute insulin deficiency. The symptoms of hyperglycaemia usually occur when the blood glucose is persistently above 15 mmol/l. The cause of the hyperglycaemia should be sought in people with an established diagnosis of diabetes and corrected to avoid the development of DKA or HHS. Hyperglycaemia, DKA and HHS are often referred to as short-term complications of diabetes. DKA develops relatively quickly. HHS is often insidious and usually evolves over several days to weeks.

Hyperglycaemia disrupts multiple organ systems and must be treated to reduce the morbidity and mortality associated with the illness and its metabolic consequences (American Association of Clinical Endocrinologists [AACE] 2011; ADS 2012; Inzucchi et al. 2012). Fluid resuscitation corrects dehydration, improves microcirculation, and reduces tissue damage during acute sepsis, which helps correct hyperglycaemia, but increased insulin doses and/or dose frequency or rescue insulin therapy in type 2 diabetes is usually required.

Hyperglycaemia is associated with adverse outcomes in hospitalised people, both with and without diabetes. Controlling blood glucose improves outcomes (Abourzik et al. 2004; Clement et al. 2004; ADA 2006; Inzucchi et al. 2012; Dhatariya and Vellanka 2018). However, higher rates of hypoglycaemia are associated with stringent control of blood glucose below 5 mmol/l, and hypoglyacaemia, especially severe hypoglycaemia, is associated with significant adverse events (Unger 2012; Unger and Parkin 2011); Chapter 6. There is still debate about whether continuous IV insulin infusion is the safest way to manage hyperglycaemia in hospital despite the well-described benefits in people with and without diabetes (van den Berghe et al. 2001; AACE 2011). Intensive insulin therapy protects renal function in critically ill patients and reduces the incidence of oliguria and the need for renal replacement therapy in surgical patients and improves lipid and endothelial profile (Schetz 2008).

Laboratory or capillary blood glucose tests are used to monitor blood glucose during hospitalisation. Capillary tests are undertaken more frequently than laboratory tests except in intensive care situations, and may give better insight into the blood glucose pattern (Cook et al. 2007).

Table 7.1 Self-management advice for managing blood glucose, ketones and fluid during illness.

	Type 1	Type 2
Blood glucose (BG)	Monitor at least two hourly Monitor ketones two hourly if >15 mmol on two consecutive occasions in a 2- to 6-hour period	Monitor two hourly If >15 mmol on two consecutive occasions in an 8- to 12-hour period increase monitoring frequency to 2–4 hourly QID testing may be adequate in people managed with diet and exercise
Blood ketones		
<1 mmol/l 1–1.4 mmol/l:	BG 4–15 mmol/l recheck in two hours BG, <8 mmol/l extra sweet fluids: >8 mmol/l extra 5% insulin	Follow the same monitoring procedure as described for Type 1 diabetes Ketones are less common in Type 2 diabetes but do occur in serious illness such as septicaemia and myocardial infarction. Monitor conscious state and other symptoms.
>1.5 mmol/l: <1 mmol/l	BG, <8 mmol/l extra sweet fluids: >8 mmol/l extra 5–10% insulin BG 15–22 mmol/l 5% extra insulin	
1–1.4 mmol/l >1.5 mmol/l <1 mmol/l 1–1.4 mmol/l >5 mol/l	10% extra insulin 15–20% extra insulin and hospitalise if ketones persist BG >22 mmol/l 10% extra insulin 15% extra insulin 20% extra insulin and hospitalise if ketones persist	
Medicines	Give supplemental doses of quick/rapid acting insulin 2–4 hours	*GLMs* Consider ceasing Metformin Increase sulphonylurea dose unless on maximal doses or on a slow release preparation when insulin is preferred[a] *GLM and insulin* Supplemental doses of quick/rapid-acting insulin *Insulin treated* Supplemental doses of quick/rapid-acting insulin
Refer to hospital	Unable to maintain fluid intake Blood glucose and ketones not falling despite supplemental insulin Unable to self-care and no support available Condition deteriorating Cognitive changes Abdominal pain.	Unable to maintain fluid intake Blood glucose and ketones not falling despite supplemental insulin Unable to self-care and no support available Condition deteriorating Cognitive
Fluids	BG <4 mmol/l usual meals and extra sweet fluids if tolerated ~10–12 mmol/l and able to tolerate food 150 ml easily digested fluid every 1–2 hours, e.g. soup, fruit juice, ice cream BG >12 mmol/l and unable to tolerate food, 100–300 ml low calorie fluids every hour, e.g. gastrolyte (contains electrolytes), low calorie soft drink, mineral water, water Unable to tolerate fluids at any BG level, refer to hospital	BG <4 mmol/l usual meals and extra sweet fluids if tolerated ~10–12 mmol/l and able to tolerate food 150 ml easily digested fluid every 1–2 hours, e.g. soup, fruit juice, ice cream BG >12 mmol and unable to tolerate food 100–300 ml low calorie fluids every hour, e.g. gastrolyte, low calorie soft drink, mineral water, water Unable to tolerate fluids at any BG level, refer to hospital

Note: These recommendations should be tailored to the individual's self-care capabilities, available assistance, and their physical condition. Ketosis can develop rapidly in people using insulin pumps. The underlying cause needs to be ascertained and treated.
[a] If the person has no experience of insulin, they will need reassurance and a careful explanation about why insulin is needed. If they are not able to manage or do not have assistance and home nursing is not available they may need to be managed in hospital.

The trend of the blood glucose pattern over time (up or down) is important information on which to base management decisions, including about medicine regimen.

Despite the evidence that insulin requirements increase during illness, insulin doses are often reduced, even in the presence of significant hyperglycaemia, because clinicians are concerned about causing hypoglycaemia, whereas the factors contributing to hypoglycaemia are only rarely investigated and addressed (Cook et al. 2007). Coughlin (2012) suggested that hospitals need to focus on patients' views of their hospital experience, which should be measured using appropriate tools rather than the ubiquitous 'patient satisfaction' questionnaires.

Diabetic ketoacidosis (DKA)

Diabetic ketoacidosis is a life-threatening complication of diabetes. Glucose is unable to enter the cells when insulin is insufficient/absent and accumulates in the blood. Insulin deficiency leads to catecholamine release, lipolysis, and the mobilisation of free fatty acids and subsequently the formation of ketone bodies, B-hydroxybutyrate, acetoacetate, and acetone, resulting in metabolic acidosis (ADA 2002).

Protein catabolism also occurs and forms the substrate for gluconeogenesis, which further increases the blood glucose. At the same time, glucose utilisation in tissues is impaired. DKA usually only occurs in people with type 1 diabetes, but can occur in people with type 2 people in the presence of severe infections or metabolic stress. The mortality rate in expert centres is <5% but is higher at the extremes of age and if coma and/or hypotension are present (Chiasson et al. 2002).

Diabetic ketoacidosis is characterised by hyperglycaemia, osmotic diuresis, metabolic acidosis, glycosuria, ketonuria, and dehydration. The definition by laboratory results differs amongst various countries; Table 7.2 outlines the main diagnostic criteria used in Australia, United Kingdom, and the United States. The signs, symptoms of, and precipitating factors for DKA are shown in Table 7.3, and Figure 7.1 outlines the physiology and the signs and symptoms that occur as a result of impaired glucose utilisation, and the biochemical manifestations found on blood testing. Early identification and management are essential to limit the adverse effects of

Table 7.2 Biochemical diagnostic criteria for DKA comparing Australia, the United Kingdom, and the United States.

Blood chemistry	Australia	UK	USA
Blood glucose	Capillary >15.0 mmol/l for >8–12 hours But can be normal	>11.0 mmol/l (200 mg/dl)	Mild, moderate or severe 13.9 mmol/l (>250 mg/dl) Anion gap >10
Ketones	0.6–1.5 mmol/l (at risk) 0.7–1.5 (at high risk)	>3.0 mmol/l blood or 2+ on urine test strip	Mild, moderate, and severe Urine or blood ketones positive
Acidosis pH	<7.35	7.3	Mild 7.25–7.90 Moderate 7.0–7.25 Severe 7.0 Anion gap >12
Sodium bicarbonate	<15	<15	Mild 15–18 Moderate 10–15 Severe <10 Anion gap >12

Note: Australia and the United Kingdom do not include the anion gap. The United States includes anion gap in their diagnostic criteria and classify DKA as mild, moderate, or severe (Dhatariya and Vellanki 2017; RACGP/ADS 2018).

Table 7.3   Early signs, symptoms, and precipitating factors of diabetic ketoacidosis (DKA).

Symptoms and signs	Precipitating factors

Thirst
Polyuria
Fatigue
Weight loss
Nausea and vomiting
Abdominal pain
Muscle cramps
Tachycardia
Kussmaul's respirations
  (early sign)
	(1) Newly diagnosed type 1 (5–30%)
	(2) Omission of insulin therapy/GLMs (33%)
	(3) Inappropriate insulin/GLM dose reduction. DKA has also been associated with inaccurate use of insulin delivery devices after changing devices in both older people and adolescents (Bhardwaj and Metcalfe 2006).
	(4) Eating disorders
	(5) Severe emotional distress, either directly or by insulin manipulation
	(6) Relative insulin deficiency due to:
	(7) Insulin pump failure
	(8) Severe morning sickness during pregnancy
	    (a) Acute illness:
	          Infection (10–20% of cases)
	          Myocardial infarction
	          Trauma, burns
	          Cerebrovascular accident
	          Surgical procedures
	    (b) Endocrine disorders (rare):
	          Hyperthyroidism
	          Pheochromocytoma
	          Acromegaly
	          Cushing's disease
	    (c) Medications:
	          SGLT-2 inhibitors in specific situations (see Chapter 5)
	          Glucocorticoids
	          Thiazide diuretics
	          Sympathomimetic agents
	          Alcohol
	          Illicit drugs
	          Brittle diabetes: life-disrupting blood glucose liability associated with frequent admission to hospital (Benbow et al. 2001) (Chapter 10)

DKA. Recent research suggests that a single episode of moderate/severe DKA in young children at diagnosis is associated with lower cognitive scores and altered brain growth (Aye et al. 2018). More research is needed to determine the significance of the findings and the longer-term implications.

Late signs of severe DKA

The initial signs and symptoms of DKA (polyuria, polydipsia, lethargy, and Kussmaul's respirations) are compensatory mechanisms to overcome the acidosis. If treatment is delayed, the compensatory mechanisms are overwhelmed. Signs of decompensation (late signs) include:

- Peripheral vasodilation with warm, dry skin
- Hypothermia
- Hypoxia and reduced conscious state
- Oliguria
- Slow respiratory rate and *absence* of Kussmaul's respirations
- Bradycardia

The signs and symptoms can be masked by intercurrent illness, especially in older people. For example, pneumonia can cause tachyapnoea, dry mouth, and dehydration; abdominal pain and vomiting are symptoms of gastrointestinal disease. Likewise, abdominal pain is usual in appendicitis and in labour. Polyuria and polydipsia can be difficult to detect in toddlers not yet toilet

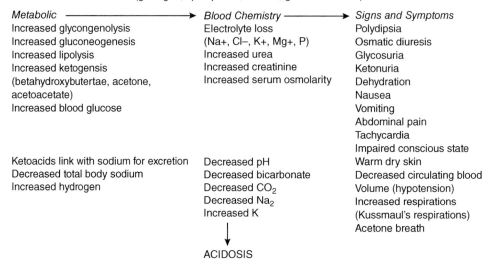

PRECIPITATING FACTORS

INSULIN DEFICIENCY

Decreased glucose uptake
Increased counter-regulatory hormone response
(glucagon, epinephrine, cortisol, growth hormone)

Metabolic	*Blood Chemistry*	*Signs and Symptoms*
Increased glycongenolysis	Electrolyte loss	Polydipsia
Increased gluconeogenesis	(Na+, Cl–, K+, Mg+, P)	Osmatic diuresis
Increased lipolysis	Increased urea	Glycosuria
Increased ketogensis	Increased creatinine	Ketonuria
(betahydroxybutertae, acetone,	Increased serum osmolarity	Dehydration
acetoacetate)		Nausea
Increased blood glucose		Vomiting
		Abdominal pain
		Tachycardia
		Impaired conscious state
Ketoacids link with sodium for excretion	Decreased pH	Warm dry skin
Decreased total body sodium	Decreased bicarbonate	Decreased circulating blood
Increased hydrogen	Decreased CO_2	Volume (hypotension)
	Decreased Na_2	Increased respirations
	Increased K	(Kussmaul's respirations)
		Acetone breath

ACIDOSIS

Late signs: coma, absence of Kussmaul's respirations, death

Figure 7.1   An outline of the physiology, signs, and symptoms and biochemical changes occurring in the development of diabetic ketoacidosis (DKA).

trained, bedwetters, and incontinent older people. Unexplained bedwetting in these groups needs to be investigated and DKA considered when the onset of incontinence and bedwetting is sudden. Hypothermia as a result of peripheral vasodilation can mask fever due to underlying infection and is associated with poor prognosis.

Differential diagnosis

- Starvation ketosis can be determined by taking a careful clinical history of the presentation.
- Alcoholic ketosis is indicated where the blood glucose is usually only mildly elevated or low.

The implications of the metabolic and physiological changes associated with DKA are shown in Table 7.4.

Assessment

The following factors should be established:

- Whether the person has known diabetes
- Usual insulin/GLM dose, dose interval and type/s of insulin/GLM
- Time the last dose was taken and dose administered
- Presence of fever, which can be a sign of myocardial infarction as well as infection
- Duration of the deteriorating control/illness
- Remedial action taken by the patient (sick-day self-care)
- Whether the person took any other medicines, complementary medicines, alcohol, or illegal drugs
- Conscious state

Table 7.4   The metabolic consequences of diabetic ketoacidosis and associated risks. Many of these changes increase the risk of falls in older people.

Metabolic consequences of ketoacidosis	Associated risk
Metabolic acidosis	Nausea and vomiting Cardiac arrest Coagulopathies Increased white cell count, which may not be a sign of infection. The white cell function is changed in hyperglycaemic states.
Hyperlipidaemia	Thrombosis/embolism Substrate for ketone formation if insulin is not replaced
Haemoconcentration and coagulation changes	Myocardial infarction, stroke, thrombosis
Dehydration	Volume depletion Renal hypoperfusion Can cause acute tubular necrosis
Gastric stasis	Inhalation of vomitus, aspiration pneumonia Delayed absorption of food and fluids given via the oral route Abdominal discomfort
Hyperkalaemia but overall deficit in total potassium due to loss in osmotic diuresis	Cardiac arrhythmias
Hyperglycaemia, which is exacerbated by glycogenolysis and gluconeogenesis	Plasma hyperosmolality Cellular dehydration Osmotic diuresis Compromised immune function leading to infection and delayed wound healing, thrombosis, low mood, and vision changes Cognitive changes and coma.
Glycosuria	Hyponatraemia and ketonaemia, which contributes to sodium, potassium, and chlorine loss
	Hyponatraemia is common but if sodium is <120 mmol/l may indicate hypertriglyceridaemia
Abdominal pain	Unnecessary surgery, inappropriate pain relief causing further respiratory distress, missed labour in women Death

A thorough physical assessment should be undertaken and blood taken to do the following:

- Establish the severity of the DKA: glucose, urea, and electrolytes, pH and blood gases, degree of ketonaemia. If severe acidosis is present, pH <7.1, and the blood glucose is not significantly elevated, alcohol, aspirin overdose or lactic acidosis need to be excluded especially in older people. Ketones in the presence of low blood glucose can indicate starvation, malnutrition, or cachexia.
- Assess the cause: full blood count, cardiac enzymes, blood cultures, ECG, chest X-ray, urine culture.

Aims of treatment of DKA

Treatment aims to correct the following:

- Dehydration
- Electrolyte imbalance
- Ketoacidosis
- Hyperglycaemia

Hyperglycaemia, relative insulin deficiency, or both, predispose people with and without diabetes to complications such as severe infection, polyneuropathy, multiorgan failure and death (van den Berghe et al. 2001; Clement et al. 2004). It is addressed by slowly reducing the blood glucose to 7–10 mmol/l.

In addition, treatment aims to do the following:

- Reverse shock.
- Ascertain the cause of DKA and treat appropriately.
- Prevent complications of treatment.
- Educate/re-educate the patient and their family/carers.

Objectives of care

The objectives are to provide interdisciplinary team care. This is facilitated through the following actions:

(1) Restore normal hydration, euglycaemia, and metabolism.
(2) Prevent complications of DKA, including complications occurring as a result of management.
(3) Pay meticulous attention to detail.
(4) Document progress of recovery, e.g. blood glucose levels, medicines administered, and vital signs.
(5) Refer to other specialist care when indicated, e.g. psychologist.
(6) Re-educate/educate the patient and their family/carers about the management of illness at home or general diabetes education if the person is newly diagnosed. Patient education about managing diabetes during illness can be found in this chapter.
(7) Ensure follow-up care is arranged after discharge. In particular: review diabetes knowledge, nutritional assessment and physical and psychological assessment.

Preparing the unit to receive the patient

When receiving a patient who has DKA, assemble the following:

(1) Oxygen and suction (Test to ensure they are in working order.)
(2) Intravenous trolley (IV) containing:
    - Dressing tray and antiseptic solution
    - Local anaesthetic
    - Selection of intravenous cannulae
    - IV fluids: normal saline, SPPS, dextrose/saline
    - IV giving sets, burette
    - Imed pump or syringe pump
    - Clear short- or rapid-acting insulin, preferably administered as an IV infusion
    - Blood gas syringe
    - Blood culture bottles
(3) Cot sides and IV pole
(4) Blood glucose testing equipment (cleaned, calibrated)
(5) Blood ketone testing equipment
(6) Appropriate charts:
    - Fluid balance
    - Blood glucose monitoring
    - Medication
    - Conscious state
(7) Urinary catheterisation equipment
(8) Nasogastric tubes, if needed

Nasogastric tubes may or may not be used. Some experts recommend passing a nasogastric tube to prevent gastric dilatation and aspiration.

Initial care in the intensive care unit is preferable for moderate to severe ketoacidosis. If the patient is admitted to the intensive care unit, central venous pressures, continuous blood gas, and electrocardiogram monitoring is usually performed.

Practice point

Rapid-acting insulin quickly promotes transport of glucose into the cells. Intravenous administration is preferred because the peripheral circulation can be compromised and absorption from an IV infusion is more predictable than by the subcutaneous route.

Care/observations

Managing DKA involves early recognition and treatment and monitoring the response to treatment.

Initial Patient Care

Initial patient care is often given in the intensive care unit. The procedure is:

- Maintain the airway.
- Nurse the patient on their side, even if the patient is conscious, because gastric stasis and inhalation of vomitus is a possible and preventable complication of DKA.
- Ensure strict aseptic technique.

Nursing Observations (One to Two Hourly)

(1) Observe 'nil orally'. Provide pressure care, especially in older people.
(2) Provide mouth care to protect oral mucous membranes and relieve the discomfort of a dry mouth.
(3) Administer IV fluid according to the treatment sheet, usually initially isotonic saline until the blood glucose is <12 mmol/l then 10% dextrose. However, the first litre of saline may be 0.45% in the presence of hypernatraemia (sodium >150 mmol/l).
(4) Administer insulin according to the treatment sheet; it is usually given via an insulin infusion and the dose adjusted according to blood glucose levels; see Chapter 7. Intensive insulin therapy maintains the blood glucose within a narrow range and thereby reduces the morbidity and mortality associated with critical illness (van den Berghe et al. 2001). In some situations, rapid- or short-acting insulin is given intramuscularly, usually in remote areas where intensive care units (ICU) are not available.
(5) Replace serum potassium. If the initial biochemical result is >5.0 mmol/l, potassium is not required initially. It should be added to the second or third litres of IV fluid or when levels fall to <4.5 mmol/l, depending on expected potassium loss, for example, from vomiting. Initially potassium levels should be monitored on an hourly basis.
(6) There is general agreement that bicarbonate replacement is not required if the pH is >7.0. There is no consensus about pH <7.0. Some experts state that bicarbonate should be given to minimise respiratory decompensation. Others believe bicarbonate automatically corrects as the acidosis resolves with fluid and insulin (Hamblin 1995). Some experts use bicarbonate if the pH is <7.1, if the patient presents with a cardiac arrest, or cardiac arrest is imminent.
(7) Estimate blood glucose levels one to two hourly and confirm biochemically in the early stages.
(8) Observe strict fluid balance. Record second hourly subtotals of input/output *from admission*. Urine output should be >30 ml/h measured hourly in a calibrated collecting device. Report a urine output of <30 ml/h. Measure specific gravity (SG). Be aware that some creatinine assays cross react with ketones and creatinine may not reflect renal function in DKA.
  - *Heavy* glycosuria invalidates SG readings.
  - Record fluid loss, for example, vomitus.
(9) Monitor central venous pressure.

(10) Monitor conscious state. In children with DKA, the level of consciousness initially is significantly associated with pH as well as age but not blood glucose or sodium levels (Edge et al. 2006). Therefore, cerebral function in DKA is related to the severity of the acidosis in children even when cerebral oedema is not present. Cerebral oedema is a serious complication of DKA and has a high morbidity rate in children and older people. If coma is prolonged heparin might be indicated to prevent thrombosis and pulmonary embolism.

(11) Record pulse, respiration, and blood pressure. Fever associated with DKA indicates sepsis. But it should be noted that an elevated white cell count can be due to metabolic abnormalities and does not necessarily indicate the presence of infection.

(12) Administer oxygen via face mask or nasal catheter.

(13) Monitor and report all laboratory results (electrolytes and blood gases).

(14) Report any deterioration of condition immediately.

(15) Physiotherapy may be helpful to prevent pneumonia and emboli due to venous stasis, and to provide passive mobilisation.

(16) Administer other medications as ordered (potassium, calciparine, broad-spectrum antibiotics to treat underlying infections, Mannitol to reduce cerebral oedema).

(17) Reposition and provide skin care to avoid pressure areas and/or venous stasis.

Subsequent care

As the patient's condition improves:

- Review the frequency of blood glucose testing, decreasing to four-hourly, including at night.
- Allow a light diet and ensure the patient is eating and drinking before the IV is removed.
- Administer subcutaneous insulin before the IV is removed. Often, the infusion is turned off before a meal but the IV line left in situ until the person can eat and drink normally and the blood glucose level is stable within the normal range.
- Continue to monitor temperature, pulse, and respiration every four hours.
- Provide support and comfort for the patient.
- Establish the duration of deteriorating control and identify any precipitating factor such as infection.

Plan for:

- Discharge and follow-up education early during the admission.
- Medical and nursing follow-up appointment after discharge.
- Evaluate the person's sick-day-care plan and decide whether it needs to be revised.
- Nutrition review.
- Educate/re-educate about appropriate management (for days when the patient is unwell); see Chapter 16.
- Undertake a general health review and assess immunisation status and any new complication/comorbidity that could trigger a future DKA event and address any issues identified.
- Review medication dosage, especially insulin. DKA can occur as a result of incorrect use of insulin delivery devices, which highlights the importance of checking insulin administration technique, particularly given hospital staff do not consider incorrect technique as a potential cause (Bhardwaj and Metcalfe 2006).
- Consider psychological review. For example, sexual assault, other abuse, and adverse family dynamics are uncommon but important cause of DKA in some people and should be considered when repeated admissions occur. This is a difficult area to assess and should be undertaken by people with the appropriate skills and with consideration of the legal implications and the effect on the individual and their family.

Practice points

- Psychiatric consultation should be considered if a patient repeatedly presents in DKA. Eating disorders complicate 20% of recurrent cases of DKA (Polonsky et al. 1994).
- People, especially young women, reduce their insulin doses to avoid weight gain and hypoglycaemia. Reducing or stopping insulin is also a form of risk taking and rebellion at having diabetes (Dunning et al. 1994).

Brittle diabetes and hyperglycaemia

Brittle diabetes is difficult to understand and manage for people with diabetes and their carers and healthcare professionals. Brittle diabetes most commonly occurs between 15 and 30 years of age and often leads to frequent hospital admissions for DKA or hypoglycaemia. However, brittle diabetes also occurs in older people. Criteria for brittle diabetes in older people are >60 years, treated with insulin, experiencing unstable blood glucose associated with frequent, often prolonged admissions to hospital (Gill et al. 1996; Benbow et al. 2001). In the older group, women are more likely to present with brittle diabetes than men, but the preponderance of women may reflect the proportion of older men and women in the population. There does not appear to be consistent underlying causative factors but cognitive behavioural factors appear to play a role (Benbow et al. 2001). See also Chapter 10.

Complications that can occur as a result of DKA

Most complications of DKA are due to complications of treatment and most are avoidable:

(1) Hypoglycaemia can be caused by inappropriate insulin replacement and rapid reduction in blood glucose.
(2) Inhalation of vomitus can cause aspiration pneumonia.
(3) Hypokalaemia may lead to cardiac arrhythmias.
(4) Cerebral oedema is rare and can be fatal. It occurs in 0.7–10% of children especially on the first presentation of diabetes, and any morbidity that occurs is permanent (Rosenbloom 1990).
(5) Cognitive scores and brain growth can be reduced in (Aye et al. 2018) young children.
(6) Myocardial infarction.
(7) Deep venous thrombosis.
(8) Adult respiratory distress syndrome.

Be extra vigilant with:

(1) Older people, especially those with established vascular and coronary disease. Risks include myocardial infarction and deep venous thrombosis.
(2) Children are at increased risk of cerebral oedema, which has a high mortality rate in this group of people.

Euglycaemic DKA

Munro et al. originally documented euglycaemic DKA in 1973 (Munro et al. 1973). Euglycaemic DKA refers to ketoacidosis in the setting of near normal blood glucose levels. Euglycaemia indicates that the blood glucose level and development of DKA do not necessarily correlate. De and Child (2001) postulated that heavy glycosuria triggered by counter-regulatory hormone activity or reduced hepatic glucose production could result in lower than expected blood glucose levels. Although euglycaemic DKA is a rare condition, it highlights the importance of monitoring serum ketones and blood gases and using low-dose IV insulin infusions in all people with diabetes during illness.

Ketosis without hyperglycaemia occasionally occurs postoperatively in the presence of repeated vomiting. Rehydration with dextrose/saline and controlling the vomiting are required to restore depleted hepatic glycogen stores. More recently, euglycaemia has been reported with some SGLT-2 inhibitors, see Chapter 5. These medicines should be stopped three days prior to surgical procedures and possibly during sick days (Dunning 2007).

Hyperosmolar hyperglycaemic states

HHS is a serious metabolic disturbance characterised by a marked increase in serum osmolality, the absence of ketones, hyperglycaemia (usually >40 mmol/l), and extreme dehydration caused by a concomitant illness (often infection) that leads to inadequate fluid intake. Coma is rare, hence the name change some years ago from hyperglycaemic hyperosmolar non-ketotic coma (HONK) to HHS. HHS most commonly occurs in people with Type 2 diabetes, usually in older people >65, however, HHS has been reported in a nine-month-old baby, toddlers (Goldman 1979; Sagarin et al. 2005), and children (Kershaw et al. 2005). HHS has a higher mortality than DKA (Dhatariya and Vellanka 2017; Hirsch and Emmett 2018).

People with type 2 diabetes usually secrete enough endogenous insulin to prevent lipolysis and ketoacidosis (Kitabchi et al. 1994) but not sufficient to prevent hyperglycaemia and hepatic glucose output. HHS has a higher mortality rate than DKA, an estimated 10–20%, although mortality rates as high as 58% are reported. The severity of the metabolic derangements, especially delay establishing the diagnosis, inadequate treatment, and the degree of dehydration contribute to the high mortality rate (Hemphill and Schraga 2012).

In addition, the hyperosmolality may limit ketogenesis and the level of free fatty acids available for ketogenesis (Sagarin et al. 2005). Type 2 diabetes is associated with progressive beta cell loss so the risk of DKA and HHS may be higher with long duration of type 2 diabetes or people with LADA; see Chapter 1. Approximately one third of cases occur in people with no previous diagnosis of diabetes. Dehydration is usually severe. The person is often confused, and focal and general neurological signs are usually present; however, despite the name, coma is rare, occurring in <10% of cases (Sagarin et al. 2005; Hemphill and Schraga 2012). Once HHS develops, it can be difficult to differentiate it from the precipitating illness (Hemphill and Schraga 2012).

Practice point

People with type 2 diabetes often have sufficient endogenous insulin production to prevent the formation of ketones.

HHS has a mortality rate of 10–20% with a slightly higher prevalence in women (Sagarin et al. 2005). The mortality could be associated with the underlying illness. The onset is associated with severe stress such as acute febrile illnesses including infection, (e.g. pneumonia and urinary tract infections), extensive burns, myocardial infarction, stroke and/or reduced fluid intake. People in aged-care facilities are at the highest risk of HHS because they are often unaware of thirst and are not always offered fluids in hot weather. However, the cause is not identifiable in many people.

Factors that increase risk of HHS

Precipitating factors include an acute illness that increases the counter-regulatory hormone response in the setting of insulin deficiency such as:

- Stroke.
- Intracranial haemorrhage.
- Silent myocardial infarct; this should be considered in all presentations of HHS until it is excluded.
- Pulmonary embolism.
- Underlying congestive heart failure and/or renal disease, although hyperosmolality can trigger rhabdomyolysis and cause acute renal failure.
- Surgery, especially cardiac surgery; some endocrine conditions such as Cushing's syndrome.
- Some medications such as diuretics, for example IV diazoxide and furosemide in the surgical setting, corticosteroids, atypical antipsychotic, beta blockers, Histamine$_2$ blockers immuno-suppressant agents.
- Dialysis.
- Parenteral nutrition solutions that contain dextrose.
- IV fluids that contain dextrose.
- Non-adherence with GLMs and other diabetes self-care.

There is a high mortality rate associated with HHS. Although the mortality rate has decreased since the 1960s, is still 10–20% (ADA 2002; Sagarin et al. 2005; Hirsch and Emmett 2018).

Presenting signs and symptoms

HHS usually develops over days to weeks. People may complain of thirst, polyuria, or increased incontinence or new onset of incontinence in people with dementia, weight loss (primarily due to fluid loss), and lethargy. Oral hydration may be compromised by lack of thirst, swallowing difficulties, dementia, vomiting, mobility deficits, and limiting fluids to avoid urine frequency/incontinence.

A thorough physical examination should be carried out to detect sources of infection and include eyes, ears, nose, throat and teeth and gums, pneumonia, UTI, skin, meningitis, pelvic infection, and triggers such as congestive cardiac failure (CCF), and acute respiratory distress syndrome. HHS is the initial presentation in 30–40% of new diabetes presentations (Kitabchi et al. 2006).

- Neurological signs include drowsiness and lethargy, delirium, seizures, visual disturbances, hemiparesis, diminished reflexes, unsteady gait, and sensory deficits.
- Dehydration is indicated by reduced skin turgor, sunken eyes, and dry mouth.
- Tachycardia is an early sign; hypotension is a late sign and indicates profound dehydration. Tachycardia could also indicate thyrotoxicosis.
- Tachypnoea is a consequence of respiratory compensation for the metabolic acidosis.
- Hypoxaemia may compound the effects of dehydration on mental function.
- Signs of infection include enlarged lymph nodes. Warm moist skin is an early indication of infection whereas cool dry skin indicates late sepsis.
- Vision changes and other sensory and speech deficits are potential symptoms.
- Focal or generalised seizures can indicate HHS.

Specific investigations depend on the results of the physical assessment. Laboratory investigations include blood glucose ketones, electrolytes, renal function (blood urea nitrogen [BUN] and creatinine, which can be elevated due to the dehydration), osmolality (≥320 mOsm/kg), creatine phosphokinase (CPK), blood cultures, coagulation studies, arterial blood gases (pH is usually >7.30), bicarbonate (≥15 mEq/l), and urine cultures. Blood glucose is usually>30 mmol/l (540 mg/dl), and ketones are absent or very low (Dhataira and Vellanka 2017; Hirsch and Emmett 2018).

Other investigations such as electrocardiogram (ECG), cardiac enzymes and troponins, lumbar puncture and cerebrospinal fluid (CSF) studies, chest X-ray, head and abdominal CT, and HbA1c as an indication of preceding metabolic control may be useful to plan future management (Kitabchi et al. 2006).

The care and objectives are similar to those for DKA, but extra vigilance and close monitoring is needed because of the age of most people presenting with HHS:

- Record strict fluid balance.
- IV fluid rate. Central venous access may be used. In some cases, a Swan-Ganz catheter is inserted to monitor intravascular volume. There is usually a large fluid deficit (~10l). Replacement: in the first two hours 1–2 l isotonic saline but the rate depends on the degree of dehydration, if severe a higher volume may be indicated; lower volumes may be used if there is no urine output. Half normal saline is used once the blood pressure and urine output are normalised and stable.
- An arterial line may be inserted in ICU settings to monitor blood gases.
- Blood glucose may fall with rehydration alone over the first one to three hours but usually insulin is indicated to correct the hyperglycaemia and is usually given as an IV insulin infusion adjusted according to the blood glucose level (monitored one to two hourly).
- ECG.
- Urine output. A urinary catheter may be required to accurately measure output and obtain a clean urine specimen to detect infection but can introduce infection.
- Neurological observations.
- Manage the airway.
- Maintain skin integrity including the feet. Compromised peripheral circulation and peripheral neuropathy increases the risk of foot ulcers, which are slow to heal and increase length of stay and the risk of amputation. Nursing on air mattresses may be indicated.
- Observe for deep venous thrombosis or embolism.
- Administer medications as indicated, which might include antibiotics, which might be administered IV. Subsequent care as for DKA.

Education may be more difficult initially because of the mental confusion associated with HHS and the age of these patients. Ensuring that the family/caregivers understand how to care for the individual and ensuring follow-up education occurs in two to three weeks is important.

Figure 7.2 outlines the factors involved in the development of HHS. There are similarities with DKA, and some important differences. Ketone production is absent or minimal because the patient is usually producing enough endogenous insulin to allow the ketone bodies to be metabolised and utilised. The degree of dehydration is often greater in HONK and the serum and urine osmolality is increased.

Lactic acidosis

Lactic acidosis is another rare condition that sometimes occurs in people with diabetes. Lactic acidosis occurs in 0.06 cases per 1000 patient years, usually those with predisposing factors (Nicks 2006). Lactate is a product of anaerobic glucose metabolism. Disordered lactate metabolism frequently occurs in critically ill people who are at risk of multiorgan failure and the mortality rate is about 70% if the serum lactate remains >2 mmol/l for >24 hours (Nicks 2006). Lactate is primarily cleared from the blood by the liver, kidneys, and skeletal muscles.

Lactic acidosis is defined as metabolic acidosis associated with serum lactate >5 mmol/l. It occurs due to either an increase in hydrogen ions or reduction in bicarbonate with increased acid production, loss of alkali and reduced renal clearance of acids. Lactic acidosis should be considered during acute illness in patients with vasoconstriction, hypotension and with underlying diseases associated with poor tissue perfusion and hypoxia such as:

- Recent myocardial infarction
- Cardiac failure and cardiogenic shock
- Pulmonary disease
- Cirrhosis

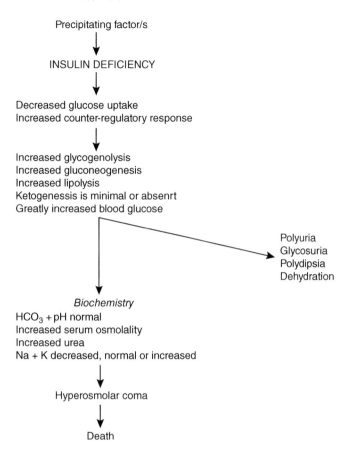

Precipitating factor/s

↓

INSULIN DEFICIENCY

↓

Decreased glucose uptake
Increased counter-regulatory response

↓

Increased glycogenolysis
Increased gluconeogenesis
Increased lipolysis
Ketogenessis is minimal or absenrt
Greatly increased blood glucose

→ Polyuria
Glycosuria
Polydipsia
Dehydration

↓

Biochemistry
HCO_3 + pH normal
Increased serum osmolality
Increased urea
Na + K decreased, normal or increased

↓

Hyperosmolar coma

↓

Death

Figure 7.2 An outline of the development of hyperosmolar hyperglycaemic states (HHS).

- Sepsis
- Renal impairment
- Medicines and toxins such as isoniazid, salicylates, beta-adrenergic agents, alcohol and biguanides especially in older people with hypoxic diseases and/or dehydration
- Surgery
- Inborn errors of metabolism such as fructose 1, 6-diphosphatase deficiency

Two types of lactic acidosis are associated with diabetes:

(1) Type A (anaerobic), which develops with tissue hypoxia or hyperfusion due to sepsis, shock heart failure or respiratory failure.
(2) Type B (aerobic) is caused by factor besides hypoxia such as DKA, renal and liver failure, malignancy, high doses of salicylates and alcohol, and, rarely using metformin when it is contraindicated (Chapter 3) (Rodríguez-Gutiérrez et al. 2017).

Excess lactate is produced in ischaemic skeletal muscle and to a lesser extent in the intestine and erythrocytes and accumulates due to a fall in lactate consumption in the liver, which overwhelms the buffering system (Nicks 2006). Lactate levels correlate with tissue hypoperfusion and mortality and the duration and degree of lactic acidosis predicts morbidity and mortality. Lactate >4 mmol/l for >24 hours carries an 11% mortality rate in critically ill patients. After 48 hours, only 14% survive.

Signs and symptoms

- Signs that the cardiovascular system is compromised, for example, cyanosis, cold extremities, tachycardia, hypotension, dyspnea
- Lethargy, confusion, stupor
- Dry mucous membranes
- Hyperapnoea (Kussmaul respirations), hypotension, and/or shock

Biochemistry shows an anion gap, lactate >5 mmol/l (normal ~1 mmol/l) low pH, usually <7.1 but only moderate, if any ketones, and mildly elevated or normal blood glucose, usually <20 mmol/l, hyperkalaemia is usually present.

Lactic acidosis must be distinguished from DKA, HHS and alcohol poisoning. Lactic acidosis should be managed in ICU settings.

Lactic acidosis associated with metformin

Patients are often treated with metformin despite having clinical conditions that place them at some risk for developing lactic acidosis (Calabrese and Turner 2002). Ninety percent of metformin is excreted unchanged via the kidneys and the half-life is prolonged when renal clearance reduced in patients with renal impairment where creatinine clearance is reduced. Renal impairment may develop slowly as a complication of diabetes or acutely. It is extremely rare: <10 events/100 000 patient years of exposure (DeFronzo et al. 2016; also see an earlier study by Emslie-Smith et al. 2001), However, it still occurs and mortality rates are reported to be 30–50%.

Management

Management consists of:

- Preventing the risk by carefully assessing individual for risk factors before prescribing metformin and following metformin prescribing guidelines. Risk factors include acute renal impairment from dehydration, vomiting and/or diahorrea, surgery, and some investigations.
- IV fluid replacement with normal saline to maintain the circulating volume and tissue perfusion.
- Oxygen therapy.
- Bicarbonate given early to correct the acidosis; it should be administered slowly to avoid causing metabolic alkalosis and ventilatory failure.
- Renal dialysis to remove metformin.
- IV insulin at a rate of 10–12 units/h in dextrose solution.
- Monitoring renal and cardiac status.
- The mental status should be monitored as well as monitoring the physical status.
- Withdrawing precipitating medicines or toxins, which might include haemodialysis in some cases.
- Antibiotics if sepsis is present.
- Medication review and discontinuing medication or reducing the dose if contraindications exist. Metformin is the medicine of choice in overweight type 2 patients but doses >500 mg per day should be used with caution in older people with renal, liver, and cardiac disease or other hypoxic diseases (Nisbet et al. 2004).
- Thiamine 50–100 mg IV followed by 50 mg orally for one to two weeks in some cases where thiamine deficiency is likely, such as malnourished older people and alcoholics.

References

Abourzik, N., Vora, C., and Verma, P. (2004). Inpatient diabetology: the new frontier. *Journal General Internal Medicine* **19**: 466–471.

American Association of Clinical Endocrinologists (AACE) (2011). Medical guidelines for clinical practice for developing a diabetes mellitus comprehensive care plan. *Endocrine Practice* **17** (Suppl. 2): 1–53.

American Diabetes Association (ADA) (2002). *Hyperglycaemic Crisis in Patients with Diabetes Mellitus*. USA: American Diabetes Association.

American Diabetes Association (2006). American College of Endocrinology and American Diabetes Association consensus statement on inpatient diabetes and glycemic control: a call to action. *Diabetes Care* **29** (8): 1955–1962.

American Diabetes Association (2017). Standards of medical care in diabetes—2017 abridged for primary care providers. *Clinical diabetes: a publication of the American Diabetes Association* 35 (1): 5.

Australian Diabetes Educators Association (ADEA) (2006). *Guidelines for Sick Day Management for People with Diabetes*. Canberra: ADEA.

Australian Diabetes Society (ADS) (2012). Guidelines for routine glucose control in hospital ADS, Canberra. www.diabetessociety.com.au/documents/ADSGuidelinesforRoutineGlucoseControlinHospitalFinal2012_000.pdf (accessed November 2012).

Australian Paediatric Endocrine Group (APEG) (2005). The Australian Clinical Practice Guidelines on the Management of Type 1 Diabetes in Children and Adolescents www.chw.edu.au/prof/services/endocrine/apeg (accessed January 2013).

Aye, T., Mazaika, P., Mauras, N. et al. (2018). Impact of early diabetic ketoacidosis on the developing brain. *Diabetes Care*: dci181405. https://doi.org/10.2337/dc18-1405.

Benbow, S., Walsh, A., and Gill, G. (2001). Brittle diabetes in the elderly. *Journal of the Royal Society of Medicine* **94**: 578–580.

Bhardwaj, V. and Metcalfe, N. (2006). Diabetic ketoacidosis after changing insulin pens: check technique to avoid complications. *British Medical Journal* 332: 1259–1260.

Calabrese, A. and Turner, R. (2002). Evaluation of prescribing practices: risk of lactic acidosis with metformin therapy. *Archives of Internal Medicine* 162: 434–437.

Chiasson, J., Josse, R., Gomis, R. et al. (2002). Acarbose treatment and the risk of cardiovascular disease and hypertension in patients with impaired glucose tolerance: the STOP-NIDDM Trial. *Lancet* **359**: 2072–2077.

Ciechanowski, P., Katon, W., and Russo, J. (2000). Depression and diabetes: impact of depressive symptoms on adherence, function and costs. *Archives of Internal Medicine* 160: 3278–3285.

Clement, S., Braithwaite, S., Magee, M. et al. (2004). Management of diabetes and hyperglycaemia in Hospitals. *Diabetes Care* **27** (2): 553–591.

Cook, C., Castro, J., Schmidt, R. et al. (2007). Diabetes care in hospitalized noncritically ill patients: More evidence for clinical inertia and negative therapeutic momentum. *Journal of Hospital Medicine* **2** (4): 203–211.

Coughlin, C. (2012). An ethnographic study of main events during hospitalization: perceptions of nurses and patients. *Journal of Clinical Nursing* https://doi.org/10.1111/j.1365-2702.2012.04083.x.

De, P. and Child, D. (2001). Euglycaemic ketoacidosis – is it on the rise? *Practical Diabetes International* **18** (7): 239–240.

DeFronzo, R., Fleming, A., Chen, K., and Bicsak, T. (2016). Metformin-associated lactic acidosis: current perspectives on causes ad risk. *Metabolism*: 26–29. www.metabolismjournal.com (accessed November 2018).

Dhatariya, K. and Vellanka, P. (2017). Treatment of diabeteic ketoacidosis (DKA)/hyperglycaemia huperosmolar state (HHS): novel advances in the management of hyperglycaemic crises (UK versus USA). *Current Diabetes Reports* **17** (5): 33. https://doi.org/10.1007/s11892-017-0857-4.

Diepersloot, R., Bouter, K., and Hoekstra, J. (1990). Influenza infection and diabetes mellitus: case for annual vaccination. *Diabetes Care* **13**: 876–882.

Dunning, P., Ward, G., and Rantzau, C. (1994). Effect of alcohol swabbing on capillary blood glucose measurements. *Practical Diabetes* **11** (4): 251–254.

Dunning, T. (2001). Depression and diabetes, summary and comment. *International Diabetes Monitor* **13** (5): 9–11.

Dunning, T. (2007). Diabetes: Managing sick days, a patient-centred approach. In: *General Practice Continuing Education Conference Proceedings. Exhibition Centre*. Melbourne: Royal Australian College of General Practitioners (RACGP).

Edge, J., Roy, Y., Bergomi, A. et al. (2006). Conscious level in children with diabetic ketoacidosis is related to severity of acidosis and not to blood glucose concentration. *Pediatric Diabetes* **7**: 11.

Emslie-Smith, A., Boyle, D., and Evans, J. (2001). Contraindications to metformin therapy in patients with Type 2 diabetes – a population based study of adherence to prescribing guidelines. *Diabetic Medicine* **18**: 483–488.

Gill, G., Lucas, S., and Kent, L. (1996). Prevalence and characteristics of brittle diabetes in Britain. *Quarterly Journal of Medicine* **89**: 839–843.

Goldman, S. (1979). Hyperglycaemic hyperosmolar coma in a 9-month-old child. *Archives of Paediatrics and Adolescent Medicine* **133** (2): 30.

Hamblin, S. (1995). Diabetic ketoacidosis. *Australian Diabetes Educator's Association Journal* **Spring**: 17.

Hemphill, R. and Schraga, E. (2012). Hyperosmolar Hyperglycaemic State. http://emedicine.medscape.com. article/1914705 (accessed October 2012).

Hirsch, B. and Emmett, M. (2018). Diabetic ketoacidosis and hyperosmolar hyperglycaemia state in adults. https://www.uptodate.com/.../diabetic-ketoacidosis-and-hyperosmolar-hyperglycemic (accessed December 2018).

Inzucchi, S., Bergenstal, R., Buse, J. et al. (2012). Management of hyperglycaemia in type 2 diabetes: a patient-centered approach. Position Statement of the American Diabetes Association (ADA) and the European Association fo the Study of Diabetes (EASD). *Diabetologia* https://doi.org/10.1007/s00125-012-2534-0.

Ismail-Beigi, F., Moghissi, A., Tiktin, M. et al. (2011). Individualising glycaemic targets in Type 2 diabetes mellitus: implications of recent clinical trials. *Annals of Internal Medicine* 54: 554–559.

Kershaw, M., Newton, T., Barrett, T. et al. (2005). Childhood diabetes presenting with hyperosmolar dehydration but without ketoacidosis. *Diabetic Medicine* 22 (5): 645–647.

Kitabchi, A., Fisher, J., Murphy, M., and Rumbak, M. (1994). Diabetic ketoacidosis and the hyperglycaemic hyperosmolar nonketotic state. In: *Joslin's Diabetes Mellitus* (eds. C. Kahn and G. Weir), 738–770. Philadelphia: Lea & Febiger.

Kitabchi, A., Umpierrez, G., Murphy, M., and Kreisberg, R. (2006). Hyperglycaemic crises in adult patients with diabetes: a consensus statement from the American Diabetes Association. *Diabetes Care* 29 (12): 2739–2748.

Kornum, J. (2007). Type 2 diabetes linked to higher pneumonia-related mortality. *Diabetes Care* 30: 2251–2257.

Laffel, L., Wentzell, K., Loughlin, C. et al. (2005). Sick day management using blood 3-hydroxybutyrate (3-OHB) compared with urine ketone monitoring reduces hospital. *Diabetes Care* 28: 1277–1281.

Munro, J., Campbell, I., McCuish, A., and Duncan, L. (1973). Euglycaemic ketoacidosis. *British Medical Journal* 2: 578–580.

National Asthma Council Australia (2005). *Roles of Influenza and Pneumococcal Vaccinations in Subgroups with Asthma, COPD, Diabetes or Heart Disease*. Canberra: CSL Pharmaceuticals.

Nicks, B. (2006). Lactic acidosis. E medicine. http://www.emedicine.com/emerg/topic291.htm (accessed January 2008).

Nisbet, J., Sturtevant, M., and Prins, J. (2004). Metformin serious adverse effects. *Medical Journal of Australia* 180 (2): 53–54.

Polonsky, W., Anderson, B., Lohrer, P. et al. (1994). Insulin omission in women with IDDM. *Diabetes Care* 17: 1178–1185.

Rodríguez-Gutiérrez, R., Velez-Viveros, A., Quintanilla-Siller, A. et al. (2017). Lactic Acidosis. In: *McMaster Textbook of Internal Medicine* (eds. V.M. Montori and J.P. Brito). Kraków: Medycyna Praktyczna https://empendium.com/mcmtextbook/chapter/B31.II.13.3.3 (accessed 19 September 2019).

Rosenbloom, A. (1990). Intracerebral crises during treatment of diabetic ketoacidosis. *Diabetes Care* 13: 22–33.

Royal Australian College of General Practitioner, and Australian Diabetes Society (2018). Joint Position Statement on Emergency Management of Hyperglycaemia in Primary Care. www.racgp.org.au (accessed November 2018).

Sagarin, M., McAfee, A., Sachter, J. et al. (2005). Hyperosmolar Hyperglycaemic Coma. *E medicine*. http://www.emedicine.com/emerg/topic24.htm (accessed January 2008).

Schetz, M. (2008). Intensive insulin therapy may protect renal function in critically ill patients. *Journal of the American Society of Nephrologists Online* (January 30) (accessed January 2008).

Smith, S. and Poland, G. (2004). American Diabetes Association: influenza and pneumococcal immunisation in diabetes. *Diabetes Care* 27 (Suppl. 1): S111–S113.

Unger, J. (2012). Uncovering undetected hypoglycaemic events. *Diabetes, Metabolic Syndrome, Obesity Targets and Therapy* 5: 57–74.

Unger, J. and Parkin, C. (2011). Hypoglycemia in insulin-treated diabetes: a case for increased vigilance. *Postgraduate Medicine* 123 (4): 81–91.

van den Berghe, M., Wouters, P., Weekers, F. et al. (2001). Intensive insulin in critically ill patients. *New England Journal of Medicine* 345: 1359–1367.

Wang, C., Wang, S., and Lai, C. (2004). Reducing major cause-specific hospitalization rates and shortening hospital stays after influenza vaccination. *Clinical Infectious Diseases* 39: 1322–1332.

Chapter 8
Long-Term Complications of Diabetes

Key points

- Diabetes is associated with devastating long-term complications that are psychologically, physically, and financially costly to the person with diabetes, society, and health services.
- Diabetes complications affect function and life expectancy.
- Maintaining euglycaemia reduces the likelihood of complications developing, however, diabetes complications are often present at diagnosis and/or trigger the diagnosis in type 2. Both hyper- and hypoglycaemia are associated with increased risk of death,
- People with diabetes, especially older people, often require assistance to perform diabetes self-care and other activities of daily living as a consequence of diabetes complications.
- People with diabetes worry about developing complications and the worry and/or actuality of complications affects their emotional wellbeing and can lead to significant diabetes-related distress and depression.
- Diabetes management requires coordinated interdisciplinary care and active self-care by the individual, which is often burdensome, and family support.
- People with diabetes often have other comorbidities in addition to diabetes complications, which increase the risk of uncoordinated care, suboptimal care, frequent hospitalisations, and polypharmacy.
- Proactive, preventative complication screening and risk and other assessment is essential and should encompass assessing the individual' risk profile to plan holistic, personalised care, including end-of-life care.
- Focusing on improving the individual's self-care capability, detecting, managing diabetes-related distress, and improving inter-professional collaboration/communication, the individual-clinician relationship, and communication is as essential as the medical aspects of care.

Care of People with Diabetes: A Manual for Healthcare Practice, Fifth Edition. Trisha Dunning and Alan Sinclair.
© 2020 John Wiley & Sons Ltd. Published 2020 by John Wiley & Sons Ltd.

Introduction

The physical long-term complications of diabetes are generally classified as:

- Macrovascular disease: cardiovascular disease, cerebrovascular disease, and peripheral vascular disease. These are common in type 2 diabetes and are often present at diagnosis. Type 2 diabetes is often preceded by the metabolic syndrome, which confers a high level of cardiovascular risk. Myocardial disease is the leading cause of death in people with type 1 diabetes. Significantly, myocardial infarction (MI) is often 'silent' and sudden (Schernthaner et al. 2018).
- Microvascular disease: nephropathy and retinopathy. These are a major concern in both type 1 and type 2 diabetes. type 2 diabetes-related nephropathy is one of most common reasons for commencing dialysis.
- Neuropathy: peripheral. This predominantly affects the feet and legs and autonomic, which can lead to gastroparesis, erectile dysfunction (ED), and hypoglycaemic unawareness. They contribute to atypical symptoms and silent disease, especially in older people.

Morbidity, mortality, and other complications are interrelated and often occur concomitantly. For example, ED has vascular and nerve components. In the long term in, the presence of persistent hyperglycaemia, diabetes can affect almost all body systems. Diabetes is associated with a number of other disease processes, especially type 2 diabetes (Chapters 4 and 10).

Diabetes is also associated with a range of musculoskeletal disorders, infections, osteoporosis, depression, dementia, and frailty, although the causal links are not clear in all cases (Chapter 10). The presence of other concomitant and age-related diseases such as arthritis contribute to reduced quality of life, significant distress and depression and inhibit self-care; thus, psychological issues are also associated with diabetes, Chapter 15.

Diabetes and complexity

Multimorbidity refers to the simultaneous occurrence of two or more chronic conditions (Bayliss et al. 2008). Multimorbidity increases the risk that services will be duplicated and inefficient (Barnett et al. 2012) the individual will not receive best practice care, will be hospitalised more frequently and for longer, use a greater range of health services at increased cost, and be prescribed more medicines (polypharmacy) (Taylor et al. 2010). Prevalence estimates for multimorbidity range from 35% to 80% (Fortin et al. 2005; Britt et al. 2008; Nagel et al. 2008), although the prevalence is difficult to determine because different data collection methods and definitions are used and many studies focus on older people. The prevalence of multimorbidity increases with age, but it also occurs in younger age groups: more than 40% of people <60 years have several comorbidities (Taylor et al. 2010).

Multimorbidity often coexists with smoking and obesity; both increase the risk the person will develop more morbidities. Multimorbidites affect self-care and can represent a significant care burden for relatives. Thus, a multifactorial approach to managing diabetes complications and other concomitant morbidities is needed and encompasses personalised care, regular systematic, individualised risk assessment processes, effective self-care, and optimising physical and mental health and diabetes education to prevent/reduce the morbidity and mortality and reduce the health costs associated with diabetes.

Diabetes is a complex condition. People with diabetes' self-care and other capacities is also complex and dynamic and can be enhanced or hindered by a range of factors (Boehmer et al. 2016). Complexity has a profound effect on the care provided and outcomes. Multimorbidity and the associated complexity challenges individuals and clinicians to identify risk factors, interpret signs and symptoms, diagnose early, and select appropriate management strategies.

The WHO International Classification of Functioning, Disability and Health (2018) categorised some dimensions of complexity as medical, situational, and system complexity. These categories reflect a more holistic approach rather than mainly focusing on the individual and their health conditions. It indicates that solving complex problems requires a broad approach, clinician training, an engaged individual, and for both to have the skills to negotiate the health system.

The Australian Commission on Safety and Quality in Health Care (2017) National Safety and Quality Standards encompass comprehensive care in standard 5. Standard 5 appears to encompass the WHO classification and contains standards for clinical governance, developing a comprehensive care plan, delivering comprehensive care, and minimising harm. The Standards are currently being implemented; thus, it is difficult to determine their effectiveness.

Pathophysiology of diabetes complications

The pathophysiology of diabetes complications is complex: glycaemic control is an important determinant of optimal mitochondrial function and therefore, long-term health outcomes (Giacco and Brownlee 2012; Zhang et al. 2007). Changes in mitochondrial function result in oxidative stress and play a key role in the development and progression of both micro and macrovascular complications associated with diabetes. Impaired glucose tolerance increases cardiovascular risk three- to eightfold. Thus, maintaining normoglycaemia to preserve normal oxidative mitochondrial function is important to delay or prevent the progression of complications (Forbes and Cooper 2007).

Increases in HbA1c from normal to 9.5% confer a 10-fold increased risk of microvascular disease. The relationship between macrovascular disease and hyperglycaemia is not as clear; for example, only a twofold increase in macrovascular disease risk at the same HbA1c was noted in the UKPDS (UKPDS 1998). This finding might be partly explained by the fact that free fatty acids (FFAs) can also be utilised as fuel for oxidative processes in the mitochrondria.

Importantly, achieving HbA1c < 6.5% (< 48 mmol/mol) for the first year after diagnosis is associated with a legacy effect and reductions in microvascular events. Reduction in cardiovascular and mortality were observed 10 years after the UKPDS ended and more recently in the Diabetes and Ageing Study (Huang et al. 2011, Laiteerapong et al. 2019). Similar findings also occurred in the DCCT in type 1 diabetes. These findings suggest early diagnosis and immediate intensive glucose lowering is important to avoid the long-term risk of complications. However, other risks such as those associated with hypoglycaemia and life expectancy need to be considered.

Some studies suggest the risk of death is increased with both hyper- and hypoglycaemia (Currie et al. 2010; Huang et al. 2011). Currie et al. 2010 found a U-shaped association with mortality risk at HbA1c < 6.1–6.6% (42–48 mmol/mol) and HbA1c 10.1–11.2% (86–97 mmol/mol) in a population of people with diabetes in the UK. It is still not clear whether excess risk of mortality associated with hypoglycaemia is a result of other underlying factors.

Hyperglycaemia initiates a cascade of pathological changes that underlie diabetes complications. Glucose is the major source of fuel for energy production by oxidative phosphorylation. Hyperglycaemia has significant effects on metabolic pathways concerned with generating cellular energy, especially in the mitochondria. Most cells have the capacity to reduce glucose transport across the plasma membrane into the cytosol to maintain glucose homeostasis in the presence of hyperglycaemia.

Some cells are not able to adapt and reduce glucose transport sufficiently to prevent intercellular changes in glucose concentration. Cells at particular risk include capillary endothelial cells in the retina, mesangial cells in renal glomeruli, and neuronal and Schwann cells in peripheral nerves (Forbes and Cooper 2007). Glycaemic variability, glucose fluctuations between high and low, is emerging as an important determinant of cardiovascular outcomes and may be a predictive indicator of midterm major adverse cardiac events in people with acute coronary syndrome and diabetes (Gerbaud et al. 2019).

An increasing body of research suggests that reactive oxygen species (ROS) initiate the development of diabetic complications (Nishikawa et al. 2000). ROS are generated by damaged or dysfunctional mitochondria. The antioxidant chain is a complex pathway involving the metabolism of oxygen and the transfer of electrons from glucose and other fuels through the respiratory chain via a complex series of reactions. When excess fuel enters the respiratory chain, the mito-chondrial membrane potential is overwhelmed and leaks electrons to oxygen to form superoxide (Nishikawa et al. 2000).

However, despite the increasing evidence that ROS plays a role in the pathogenesis of diabetes complications, the exact mechanisms are still being determined. Maintaining optimal mitochon-drial function appears to be important to reduce the progression of diabetes complications. More recent research suggests preventing glucose variability might also be important (Weber and Schnell 2009; Wen et al. 2012; Piccone 2012).

The role of antioxidant agents in managing diabetes complications and reducing oxidative damage is controversial, although it is widely promoted. Folic acid has been shown to reduce oxidative damage in type 2 diabetes (Lazalde-Ramos et al. 2012). Likewise, Coenzyme Q10 (CQ-10) is essential for all energy-dependent processes in the heart; consequently, the heart is very sensitive to CQ-10 deficiencies (Kumar et al. 2009). CQ-10 is often deficient in diabetes and cardiac disease. CQ-10 is available in foods such as beef, poultry, broccoli, fish oils, and peanuts, but dietary intake is inadequate to achieve optimal CQ-10 levels in the blood. Supplements may reduce the progression of atherosclerosis, proinflammatory cytokines, and blood viscosity (Kumar et al. 2009).

A small randomised crossover study (26 males and 5 females, mean age 68 and mean diabetes duration 6.8 years) examined the effects of 4 months supplementation with ascorbic acid (vita-min C). The researchers reported significant reductions in daily post-prandial glucose and in systolic and diastolic blood pressure (Mason et al. 2019). The clinical applications of the find-ings are unclear.

Hyperglycaemia contributes to cell death, thickened basement membranes in blood vessels, and stiffened vessels. It reduces the functionality and structure of resistance vessels (proximal vessels before the blood flows into the capillaries). Calcium-regulated potassium channels are disrupted, which affects smooth muscle cell contraction, which contributes to hypertension. As a result, both under-perfusion and over-perfusion occur. The myogenic response is lost, so the resistance vessels no longer have the capacity to cope with the increased blood flow. Increased basement membrane dysfunction and reduced nerve fibre density is apparent in impaired glu-cose tolerance. Micro- and macrovascular and endothelial cell damage and reduced lumenal size also occur.

Giacco and Brownlee (2012) suggested that no 'unifying hypothesis' links the four main hypotheses proposed to explain the pathogenesis of diabetic complications shown below, but suggested either redox changes in the polyol pathway or hyperglycaemia-induced formation of ROS might account for all the underlying biochemical changes.

(1) Formation of advanced glycation endproducts (AGE). Products of glucose metabolism from glycolysis and the tricarboxylic acid cycle initiate protein glycosylation more rapidly than glucose. The protein–glucose complex is broken down by proteosomes or form AGE that become cross-linked and resistant to proteosome activity. Tissues become stiffened and func-tion is compromised. AGE formation may be due to the effects of glucose metabolites rather than glucose itself (Wells-Knecht et al. 1995; Dantas et al. 2012). The interaction of AGEs with their receptor (RAGE) triggers a variety of cellular signalling processes that mediate gene expression and enhance the release of proinflammatory molecules and oxidative stress (Farmer and Kennedy 2009).

(2) Activation of protein kinase C (PKC) isoforms. Hyperglycaemia stimulates diacylglycerol, the lipid second messenger, which activates isoforms of PKC and alters gene and protein expression in organs prone to complications. Inhibiting PKC prevents renal and retinal dam-age in animal models, and a number of clinical trials are in progress involving ruboxisatau-rin (Forbes and Cooper 2007).

(3) Increased flux through the polyol pathway. In the polyol pathway, glucose is converted into sorbitol via aldose reductase and subsequently oxidised to fructose, which eventu-ally contributes to the mitochondrial respiratory chain. Intracellular hyperglycaemia

results in increased production of sorbitol and reduces the level of other important enzymes involved in detoxifying toxic aldehydes such as glutathione and adenine dinucleotide phosphate, and compounds oxidative stress. Sorbitol does not cross cell membranes and causes osmotic stress. Inhibiting aldose reductase delays or prevents diabetes complications especially neuropathy (Kaiser et al. 1993). To date, aldose reductase inhibitor medications have been disappointing despite improvements in nerve physiology and nerve fibre density, largely due to poor tissue penetration and side effects (Hotta et al. 2001).

(4) Increased flux through the hexosamine pathway. When intracellular glucose is high, the normal glucose-6-phosphate metabolic cascade is disrupted and a series of moieties are produced that bind to transcription factors and increase the synthesis of some proteins such as transforming growth factor-b_1 and plasminogen activator inhibitor type 1, both of which have adverse effects on blood vessels (Du et al. 2000). The role of the hexosamine pathway in the pathogenesis of diabetic complications is still evolving.

Cardiovascular disease and diabetes

Key points

- Cardiovascular disease is often 'silent' in people with diabetes.
- Cardiovascular disease (unstable angina, coronary artery disease, acute myocardial infarct, and sudden death) is a leading cause of death in people with diabetes.
- Heart failure is common in people with diabetes. Hypertension is often a precursor for heart failure and heart failure often coexists with other cardiovascular disease (Rosano et al. 2017).
- Excess mortality from cardiovascular disease is evident in all age groups including young people with type 1 diabetes.
- People with diabetes and no heart disease need to be treated as if they have heart disease, especially people with type 2 diabetes.
- Chest pain may be atypical in people with diabetes, and may present as weakness, fatigue, hyperglycaemia, or congestive cardiac failure (CCF).
- Women with diabetes have a higher relative risk (RR) of death from cardiovascular disease than men, but the absolute risk is lower.
- Primary prevention through healthy eating and regular activity, managing dyslipidaemia, hypertension, and hyperglycaemia is imperative to reduce the risk of heart disease and stroke (Sindone 2019).
- Family history of cardiovascular disease increases cardiovascular risk.
- Smoking increases micro- and macrovascular damage. Smoking cessation is imperative.
- Depression is common in people with diabetes and cardiac disease.
- Transient ischaemic attacks (TIA) may indicate impending stroke.

Rationale

Diabetes is a significant risk factor for cardiovascular disease, for example, coronary heart disease, cardiomyopathy, peripheral vascular disease, and stroke (Australian Institute of Health and Welfare (AIHW) 2007; Dantas et al. 2012; American Diabetes Association 2019). Cardiovascular disease is a major cause of hospital admissions, reduced life expectancy, and mortality in people with diabetes. It is often associated with other vascular disease and depression.

Heart failure

People with diabetes are at increased risk of heart failure and people with heart failure, especially those with preserved ejection fraction, are at increased risk of diabetes. (Rosano et al. 2017; Baker IDI 2019). Heart failure reduces quality of life and is associated with more hospital admissions, longer length of stay, more readmissions, and is a leading cause of cardiovascular death in adults with type 2 diabetes (Newton et al. 2016).

Hyperglycaemia and insulin resistance contribute to heart failure. Heart failure has a worse prognosis than diabetes (Metra et al. 2011) and reduces life expectancy (White et al. 2016). Significantly meta-analysis suggests that intensive glucose lowering is not associated with significant reduction in cardiovascular risk but it does result in increased risk of heart failure (Rosano et al. 2017). Atrial fibrillation increases the risk of heart failure approximately threefold.

Heart failure is characterised by symptoms such as dyspnoe and fatigue. The increased risk of heart failure in people with diabetes is due to abnormal glucose and FFA handling in cardiac muscle. Glucose is switched to FFA oxidation, which has an effect of cardiac contractility and functioning that induces left ventricular systolic and diastolic dysfunction, even when coronary disease is not present. These functional changes occur due to a number of mechanisms, including reduced glucose transport and carbohydrate oxidation, increased FFA utilisation, reduced sarcolemmal calcium transport, and changes in myofibrillar regulatory proteins (Rosano et al. 2017).

Treatment includes managing hypertension using beta blockers, especially selective beta blockers that have less effect on glycaemia, and angiotensin-converting enzyme inhibitors (ACE), mineralocorticoid receptor antagonists, except in people with nephropathy and more recently, LCZ696 and ivabradine (Ponikowski et al. 2016). Some glucose-lowering medicines (GLMs) can increase risk of heart failure and hospital admission (Chapter 5). Independent risk factors for heart disease include age, diabetes duration, insulin use, presence of coronary artery disease, and high serum creatinine (Wang et al. 2017). However, some GLP-1 receptor agonists and SGLT-2 inhibitors have cardiovascular benefits as well as glucose lowering effects (Alzaid 2019; Clemens et al. 2019).

Hypoglycaemia and cardiac disease

Hypoglycaemia is a strong predictor of macrovascular events, adverse outcomes, and death in people with type 2 diabetes. It is not clear whether there is a direct pathophysiological connect or whether hypoglycaemia indicate vulnerability to cardiovascular events (Hanefield et al. 2016). No such association has been demonstrated in type 1 diabetes. Hypoglycaemia may trigger cardiovascular events in people with preexisting cardiovascular disease and those with risk factors for cardiovascular disease.

Hypoglycaemia is associated with neuroglycopenia and low supplies of energy that activate the sympathoadrenal response and release of catecholamines, which increase the heart rate, cardiac stroke volume, and peripheral resistance and cause arrhythmias (Laitinen et al. 2003). These changes contribute to a prothrombotic state and the release of inflammatory markers. They can lead to sudden death.

Manifestations of cardiovascular disease

Cardiovascular disease involves:

- Heart and coronary circulation
- Brain and cerebral circulation
- Lower limbs: peripheral vascular disease

Cardiovascular disease leads to a cascade of symptoms and pathological events that lead to myocardial necrosis. If early disease is not treated, the pathology progresses and plaque accumulates in the coronary arteries and partially occlude the vessels, causing unstable angina, or the vessel can be totally occluded and lead to infarction and/or sudden cardiac death (Baker IDI 2019).

At risk populations include older people, Aboriginal and Torres Strait Islander peoples, those from lower socioeconomic groups, and younger onset of type 2 diabetes diagnosed before age 40. The increased risk for people with diabetes reflects cardiovascular pathophysiology:

- Increased plaque, complex lesions and coronary calcification.
- Coronary ischaemia is more diffuse.
- Several vessels are usually involved and there are fewer normal vessels.
- Reduced coronary vessel recruitment.
- Reduced coronary vasodilatory response.
- Abnormal cardiac handling of glucose and FFAs.

Cardiac disease is a common complication of diabetes, and it carries a higher mortality rate than for people without diabetes. Half of the people who have a cardiac event die before they reach the hospital. The mortality rate has not been reduced despite new therapeutic measures and preventative health programmes. As indicated, MI infarction may be a diabetes risk equivalent in people without diabetes. Diabetes often occurs within 3.5 years of a MI, particularly in older people, smokers, and those with a high BMI, hypertension. The risk is lower in people consuming a Mediterranean diet and those on lipid-lowering medicines (Mozaffarian 2007).

There is an association among increasing age, duration of diabetes, the presence of other complications and mortality. Cardiac disease is associated with diffuse atherosclerosis, coexisting cardiomyopathy, autonomic neuropathy, hyperglycaemia, and hyperlipidaemia, the metabolic consequences being hypercoagulability, elevated catecholamines, and insulin resistance. Atherosclerosis is more frequent and more severe in people with diabetes. It occurs at a younger age than in people without diabetes and is more prevalent in women, especially after menopause. Female sex hormones, especially oestrogen, have many haemodynamic, vascular, and metabolic effects, which are associated with cardiovascular protection in women (Dantas et al. 2012).

The protective effects of oestrogen include:

- Influencing the metabolism of lipoproteins.
- Controlling blood pressure.
- Reducing formation of atheromatous plaques.
- Increasing NO bioavailability.
- Regulating the production of endothelium-derived relaxing factors and endothelium-derived hyperpolarizing factors, which affect vascular relaxation and resistance. Oestrogen also has an effect on vascular constrictor factors.
- Suppressing vascular inflammation by down-regulating proinflammatory molecules, including cytokines and adhesion molecules.
- Regulating energy balance, fat distribution, and insulin sensitivity, which is largely lost after the menopause. Oestrogen replacement therapy in postmenopausal women has beneficial effects on diabetes and cardiovascular risk (Margolis et al. 2004) but the benefits must be weighed against the risks for each individual woman.

A number of clinical trials and guidelines emphasise the importance of reducing lipids, blood pressure, and blood glucose to reduce the risk of cardiovascular disease (Hansson et al. 1998; UKPDS 1998; NICE 2009; SIGN 2010; ADA 2013, 2019). Hypertension leads to thicker, less elastic blood vessel walls and increases the strain on the heart. There is a linear relationship between the diastolic blood pressure and the eventual outcome of type 2 diabetes. Reducing the blood pressure below 90 mmHg significantly improves the outcome (UKPDS 1998).

Subtle changes occur in the heart as a result of ischaemia-induced remodelling and the effects of hyperglycaemia on the endothelium of large blood vessels that predispose the individual to heart failure (Standl and Schnell 2000). Heart muscle metabolism is critically dependent on glucose during ischaemia, and heart muscle performance is improved in the presence of insulin, which stimulates glucose uptake, which support the use of IV insulin in acute MI (Malmberg et al. 1995). However, impaired heart performance is multifactorial, and blood pressure, lipids, and prothrombin imbalance all play a part. Table 8.1 outlines some of the diabetes-specific abnormalities linked to the development of cardiovascular disease.

Silent myocardial disease

> People do not report chest pain. They think they are bulletproof. They do not react quickly enough to the signs and are often embarrassed to call an ambulance.
>
> (Channel 9 news Sunday 29 April 2007)

Autonomic neuropathy can contribute to atypical presentations (silent) of cardiovascular disease and MI and lead to delayed treatment in one in three people with type 2 diabetes. Atypical symptoms include shortness of breath, fatigue, gastrointestinal symptoms, and glucose variability (Mayer and Rosenfeld 2006). Experts recommend that all people with diabetes be treated as if they have cardiovascular disease, given that diabetes is a 'coronary risk equivalent'.

Angina pectoris appears to be a poor indicator of MI, especially in people with diabetes and older people. The ADA (2019) recommends that people with proteinuria, microalbuminuria, peripheral vascular disease, carotid occlusive disease, or an abnormal ECG should have an exercise stress test. It is also important that people with diabetes, families, and clinicians receive education about atypical MI symptoms and the importance of undertaking appropriate steps to identify and manage it early.

MI is silent in 32% of people with diabetes, which leads to delay in seeking medical attention and may be a factor in the increased mortality rate. 'Silent' infarct means that the classic pain across the chest, down the arm and into the jaw is absent. Only mild discomfort, often mistaken for heartburn, may be present. The atypical nature of the chest pain may make it difficult for people to accept that they have had a heart attack. Risk factor modification may not be seen as essential. The person may present with hypertension, heart failure, cardiogenic shock, or, in older people with diabetes, ketoacidosis or hyperosmolar states (Chapter 7).

Diabetes may be diagnosed at the time an infarct occurs or during cardiac surgery. Emotional stress, and the associated catecholamine response, leads to increased blood glucose levels in 5% of patients admitted to coronary care units (CCU). The blood glucose may normalise during convalescence; however, counselling about diabetes and its management is important, especially if other diabetes risk factors are present. Tact and sympathy are necessary when informing the patient about the diagnosis of diabetes in these situations.

Women with cardiovascular disease have poorer outcomes than men, regardless of other comorbidities and management (Davidson et al. 2011). As discussed earlier, low female sex hormone levels after menopause, especially oestrogen, may play a role in cardiovascular disease in women. Atrial fibrillation in women confers a greater risk of stroke than in men and anticoagulation therapy is associated with a higher risk of bleeding problems (Davidson et al. 2011).

Cardiac markers

- Symptoms, but these are not reliable.
- 12-lead ECG helps stratify risk, e.g. ST elevation suggests MI.
- Markers of cardiac necrosis, which may not detect minor myocardial injury such as troponin and cardiac-specific troponin, myoglobin, C-reactive protein (CRP, brain natriuretic peptide (BNP). The sensitivity of these markers depends on the time of onset of the event to the time the person presents for care and the rise and fall of the specific marker (Casey 2004).

Several cardiac risk calculators are available for people to calculate their 10-year risk and/or for clinicians. Risk calculators generally determine 5- or 10-year risk. It is important to consider absolute risk rather than only managing individual risk factors. Algorithms help rank individuals

Table 8.1 Some diabetes-specific cardiovascular abnormalities that predispose an individual to heart disease.

Abnormality	Relevance to cardiovascular disease
Insulin resistance	Increases cardiovascular mortality
Chronic hyperglycaemia	Every 1% (11 mmol/mol) increase in HbA1c is associated with a 15% increase in hazard of all-cause mortality, 25% for cardiovascular mortality, and 17% fatal coronary heart disease (Zhang et al. 2007).
	In the UKPDS, each 1% (11 mmol/mol) reduction in HbA_{1c} was associated with a 21% lower risk of diabetes-related death and 14% lower risk of MI over 10 years.
	Contributes to microvascular disease.
Microvascular disease with microalbuminuria	May be detected earlier than macrovascular disease and often occurs concomitantly with macrovascular disease.
	Affects nutrient and oxygen exchange. Nephropathy, frequently in association with retinopathy. Nephropathy doubles the risk cardiac disease in people with type 1 diabetes (Lehto et al. 1999) but it is not clear whether reducing microalbuminuria reduces cardiovascular risk.
Autonomic neuropathy	Postural hypotension Abnormal cardiovascular reflexes Loss of sinus rhythm Resting sinus tachycardia Painless myocardial ischaemia and infarction 'silent MI' Delayed recognition and treatment Increased anaesthetic risk Increased risk in critical care situations Sudden death
Endothelial damage in basement membrane or outer lining of large blood vessels	Weak vessel walls, stiffened vessels contributing to hypertension Calcified vessels Impaired blood flow Reduced tissue oxygenation and nourishment
Hypertension	Thickening of blood vessel walls. Increased strain on the heart. Risk of cardiovascular disease increases progressively with increasing systolic blood pressure. Each 10 mmHg reduction in systolic blood pressure is associated with 15% reduction in risk of cardiovascular death over 10 years.
Hyperlipidaemia Obesity predisposes the individual to insulin resistance, dyslipidaemia and high circulating free fatty acids (FFA) but does not appear to be an independent risk factor for cardiovascular disease. Ethnicity needs to be considered when determining obesity.	Increased LDL cholesterol or total cholesterol is an independent risk factor for cardiovascular death. Type 2 diabetes is associated with high triglycerides, low HDL, and small dense LDL. A 1 mmol/l reduction in LDL represents a 21% reduction in risk. Hypertriglyceridaemia is an independent marker of increased cardiovascular risk in type 2 diabetes. Increased lipolysis as FFA are liberated from adipose tissue. Increased mediators of vascular function such as angiotensinogen, adiponectin, IL-6, prostaglandins and TNF∂. Statins are useful in people with diabetes used with healthy lifestyle recommendations. Some people require additional therapies such as ezetimibe and PCsK9 inhibitors (ADA 2019).
Adiponectin and adipocyte-derived protein C-reactive protein (CRP) Homocysteine Glutathione peroxidase 1 (GP1) is present in atherosclerotic plaques.	Associated with metabolic derangements, including type 2 diabetes via their role in glucose regulation and catabolism of fatty acids. Adiponectin levels correlate with the development of insulin resistance, progression of type 2 diabetes, and hypertension. High adiponectin is related to higher all-cause mortality after controlling for other confounders (Singer et al. 2012). High baseline GP1 is associated with lower rates of cardiovascular events after adjusting for other risk factors. High homocysteine and interleukin-6 and low GP1are associated with adverse outcomes.

SgLT-2 inhibitors reduce cardiovascular risk as well as blood glucose (Chapter 5).

for treatment priority and a cut point for action. Most risk calculators can under- or over-estimate risk (Nelson and Woodward 2019). Australian and New Zealand guidelines recommend using five-year risk estimates, consistent with most clinical trials and patient preferences (Nelson and Woodward 2019). Some cardiovascular risk calculators are:

- American College of cardiology/American Heart Foundation ASCVD risk calculator http://tools.acc.org/ASCVD-Risk-Estimator-Plus
- Australian Risk Calculator www.cvdcheck.org.au
- Coronary Artery Calcification Calcium Calculator https://www.mesa-nhlbi.org/calcium/input.aspx (Calcium contributes to stiffening in coronary arteries compounding the narrowing caused by plaque). The calcium score is useful for deciding statin management (Lee et al. 2017).
- Coronary Artery Calcium Scoring – Position Statement – csanz https://www.csanz.edu.au/wp-content/uploads/2017/07/CAC_Position-Statement_2017_ratified-26-May-2017.pdf

A Coronary Artery Calcium (CAC) score of zero excludes significant cardiovascular disease. CAC could be a useful complement to other tools to assess cardiovascular risk and the level of risk and to individualise lifestyle and statin therapy in asymptomatic people who require intensive statin therapy (Lee et al. 2017). A CAC score of 0–1 indicates low 10-year risk; > 1 represents high risk. It has good negative predictive value for excluding presence of significant coronary disease and provides important prognostic information to stratify cardiovascular risk than other biomarkers (Lee et al. 2017).

- The Heart Foundation Absolute Risk Indicator (2019)
  http://www.heartfoundation.org.au/for-professionals/clinical…/absolute-risk
- Framingham Risk Score for Hard Coronary Heart Disease
  https://www.mdcalc.com/framingham-risk-score-hard-coronary-heart-disease
- Cardiac Risk Score Calculator
  https://www.csanz.edu.au/wp-content/uploads/2017/07/CAC_Position-Statement_2017_ratified-26-May-2017.pdf
- The QRISK®2 calculator
  www.riskscore.org.uk

Medicines and cardiovascular disease

Many types of medicines may be needed to prevent and/or manage cardiovascular disease (Chapter 5). The choice of medicines depends on the clinical indications, patient factors such as cardiovascular risk, contraindications/precautions, risk of medicine interactions, availability, and cost.

Generally, management targets address hypertension, hyperglycaemia, coagulopathies, and hyperlipidaemia. Most modern guidelines recommend individualising targets and commonly recommend:

- Blood pressure 130/80 mmHg including in people with albuminuria, if it can be achieved without hypotension. People at low risk <140/90 mmHg and pregnant women with pre-existing hypertension treated with antihypertensive therapy 120–60/80–105.
- LDL cholesterol <2 mmol/l.
- HbA_{1c}:
  - Diabetes short duration and no cardiovascular risk <6% (<42 mmol/mol);
  - Lifestyle management with or without metformin <6.5% (<48 mmol/mol);
  - Requiring any glucose lowering medicine besides Metformin or insulin <7% (< 53 mmol/mol);
  - Requiring insulin <7% (< 53 mmol/mol);
  - Diabetes of long duration and/or presence of cardiovascular disease, because these people do not benefit from tight blood glucose control <7% (<53 mol/mol) (Accord Study Group 2011);

○ If the person has severe hypoglycaemia or hypoglycaemic unawareness and older people <8% (<64 mmol/mol) (ADA 2019).

The Accord Study Group (2011) found that tight blood glucose control (<6% <42 mmol/mol) resulted in 10 extra deaths per 1000 people over 3.5 years. Likewise, severe hypoglycaemia is associated with increased morbidity and mortality (Chapter 6). It is also associated with long duration of diabetes and microalbuminuria (Yun et al. 2012). These significant adverse events highlight the importance of determining individual risk for cardiovascular disease and the risks associated with treatment.

Estimating cardiovascular risk in people with diabetes is complicated: see the currently available risk calculators discussed previously. The Framingham and UKPDS risk calculators are inaccurate in people with diabetes (Coleman et al. 2007), and people should be informed that the risk calculation is only an estimate of their actual risk (NICE 2009). However, the likelihood of error is reduced if the person has several cardiovascular risk factors (NICE 2009). Risk calculators can underestimate risk in South Asian, Maori, Pacific Islanders, and Middle Eastern peoples (NPS 2012).

In addition to medicines, stopping smoking, eating a healthy diet, and enaging in regular exercise and effective self-care are essential to achieving optimal control. A recent study suggests that eating nuts may reduce cardiovascular risk and associated death in people with type 2 diabetes (Liu et al. 2019). Nuts are a source of unsaturated fatty acids, plant proteins, fibre, minerals, vitamins and anti-inflammatory phytochemicals. Eating five or more servings of 28 g of nuts per week is associated with lowering the risk of cardiovascular disease, cancer, and all-cause death. It is important to not note that despite their name, peanuts are not nuts; they are legumes.

Sedentary time is associated with increased risk of type 2 diabetes (112% increased RR), cardiovascular disease (90% RR), and all-cause mortality (40% RR) (NPS 2012; Wilmot et al. 2012). Sedentary time includes occupational sitting and watching TV. Medicines may be required to manage cardiovascular risk or treat cardiovascular disease.

Medicine commonly used to manage cardiovascular disease include:

- Antithrombotic medicines to prevent thromboembolism generally and during coronary procedures and surgery, prevent stroke in patients with atrial fibrillation, prevent thromboembolism in patients with prosthetic heart valves, and treat acute MI. Types of medicines include Vitamin K antagonists (warfarin), heparin (enoxaparin), platelet aggregation inhibitors (aspirin), and thrombolytic enzymes (alteplase). These medicines require frequent monitoring and interact with many other medicines including complementary medicines (CA). The benefits of low-dose aspirin (75–150 mg/day) outweigh the risks in adults with diabetes and existing cardiovascular disease. However, evidence for the benefits for people without existing cardiovascular disease, including people with diabetes, is weak (NPS 2012). Thus, aspirin is not recommended for primary prevention (SIGN 2010). The risks of major bleeds and macular degeneration are significant. Consequently, the NPS, the National Vascular Disease Prevention Alliance Guidelines, and SIGN 2010 do not recommend routine use of low-dose aspirin in people without existing cardiovascular disease. (NICE 2009) recommends offering 75 mg aspirin/day to anybody with blood pressure <145/90 mmHg, and the American Diabetes Association (ADA) (2012) recommends people with 10-year cardiovascular disease risk 10% should take 75 mg aspirin/day. ADA does not advocate using aspirin for people whose cardiovascular risk is <5% and recommends that clinical judgement be used for people whose 10-year risk is 5%–10%.
- Cardiac medicines to treat arrhythmias (cardiac glycosides such as digoxin), heart failure antiarrythmics such as amiodarone), relieve cardiac symptoms such as angina (vasodilators such as isorbide), treat high and low blood pressure, cardiogenic shock, and MI (cardiac stimulants such as adrenaline).
- Antihypertensive agents often used as primary prevention to reduce the risk of microvascular disease. Blood pressure should be measured with patients seated and their feet flat on the floor, their arm level, and using the right size cuff (ADA 2019). Ambulatory blood pressure monitoring can be useful. Antihypertensive agents include low-dose diuretics as first-line

treatment (frusemide), peripheral vasodilators (oxpentifylline), and calcium channel blockers (amlodipine). Antihypertensive therapy is usually selected according to the comorbidities present to achieve blood pressure 130/80 in people with cardiovascular disease. The first-line medicine for people with diabetes and hypertension is an ACEI or an ARB; the most appropriate choice in an older person following a MI is a calcium channel blocker to reduce the risk of stroke. However, most people require several antihypertensive medicines (European Society of Hypertension 2007; ADA 2019) Doses may need to be adjusted to avoid postural hypotension in people with acute nephropathy an education about the risk is important.

- Beta blocking agents (Atenolol, Metorpolol, Propanolol), which can be used with a diuretic and an ACE inhibitor. Beta blockers confer benefit in the medium- to long-term but can cause decompensation and worsen heart failure and hypotension in the short term. They should be started at a low dose and gradually increased. Contraindications include asthma, heart block and symptomatic hypotension.

- Medicines acting on the renin–angiotensin system such as ACEI, which are first-line treatment in heart failure, left ventricular dysfunction following MI, and diabetes in the presence of microalbuminuria (Ramipril); angiotensin 11 antagonists (Irbesartin), which are used if the person cannot tolerate ACE. For example, ACE inhibitors are associated with a three-times-higher rate of cough. SIGN (2010) recommends ACEI be considered in people with all New York Heart Association (NYHA) functional classes of heart failure due to left ventricular systolic dysfunction.

- Lipid-lowering agents such as HMG-CoA reductase inhibitors (statins, e.g. Atorvastatin), which reduces LDL cholesterol, fibrates, which are first choice if triglycerides are elevated, nicotinic acid, which lowers both cholesterol and triglycerides but is not tolerated very well (Rossi 2006). However, there is not enough evidence to recommend fibrates, Ezetimibe, or nicotinic acid for primary prevention (SIGN 2010).

- Glucose-lowering medicines are discussed in Chapter 5. Some also have cardiovascular benefits, e.g. SGLT-2 (canaglozin, dapagflozin, sotagliflozin) GLP-1 (liraglutide) (Cefalo et al. 2019).

However, these medicines are not always prescribed optimally. For example, antithrombotic medicines, ACE inhibitors, ACE, beta blocker combinations, and antihypertensive agents are underutilised (National Institute of Clinical Studies 2005). Patient nonadherence with many medicines is high and is a significant limiting factor in achieving optimal outcomes.

Complementary medicines (CM)
CM should not replace evidence-based conventional medicines in most circumstances. There is evidence for some CM; for example WS 1442, a formula of *Crateaegus monogyna* (hawthorn), was shown to increase intracellular calcium concentration, contractile force, action potential, and the refractory period, improve coronary blood flow and reduce preload and after load (Pittler et al. 2008). Animal studies also demonstrate a smaller area of infarction after induced MI using *C. monogyna*. These findings suggest that WS 1442 *might* have a place in managing cardiovascular disease, but that place is not yet defined.

CQ-10 lowers systolic and diastolic blood pressure and reduces inflammation. Individuals with mild-to-moderate hypertension and cardiac disease might benefit from CQ_{10} supplements (Rosenfeldt et al. 2007), but like W1442, its place is under-researched. CQ-10 is an antioxidant and is present in LDL-c, where it reduces the potential for LDL-c to be oxidised and become atherogenic. Some experts suggested CQ_{10} might be a useful addition to statins to reduce myotoxicity. However, while it may have a place, at present there is no recommendation to use CQ-10 in people taking statins (Barenholtz and Kohlhaas 2006). If people do elect to use CQ-10, the effects on their conventional medicines need to be monitored.

Other CM such as massage, meditation, and Tai Chi can help reduce stress, improve quality of life, and manage pain but should be used within a Quality Use of Medicine framework (Chapter 18).

Other management considerations

Hyperglycaemia is common in MI, and there is an association between initial blood glucose level and outcomes, including mortality, even if the blood glucose is only mildly elevated (ADS 2012). However, hyperglycaemia is also associated with adverse outcomes (Chapter 6). Various guidelines suggest different blood glucose targets in acute MI; generally, the aims should be blood glucose <10 mmol/l, and IV infusions are recommended when resources permit (ADS 2012). The International Diabetes Federation (IDF) (2011) suggested a two-hour postprandial blood glucose >7.8 mmol/l is a stronger predictor of cardiovascular events than fasting blood glucose and recommended monitoring postprandial blood glucose and to aim for <7.5 mmol/l.

People with an acute cardiovascular event are usually cared for in CCUs, but patients in other wards and in the community may develop cardiovascular problems, including silent MI. A longer stay in CCU may be indicated for people with diabetes, because 35% of patients die, often in the second week after the infarct (Karlson et al. 1993). People with diabetes and unstable angina, MI without ST elevation or STEMI, have a higher mortality risk within one year of the onset of acute coronary syndrome than nondiabetics (Donahoe et al. 2007).

Silent MI may be relatively common in common critical care settings, the diagnosis can be difficult to establish, and the MI is often missed due to analgesia used to control chest pain, intubation, sedation, and coma (Lim et al. 2008). Lim et al. (2008) suggested screening for elevated troponin levels in critically ill patients and performing an ECG could reduce mortality, and that elevated troponins might be predicative of mortality. Although more research is needed, these findings might be particularly relevant to people with diabetes where the risk of cardiovascular disease is likely to be high.

Short- and long-term morbidity and mortality can be improved by IV insulin/glucose infusion followed by multidose subcutaneous insulin injections (Malmberg et al. 1995). Acute myocardial infarction causes a rapid increase in catecholamines, cortisol, and glucagon. Insulin levels fall in the ischaemic myocardium and tissue sensitivity to insulin falls and impairs glucose utilisation by cardiac muscle. Free fatty acids are mobilised as fuel substrates and potentiate ischaemic injury by direct toxicity or by increasing the demand for oxygen and inhibiting glucose oxidation. IV insulin during acute episodes and subcutaneous insulin for three months after the infarct may restore platelet function, correct lipoprotein imbalance, reduce plasminogen activator inhibitor-1 activity, and improve metabolism in noninfarcted areas of the heart.

The need for invasive procedures depends on the severity at presentation and the results of relevant investigations. Pfisterer (2004) showed that invasive treatment provided short-term symptomatic relief and reduced the rate of revascularisation and hospitalisation and use of antianginal medicines, compared to medicine treatment. In the longer term, both strategies were effective in older patients with angina. Mortality risk factors included age >80 years, prior heart failure, left ventricular ejection <45%, and the presence of two or more comorbidities.

Objectives of care in hospital

Care should be planned to avoid constantly disturbing the patient and allow adequate rest and sleep. The following are the objectives of care:

- Treat the acute attack according to medical orders, guidelines, and standard protocols.
- Stabilise cardiac status and relieve symptoms.
- Prevent extension of the cardiac abnormality and limit further episodes.
- Retain independence as far as possible.
- Achieve and maintain euglycaemia but prevent hypoglycaemic events; thus, blood glucose monitoring is important.
- Provide psychological support.
- Prevent complications while in hospital.
- Counsel about risk factor modification.
- Educate/re-educate about diabetes, including how to recognise and manage cardiovascular events.

Mental health and cardiovascular disease

Anxiety is common among people with cardiac disease and can have serious consequences for self-care and long-term outcomes if it is not recognised and managed to prevent depression. However, anxiety can be life-saving if it prompts the person to seek help early (Moser et al. 2007). Significantly, depression is an independent risk factor for cardiovascular disease and its prognosis. Both depression and heart disease are associated with social isolation and lack of social support (Bunker et al. 2003). These factors need to be considered when estimating cardiovascular risk.

Several trials have investigated the cardiovascular benefit of treating depression. These include ENRICH (cognitive behaviour therapy and SSRI medicines), which is difficult to interpret but which showed no significant difference between treatment and usual care. SADHART (SSRI), showed improvements in mild-to-moderate depression but no significant differences in cardiac events. The results of CREATE (SSRI [Citalopram] and interpersonal psychotherapy) are not yet available but suggest that depression improves but HbA1c does not significantly improve (Reddy 2008).

The effects on mental health may change; for example, Gudjhar et al. (2003) found that people with diabetes were most concerned about the implications of the MI immediately after the event and less concerned about the impact of diabetes on their long-term physical health, mental health, and quality of life. Patient-generated quality-of-life tools were used. As people recovered and realised they would survive, about four months after the MI, concern about the MI began to diminish and pre-MI worry about diabetes and its complications reemerged.

Depression may increase cardiovascular risk and vice versa via several mechanisms:

- Risk behaviours such as inadequate diet and inactivity, smoking, and non-compliance with medicines.
- Effects on autonomic function by enhancing sympathetic nervous system activity and heart rate variability.
- Consequence model: inflammatory processes with sub-chronic elevation of cytokines activate the stress response and inhibit serotonin. MI might also induce physical changes in the brain that are mediated by the inflammatory response and cause depression.
- Coincidence model: autonomic dysregulation decreased heart rate variability and increased risk of ventricular arrhythmias, changes in platelets, inflammation, and changes in endothelial function, some of which might be linked to dietary factors. For example, increasing omega-3 fatty acids improves cardiac function (Lesperance and Frasure-Smith 2007).

Clinician responsibilities

(1) To be aware that myocardial infarction can present atypically in people with diabetes and may present as CCF, syncope, vomiting, abdominal pain, and fatigue that improves with rest. An ECG should be performed urgently if any of these symptoms are present. A high resting heart rate is associated with mortality in people with diabetes. Sanchis (2007) developed a risk assessment process for patients without increased troponins or ST deviation that was able to identify patients with a similar prognosis to patients with elevated troponins and ST depression that might be useful in people with diabetes.
(2) To provide psychological, educational, and physical care.
(3) To monitor blood glucose, two to four hourly depending on stability and route of insulin administration.
(4) To provide adequate pain relief, and to control vomiting, which contribute to/exacerbate high blood glucose levels.
(5) To deliver care according to the medical orders for the specific cardiac abnormality.
(6) To administer insulin:
    - Many patients on GLMs are changed to insulin during the acute phase to improve blood glucose control.

- Insulin is usually administered via an infusion at least for the first 48 hours. Only clear insulin is used. Insulin infusions are discussed in Chapter 7. The patient should be eating and drinking normally before the infusion is removed, and a dose of subcutaneous insulin given to prevent hyperglycaemia.

Some endocrinologist/cardiologist teams adopted Malmberg et al.'s recommendations, the so-called DIGAMI protocol, or some variation of it, which usually involves commencing an IV insulin infusion for people with diabetes presenting with MI from the time of presentation in the emergency room. IV insulin is usually continued for 24 hours, after which time subcutaneous insulin is commenced and maintained for three months.

The aim of the IV insulin is to normalise glucose utilisation in the myocardium, achieve normoglycaemia, and reduce morbidity and mortality (Chapter 5).

(7) Other medications: GLMs should be stopped while the patient is having IV insulin to reduce the risk of hypoglycaemia:
- Thiazide diuretics can increase blood glucose levels and cause hypokalaemia.
- Beta blockers reduce mortality by >30%. ACE inhibitors improve blood pressure and cardiac remodelling and stabilise the rate of progression of renal disease. There is a close association between cardiac and renal disease in diabetes.

Non-cardiac-specific beta-blocking agents may mask the signs of hypoglycaemia. Peoples who are normally on oral GLMs will require support and education about the use of insulin. It should be explained that insulin is being given to increase the glucose available to the myocardium and decrease FFAs in the blood. Units where IV insulin infusions are used often discharge the patient on subcutaneous insulin, which is continued for three months then reassessed the individual's medicine needs are reassessed.

(8) Physical status:
- Monitor fluid balance and maintain accurate documentation to help assess kidney function.
- Monitor blood pressure, lying, and standing. Some antihypertensive medications can cause orthostatic hypotension. Counsel the patient to change position gradually, especially on getting out of bed or out of a chair. Postural hypotension is a risk factor for falls, especially in older people.
- Monitor ECG.
- Observe for weakness, fatigue, CCF, or unexplained hyperglycaemia, which could indicate another infarct or extension of the original infarct.
- Provide appropriate skin care to prevent dryness and pressure areas.
- Provide adequate pain relief.

(9) Investigative procedures:
- Monitor serum electrolytes, cardiac enzymes, blood gases, and potassium levels. Report abnormalities to the doctor promptly. Fluctuating potassium levels can cause or exacerbate cardiac arrhythmias.
- Prevent hypoglycaemia by carefully monitoring the blood glucose and carbohydrate intake.
- Prepare the individual for investigative procedures appropriately, and inform them what to expect (Chapter 9).

(10) Thrombolytics are beneficial to reduce plaque. Low-dose aspirin reduces emboli and reduces the risk of cardiac disease and stroke in people with existing cardiovascular disease; see the previous section.

(11) If relevant, consider end-of-life care (Chapter 18) and support the family to cope with the crisis.

In many cases, metabolic control prior to the MI was suboptimal and insulin therapy was indicated for some time before the infarct occurred.

Some GLMs are contraindicated if cardiac, renal, and/or liver disease is present (see Chapter 5).

Practice points

(1) The person may not recognise the signs of hypoglycaemia if:
- Autonomic neuropathy is present.
- Nonselective beta-blocking agents are used.

(2) Neuroglycopenic signs of hypoglycaemia (confusion, slurred speech, or behaviour change) may predominate. Alternatively, these signs may indicate a cardiovascular event.

Medical tests/procedures (see chapter 9)

(1) The eyes should be assessed *before* thrombolytic medications are commenced. If proliferative retinopathy is present, bleeding into the back of the eye may occur, requiring urgent treatment.

(2) Diagnostic procedures that require the use of contrast dyes, for example, angiograms, have been associated with renal complications. Ensure adequate hydration before and after procedures and monitor urine output, especially in older people and people with renal disease.

(3) There is a high prevalence of cardiovascular disease in people with renal disease (Levin et al. 2000). Renal disease is a predictor of MI risk on some modern cardiovascular disease risk calculators.

Rehabilitation

Structured rehabilitation after an acute cardiovascular event and heart failure improves long-term outcomes, reduces social isolation, and improves function and quality of life.

(1) Encourage activity within tolerance limits. Refer for physiotherapy/occupational therapy.

(2) Encourage independence.

(3) Counsel about resumption of normal activity, including sexual intercourse, after discharge home.

(4) Explain restrictions on driving after cardiac surgery.

(5) Ensure diabetes education/re-education is available. Refer to diabetes nurse specialist/ diabetes educator, dietitian, and physiotherapist. Education should include the need to protect kidney function and also address the risk factors involved in the development of cardiac disease. The following are particular concerns to address:
- Recognise hypoglycaemia.
- Correct insulin technique.
- Correct blood glucose monitoring technique.
- Note possible indicators of further cardiac problems.
- Provide dietary assessment and advice.
- Modify risk factor modification.

(6) Explain the need for multi-medicine therapy and the importance of adhering to the medicine regimen.

(7) Monitor to detect anxiety and depression and treat early.

Modifying risk factors associated with the development of cardiac disease

Current cardiovascular management guidelines focus on reducing global cardiovascular risk, which requires a proactive approach and attention to multiple risk factors taking age into account: cardiovascular risk, which can be stratified and individualised to enable personalised teaching using tools such as the QRISK and ASSIGN in the UK and the Framingham algorithm, which is gender-specific and is based on the presence of hypertension, dyslipidaemia, and smoking. The Systematic Coronary Risk Evaluation (SCORE) based on cholesterol, blood pressure, and age was developed for European countries (Zannad 2008). Note the discussion about the limitations of risk scores in a previous section of this chapter.

Significantly, research suggests that doctors do not adequately assess cardiovascular risk and this contributes to people not achieving management targets (Bohm 2008; Mulnier 2012). Other researchers found general practitioners overestimate the risk of diabetes complications but the impact on patient care and service utilisation or outcomes was not reported (Haussler et al. 2007).

People with diabetes require both information and support to manage diabetes and reduce the risk of adverse health outcomes. Personalised information is more effective than generalised information. Management targets are described in this chapter and Chapter 2. As indicated in Chapter 16, helping people determine their cardiovascular age could be a useful way to help people understand their cardiovascular risk and help them adhere to their risk reduction strategies.

Key messages are to:

- Start in early childhood and encourage parents to be appropriate role models. Clinicians also need to be appropriate role models for people with diabetes.
- Stop smoking.
- Avoid high-calorie foods and high fat intake, especially transfats, to achieve sensible weight reduction. Include omega-3 fatty acids in the diet. Reduce salt intake. Suitable diets are described in Chapter 4 and include the DASH and Mediterranean diets.
- Limit alcohol intake.
- Maintain a healthy weight range suitable to age and developmental stage. In particular, reduce abdominal obesity.
- Increase regular exercise/activities.
- Achieve acceptable blood glucose levels.
- Reduce blood lipids. If this is not achieved by diet and exercise, lipid-lowering agents are needed; see Chapter 5. High LDL-c, low HDL-c, and mixed hyperlipidaemia significantly increase the risk of developing cardiovascular disease (Bruckert and Hansel 2007; Hansel et al. 2004).
- Reduce blood pressure by appropriate diet, exercise, and stopping smoking. Optimal blood pressure control is important and people are often prescribed three or more antihypertensive agents. The choice of medication is individualised and includes reducing blood glucose as part of a comprehensive cardiovascular risk management plan (Lowe 2002). Hypertension is also a risk factor for poorer performance on verbal and concept formation tests in type 2 diabetes (Elias et al. 1997), which has implications for self-care and activities of daily living.
- Manage hypertension and monitor the day–night dip. A blunted day–night dip is associated with a blunted morning BP surge and vice versa. A blunted morning BP surge could be an independent predictor of cardiovascular events (Verdecchia et al. 2012).
- Secondary prevention programmes such as cardiac rehabilitation are important to help individuals regain the best possible functioning.
- Manage stress. Long-term stress is associated with increased risk of cardiovascular disease in both men and women, and a high level of trait anger in middle aged men with hypertension is associated with increased risk of hypertension progression to a cardiovascular event (Player et al. 2007).
- Seek treatment for depression.
- People with known cardiac disease should have a written action to plan to follow if they experience chest pain. They should know early management is important and not to delay presenting to hospital. The plan might include using short-acting nitrate medicines, resting, taking aspirin if they are not already prescribed this medicine, calling an ambulance, notifying their doctor, and wearing medic alert information.

Telephone coaching for people with coronary heart disease and suboptimal lipid levels improves adherence to medication therapy and dietary advice. It contributes to an improved lipid profile and could be an important aspect of cardiac rehabilitation programmes (Vale et al. 2003). The COACH protocol is currently under investigation in a general practice setting with practice nurses providing coaching with support from the COACH investigators (Young et al. 2007).

Cerebrovascular disease

The incidence of stroke associated with diabetes is high and mortality following a stroke is higher in people with diabetes than nondiabetics. The brain is supplied with blood by four main arteries: two carotids and two vertebral arteries. The clinical consequences of cerebrovascular disease depend on the vessels or combination of vessels involved. TIAs arise when the blood supply to a part of the brain is temporarily interrupted without permanent damage. Recovery from a TIA usually occurs within 24 hours. If TIAs occur frequently they can indicate impending stroke. Small repeated strokes that cause progressive brain damage can lead to multi-infarct dementia, which is common in diabetes. Signs of multi-infarct dementia include:

- Gradual memory loss
- Diminished intellectual capacity
- Loss of motor function
- Incontinence (Chapter 10)

Strokes are classified as thrombotic or haemorrhagic and occur when a major vessel is blocked. They frequently cause permanent damage requiring prolonged rehabilitation and often significantly reduced self-care potential and quality of life. In these cases, diabetes management should be discussed with the family or carers who will be responsible for assisting the person with diabetes.

The risk factors for cerebrovascular disease are similar to those for cardiovascular disease. High BMI >25 kg/m^2 and systolic hypertension increase risk of death after a stroke among men (Chen 2008). However, there appear to be some significant differences between men and women. Women may have worse outcomes after acute stroke than men if they do not receive thrombolytic therapy, and women are more likely to benefit from thrombolytic therapy than men (Lutsep 2008). Likewise, healthy women over age 65 benefit from alternate day aspirin (100 mg) to prevent stroke, but aspirin has not been shown to prevent strokes in healthy men (Ridker et al. 2005). However, the NPS, SIGN, NICE, and ADA guidelines regarding aspirin use should be considered.

There are also gender differences in response to treatment and outcome following acute stroke. Women with carotid artery stenosis have a lower risk of recurrent stroke than men and receive less benefit from surgical treatment of moderate carotid artery stenosis than men (Alamowitch et al. 2005). Women with intracranial stenosis are at higher risk of recurrent stroke than men (Williams et al. 2007).

Poor sleep quality is linked to increased risk of vascular events including stroke; and daytime sleepiness could be an independent risk factor for stroke conferring a 4.5-fold increased risk (Boden-Albala 2008) (Chapter 10).

- A careful history will elicit failing mental function and sleep issues.
- Carotid bruits are usually present and can be evaluated using Doppler studies.
- Angiography is required in symptomatic cases.
- Various degrees of paralysis and effects on speech depending on the site and extent of the stroke.

Management

There is limited evidence concerning managing stroke in people with diabetes. The preventative measures outlined for cardiovascular disease apply to cerebrovascular disease. Acute stroke is managed as for people without diabetes, but hyperglycaemia and hyoglycaemia should be avoided. Blood glucose monitoring will aid decisions about titrating GLM medicine doses and the dose regimen.

Carotid endarterectomy is indicated if the carotid arteries are significantly narrowed. Low-dose aspirin may be beneficial, considering the risks and benefits.

Management in a stroke unit improves outcomes, and optimal collaboration among care providers in the emergency department and stroke unit is essential. Nursing responsibilities include care during investigative procedures (see Chapter 9). Rehabilitation focuses on returning the person to optimal functioning and independence within their capabilities. Observational data suggests there is an association between blood glucose in the first 24 hours and mortality and infarct size. ADS (2012) recommends maintaining blood glucose ~ 10 mmol/l and avoiding hypoglycaemia <5 mmol/l.

Middleton et al. (2011) developed a treatment protocol, Fever, Hyperglycaemia Swallowing (FeSS), for managing stroke in the first 72 hours following an acute stroke. The protocol involves the following:

- Monitor and document fever every four hours and treating fever >37.5 with paracetamol, IV, rectally or orally unless contraindicated.
- Monitor venous blood glucose on admission and capillary glucose every one to six hours.
- Commence an IV saline infusion and deliver for six hours when blood glucose is between 8 and 11 mmol/l in people with diabetes or 8 and 16 mmol/l in people without diabetes.
- Commence an IV insulin infusion if the blood glucose is >11 mmol/l in people with diabetes and if the blood glucose is >16 mmol/l in nondiabetics.
- Screen for dysphagia and clearly documenting the findings in the person's medical record. Middleton et al. developed an education programme to train nurses to undertake dysphagia screening. Speech therapists usually undertake such assessments. People who were managed using the FeSS protocol had better outcomes after discharge.

Middleton et al. like other stroke researchers, used a combination of strategies, and it is difficult to separate the different contribution of the IV insulin infusion. The *combination* may be the important element. However, ADS (2012) choose not to include the FeSS study in their review when developing guidelines for managing hyperglycaemia in hospital.

Other important assessments after the acute phase include functional ability and mental health as well as social support and whether the home environment requires modification. Rehabilitation programmes can help people improve physical functioning and independence. Driving assessment needs to be undertaken following a stroke and assessed regularly; see Chapter 10.

Diabetes and eye disease

Key points

- Retinopathy occurs in type 1 and type 2 diabetes and is related to the duration of diabetes and glycaemic control. It is a frequent cause of new blindness in people aged 20–74.
- Regular screening is essential to detect and treat changes early, and optimising glycaemic control and managing hypertension are essential aspects of treatment
- Glaucoma, cataracts, and other eye disorders occur earlier and more frequently in people with diabetes than the general population (ADA 2019).

- Encourage independence. People with visual loss are capable of caring for themselves if they are provided with appropriate sight aids and information. However, vision impairment has a profound impact on an individual's ability to learn diabetes self-care tasks and on their psychological wellbeing.
- Becoming blind is a significant fear for people with diabetes.
- Maintain a safe environment.
- Orient patient to the environment and staff.
- Explain procedures carefully, fully recognising that the person is probably not a visual learner.
- Return belongings to the same place.
- Use appropriate teaching style to the individual's learning style.

Rationale

Retinopathy is a significant complication of diabetes. Prevention and early identification of people at risk are essential. Nurses need to be aware of the impact of visual loss on the self-care and psychological wellbeing of people with diabetes and their role in preventative care. Other vision changes occur in people with diabetes in addition to diabetic retinopathy, for example macular degeneration is common in older people. Age-related macular degeneration might be related to elevated levels of high-sensitivity CRP. Cataracts and glaucoma are common in people with diabetes but also occur in nondiabetics.

Introduction

Vision impairment and blindness are significant complications of diabetes. Blindness occurs in 50–60 people/100 000 people with diabetes (Cormack et al. 2001). Most people with diabetes do not have sight-threatening retinopathy, but if they have macular oedema and/or proliferative retinopathy it must be treated to reduce the progression to vision impairment. Screening programmes have enabled early identification and treatment of early retinal changes and reduced the progression to sight-threatening retinopathy.

The specific cellular mechanisms that lead to reduced visual acuity have not been defined. Antonetti et al. (2006) proposed a combined nerve and vascular mechanism that causes loss of neurons, which compromises neurotransmission and alters structure and function of retinal cells types. Macular cysts could scatter light and reduce the quality of the image and/or visual function could decline as a result of fluid accumulation in the retina. The neurons are susceptible to circulating amino acids, antibodies, and/or inflammatory cells that reach the retina through leaking capillaries. The vascular leakage can affect vision even when macular oedema is not present (Antonetti et al. 2006).

Kim et al. (2012) found an association between 1,5-anhydroglucitol (1,5-AG), a marker of postprandial hyperglycaemia, and diabetic retinopathy especially in people with 'moderate' glucose control but not albuminuria. The authors suggested 1,5-AG could be used as a marker to target people at risk of retinopathy. There is also evidence that cognitive ability declines over time in people with diabetes and may be linked to complications such as proliferative retinopathy (Ryan et al. 2003).

Key changes in the eye include:

- Maculopathy: macular oedema and macular ischaemia. The macular may be distorted or elevated or vitreous haemorrhages may occur and distort the ocular media (Antonetti et al. 2006).
- Retinopathy: stages of retinopathy have been described based on a system of photographic grading that requires comparison with a standard set of photographs showing different features and stages of retinopathy (DRS 1981; EDTRS 1991).

- Generalised ocular oedema.
- Lens opacity: cataract.
- Papillopathy: optic disc swelling that occurs in type 1 diabetes.

Some degree of retinopathy occurs in almost all people with type 1 diabetes after 20 years duration of diabetes and 70% of people with type 2 diabetes (DRS 1981; DCCT 1993). Retinopathy occurs as a result of microvascular disease that manifests as increased capillary permeability and closure of the retinal capillaries, which causes vascular leakage, retinal oedema, and accumulation of lipids that is seen as hard exudates in the retina and retinal ischaemia.

Risk factors for retinopathy

The factors that lead to an increased risk of retinopathy are similar to the risk factors for other complications and include:

- Long duration of diabetes.
- Poor metabolic control.
- Renal disease with microalbuminuria and proteinuria.
- Hyperlipidaemia, especially hypertriglyceridaemia, which contribute to macular exudates and oedema.
- Low haematocrit.
- Pregnancy in people with diagnosed diabetes. Pregnancy may exacerbate existing retinopathy (see Chapter 14), but it does not usually develop in women with gestational diabetes.
- Smoking, although the effect of smoking on the development and progression of retinopathy is unclear.
- Hypertension.

People with diabetic eye disease are at greater risk of developing other diabetes-related complications, especially nephropathy, unless they are screened regularly, take appropriate preventative action and treatment is commenced early.

Vision impairment from nondiabetic causes can coexist with diabetes. People with diabetes also have an increased incidence of glaucoma and cataracts and there is an increasing correlation with age-related macular degeneration. Many of the underlying causes that lead to macular degeneration are also associated with diabetes; see Table 8.2, which depicts risk factors for age-related macular degeneration (Lim 2006). Many of these risk factors are similar to the risk factors for diabetic retinopathy and the same risk reduction strategies apply to both conditions. Table 8.2 shows modifiable and nonmodifiable factors. Sun exposure, and iris and hair colour do not appear to be associated with AMD (Khan et al. 2006).

Poor vision can be a significant disadvantage during diabetes education and general living because most diabetic and general health information contains essential visual components.

Practice points

(1) The shape of the lens changes with changes in blood glucose concentrations, leading to refractive changes and blurred vision. This usually corrects as the blood glucose is normalised, but may take some time if the blood glucose has been high for a long time.

(2) Vision can worsen in the short term when blood glucose control begins to improve, for example, when commencing insulin and during pregnancy.

(3) The temporary vision disturbance creates significant stress for the person with diabetes and a careful explanation is needed.

Table 8.2   Risk factors for age-related macular degeneration based on Lim (2006).

Modifiable factors	Nonmodifiable factors
Cigarette smoking; the risk increases with long duration of smoking	Increasing age: for both exudative and nonexudative AMD
Diet high in fats especially monounsaturated and polyunsaturated fats. Linoleic acid increases the risk for advanced AMD.	Ethnicity. AMD is more prevalent in Whites. Especially for the components of late AMD, increased retinal pigmentation and retinal pigment epithelial depigmentation. Cataracts and glaucoma are more common in Blacks.
Omega-3 fatty acids are associated with lower risk High GI food is related to the development of retinal pigmentation abnormalities (Chui et al. 2006). Emerging research suggests a diet rich in fruit and vegetables, especially carotenoids, may help prevent AMD. Vitamins C and E and zinc (van Leeuwen et al. 2005)	
High BMI. The risk of developing AMD increases with increasing BMI, and geographic atrophy could be associated with high BMI, low education, and antacid use (Clemons et al. 2005).	Genetic inheritance
Hypertension is associated with exudative AMD but not non-exudative AMD.	
Hypercholesteraemia is also associated with exudative AMD.	
Inflammation. Recent studies suggest C-reactive protein is associated with intermediate and advanced AMD (Seddon et al. 2004).	

AMD: age-related macular degeneration; GI: glycaemic index; BMI: body mass index.

Eye problems associated with diabetes

(1) One-third of people with diabetes have retinopathy as a result of microvascular disease. The incidence is related to the duration of diabetes. Sixty percent of people with diabetes and duration of more than 15 years have some degree of retinopathy, especially women. Up to 30% people with type 2 diabetes have retinopathy at diagnosis (4–8% is sight-threatening). There is increasing evidence that ACE inhibitors can reduce the risk of microvascular disease (see Chapter 5).

(2) People can have severe eye damage without being aware of it. Vision is not always affected and there is usually no pain or discomfort.

(3) Cataracts are more common in people with diabetes.

(4) Maculopathy is the most common cause of visual loss in people with diabetes.

(5) Sudden loss of vision is normally an emergency. It may be due to:
  - vitreous haemorrhage;
  - retinal detachment;
  - retinal artery occlusion.

Reassurance, avoidance of stress and sudden movement, and urgent ophthalmological assessment are required.

(6) Prevention and early detection are important aspects in the management of visual impairment. It involves:
  - Good blood glucose control can slow the rate of progression in type 1 diabetes (DCCT 1993).
  - Regular eye examinations commencing at diagnosis in type 2 and from age 12 in type 1. Screening should be undertaken annually if retinopathy is present of every two years it there is no retinopathy (SIGN 2010). Screening consists of comprehensive eye examinations, which should be undertaken at diagnosis in people with type 2 diabetes and within

5 years of onset in type 1 (ADA 2019). Then every 1–2 years if there is no sign of retinopathy and more frequently if changes are noted. Ideally, eye examinations should be undertaken during prepregnancy planning or in the first trimester in women with preexisting diabetes.

- Using an ophthalmoscope opportunistically during regular appointments.
- Seven-field stereoscopic photography with the pupils dilated to investigate macula oedema and proliferative retiopathy.
- Retinal photography or slit lamp biomicroscopy.
- Confocal microscopy is increasingly being applied to diabetes complication screening, especially to detect eye changes and neuropathy. Confocal microscopy enables greater contrast to be achieved and three-dimensional images to be created that show great detail. The technique uses a spatial pinhole to eliminate out of focus light and flare. It enables faster diagnosis, is noninvasive and painless.
- Telemedicine using valid retinal photography have improved access and outcomes for people in rural areas.
- Artificial intelligence image processing algorithm that can detect fluid on the retina with and accuracy of 98% (Kumar et al. 2019; Khojasteh 2019). The technique relies on retinal images generated with usual optometry equipment or taken with fundus cameras. The clinical use has not yet been tested.
- Fluorescein angiography is still sometimes used.

(7) Coagulation or laser treatment is very effective in preventing further visual loss in people with high-risk proliferative retinopathy. Vitrectomy may be indicated if there is evidence of persistent vitreous haemorrhage. Cataract extraction should not be delayed when indicated. Advanced cataracts need to be removed or stabilised prior to surgery and reviewed closely in the postoperative period (SIGN 2010).

(8) Intravitreous injections of antivascular endothelial growth factor (VEG-F) may be indicated to manage macular oedema beneath the fovea.

(9) Medicines include intravitreal Triamcinolone, which reduces retinal thickness in the short term and improves visual acuity but may not have long-term benefits. Small studies suggest Simvaststin reduces oedema and improves visual acuity (Sen et al. 2002) and Atorvastation reduces the severity of hard exudates after laser treatment in people with type 2 diabetes and high lipids (Gupta et al. 2004). Generally, aspirin for cardiovascular protection can be continued in people with retinopathy and does not increase the risk of retinal haemorrhage (ADA 2019).

Clinical observation

Eye drops occasionally cause pain and increased pressure in the eye some hours after they were instilled. If this occurs the patient should be advised to call the doctor.

Resources for people with visual impairment

People with significant visual loss often require assistance to perform blood glucose monitoring and to administer their own insulin. It is important to encourage independence as far as possible. Careful assessment is important and should include assessment of the home situation.

Vision Australia and the Royal National Institute for the Blind in the UK and similar organisations in other countries offer a variety of services for people who have degrees of visual loss. These services include:

- Assessing the home situation to determine whether modifications are necessary to ensure safety at home.
- Low-vision clinics.
- Talking library and books in Braille.

- Training on how to cope in the community with deteriorating vision.
- Assistance dogs. It takes time to train a dog to guide a blind person and time for a person to learn to work with a guide dog, usually through a harness, and for the person to recognise tactile and sound clues to complement their knowledge of the environment. Several factors can affect the individual's ability to work with a guide dog, including loss of sensitivity in hands or feet and hypoglycaemia, which affects concentration and sometimes behaviour (Stanway 2012). Interestingly, dogs can perform more than one kind of medical assistance and actually enjoy the extra work (medical detection dogs). For example, they can be trained to become familiar with chemical markers associated with diabetes and can detect hypoglycaemia and fetch the person's hypo kit or alert another person. A recent report in the author's local newspaper described how a blue heeler dog, which was deaf, was learning to recognise sign language.

Other help includes:

- Services such as pensions, which may be available from the government.
- A range of diabetes products are available that can help vision impaired people remain independent (see next section).

The community nurses and home-based services play a major role in maintaining vision-impaired people in their own homes, especially when they are older.

Aids for people with low vision

Various magnifying devices are available to help people continue to care for themselves. They can be obtained from diabetes associations and some pharmacies specialising in diabetes products. Other aids include:

(1) Insulin administration:
   - Instaject devices, clicking insulin pens.
   - Chest magnifying glass (available from some opticians); Magniguide fits both 50 and 100 unit syringes and enlarges the markings.
   - Location tray for drawing up insulin if syringes are used.
(2) Blood glucose monitoring:
   - Strip guides for accurate placement of the blood on to the strips.
   - Talking blood glucose meters, blood pressure monitors, and talking weight scales.
   - Meters with large result display areas.
(3) Medications:
   - Dosette boxes, which can be prefilled with the correct medicines;

Care of people who have vision impairments

Aims of Care
- To encourage independence as far as possible.
- To ensure the environment is safe when the patient is mobile.

People Confined to Bed
(1) Introduce yourself and address the patient by name, so the patient is aware that you are talking to them.
(2) Ascertain how much the patient is able to see (few people are totally blind). Assess whether the blood glucose fluctuates at certain times. High and low levels can interfere with clear vision. Plan education to avoid these times and determine measures that can avoid such fluctuations, for example, appropriate timing of meals and medications. Dexterity and cognitive function may also be impaired especially in the elderly and hamper diabetes education. Visual impairment increases the risk of falls in elderly patients (see Chapter 12).

(3) Some people prefer a corner bed because it makes location easier, avoids confusion with equipment belonging to other patients and enables greater ease in setting up personal belongings.

(4) Introduce the patient to other people in their ward or close by.

(5) If you move the patient's belongings, they must be returned to the same place.

(6) Explain all procedures carefully and fully before commencing. An injection when you can't see it and don't expect it can be very unnerving.

(7) If eye bandages are required, make sure the ears and other sensory organs are not covered as well.

(8) Consider extra adjustable lighting for those patients with useful residual vision.

(9) Mark the person's medication with large print labels or use a dosette.

(10) A radio, talking clock, talking watch, Braille watch, or a large figured watch, helps the patient keep orientated to time and place.

(11) Indicate when you are leaving the room and concluding a conversation.

People Who Are Mobile

(1) A central point like the person's bed helps them orient around the room.

(2) When orientating a person to a new area, walk with them until they become familiar with the route.

(3) Keep obstacles (trolleys, etc.) clear of pathways where possible.

Meals

(1) Describe the menu and let the person make a choice.

(2) Ensure the person knows that the meal has been delivered.

(3) Ask, 'Do you need assistance with your meal?' rather than say, 'I will cut your meat for you'.

(4) Colour contrast is important for some patients. A white plate on a red tray-cloth may assist with location of place setting.

When the person has a guide dog, provide water in hot weather bur remember the dog is doing a job. Ask the owner's permission before patting the dog or offering treats, which can distract the dog and confuse it.

Diabetes and renal disease

Key points

- Obesity is a strong predictor of renal disease, renal calculi, and cancer (Kovesdy et al. 2017).
- Diabetes is the most common cause of renal disease. Regular screening, usually at least annually, is important in all people with type 2 diabetes and those with type 1 diabetes <5 years duration. Screening includes spot urine-to-creatinine ratio (ACR) and estimated GFR (eGFR).
- Measuring microalbuminuria is a useful method of detecting abnormal renal function. Microalbuminuria indicates early renal disease and predicts cardiovascular disease in people with diabetes.
- Microalbuminuria predicts severe hypoglycaemia in people with type 2 diabetes.
- Hypertension is an early indicator of renal disease.
- There is a strong association between retinopathy and renal disease in people with type 1 diabetes. Women with diabetes have greater prevalence of advanced kidney disease than men with diabetes, especially among older people.
- People with diabetes and nephropathy are at increased risk of cardiovascular disease.
- Older people with diabetes and CKD require careful monitoring and management.

Introduction

Diabetic nephropathy is a significant microvascular complication of diabetes, and diabetes is the second most common cause of end-stage renal disease globally. There is a similar initial disease progression in both type 1 and type 2 diabetes. Eventually, microalbuminuria occurs in up to 20% of people with type 1 diabetes and in a similar percentage of people with type 2. Some cultural groups are at significant risk – for example, Aboriginal and Torres Strait Islander Peoples and Afro-Caribbean people.

Obesity prevalence is increasing worldwide. Visceral fat associated with increased BMI and waist hip ratio (WHR) increase the risk of cardiovascular disease. There is an association between obesity and poor renal outcomes, even when possible modulators of cardiac and the metabolic effects of obesity are considered (Scales et al. 2012). WHR more useful than BMI to classify obesity in people with chronic renal disease (> 102 cm 0.9 cm in males and >88 cm and 0.8 cm in females) (Scales et al. 2012).

Treatment of CKD-related obesity is unclear. Treatment may involve managing energy intake, which with activity reduces risk of CKD by 30% (Look Ahead Study Group 2013). Medicines may be required to manage glycaemia, hypertension, and dyslipidaemia. It is clear that it is important to detect and treat CKD early.

Interestingly, obesity, especially subcutaneous fat is associated with lower mortality and better outcomes in people with significant kidney disease (Kalantar-Zadeh et al. 2006) as well as those with frailty and cerebrovascular disease.

Stages of chronic kidney disease

Kidney disease is progressive unless it can be prevented and is usually classified as shown in Table 8.3 (Kidney Health 2019).

Proteinuria must be present to diagnose stages 1 and 2. People on dialysis are classified as stage 5D and people with a functioning renal transplant are denoted by the suffix 'T.'

Proteinuria is an important marker for cardiovascular disease in type 2 diabetes.

Prediction equations that improve the inverse correlation between serum creatinine and GFR have been developed and take account of variables that affect the relationship, but they were not specifically developed in older adults (Clemmens et al. 2019), for example:

- Kidney filtration and secretion (GFR) is a measure of functioning neurons.
- Cockcroft-Gault equation, which estimates creatinine clearance, which encompasses age, gender, weight, and creatinine. Creatinine production depends on muscle mass: production of creatinine in older people can be variable and the results can be misleading (concealed renal failure). People with nephrotic syndrome can also have variable creatinine secretion.
- Four variable formula used in the modification of diet in renal disease (MDRD) study, which encompasses age, gender and ethnicity.
- Chronic Kidney Disease Epidemiology Collaboration equation (CKD-EPI).

Table 8.3   Stages of kidney disease

Stage	GFR ml/min/1.73 m²
(1) Kidney damage with normal glomerular filtration rate (GFR)	> 90
(2) Kidney damage with mild reduction in GFR	60–89
(3) Moderately reduced GFR:	
(a) 3A	45–59
(b) 3B	30–44
(4) Severe reduced GFR	15–29
(5) End-stage renal failure	< 15

- Berlin Initiative Study 2 equation is a new eGFR equation that uses cystatin C and creatinine and appears to be more reliable, but requires further study (Clemens et al. 2019).

All equations appear to provide similar estimates when the eGFR is <30 ml/min/1.73m^2, the cut point for deciding medicine doses. In cases where highly toxic medicines are indicated and kidney function needs to be accurately quantified nuclear GFR or 24 hour using creatinine measurement (National Kidney Foundation 2018). However, collecting 24-hour urine is likely fraught, especially in older people with cognitive changes and those with urinary incontinence.

New research suggests that Galectin-3 could be a prognostic biomarker of diabetic nephropathy in people with type 2 diabetes (Hodeib et al. 2019). Galectin-3 is a glycoprotein in the lectin family found in the intra- and extracellular spaces that is involved in cell adhesion, cell growth, and deferentiation, apoptosis, and angiogenesis. It is involved in the development and progression of many pathophysiological responses including inflammatory process. Its role in kidney disease is unclear, but it contributes to renal fibrosis (Hodeib et al. 2019).

Risk factors for renal disease

There is a strong link between hypertension and the progression of renal disease. The risk of end-stage renal failure increases as the diastolic blood pressure increases to >90–120 mmHg. Other risk factors include:

- Smoking, which represents a significant and dose-dependent risk.
- Hyperglycaemia, predialysis control is an independent predictor of the outcome in people with type 2 diabetes on haemodialysis (Wu et al. 1997). The Diabetes Control and Complications Trial (DCCT) demonstrated that good control of blood glucose delayed the rate and progression of microvascular disease including renal disease (DCCT 1993).
- The presence of microalbuminuria and proteinuria are independent risk factors for the development and progression of renal disease in people with diabetes (Keane 2001). People with diabetes are at risk of renal disease if they have any of the following. The more of these factors present the greater the risk:
  - A urine albumin excretion rate in the upper range of normal (20–30 mg/day).
  - Systolic blood pressure >130 mmHg.
  - HbA$_{1c}$ >9%. Preventing and managing hyperglycaemia reduces the development of renal disease.
  - Total cholesterol >5.2 mmol/l. Duration of diabetes exceeding five years (Kerr 2008). Treatment includes minimising proteinuria using ACEIs and ARBs, often in combination. Hyperkalaemia is a risk when ACEI and ARBs are combined but may not be significant.
  - Tests for microalbuminuria include timed urine collections (12- or 24-hour collections) usually on an outpatient basis, but compliance is poor. The spot albumin–creatinine urine test, which corrects the albumin level for the urine concentration, is the optimal screening test for early renal disease. A level > 3.5 mg/mmol most likely indicates early renal disease (Kerr 2008). However, alternative causes of proteinuria such as nephrosclerosis and hypertensive renal disease should be considered: The eGFR, which approximates the GFR rate and is based primarily on serum creatinine as well as age and gender, gives a reasonable approximation of the GFR (Kerr 2008). However, renal function declines with age by approximately one ml/min/year after age 25. Thus, approximately 60% of people over age 65 will have an eGR in the normal range (60–90 ml/min).
  - Hypertension is a risk factor for cardiovascular disease and kidney disease, and the risk is continuous and independent of other cardiovascular risk factors (Committee on the Prevention, Detection, Evaluation, and Treatment of High Blood Pressure: Chobanian et al. 2003). Most people with advanced renal disease develop hypertension. If not controlled, hypertension can accelerate the rate of decline in renal function. If the cycle from hypertension to renal impairment can be halted, fewer people would require dialysis (Nurko 2006). Thus, good blood pressure control is important and is the single-most effective measure to

slow the progression of renal disease. The Australian and New Zealand Society of Nephrology and Diabetes recommends that everybody with diabetes and microalbuminuria or nephropathy be treated with an ACE-inhibitor and recommend a general target 140/90; of 130/90 in people over 50 years; and 120/70–75 in people younger than 50 years (ADA 2019). The guidelines also advise that multiple antihypertensive agents might be needed.

- Presence of retinopathy (Gilbert et al. 1998).
- Long duration of diabetes.
- Male gender, although a recent study suggests women are more at risk of diabetes-related renal disease than men with diabetes, especially in the older age group (Yu et al. 2012).
- Increasing age.

People with type 2 diabetes often have microalbuminuria at diagnosis, which is consistent with the fact that impaired glucose tolerance or diabetes is often present for many years before it is diagnosed. Thus, screening should begin at diagnosis in type 2 diabetes. Microalbuminuria is rarely present in type 1 diabetes at diagnosis so screening usually begins at about five years' duration of diabetes. However, people with LADA may present differently and screening might need to be commenced earlier in these patients.

Practice points

(1) False-positive results can occur after heavy exercise or if the person has an UTI.
(2) Women with diabetes may develop proteinuria during pregnancy and the cause should be investigated to ensure the protein is not an early sign or preeclampsia especially if they also present with hypertension.
(3) If a person develops heavy proteinuria in a short period of time other cause should be investigated.
(4) Serum creatinine alone is a poor indicator of renal status in older people. Underweight and overweight are risk factors for misclassifying the degree of renal dysfunction (Giannelli et al. 2007).
(5) Some GLMs have benefits as well as glucose lowering. These include some SGLT-2 inhibitors reduce glucose renal glucose reabsorption, weight, and blood pressure, which have positive effects for renal disease. Some GLP-1 receptor agonists have direct effects on the kidney; see Chapter 5.

Renal failure

Early referral to a nephrologist is imperative to improve the long-term outcomes especially when dialysis or transplantation may be needed, e.g. when the eGFR is 60 ml/min/1.73 m^2. However, collaboration with diabetes and other relevant experts must still occur. Late referral is associated with higher morbidity and mortality rates in people on dialysis even when they survive the first year on dialysis (Cass et al. 2002; ADA 2019). Nephrologists can advise about managing issues associated with renal failures:

- Recognize calcium and phosphate abnormalities.
- Calcific medial stenosis contributes to cardiovascular disease. Phosphate binders might be prescribed to manage the problem if the phosphate is >1.6 mmol/l.
- Anaemia might include erythropoietin as well as iron and vitamin B$_{12}$.
- Prepare the person for dialysis.

Renal failure, often requiring dialysis, occurs in 25% of people diagnosed with diabetes before the age of 30. The presence of mild renal disease increases the risk of cardiovascular disease even with only small elevations of urinary protein, but the relationship is not clear. The presence of other cardiovascular risk factors increases the risk, and endothelial cell dysfunction may play a part. ACE inhibitors have been shown to delay or stabilise the rate of progression of renal disease and to decrease cardiac events (Keane 2001; Kerr 2008).

The development of renal problems is insidious, and frank proteinuria may not be present for 7–10 years after the onset of renal disease. Microalbuminuria, on the other hand, is detectable up to 5–10 years before protein is found in the urine. Regular urine collections to screen for micro-albuminuria are still used in some places controlling blood glucose and blood pressure, the use of ACE inhibitors (type 1) and angiotensin receptor blockers (type 2) and avoiding nephrotoxic agents can attenuate renal and cardiac disease (Gilbert and Kelly 2001).

ACE inhibitors have been shown to be more effective than other antihypertensive agents in reducing the time-related increase in urinary albumin excretion and plasma creatinine in type 2 diabetes and in people with other cardiovascular risk factors, heart failure, and myocardial infarction (Ravid et al. 1993). Likewise, the HOPE and MICRO-HOPE studies demonstrated that ACE inhibitors reduced cardiovascular events and overt nephropathy whether or not micro-albuminuria was present (HOPE 2000). An ARB can be used in people with type 1 diabetes do not tolerate ACE and people with type 2 should be treated with ACE and/or ARB (SIGN 2010). However, ACE and ARBs are more effective in Caucasians than in black people of African descent, and the benefits need to be assessed in these people.

Great care should be taken if IV contrast media are required for diagnostic purposes; see Chapter 9. Contrast-induced nephropathy (CIN) is defined as renal dysfunction following any investigative procedure where radi-opaque contrast media were used (Rudnick et al. 2006). Most episodes of CIN do not cause oliguria but result in a rise in serum creatinine ~2 days after the procedure, which usually returns to pre-procedure levels within a week. CIN occurs in 7–15% of patients and up to 50% in high-risk groups such as people with diabetes, with a mortality rate of 14% (Rudnick et al. 2006).

Risk factors for CIN are:

- Preexisting renal disease
- Increasing age
- Congestive heart failure
- Hypotension
- Using large volumes of contrast media
- The type of contrast media used
- Presence of anaemia
- Diabetes

In addition to diabetes per se, people with diabetes are likely to have greater than two other risk factors for CIN, which puts them in a very-high-risk group. A rise in serum creatinine by 25% is an indicator of CIN but the inaccuracy of creatinine in various states has been outlined. Therefore, eGFR may be a better marker.

The Australian Adverse Drug Reactions Bulletin (2008) issued a warning about using gadolinium-containing contrast agents in people with renal impairment because of the risk of nephrogenic systemic fibrosis (NSF). The incidence of NSF may vary between the different gadolinium agents available. Renal function should be assessed in all patients before using gadolinium, especially if they are in a high-risk category and the risks and benefits of using gadolinium carefully considered.

Using as low a volume of contrast media as possible and ensuring the person is well hydrated are important preventative measures (Meschi et al. 2006). However, recent research suggests that IV sodium bicarbonate administered seven hours before procedures involving radio contrast media reduces the incidence of CIN from 15% to 2% (Briguori 2007). Research is currently underway to determine whether oral sodium bicarbonate will be effective.

Renal function can decline in critically ill patients especially people with diabetes and is associated with high morbidity and mortality (Schetz et al. 2008). For example, hyperglycaemia and insulin resistance are common in critically ill patients with and without diabetes. Associations between interoperative hyperglycaemia during cardiac surgery, cardiac catherisation, total parenteral nutrition, and acute kidney injury have been noted. Intensive insulin therapy in these settings is renoprotective. The incidence of oliguria, and the need for renal replacement therapies (dialysis), is reduced (Schetz et al. 2008). The authors suggested that insulin improves the lipid profile and reduces nitric oxide levels and oxidative damage, as well as controlling hyperglycaemia.

Over 50% of patients on GLMs with significant renal disease require insulin therapy. Insulin requirements often reduce in people already on insulin because insulin, like many other medicines, is degraded and excreted by the kidney. Kidney damage can delay degradation and excretion of many medicines and prolong their half-life, increasing the risk of unwanted side effects and medicine interactions. The medicine/s dose, or dose interval may need to be altered.

The American Society of Nephrology (2012) released new recommendations to avoid unnecessary testing and reduce costs as part of the 'Choosing Wisely' campaign. The recommendations are not specific for diabetes, and they stress the need for close collaboration between the patient and their doctors and the following key recommendations:

- Avoid cancer screening in people receiving dialysis who have limited life expectancy unless they have signs and symptoms of cancer.
- Do not administer erthropoiesis-stimulating medicines if the person had haemoglobin >10 g/dl unless they have symptoms of anaemia.
- Avoid nonsteroidal anti-inflammatory agents in people with hypertension, heart failure, or chronic kidney disease from all causes including diabetes.
- Avoid placing peripherally inserted central catheters in people with stages 3–5 renal disease without consulting a nephrologist.
- Avoid initiating chronic dialysis without discussing all the issues with the person concerned and their carers and other health professionals.

Renal disease and anaemia

Anaemia occurs as a consequence of chronic renal insufficiency. Renal anaemia occurs earlier in people with diabetes than in people without diabetes. It is more severe and is associated with other factors such as erythrocyte abnormalities and increased osmotic stress that are associated with decreased erythropoietin production (Bosman et al. 2001; Ritz 2001). As renal function declines the anaemia becomes more marked. Anaemia is associated with fatigue, decreased quality of life, depression, left ventricular hypertrophy, decreased exercise capacity, malaise, and malnutrition. Annual testing is recommended on people with renal disease stages 3–5. Anaemia is treated with recombinant human erythropoietin (rhEPO) in conjunction with intravenous iron.

Clinical observation

To date there has been little, if any, focus on monitoring haemoglobin (Hb) as part of routine biochemical monitoring or diabetes complication screening in patients with renal impairment. Dunning et al. (2012) demonstrated Hb can be determined in point of care testing at the same time as blood glucose tests are performed, provided staff are trained to use the equipment.

Diet and renal disease

Improving nutritional status can delay end-stage renal failure (Chan 2001, 2008). Nutritional needs are individual and depend on the stage and type of renal disease. The aim is to maintain homeostasis and electrolyte balance, decrease uraemic symptoms, and regularly reassess dietary requirements to ensure changing needs are addressed (National Kidney Foundation 2002).

The nutritional goals for people with renal disease need to be individualised and assessed regularly to ensure they are appropriate for the degree of renal damage and maintain health and wellbeing. The goals focus on the following:

- Maintaining a desirable body weight, body composition, and nutritional status and prevent protein loss (protein energy wasting). Control accumulation of uraemic toxins.
- Control uraemic symptoms and its consequences such as nausea.
- Manage blood glucose and lipids.
- Maintain fluid and electrolyte balance, which may involve fluid restriction.
- Manage comorbidities such as blood glucose, reducing salt intake or omitting salt (hypertension), maintaining calcium, phosphate, and vitamin D balance (bone disease and hyperparathyroidism, calcific medial arteriosclerosis), reducing lipids (cardiovascular disease), maintaining iron, folate, and vitamin B12 (anaemia).
- Improve graft survival if the person receives a transplant.

Specific goals apply to the stages of CK:

- Stages 1–4, the predialysis stages. The aim is to slow the progression of renal disease and preserve remaining renal function.
- Stage 5, end-stage renal disease. Conservative management; control symptoms and provide nutritional support.
- Stage 5 on dialysis. Replace dialysis nutrient losses, which include protein and water-soluble vitamins.
- Stage 5, transplant. Manage side effects of immunosuppressant medicines, manage. Monitor dietary needs (Chan 2012).

Conversations about management options, preparing for end-of-life care and preparing advanced care directive may be appropriate in any of these stages but especially stage 5.
    The diet generally comprises:

- Carbohydrates should contribute 50–60% of the total daily energy. When protein requirements change in advanced renal disease, extra carbohydrates are sometimes needed.
- People who do not require dialysis should have the recommended daily allowance of protein: 0.8 g/Kg body weight/day people on dialysis may require more protein than the recommended daily allowance (ADA 2019).
- Fat intake should be about 30% of daily total energy and where possible should come from unsaturated fat, but the proportion may increase in advanced kidney disease. Mono- and poly-unsaturated fats are preferred. People on dialysis and those who have a renal transplant require a low-fat diet.
- Vitamin and mineral supplements may be required, especially when dialysis commences, for example iron, and water-soluble vitamins (e.g., B_{12} and C as well as vitamin D).

Protein and energy malnutrition are common and need to be corrected to prevent catabolism, lipid metabolism, and anaemia. Sodium restriction is often recommended, but salt substitutes should not be used because they are usually high in potassium and can increase the serum potassium, usually already elevated in renal disease.
    Anorexia is often a feature of renal disease, and food smells can further reduce appetite and predispose the patient to malnutrition. Small frequent meals may be more appealing. Malnutrition has implications for the individual's immune status and phagocyte function and increases the risk of infection (Churchill 1996). Referral to a dietitian is essential.
    Malnutrition is prevalent in people on haemodialysis and has a high mortality rate (Lopes et al. 2007). Lack of appetite is a significant predictor of malnutrition and is related to inflammation and may link protein-energy malnutrition in these patients. However, appetite varies and is often lower on haemodialysis days. This predisposes the person to hypoglycaemia in the short

term and malnutrition in the long term. Lopes et al. (2007) suggested asking people with diabetes on haemodialysis about their appetite in the past four weeks or asking them to keep a food and appetite diary for three to four days is helpful. The Kidney Disease Quality of Life-Short Form (KDQOL-SF) (Hays et al. 1994) includes questions about appetite.

Depression, the presence of several coexisting comorbidites, cachexia, using oral medicines, being older, and women on haemodialysis are particularly at risk of malnutrition. As anorexia increases markers of malnutrition decreases (serum albumin, creatinine, nPCR, and BMI) (Lopes et al. 2007) (see also Chapters 4 and 12).

Renal disease and older people

Older people with renal disease are at increased risk unrecognised renal disease due to changed creatinine production (Clemens et al. 2019) and of adverse medicine events due to changed medicine excretion through the kidney, e.g. sulphonylurea-related hypoglycaemia. A wide range of medicines are used in older people and some may need dose adjustments especially digoxin, ACE inhibitors, narcotics, antimicrobials, and GLMs (Howes 2001). Long-acting agents are contraindicated because of the risk of hypoglycaemia (see Chapters 5 and 6). Medicine therapy needs to be closely monitored, along with monitoring renal function and nutritional status and nonmedicine alternatives used where possible.

Practice points

(1) Lower rates of creatinine are produced by older people, and creatinine clearance rates can be misleading, especially in people with low muscle mass due to sarcopenia and frailty or other causes of malnutrition.
(2) Renal disease is an important cause of medicine toxicity in older people, often necessitating a hospital admission.

Kidney biopsy

Extra care is required for people with renal disease undergoing renal biopsy; see Chapter 9. A pressure dressing should be applied to the site and the patient should lie supine after the procedure for six hours. The blood pressure should be monitored and fluids are encouraged to maintain urine output unless fluid is restricted. Activity should be reduced for two weeks.

Renal dialysis

Dialysis can be used in the management of diabetic kidney disease. Dialysis is a filtering process that removes excess fluid and accumulated waste products from the blood. It may be required on a temporary basis or for extended periods of time. Some patients may eventually receive a kidney transplant. Several forms of dialysis are in use.

Haemodialysis

Blood is pumped through an artificial membrane and then returned to the circulation. Good venous access is required and special training in management. Haemodialysis is usually administered three times per week. A recent Canadian study suggests frequent nocturnal haemodialysis (six times per week) is associated with improved left ventricular mass, fewer antihypertensive agents, improved mineral metabolism and improvements in some aspects of quality of life (Culleton 2007).

Hypotension is common when haemodialysis therapy is first commenced. Management consists of:

- An appropriate haemodialysis prescription.
- Minimising interdialytic fluid gains by setting limits on fluid intake.
- Elevating the foot of the bed.
- Differentiating between disequilibrium syndrome and hypoglycaemia.
- Advising the patient to sit on the edge of the bed or chair to allow the blood pressure to stabilise before standing (Terrill 2002).
- Maintaining good glycaemic control. Significantly, >50% of people with diabetes on haemodialysis have HbA1c > 7%, especially those with long duration of diabetes, microvascular disease and on insulin (Iliescu 2006). These findings probably reflect advanced diabetes and may not be due to haemodialysis. However, given the amount of glucose in dialysate, it is imperative that HbA1c be as close to normal as possible without causing excess hypoglycaemia to reduce the risk of infection and other complications. Iliescu (2006) suggested it may not be possible to achieve good control with medicines and suggested insulin pumps might be a useful strategy. Significantly, poor glycaemic control is linked to lower survival rates in patients on haemodialysis (Oomichi et al. 2007).

Strict aseptic technique and careful patient education are essential when managing dialysis therapies. Patients with CKD are susceptible to infections due to abnormal immune function, which is likely to be worse in people with diabetes and hyperglycaemia where neurophil function is abnormal and malignancies (Choudhury and Luna-Salazar 2008). Mucocutaneous barriers are often disrupted secondary to skin excoriation from pruritis, xerosi, and sweat gland atrophy. Common bacterial infections include *Staphylococcus species, Escherichia coli, Klebsiella,* and *Mycobacterium tuberculosis.* Viral infections are also common. Strict aseptic technique and careful patient education are essential when managing dialysis therapies.

Peritoneal dialysis

The filtering occurs across the peritoneum. This form of dialysis is an excellent method of treating kidney failure, in people with and without diabetes. The uraemia, hypertension, and blood glucose can be well controlled without increasing the risk of infection, if aseptic techniques are adhered to. However, infection is a significant risk and is often the reason people change to haemodialysis.

Continuous ambulatory peritoneal dialysis (CAPD)

CAPD is a form of peritoneal dialysis in which dialysate is continually present in the abdominal cavity. The fluid is drained and replaced four to five times each day or overnight if the patient is on automated peritoneal dialysis (APD). The person can be managed at home, which has psychological advantages once the care of equipment is understood and the person is metabolically stable. CAPD can also be used postoperatively to control uraemia related to acute tubular necrosis or early transplant rejection.

Insulin added to the dialysate bags achieves smoother blood glucose control because the insulin is delivered directly into the portal circulation and is absorbed in the dwell phase, which is closer to the way insulin is normally secreted after a glucose load. However, it also has disadvantages and is an infection risk and is not always recommended.

The usual insulin dose may need to be increased because of glucose absorption from the dialysate fluid (and to account for insulin binding to the plastic of the dialysate bags and tubing if it is added to the dialysate bag). The continuous supply of glucose and lactate in the dialysate fluid are calorie-rich energy sources and can lead to weight gain and hyperglycaemia. The art is to calculate insulin requirements to avoid hyperinsulinaemia, which carries its own complication risks. Glucose-free solutions such as Nutrimeal and glucose polymers may help reduce complications associated with high insulin and glucose levels (Rutecki and Whittier 1993). Insulin is usually administered subcutaneously if the person is on APD. Many renal dialysis units do not advocate adding insulin to dialysate bags due to the increased risk of infection.

Priorities of dialysis treatment

(1) Remove waste products and excess fluids from the blood (urea and creatinine).
(2) Provide adequate nutrition and safe serum electrolytes, and to prevent acidosis.
(3) Provide patient comfort.
(4) Prevent complications of treatment.
(5) Provide information and support to the patient.
(6) Ensure privacy.

Objectives of care

The individual's ability to carry out self-care tasks needs to be assessed early when considering renal replacement therapies. Changed joint structure due to oedema and tissue glycosylation (e.g. carpel tunnel syndrome) can limit the fine motor skills required to manage CAPD. Visual impairment due to retinopathy frequently accompanies renal disease and if present, can limit self-care abilities.

(1) Assess the patient carefully in relation to:
  - Knowledge of diabetes
  - Preventative health-care practices
  - Ability to use aseptic technique
  - Usual diabetic control
  - Presence of other diabetic complications
  - Support available (family, relatives)
  - Mental health and wellbeing and motivation for self-care
  - Uraemic state
(2) Ensure thorough instruction about administration of dialysate and intraperitoneal medication (insulin).
(3) Ensure a regular meal pattern with appropriate carbohydrate in relation to dialysate fluid.
(4) Maintain skin integrity by ensuring technique is aseptic, especially in relation to catheter exit site and skin care.
(5) Monitor urea, creatinine, and electrolytes carefully.
(6) Provide psychological support.
(7) Encourage simple appropriate exercise.
(8) Ensure adequate dental care and regular dental assessments. Poor oral health causes chronic inflammation and is a site of infection. Untreated uraemia is associated with stomatitis, and patients on dialysis are prone to gingivitis and peridontitis. Prophylactic antibiotics for dental procedure may be advisable (Choudhury and Luna-Salazar 2008).
(9) Prevent pain and discomfort, especially associated with the weight of the dialysate.
(10) Ensure that the patient reports illness or high temperatures immediately.
(11) Monitor for infections and advise people to have preventative vaccines such as influenza and pneumococcal vaccination and an annual screen for tuberculosis. Regular screening for nasal *staphylococcal* infections and certain types of malignancy may also be indicated, for example, renal cell carcinoma, and prostate, breast, and cervical cancer.

Clinician responsibilities

(1) Follow the guidelines, policies, and procedures used in the care setting.
(2) Provide meticulous skin care.
(3) Inspect catheter exit site daily, report any redness, swelling, pain, or discharge.
(4) Monitor fluid balance carefully:
  - Measure all drainage.
  - Maintain progressive total of input and output.

- Report a positive balance of more than 1 l: the aim generally is to achieve a negative balance to maintain the dry weight.
(5) Monitor blood glucose.
(6) Monitor temperature, pulse, and respiration, and report abnormalities.
(7) Monitor nutritional status – intake and biochemistry results.
(8) Weigh daily to monitor fluid intake and nutritional status.
(9) Ensure patency of tubes and monitor colour of outflow. Report if:
  - Cloudy
  - Faecal contamination
  - Very little outflow (tube blocked)
(10) Report lethargy and malaise that can be due to uraemia or high blood glucose levels.
(11) Warm dialysate before the addition of prescribed drugs and before administration to decrease the possibility of abdominal cramps.
(12) Oral fluid intake may be restricted – provide mouth care and ice to suck.
(13) Assess self-care potential:
  - Blood glucose testing
  - Adding medication to bags
  - Aseptic technique
  - Psychological ability to cope
(14) Protect the kidney during routine tests and procedures by avoiding dehydration and infection (Chapter 9).

Commencing CAPD in people on insulin

A 24-hour blood glucose profile is often undertaken prior to commencing intraperitoneal insulin to assess the degree of glycaemia and calculate insulin requirements. The glucose profile should be carried out following catheter implantation, with the patient stabilised on a CAPD regimen. One method consists of these steps:

(1) Obtain venous access for drawing blood samples.
(2) Obtain hourly blood glucose levels for 24 hours.
(3) Send at each bag change:
  - 10 ml new dianeal fluid for glucose analysis
  - 10 ml drained dianeal fluid for glucose and insulin analysis to the appropriate laboratory

Here is one protocol for administering insulin to people with diabetes on CAPD based on four bag changes each day:

(1) Calculate usual daily requirement of insulin and double it.
(2) Divide this amount between the four bag changes.
(3) The overnight bag should contain half the daytime dose. Some centres only administer 10% of the total daily dose at night.

Example:

Usual total insulin units	= 60 units.
Multiply this amount by 2	= 120 units.
Divide 120 units by 4 exchanges	= 30 units.
3 daily exchanges	= 30 units/bag.
Overnight exchange	= 15 units/bag.

Adjustments for the dextrose concentration of the dialysate may be necessary. Intraperitoneal insulin requirements are usually one-third higher than the amount needed before CAPD.

Practice point

Many renal units no longer recommend adding insulin to dialysis bags because of the risk of infection.

Subcutaneous insulin via an insulin pump using a basal bolous regimen could be an effective way of administering insulin to people receiving dialysis providing absorption was affected and the individual has the knowledge and skills to manage the insulin pump.

Educating the patient about CAPD

The patient should be instructed to do the following:
 (1) Not have a shower or bath for the first five days after the catheter is inserted.
 (2) Always carefully wash hands prior to changing the bags.
 (3) Wear loose-fitting clothes over exit site.
 (4) Examine feet daily for signs of bruising, blisters, cuts, or swelling.
 (5) Wear gloves when gardening or using caustic cleaners.
 (6) Avoid hot water bottles and electric blankets because sensory neuropathy can diminish pain perception and result in burns.
 (7) Avoid constrictive stockings or wearing new shoes for a long period of time.
 (8) Wash cuts or scratches immediately with soap and water and apply a mild antiseptic (e.g. betadine ointment). Any wound that does not improve within 24–36 hours or shows signs of infection (redness, pain, tenderness) must be reported promptly.
 (9) Bag exchanges should be carried out four to six hours apart. The person may be on APD having overnight exchanges.
 (10) Only short-acting clear insulin must be used in bags.
 (11) Adjust insulin doses according to diet, activity, and blood glucose levels and at the physician's discretion.
 (12) Accurately monitor blood glucose 4-hourly. A blood glucose meter may be required.
 (13) Provide written information.

Immediate help should be sought if any of the following occur:

- Decreased appetite
- Bad breath/taste in mouth
- Muscle cramps
- Generalised itch
- Nausea and vomiting, especially in the morning
- Decreased urine output
- Signs of urinary infection such as burning or scalding

Palliative supportive care

Some people, especially older people, may require supportive care if they are not suitable for or choose not to have dialysis or a renal transplant. Palliative supportive care refers to care that aims to achieve comfort and quality of life consistent with the person's values and care goals (Moustakas et al. 2012; Dunning and Martin 2018). Palliative encompasses shared decision-making, promoting autonomy, optimal functioning within the person's capabilities, maintaining quality of life and comfort. End-of-life care should be part of shared decision-making when a person has end-stage renal disease and documented in an Advanced Care Plan (Chapter 17).

Renal disease and herbal medicine (see also chapter 18)

People with end-stage renal failure often try complementary therapies (CM) to alleviate the unpleasant symptoms of their disease. Some therapies, for example, aromatherapy to reduce stress and maintain skin condition, or counselling for depression, are beneficial and usually safe. Herbal medicines are popular with the general public (Duncan et al. 2007), but they may not be appropriate or safe for people with renal disease (Myhre 2000).

The kidneys play a key role in eliminating medicines and herbal products from the system. Some of these medicines and herbs can cause kidney damage that may be irreversible and put already compromised renal function at great risk. In addition, some herbal products, particularly those used in traditional Chinese medicine (TCM) are often contaminated with drugs, heavy metals, and other potentially nephrotoxic products (Ko 1998). Frequently, these contaminants are not recorded in the list of ingredients in the product. As well as the direct effect of the herbs on the kidney, the intended action of particular herbs can complicate conventional treatment.

One herb, *Taxus celebica*, used in TCM to treat diabetes, contains a potentially harmful flavonoid and has been associated with acute renal failure and other vascular and hepatic effects (Ernst 1998). Kidney damage can be present with few specific overt renal symptoms; therefore, it is vital that kidney and liver function is closely monitored in people taking herbs, especially if kidney function is already compromised by diabetes.

Potentially adverse renal effects include:

- Electrolyte imbalances, for example, *Aloe barbedensis*
- Fluid imbalances, for example, *liquorice root*
- Hypokalaemia, for example, *Aloe, Senna*
- Kidney damage, for example, *Aristolochia*

Herbal and conventional medicine interactions may occur; see Chapter 17. However, a recent small study suggested the long chain omega-3 polyunsaturated fatty acids eicosapentaenoic acid (EPA) and docosahexaenoic acid (DHA) in early renal disease (ACR < 30 µ/mg) and those with microalbuminuria (ACR > 30 µ/mg) can slow progress of early-stage albuminuria (Aroda and Getaneh 2019). The clinical implications of the findings are not yet clear.

Practice points

(1) Nurses must know when their renal patients are taking herbal medicines so that their kidney function can be closely monitored. People should be asked about the use of CM periodically.

(2) Conventional medicines can also cause significant renal damage, and dose adjustments may be needed or alternative medicines used, for example, NSAID, statins, OHA.

Peripheral and autonomic neuropathy

Key points

- Lower-limb problems represent a significant physical, psychological, social, and economic burden for people with diabetes and the health system.
- Up to 50% of people with peripheral neuropathy may not have symptoms, which puts them at significant risk of significant adverse events.
- All people with diabetes should be assessed for peripheral neuropathy at diagnosis for those with type 2 and within five years of diagnosis for those with type 1 diabetes.
- Lower-limb amputations are a concern; 40–70% of amputations occur in people with diabetes.

- Peripheral neuropathy, vascular disease, infection, foot deformity, and inappropriate footwear predispose people to foot disease.
- Screening for foot disease and preventative self-care practices is essential.
- Foot complications are common in older people.
- A multidisciplinary team approach and good communication are essential to optimal management.
- Many subgroups of neuropathy occur, including mononeuropathy, peripheral, and autonomic neuropathy. The two most common forms are discussed in this chapter: peripheral and autonomic neuropathy.

Introduction

Peripheral neuropathy is present in >20% of people with type 1 diabetes after 20 years duration of diabetes and is already present at diagnosis in 10% of people with type 2 at diagnosis and 50% by 20 years duration of diabetes. Peripheral neuropathy leads to inability to sense pressure and pain in the feet, dry skin, reduced joint mobility, bony deformity, and problems with balance, which increases the risk of falling. Common foot deformities associated with diabetes are claw toes, hammer toes, *hallus valgus, haalus rigidus* callus, flattened or high foot arches, Charcot's feet, and amputation sites. These changes mean the normal cushioning that protects the feet during usual activities are deficient and the foot is at high risk of injury.

Foot ulcers occur in ~25% of people with diabetes: ~25% develop an infection, 20–60% of ulcers involve bone (osteomyelitis), and 34% present with a recurrent ulcer/year. Careful assessment, consideration of the causative factors, and managing the existing problems can limit further exacerbation of diabetic foot disease. Appropriate care can prevent foot problems from occurring in hospital and aged-care facilities.

Diabetic foot disease is a common cause of hospital admissions and is associated with long length of stay: 59% longer than for non-foot admissions, and significant morbidity and mortality. Significantly, foot ulcers also occur during hospital admissions. Diabetic foot disease is a heterogeneous disease entity, defined as a group of syndromes that lead to tissue breakdown. Infection, neuropathy, and ischaemia are usually present and increase the risk of infection and falls (Apelqvist and Larsson 2000).

Foot disease and its management have an adverse impact on the wellbeing and quality of life of people with diabetes (Brod 1998). The disease itself and some management practices, such as non-weight-bearing regimens restrict physical activity and social interaction and often result in nonadherence. They might also increase frailty-associated adverse outcomes.

Foot care self-care and foot care in hospital is an extremely important aspect of the nursing care of people with diabetes in any setting. Significantly, preventative foot care is often neglected in acute care settings. The combination of mechanical factors and vascular and nerve damage as a complication of diabetes leads to an increased risk of ulceration, infection, and amputation. In older people, these factors increase the risk of falling. An estimated 40% of people with diabetes have peripheral neuropathy, but it occurs in up to 50% of older people (Boulton et al. 2005), and 20% of hospital admissions are for foot-related problems. Not surprisingly, peripheral neuropathy is associated with significantly impaired quality of life and effects on energy, pain, mobility, and sleep (Papas et al. 2013) and neuropathic pain, which is challenging to manage, impacts on quality of life as well (ADA 2019).

As previously noted, 40-70% of lower-limb amputations occur in people with diabetes, and most begin with an ulcer. The amputation rate can be reduced by preventative foot care. The spectrum of diabetic foot disease varies globally, depending on socioeconomic circumstances, but the basic underlying pathophysiology is the same (Bakker 2000). Charcot's deformity is a severe form of diabetic foot disease that is often missed through misdiagnosis in the early stages and delay in appropriate management. The possibility of Charcot's deformity should be considered in any person with long-standing diabetes, neuropathy, and foot disease.

Vascular changes

People with diabetes and peripheral vascular disease are predisposed to atherosclerosis, which is exacerbated by chronic hyperglycaemia, endothelial damage, nonenzymatic tissue glycosylation, and polyneuropathy. These conditions impair vascular remodelling. The risk increases when the individual smokes, has hypertension, or has hypelipidaemia:

(1) *Macrovascular* (major vessel) disease may lead to:
- Intermittent claudication and rest pain.
- Poor circulation to the lower limbs, which leads to malnutrition, tissue hypoxia, and delayed healing if any trauma occurs in this area. The injured tissue is prone to infection, and gangrene can result.
(2) *Microvascular* (small vessel) disease leads to thickening of capillary basement membranes, poor blood supply to the skin, and tissue hypoxia, predisposing the feet to infection and slow healing.

Infection

Foot infections are a common and serious problem in people with diabetes. They are prone to infections and nonhealing wounds. Foot infection occurs as a result of skin ulceration or deep penetrating injuries, such as standing on a drawing pin. These injuries can go unnoticed for days because people with peripheral neuropathy do not feel pain from the penetrating object. This acts as a portal for infection that can involve tissues at all levels and foot structures, including bone.

The diagnosis of an infected wound is based on clinical signs. These include purulent discharge or two or more of erythemia, swelling, local heat, and pain. These signs may also indicate the presence of Charcot's foot rather than infection, and alkaline phosphatase, ESR, X-ray, and/or MRI may be indicated (Papas et al. 2013). Samples should also be collected to determine what organisms are present in the wound. The samples need to be collected from deep within the wound after the wound has been debrided or biopsy samples from the base of the wound rather than superficial swabs.

Acute infections are usually due to aerobic Gram-positive cocci such as *Staphylococcus aureus* or β-*haemolytic streptococci,* especially if the individual has limited exposure to antibiotics previously. Chronic ulcers and deep infections are often due to Gram-negative bacilli and anaerobic organisms such as *E. coli, Klebsiella, Proteus, Bacteroides*, and *Peptostreptococcus* with *S. aureus* is also likely to be present, sometimes as the only pathogen but usually in combination with other pathogens (Lipsky and Berendt 2000; Papas et al. 2013).

Charcot's foot is a relatively common, underdiagnosed condition that complicates management of the neuropathic foot and can lead to significant pain, mobility deficits, and amputation (Piaggesi et al. 2005). Charcot's foot is due to the progressive destruction of the bones and joints in neuropathic diabetic feet secondary to inflammation following trauma, which is usually not recognised by the person with diabetes. Inflammation is followed by sclerosis, which leads to changes in the bony architecture of the foot and reduces the capacity to reduce subsequent everyday stress such as walking. Reactivation of the inflammatory process increases bone reabsorption and increases the risk of further trauma. Higher rates of foot fractures and Charcot's feet have been observed in patients following successful pancreas transplants and those on long-term corticosteroid therapy, possibly because these medicines reduce bone resistance to minor trauma. Regular assessment of bone densitometry may be indicated in people on long-term corticosteroids.

Managing diabetic foot pathology requires a collaborative team approach and includes:

- Admission to hospital for a thorough foot and clinical assessment including self-care ability, bed rest, administration of broad-spectrum antibiotics, which needs to be continued after the acute phase resolves and surgical procedures if indicated.
- Broad-spectrum antibiotics are usually commenced initially until the results of the wound swabs are known and may be given IV for severe infections. Antibiotic therapy may be required

for one to two weeks and up to six weeks if osteomyelitis is present. The risk of the person developing antibiotic resistance must be considered and every effort made help them to prevent recurrent foot infections. The person should be asked whether they are allergic to penicillin before commencing antibiotic therapy. Flucloxacillin can be used for superficial infections and cellulitis if the person is not allergic to penicillin. Cephalexin can be used for minor infections and Clindamycin for severe infections. If the infection is deep, Augmentin or a combination of ciprofloxacin and Clindamycin may be indicated.

- X-ray (although the classical finding of osteomyelitis are not usually seen on plain X-ray until 10–21 days after the onset of bone infection) or MRI bone scans can be used to determine whether osteomyelitis is present and determine the extent of the soft-tissue injury and whether a long course of antibiotics and/or amputation is indicated. Alkaline phosphatase 135 U/L, ESR >70 mm/hour and/or being able to feel bone when probing the base of the wound are suggestive of osteomyelitis.

Risk of amputation is increased with the following:

- Persistent hyperglycaemia.
- Peripheral neuropathy and loss of pain sensation.
- Foot deformity.
- Callus or corns.
- History of foot ulcer/s.
- Previous amputation.
- Vision impairment, which affects self-care.
- Chronic kidney disease, especially people on dialysis.
- Smoking.
- Bone densitometry or ultrasound may be indicated.
- Surgical débridement to clean the wound and appropriate dressings. Referral to the wound care nurse and/or infectious disease team may be warranted.
- Revascularisation, for example, femoral/popliteal bypass, or amputation if indicated.
- Selection and application of appropriate wound dressings (Edmonds et al. 2000; Harding et al. 2000).
- Pressure off-loading to improve blood supply to the foot. Biomechanical measures such as total contact casts to relieve pressure in high-pressure ulcers and Charcot's foot deformity. Casts enable the person to remain mobile, thus improving their social and psychological well-being. Infection and subsequent oedema must be managed because they aggravate the pressure on muscles and can lead to muscle necrosis. In hospital settings high specification foam mattresses make a significant difference in preventing neuropathic foot ulcers. Prefabricated walkers are also used but must be correctly fitted.
- Improving blood glucose control and diet to ensure optimal neutrophil functioning and nutrition to promote wound healing.
- Dietetic assessment.
- Frailty assessment in older people and risk of falls.
- Counselling to stop smoking if relevant.
- Rehabilitation including regular podiatric assessment. Footwear and orthotics may need to be modified.
- Consider mental health effects of constant pain, body changes, and functional limitations (Chapter 15).

Practice points

(1) Swabs need to be taken from deep in the ulcer cavity, which can be painful, and analgesia may be required. Superficial swabs often do not identify all the organisms present, particularly anaerobes.

(2) Hyperglycaemia inhibits wound healing. Thus, people undergoing amputations and other surgical procedures are at high risk of postoperative infections. Good metabolic control, optimal nutrition, and aseptic technique reduce the risk.

Diabetes-related peripheral neuropathy

Diabetic neuropathy is defined as the presence of clinical or subclinical evidence of peripheral nerve damage, which cannot be attributed to any other disease process (Boulton et al. 1998). Neuropathy can affect the sensory nerves resulting in pain, tingling, pins and needles, or numbness. These symptoms are often worse at night. The sensory loss results in insensitivity to pain, cold, heat, touch, and vibration. The patient may not detect trauma, pressure areas, sores, blisters, cuts, and burns. Callous formation, ulceration, and bone involvement can occur.

The motor nerves can also be affected, resulting in weakness, loss of muscle fibres and diminished reflexes. Both types of nerves can be affected at the same time. Medications may not be effective in the treatment of neuropathic pain, but some commonly used medicines prescribed to manage discomfort are shown in Table 8.4.

Table 8.4 Medicines used to manage diabetic peripheral neuropathy.

Medicine	Dose range and frequency	Side effects	Cautions and contraindications
Antidepressants Tricyclic Amitriprylline[a] Desipramine[b] Doxepin[a] Impramine[a] Nortriptyline[b]	10–25 mg QID maximum dose 300 mg/day When ceasing these medicines, the dose should be reduced slowly over 2–4 weeks to prevent withdrawal syndrome.	Constipation, dry mouth, blurred vision, cognitive changes, tachycardia, urinary hesitation, sedation Secondary amines have fewer effects. Older people are more likely to experience side effects and lower doses, and slower titration is recommended.	**Cautions**: angle-closure glaucoma, benign prostatic hyperplasia, urinary retention, constipation, cardiovascular disease, impaired liver function. **Contraindications**: second- or third-degree heart block, arrhythmias, prolonged QT interval, severe liver disease, recent acute MI.
Venlafaxine Anticonvulsants Carbamazepine Gabapentin Approved for people over 18 years Lamotrigine	75 mg 100 mg BD or QID maximum 1200 mg/day 300 mg QID maximum 3600 mg/day Pain relief may only occur at higher doses 50 mg QID maximum 700 mg/day.	Nausea Somnolence, dizziness, ataxia, fatigue, occasionally tremor, diplopia, nystagmus Ataxia, blurred vision, incoordination, diplopia Rarely Stevens–Johnson syndrome, angioedema	**Cautions**: liver function tests and full blood count before commencing and repeat 2-monthly for two months then annually **Contraindication**: bone marrow depression **Caution**: renal dysfunction
Miscellaneous medicines Clonidine Oral or Weekly transdermal patch Mexiletine	0.1 mg maximum 2.4 mg/day Usually a last resort 200 mg 8 hourly Maximum 1200 mg/day An IV 'lidocaine test' may be performed to predict the response to mexiletine (an oral congener of lidocaine). It targets superficial pain: allodynia, burning and tingling.	Hypotension, dry mouth, dizziness, sedation, constipation, sexual dysfunction Local skin irritation with patches Gastrointestinal symptoms, dizziness, tremor, irritability, nervousness and headache, seizures at high doses	**Cautions**: cardiac abnormalities, cardiac symptoms should be evaluated before commencing **Contraindication**: second- or third-degree heart block

Table 8.4   (Continued)

Medicine	Dose range and frequency	Side effects	Cautions and contraindications
Topical agents Lidocaine patch Topical nitrate to the feet may relieve burning Capsaicin	5% maximum 4 patches/day Depletes substance P and may be most effective for localised pain Wear gloves to apply.		
Opoid analgesics Recent trials support some efficacy and they may have a role as add-on therapy. Tramadol Controlled-release oxycodone	Sustained relief for up to six months.	Somnolence, nausea, constipation, dependence	

Source: Data from Semla (2002), Boulton et al. (2005), ADA (2019).
Usually medicines are started at a low dose and are titrated up to maximal doses over a few weeks, depending on symptoms.
[a] Secondary amines.
[b] Tertiary amines.
Pregabalin, duloxetine or gabapentin are the first line recommended medicines for neuropathic pain.
PN: peripheral neuropathy; QID: four times per day; BD: twice per day.

Differentiating between the different types of nerve fibres involved allows a more targeted approach to pain management. Where unmyelinated C-fibres are affected, characterised by burning or dysthetic pain, capsaicin or Clonidine may be effective. Where the alpha fibres are involved, the pain is often deep and boring, and insulin infusion, lignocaine, or gabapentin may be effective (Vinik et al. 2000). Often, both types of fibres are affected.

Medicines under study include a-Lipoic acid, an antioxidant that scavenges free radicals and has been shown to reduce pain when administered parenterally (Ziegler et al. 2004). Preliminary studies suggest the protein kinase C inhibitor (LY33531) improves allodynia, and prickling pain (Litchy et al. 2002). C-peptide has recently been shown to improve early neurological abnormalities in people with type 1 diabetes with established clinical neuropathy (Brismar et al. 2007). It is given subcutaneously QID and appears to be most effective when baseline neuropathy is mild. Aldose reductase inhibitors have been under study for many years with various degrees of success. Recent research suggests Epalrestat improves objective and subjective measures of peripheral neuropathy and might slow the progression of retinopathy (Hotta 2006).

Stages of peripheral neuropathy
- Chronic and painful – improve metabolic control.
- Acute and painful – analgesia.
- Painless – education, orthoses, regular assessment.
- Late complications (Vinik et al. 2000).

Risk factors for developing foot problems
(1) Diabetes, especially if blood glucose is continually high.
(2) Smoking: people with chronic neuropathic pain are twice as likely to smoke as those with chronic nociceptive pain, but this might not represent a causative effect (Todd et al. 2008). Some studies suggest nicotine has a mild analgesic effect.
(3) Obesity.
(4) High blood pressure.
(5) Cardiovascular disease.

(6) Lack of or inadequate foot care, which is likely to be multifactorial including inability to reach the feet and lack of knowledge.
(7) Vision impairment.
(8) Inappropriate footwear.
(9) Delay in seeking help.
(10) Previous foot problems and amputation.
(11) Depression.

These factors should be part of the nursing assessment. The more risk factors present, the greater the likelihood of amputation (Pecorara 1990). Routine assessment to detect neuropathy and associated foot changes should be part of regular health assessment in primary care.

Objectives of care

(1) Assess the individual's risk of developing a foot ulcer by screening at least annually. The result of a structured foot examination can be entered into online screening tools such as the SCI-DC, which automatically stratifies the risk and recommends a management plan. Risk stages and key factors entered into the SCI-DC are:
- High risk: there is active ulcer, infection, ischaemia, and/or gangrene.
- Moderate risk: previous ulcer and/or amputation; more than one risk factor is present, such as reduced sensation, callous.
- Moderate risk: there is one risk factor such as peripheral vascular disease.
- High risk: no risk factors are present.
(2) Identify feet most at risk of trauma, ulceration, and infection in aged care, rehabilitation, and hospital settings by assessing vascular, nerve, and diabetic status:
- *Sensation* using 10 g Semmes–Weinstein monofilaments, 128 Hz tuning forks and disposable pin prickers (Apelqvist and Larsson 2000); recently, a new noninvasive test that can be undertaken by the person with diabetes was developed and is said to have 87% sensitivity and 66% specificity (Papas et al. 2013). The test, the indicator plaster neuropad (IPN) can be performed in 10 minutes and might be a useful screening tool to incorporate into the individual's foot self-care regimen.
- *Presence of vascular insufficiency* by checking capillary return and the presence of foot and peripheral pulses; Doppler ultrasound, toe pressures, and transcutaneous oxygen measurement are used in some centres.
- *Foot deformity*.
(3) Assess patient knowledge of foot care.
(4) Reinforce appropriate preventative foot care.
(5) Prevent trauma, infection, and pressure ulcers.
(6) Treat any problem detected.
(7) Refer to podiatry, orthotics, physiotherapy, rehabilitation, diabetes nurse specialist/diabetes educator, or specialist foot clinic as necessary.
(8) Control or eliminate any factors which predispose the patient to the risk of foot problems in hospital.
(9) Note risk of falls in the elderly (see Chapter 12).
(10) Manage pain.

Clinician responsibilities

(1) Prevent neuropathic ulcers occurring in people with diabetes and peripheral neuropathy during a hospital admission.
(2) Assess the feet carefully on admission. Assess self-care potential (can the patient reach the feet, see clearly?). When assessing the feet, obtain information about:
a. Past medical history:
- Glycaemic control
- Previous foot-related problems/deformities
- Smoking habits
- Nerve and vascular related risk factors

- Claudication, rest pain
- Previous foot ulcer/amputation
- Alcohol intake

    b. Type of footwear (socks, shoes):
- Hygiene
- Activity level

    c. Social factors:
- Living alone
- Older

(3) When examining the feet:
- Check both feet.
- Check pulses, dorsalis pedis, posterior tibial.
- Assess toenails: thick, layered, curved, ingrown toenails will need attention.
- Note foot structure; overlapping toes, prominent metatarsal heads on the sole of the foot.
- Check for callous, cracks, and fungal infections that can indicate inadequate foot care and poor hygiene.

(4) Note also:
- Pallor on elevation of leg
- Capillary return (normally one to two seconds)
- Any discoloration of legs
- Hair loss on the feet

(5) To ensure appropriate foot hygiene:
- Wash in lukewarm water. Use pH-neutral soap products that do not dry the skin, especially in older people or people on steroid medications and those with atopic skin.
- Check water temperature with wrist before putting the patient into a bath.
- Dry thoroughly, including between toes.
- Apply cream to prevent dryness and cracks (urea cream, sorbelene).

(6) Ensure Elastoplast/Band Aids, bandages do *not* encircle toes as they can act like tourniquets and reduce the circulation, which could result in gangrene. Apply elastic support stockings correctly.

(7) Maintain a safe environment:
- Use a bed cradle.
- Ensure shoes are worn if walking around the ward.
- Strict bed rest may be necessary while the ulcer is healing.
- Maintain aseptic technique.

(8) Check feet daily and report any changes or the development of any callus, abrasion, or trauma.

(9) Monitor blood glucose.

(10) Attend to dressings and administer antibiotics according to treatment order. Antibiotics are often given intravenously if foot infection is present.

(11) Take the opportunity to ensure self-care knowledge is current and that complication screening has been attended to. Ensure preventative foot-care education is provided, to help the patient with diabetes with these issues:
- Understand effects of diabetes on the feet.
- Know appropriate footwear.
- Be able to identify foot risk factors.
- Understand the principal effects of poor control (continual hyperglycaemia) on foot health.
- Know the services available for assistance with their diabetes care and how to obtain advice about foot care.
- Know about appropriate foot care practices – in particular, patients must inspect their feet daily and seek help early if any problems are found.

- Odour control can be an issue when infection and gangrene are present. Some wound dressings have an absorbent layer that eliminates odour by absorbing bacteria. Good foot hygiene helps reduce the odour.

Classification of foot ulcers

A number of ulcer classification systems are in existence, and nurses are advised to follow the system in their place of employment. In 2002, an international working party was established to develop an international consensus foot ulcer classification system. Foot ulcers can be loosely classified as:

(1) Clean, superficial ulcer
(2) Deep ulcer, possibly infected, but no bone involvement
(3) Deep ulcer, tracking infection, and bone involvement
(4) Localised gangrene and necrosis (usually forefoot, heel)
(5) Extensive gangrene of foot

The depth and width of the ulcer should be recorded regularly; a plastic template, dated, and filed in the patient's history, aids in the assessment of changes in ulcer size. The presence, amount, and type of exudate must be recorded.

Clinical observation

Aromatherapy essential oils on the *surface of the secondary dressing* can help reduce wound odour. They should not be applied directly to the wound. They can be used in a vapouriser for environmental fragrancing. Some essential oils can help improve mood.

Wound management

Dressings may be needed to absorb the exudate and protect the foot. No dressing is appropriate for all wound types. Surgical débridement, amputation, or an occlusive dressing may be required. It is important to keep the temperature at 37°C, the dressing moist, and the pH acidic to promote healing. Choose a dressing that does not cause tissue damage when it is removed, that is, does not stick to the wound and protects the wound from infection. The moisture aids in pain relief, decreases the healing time and gives a better cosmetic result. An acidic environment promotes granulation tissue. The management of ulcers in hospital and other specific foot problems are listed in Table 8.5.

A recent Cochrane systematic review (Wang et al. 2017) suggested phototherapy compared to placebo could increase the proportion of wound that heal and reduce wound size in people with diabetes. The effect on quality of life was unclear. More and less flawed studies are needed to determine the usefulness in clinical practice.

Practice point

Painting the area with a betadine or other skin antiseptic is of little value.
  Coloured antiseptics can obscure some of the signs of infection.

Diabetic foot ulcers heal slowly and bed rest is important. The patient may be otherwise well. Follow these procedures:

• Encourage independence with blood glucose testing and insulin administration.
• Refer for occupational therapy. The person may benefit from counselling if depressed.
• Careful discharge planning is imperative to ensure mobilisation and rehabilitation and that there is a safe environment at home.
• Interim placement in an extended care facility may be necessary.
• Assess the physical and social support available after discharge.

Table 8.5   Managing of specific foot problems while the person is in hospital or community settings.

Problem	Treatment
Burning, paraesthesia, aching	Assess neuropathic status. Encourage person to walk. Maintain euglycaemia. Administer appropriate analgesia. Manage depression if present.
Pain	Foot cradle, sheepskin. Administer appropriate analgesia.
Dry skin, cracks	Clean, dry carefully, apply moisturiser, for example, urea cream, sorbelene. A duromet can be used to evaluate skin hardness and identify areas of where plantar hyperkeratosis is likely to develop. Plantar pressures, which can indicate force and workload.
Claudication	Medications as ordered. Rest. Elevate feet. Cardiovascular assessment; peripheral pulses, ankle/brachial pressure index (APBI), transcutaneous oxygen tension (Tcp O2). Angiography.
Foot deformity	Clinically evaluate and describe. Estimate joint mobility. Refer to podiatrist. Provide physiotherapy. Orthotist.
Charcot's deformity	
Ulcers, infection	The presence of a lesion transforms an at-risk foot into an acute clinical emergency. Grade the ulcer; for example, University of Texas Staging System for Diabetic foot ulcers. X-ray and MRI may be indicated to assess the depth Record the width and depth, for example, using a polyurethane sheet Refer to specific medical order. Assess daily. Make template to note change in size of ulcer. Administer antibiotics. If necessary, provide débridement, amputation.

ABPI >0.9 normal; 0.9–0.5 indicates peripheral vascular disease is present; <0.5 indicates critical limb ischaemia. ABPI >1.3 usually indicates medial artery calcification (Monckerberg sclerosis), an indirect sign of autonomic neuropathy (Bianchi et al. 2007).
TcpO$_2$ pressure <60 mmHg indicates local ischaemia; <40 mmHg indicates critical ischaemia (Piaggesi et al. 2005).

Practice point

Orthopaedic patients with diabetes and foot or leg plasters should be encouraged *not* to scratch under the plaster, especially if they have 'at-risk' feet. Damage can occur and remain undetected until the plaster is removed.

Wound management techniques under study
Several new wound management products for hard-to-heal ulcers are under study:

- Platelet-derived growth factor applied topically to increase granulation
- Hyaff
- Dermagraft
- Apilgraf
- Granulocyte-colony stimulating factor (Edmonds et al. 2000)

Hyperbaric oxygen may be beneficial in some serious ulcers. Oxygen is necessary for wound healing, and hyperbaric oxygen can increase tissue oxygen levels and improves the killing power of phagocytes (Bakker 2000).

Pain management strategies
Nonmedicine options with varying degrees of evidence to support their benefits include:

- Physiotherapy and exercise such as tai chi to maintain muscle tone and strength.
- Percutaneous nerve stimulation, static magnetic field therapy, low-intensive laser therapy, body flow technology, and monochromatic infrared light. These techniques might improve peripheral circulation and reduce local oedema, which reduces some of the local pressure and relieves local pain.
- Acupuncture, which has benefits up to six months (Abusaisha et al. 1998).
- Other nonmedicine measures include improving blood glucose control, stopping smoking, reducing alcohol intake, and eating a healthy diet.

The autonomic nervous system may also be affected by diabetes. Autonomic nervous system involvement may lead to an absence of sweating, which causes dry, cracked skin, and increases the risk of infection. Other effects of autonomic neuropathy include gastric stasis, ED, hypogly-caemic unawareness, and incontinence. The small muscle wasting secondary to longstanding neuropathy can lead to abnormal foot shapes (e.g., clawing of the toes), making the purchase of well-fitting shoes difficult.

Vascular disease, neuropathy, and infection are more likely to develop if there is longstanding hyperglycaemia, which contributes to the accumulation of sorbitol through the polyol pathway, leading to damage to the nerves and small blood vessels. Figure 8.1 illustrates the interrelated factors that lead to foot problems in people with diabetes.

Table 8.6 lists changes in feet due to the normal aging process. These factors should all be incorporated in the nursing assessment to ensure that appropriate foot care is part of the overall management of the patient.

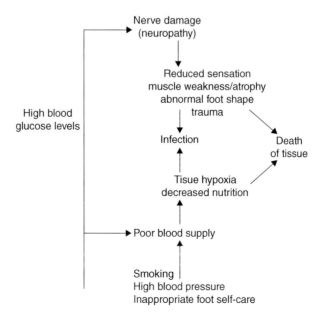

Figure 8.1   Factors leading to foot problems in people with diabetes.

Table 8.6   Changes in feet due to normal ageing.

(1) Skin becomes thin, fragile.
(2) Nails are thick and often deformed.
(3) Blood supply is reduced.
(4) Nerve function is often impaired.
(5) Muscle weakness and wasting occurs.
(6) Arthritis, may lead to pain and deformity.

Rehabilitation

Despite the best care, amputations are required in 5–15% of people with diabetes presenting with a foot problem, particularly in the presence of gangrene or nonhealing ulcers, which may be associated with osteomyelitis and severe foot infection. A rehabilitation process is necessary once the acute stage has settled. Below-knee amputations give a favourable result even if the popliteal pulses are diminished (Steinberg 1991). The goals of rehabilitation are as follows:

- Appropriate stump care. In the early stages, this may involve bandaging to reduce oedema. Circular bandages should be avoided because they tend to act like tourniquets and reduce the blood supply to the stump. Analgesia should be available. Later, correctly fitting the stump into the socket of the prosthesis and regular inspection for the presence of infection or pressure areas.
- Prevent muscle contracture with regular physiotherapy.
- Help the person be as independent and active as possible.
- Ambulation with a prosthesis or wheelchair, depending on the individual assessment. However, not all people with diabetes benefit from having a prosthesis. People who have advanced neurological disease such as stroke, Parkinson's disease, CCF, obstructive pulmonary disease, unstable angina, or knee and hip contractures may not be suitable for a prosthesis. These people often have limited ability to mobilise even before an amputation. High risk of gangrene or infection in the other limb may warrant delaying an amputation.
- Early mobilisation in whatever capacity is usually desirable after amputation to reduce postoperative complications. The person will need to learn how to manage whatever mobilisation method is appropriate.
- Care of the stump is important to prevent wound contractures.

Practice points

(1) Amputation should not always be seen as treatment failure. It can relieve pain, enable the person to return home, and enjoy an improved quality of life. Amputation is distressing for the person with diabetes and their family, and careful explanation, support, and counselling are essential. The patient should be included in the decision-making process and make the final decision. Their social and psychological situation should be considered as well as their physical needs.
(2) Amputation increases the risk of a second amputation.

Autonomic neuropathy

Key points

- Often several organs are involved.
- Signs and symptoms are often nonspecific.
- Autonomic neuropathy is often undiagnosed.

- Postural hypotension is the most significant sign of autonomic neuropathy.
- People with postural hypotension and nocturnal diarrhoea should be investigated for autonomic neuropathy.
- The progression to autonomic neuropathy is related to poor metabolic control.
- It is more common in people over 65, but it can occur in the first year after diagnosis.

Introduction

Autonomic neuropathy is a distressing condition for people with diabetes. It can cause erratic blood glucose readings. People are often accused of manipulating their food and/or diabetic medications, which causes stress and anxiety. The symptoms associated with the various manifestations of autonomic neuropathy can be uncomfortable, painful, and have an adverse impact on the individual's quality of life. The autonomic nervous system plays an important role in the regulation of carbohydrate metabolism. Many processes are affected by autonomic neuropathy – for example it both facilitates and inhibits insulin secretion:

(1) It stimulates the right vagus nerve, which innervates the pancreatic islet cells, or the beta-adrenergic receptors in the islet cells, stimulates insulin secretion.
(2) It stimulates the alpha-adrenergic receptors in the islet cells decreases insulin secretion, which is an essential aspect of blood glucose regulation and to maintaining glucose homeostasis.

The autonomic nervous system also has a role in the conversion of glycogen into glucose in the liver where FFAs undergo further metabolism to ketones. Neurogenic stimulation of the hypo-pituitary axis results in cortisol secretion, one of the counter-regulatory hormones that have a role in correcting hypoglycaemia. In stress situations, especially prolonged stress, hyperglycaemia results.

Diabetes is the commonest cause of autonomic neuropathy but it also occurs in association with other diseases such as advanced Parkinson's disease and Guillain–Barre syndrome. Autonomic neuropathy is a common, underdiagnosed condition associated with a range of signs and symptoms, depending on the specific nerves and organs affected (Vinik et al. 2000; Aly and Weston 2002). It has a slow onset and affects up to 30–40% of people with diabetes, and although many people only have mild, often subclinical features, significant functional abnormalities can be present.

Rarely, in <5% of cases, overt clinical features develop. Autonomic neuropathy can involve any system, but commonly affects the heart, gastrointestinal tract (GIT), and genitourinary systems (Spallone and Menzinger 1997). The GIT is one of the most frequently affected systems but GIT problems, not associated with autonomic neuropathy, occur in 50% of the general population and are more common in people with diabetes (Locke et al. 2000). Older people are at risk of having many neuropathic GIT changes but some GIT changes are age-related or associated with the use of vasoconstrictive drugs (Aly and Weston 2002).

Delayed gastric emptying is present in 25–55% of people with type 1 and 30% with type 2 (Wegener et al. 1990). Consequences of gastrointestinal autonomic neuropathy include early satiety, abdominal distension, reflux, stomach spasm, postprandial nausea, vomiting, altered medicine absorption and food absorption, malnutrition, and glucose variability. In addition, it causes significant diabetes-related distress and reduces quality of life.

Practice points

(1) Autonomic neuropathy is physically uncomfortable and treatment options are limited. Where the GIT is involved, frequent adjustment to the food and medication regimen is often needed. Blood glucose monitoring is important to allow such changes to be made appropriately.
(2) Psychological distress is common. Support and understanding are important aspects of management.

Table 8.7   Organs commonly affected by diabetic autonomic neuropathy and the resultant clinical features.

Affected organ	Main clinical features	Consequences
Gastrointestinal tract (gastroparesis)	Decreased peristalsis Abdominal distension and feeling of fullness Early satiety Postprandial nausea Vomiting undigested food Diarrhoea, especially at night Depression	Weight loss Erratic blood glucose control Stomach not be empty even after fasting, for example, for procedures
Urinary tract	Distended bladder Urine overflow Feeling of incomplete bladder emptying Stress incontinence Nocturia Vaginal mucous membrane excoriation in women	Silent urinary tract infection Falls in elderly people Sleep disturbance Uncomfortable sexual intercourse
Genitals	Erectile dysfunction (ED) in men. Indeterminate, if any effect in women Possibly vaginal dryness in older women	Psychological sequelae including depression Negative impact on sexual health
Cardiovascular system	Blood pressure: Postural hypotension Loss of diurnal variation Dizziness when standing Resting tachycardia Reduced sympathetic tone Decreased beta-adrenergic responsiveness	Silent myocardial infarction Stroke Falls
Lower limbs	Reduced sweating Reduced blood flow Reduced pain Redness Defective thermoregulation	Foot ulcers and infection Sleep disturbance
Brain	Cognitive impairment	Reduced self-care ability
General	Excessive sweating, especially of the upper body, resembling a hot flush and sometimes mistaken for hypoglycaemia Slow pupillary reaction Heat intolerance	Trauma Depression

Note: Many of these conditions predispose elderly people to falls (see Chapter 12).

The commonly affected systems and associated clinical manifestations are shown in Table 8.7.

Diagnosis and management

Special tests are required to make a definitive diagnosis. The particular test depends on which organs are being tested; for example, gastric emptying times for the GIT, Valsalva manoeuvre for the cardiovascular system, and voiding cystourethrogram to determine the effects on the bladder. In many cases, specific treatment is commenced on the basis of the clinical history and assessment.

Management consists of two phases:

(1) Adopt preventative strategies early by doing the following:
  • Improve blood glucose control and lipid levels.
  • Treat hypertension.

- Screen regularly for complications.
- Ensure adequate self-care.
- Be aware that antioxidants may have a role in preventing oxidative tissue damage and pre- and probiotics may have a role in maintaining normal gut flora and reducing inflammation, although evidence specify to gastric autonomic neuropathy is limited (Chapter 1).

(2) Provide direction when present.

Treatment is often by trial and error and is aimed at alleviating the unpleasant symptoms. Preventative measures should be continued. Treatment for specific autonomic neuropathic conditions consists of:

a. Gastrointestinal tract
- Dietary management depends on the degree of malnutrition present and the symptoms. Frequent small, light, easily digested, or fluid meals that are low in fat and fibre and contain a consistent proportion of carbohydrate place less burden on the gastrointestinal tract and reduce glucose variability (Sadiya 2012). Large meals and fat delay gastric emptying and exacerbates the already-slow gastric emptying time. It is imperative to ensure that essential protein, vitamins, and minerals are consumed; thus, people with severe malnutrition might need supplements and/or enteral feeding (Chapter 4). Consuming a liquid diet when the symptoms are worse sometimes helps.
- Manage distress and depression.
- GLM medicine doses usually need to be adjusted frequently; thus, a basal bolous or insulin pump provides the greatest flexibility.
- Stimulants such as caffeine, alcohol, and tobacco should be avoided. Likewise, chewing gum increases air swallowing and contributes to bloating, and foods that contain mint, chocolate, fat, and caffeine lower oesophagal sphincter pressure.
- Medications such as metoclopramide and cisapride may give some relief but should not be used continuously.
- Antibiotics such as tetracycline or trimethoprim may be required to treat bacterial overgrowth that occurs as a consequence of gastric stasis.
- Cholestyramine can be used to chelate bile salts, which immobilise the gut.
- Treat constipation, nausea, and vomiting as they occur.
- Elevate the head of the bed to use gravity to assist gastric emptying.
- Anecdotally gentle abdominal massage and compresses help reduce spasm and relieve bloating and constipation.
- Jejunostomy is a last resort.

b. Cardiovascular system:
- Support garments such as stockings or a body stocking support venous return and relieve stress on the heart. They should be put on while the person is lying down.
- Manage postural hypotension – find a balance between increasing the pressure on standing and preventing hypertension when lying. Fludrocortisone or midodrine can be used. Medications should be reviewed to exclude drugs that precipitate postural hypotension.

c. Genitourinary:
- Urinary catheterisation and self-catheterisation. Sometimes parasympathomimetic drugs are also used.
- Manage ED with drugs such as sildenafil, intracavernosal injections, or mechanical and implanted devices and counselling (see Chapter 17).

d. General measures
- Adjust insulin or GLMs and diet to manage the erratic blood glucose profile.
- Apply topical glycopyrrolate to alleviate gustatory sweating.
- Patient should stop smoking.
- Provide careful explanations about autonomic neuropathy and counselling to address the psychological consequences and treatment options.
- Encourage activity.
- Monitor mental health and diabetes distress (Chapter 15).

Clinical care

Palliative and supportive care is required (see Chapter 18). Providing a safe environment and reducing the risk of falls is essential, especially in older people, to prevent trauma, for example, fractures. This could involve ensuring the home environment is safe before discharging patients.

Clinicians can have a role in the early identification of autonomic neuropathy by having a level of suspicion and taking a careful history.

Important nursing responsibilities include the following:

(1) The prevention, early recognition, and management of hypoglycaemia is essential.
(2) Take care when moving the patient from a lying to a sitting position, and from sitting to standing. Give them time for the blood pressure to adjust. Ensure their footwear will not contribute to the risk of falling.
(3) Provide adequate foot care and appropriate advice to minimise the risk of ulcers, including advice about footwear.
(4) Arrange counselling if indicated.
(5) Use aseptic technique.
(6) Be alert to the possibility of silent pathology – myocardial infarction, urinary tract infection.
(7) Encourage people to remain physically active within their individual limits. Physical activity aids many body systems and improves mental outlook.

Clinical observation

Gentle abdominal massage and warm compresses can help alleviate the discomfort of gastroparesis. Aromatherapy essential oils can be added to the compress. The abdomen is a vulnerable part of the body, and this needs to be taken into consideration when offering an abdominal massage (see Chapter 18).

References

ACCORD Study Group (2011). Long term effects of intensive glucose lowering on cardiovascular outcomes. *New England Journal of Medicine* **364**: 11–63.

Alamowitch, S., Eliasziw, M., and Barnett, H. (2005). The risk and benefit of endarterectomy in women with symptomatic internal carotid artery disease. *Stroke* **36**: 27–31.

Alzaid, A. (2019). Managing hyperglycaemia in type 2 diabetes: where's the proof in the pudding? Medscape (7 January). https://www.medscape.com/viewarticle/907105_print.

American Diabetes Association (2019). Standers of medical care in diabetes.10 cardiovascular disease. *Diabetes Care* **42** (Suppl.1): S103–S123.

American Diabetes Association (ADA) (2012). Standards of medical care in diabetes 2012. *Diabetes Care* **35** (Suppl 1): 11–63.

American Diabetes Association (ADA) (2013). Standards of Medical Care in Diabetes. *Diabetes Care* **36** (1): S11–S66. (January), https://care.diabetesjournals.org/content/36/Supplement_1/S11.

Aroda, V. and Getaneh, A. (2019). Macrovascular complications and diabetes. *Current Diabetes Reports* **19** (6) https://link.springer.com/articale/10/1007/s11892-019-1126-5?wt_mc=alerts.TOCjournals&utm_source.

Australian Commission on Safety and Quality in Health Care (2017). *National Safety and Quality Health Service Standards*, 2e. Australian Commission on Safety and Quality in Health Care.

Australian Diabetes Society (ADS) (2012). *Guidelines for Routine Glucose Control in Hospital*. Canberra: ADS.

Australian Institute Health and Welfare (AIHW) (2007). *Medicines for Cardiovascular Health*, AIHW Cardiovascular Series No. 27. Canberra: AIHW.

Rossi, S. (ed.) (2006). *Australian Medicines Handbook*. Adelaide, Australia: Australian Medicines Handbook TY Ltd.

Baker IDI (2019). The dark heart of type 2 diabetes. Baker IDI Heart and Diabetes Institute, Melbourne, Australia.

Barnett, K., Mercer, S.W., Norbury, M. et al. (2012). Epidemiology of multimorbidity and implications for health care, research, and medical education: a cross-sectional study. *The Lancet* **380** (9836): 37–43.

Barenholtz, H. and Kohlhaas, H. (2006). Considerations for supplementing with coenzyme Q_{10} during satin therapy. *Annals of Pharmacotherapy* **40**: 290–294.

Bayliss, E., Edwards, A., Steiner, J., and Main, D. (2008). Processes of care desired by elderly patients with multimorbidities. *Family Practice* **25** (4): 287–293.

Boden-Albala, B. (2008). Daytime sleepiness is an independent risk factor for stroke. In: *Proceedings of the American Stroke Association International Stroke Conference*. Abstract 94. (20-22 February 2008). New Orleans, LA: American Stroke Association.

Boehmer, K.R., Hargraves, I.G., Allen, S.V. et al. (2016). Meaningful conversations in living with and treating chronic conditions: development of the ICAN discussion aid. *BMC Health Services Research* **16** (1): 514.

Bohm, M. (2008). Treating to protect: current cardiovascular treatment approaches and remaining needs. *Medscape Journal Medicine* **10** (Suppl. 3): 1–13.

Britt, H.C., Harrison, C.M., Miller, G.C., and Knox, S.A. (2008). Prevalence and patterns of multimorbidity in Australia. *Medical Journal of Australia* **189** (2): 72–77.

Bruckert, E. and Hansel, B. (2007). HDL-c is a powerful lipid predictor of cardiovascular disease. *International Journal of Clinical Practice* **61** (11): 1905–1913.

Bunker, S., Colquhoun, D., Esler, M. et al. (2003). 'Stress' and coronary heart disease: psychosocial risk factors. *Medical Journal of Australia* **178**: 271–276.

Casey, P. (2004). Markers of myocardial injury and dysfunction. *AACN Clinical Issues* **15** (4): 547–557.

Cefalo, C., Cinti, F., Moffa, S. et al. (2019). Sotagliflozin, the first dual SGLT inhibitoe: current outlook and perspective. *Cardiovascular Diabetology* **18**: 20. https://doi.org/10.1186/s12933-019-0828-y.

Chen, Z. (2008). High BMI linked with stroke mortality in obese, overweight men. *Stroke Online* (31 January). http://www.medscape.com/viewarticle/569864?src=mp (accessed February 2008).

Chiu, C., Hubbard, I., and Armstrong, J. (2006). Dietary glycaemic index and carbohydrate in relation to early age-related macular degeneration. *American Journal of Nutrition* **63**: 880–886.

Clemens, K., O'Regan, N., and Rhee, J. (2019). Diabetes management in older adults with chronic kidney disease. *Current Diabetes Reports* **19**: 11. https://doi.org/10.1007/s11892-019-1128-3.

Coleman, R., Stevens, R., Retnakaran, R., and Holman, R. (2007). Framingham SCORE and DECODE risk equations do not provide reliable cardiovascular risk estimates in type 2 diabetes. *Diabetes Care* **30**: 1292–1293.

Cormack, T., Grant, B., Macdonald, M. et al. (2001). Incidence of blindness due to diabetic eye disease in Fife 1990–9. *British Journal of Ophthalmology* **85** (3): 354–356.

Currie, C.J., Peters, J.R., Tynan, A. et al. (2010). Survival as a function of HbA1c in people with type 2 diabetes: a retrospective cohort study. *The Lancet* **375** (9713): 481–489.

Dantas, P., Fortes, B., and Catelli de Carvalho, H. (2012). Vascular disease in diabetic women: why do they miss the female protection? *Experimental Diabetes Research* https://doi.org/10.1155/2012/570598.

Davidson, P., Mitchell, J., DiGiacomo, M. et al. (2011). Cardiovascular disease in women: implications for improving cardiovascular health outcomes. *Collegian* **19**: 5–13.

Donahoe, S., Stewart, G., McCabe, C. et al. (2007). Diabetes mortality following acute coronary syndromes. *Journal American Medical Association* **298** (7): 765–775.

Du, X., Edelstein, D., and Rossetti, L. (2000). Hyperglycaemia induced mitochondrial superoxide overproduction activates the hexosamine pathway and induces plasminogen activator inhibitor-1 expression by increasing Sp1 glycosylation. *Proceedings of the National Academy of Science USA* **97**: 1222–1226.

Elias, P., Elias, M., D'sgostino, R. et al. (1997). NIDDM and blood pressure as risk factors for poor cognitive performance. The Framingham Study. *Diabetes Care* **20** (9): 138–139.

European Society of Hypertension (2007). Guidelines on treatment of hypertension. *Journal of Hypertension* **25**: 1105–1187.

Farmer, D. and Kennedy, S. (2009). RAGE vascular changes tone ans vascular diseaase. *Pharmacology and Therapeutics* **124** (2): 185–194.

Forbes, J. and Cooper, M. (2007). The role of mitochondrial dysfunction in diabetic complications. *International Diabetes Monitor* **19** (6): 9–15.

Fortin, M., Lapointe, L., Hudon, C., and Vanasse, A. (2005). Multimorbidity is common to family practice: is it commonly researched? *Canadian Family Physician* **51**: 244–245.

Gerbaud, E., Darier, R., Montaudon, M. et al. (2019). Glycemic variability is a powerful independent predictive factor of midterm major adverse cardiac events in patients with diabetes with acute coronary syndrome. *Diabetes Care* **42** (4): 674–681.

Giacco, F. and Brownlee, M. (2012). Mechanisms of hyperglycaemic damage in diabetes. In: *Atlas of Diabetes*, 4e (ed. J. Skyler). New York: Springer https://www.csanz.edu.au/wp-content/uploads/2017/07/CAC_Position-Statement_2017_ratified-26-May-2017.pdf.

Giannelli, S., Patel, K., Windham, G. et al. (2007). Magnitude of underascertainment of impaired kidney function in old: normal serum creatine. *Journal America Geriatric Society* **55** (6): 816–823.

Gudjhar, A., Dunning, T., and Alford, F. (2003). Metabolic and cardiac outcomes after acute myocardial infarction. *Journal of Diabetes Nursing* **7** (6): 208–212.

Hanefield, M., Frier, B.M., and Pistrosch, F. (2016). Hypoglycemia and cardiovascular risk: is there a major link? *Diabetes Care* **39** (Supplement 2): S205–S209.

Hansel, B., Giral, P., and Nobecourt, E. (2004). Metabolic syndrome is associated with elevated oxidative stress and dysfunctional dense high-density lipoprotein particles displaying impaired antioxidative activity. *Journal Clinical Endocrinology and Metabolism.* 89 (10): 4963–4971.

Hansson, L., Zanchetti, A., Carruthers, S. et al. (1998). Effects of intensive blood pressure lowering and low dose aspirin in patients with hypertension: principal results of the hypertension optimal treatment (HOT) randomised trial. *Lancet* 351 (9118): 1755–1762.

Haussler, B., Fischer, G., Meyer, S., and Sturm, D. (2007). Risk assessment in diabetes management: how do general practitioners estimate risks due to diabetes? *Quality and Safety in Health Care* 16: 208–212.

Hotta, N., Toyota, T., and Matsuoka, K. (2001). Clinical efficacy of fidarestat, a novel aldose reductase inhibitor, for diabetic peripheral neuropathy: a 52-week multicenter placebo-controlled double blind parallel group study. *Diabetes Care* 24: 1176–1182.

Huang, E., Liu, J., Moffet, H. et al. (2011). Glycaemic control, complications, and death in older diabetic patients. *Diabetes Care* 34: 1329–1336.

International Diabetes Federation (IDF) (2011). *Guideline for Management of Post Meal Glucose in Diabetes.* Brussels: IDF.

Kaiser, N., Sasson, S., and Feener, E. (1993). Differential regulation of glucose transports by glucose in vascular endothelial and smooth muscle cells. *Diabetes* 42: 80–89.

Khojasteh, P. (2019). Saving sight using AI to diagnose diabetic eye disease. *Computers in Biology and Medicine* https://doi.org/10.1016/j.compbiomed.2018.10.031.

Kidney Health (2019). Estimated glomerular filtration rate (eGFR) fact sheet. www.kidney.org.au.

Kim, C.-Y., Lee, K.-B., ark, S.-E. et al. (2012). Serum 1,5-Anhydroglucitol concentrations are a reliable index of Glycemic control in type 2 diabetes with mild or moderate renal dysfunction. *Diabetes Care* 35 (2): 281–286.

Kumar, A., Kuar, H., Devi, P., and Mohan, V. (2009). Role of coenzyme Q10 (coQ10) in cardiac disease, hypertension and Meniere-like syndrome. *Pharmacology and Therapeutics* 124: 259–268.

Kumar, S., Pathak, S., and Kumar, B. (2019). Automated detection of eye-related diseases using digital image processing. In: *Handbook of Multimedia Information Security: Techniques and Applications* (eds. A.K. Singh and A. Mohan), 513–544. Springer: Cham.

Laiteerapong, N., Ham, S.A., Gao, Y. et al. (2019). The legacy effect in type 2 diabetes: impact of early glycemic control on future complications (the Diabetes & Aging Study). *Diabetes Care* 42 (3): 416–426.

Laitinen, T., Huopio, H., Vauhkonen, I. et al. (2003). Effects of euglycaemic and hypoglycaemic hyperinsulinaemia on sympathetic and parasympathetic regulation of haemodynamics in healthy subjects. *Clinical Science* 105 (3): 315–322.

Lazalde-Ramos, B., Zanoura-Perez, A., Sosa-Macia, M. et al. (2012). DNA and oxidative damages decrease after ingestion of folic acid in patients with type 2 diabetes. *Archives of Medical Research* 43 (6): 476–481.

Lee, D.H., Youn, H.J., Jung, H.O. et al. (2017). Coronary artery calcium score plays an important role for cardiovascular risk stratification in the statin benefit groups of asymptomatic individuals. *Lipids in Health and Disease* 16 (1): 172.

Lesperance, F. and Frasure-Smith, N. (2007). Depression and heart disease. *Cleveland Clinic Journal of Medicine* 74 (Suppl. 1): S63–S66.

Lim, W., Holinski, H., Devereaux, P. et al. (2008). Detecting myocardial infarction in critical illness using screening troponin measurements and ECG recordings. *Critical Care* 12: R36. https://doi.org/10.1186/cc6815.

Liu, G., Guasch-Ferre, M., Hu, Y. et al. (2019). Nut consumption in relation to cardiovascular disease incidence and mortality among patients with diabetes mellitus. *Circulation Research* https://doi.org/10.1161/CIRCRESAHA.118.314316.

Lutsep, H. (2008). Stroke treatment and prevention are not the same in men and women. *Medscape Medical Journal* 10 (2): 26–27.

Margolis, K., Bonds, D., and Rodnbough, R. (2004). Effect of oestrogen plus progestin on the incidence of diabetes in postmenopausal women: results of the women's health initiative hormone trial. *Diabetologia* 47 (7): 1175–1187.

Mason, S., Rasmussen, B., van Loon, L. et al. (2019). Ascorbic acid supplementation improves postprandial glycaemic control and blood pressure in individuals with type 2 diabetes: findings of a randomized cross-over trial. *Diabetes Obesity and Metabolism* https://doi.org/10.1111/dom.13571.

Mayer, D.D. and Rosenfeld, A. (2006). Symptom interpretation in women with diabetes and myocardial infarction. *The Diabetes Educator* 32 (6): 918–924.

Metra, M., Zaca, V., Parati, G. et al. (2011). Cardiovascular and noncardiovascular comorbidities in patients with chronic heart failure. *Journal of Cardiovascular Medicine* 12 (2): 76–84.

Middleton, S., Ward, J., Grimshaw, M. et al. (2011). Implementation of evidence-based treatment protocols to manage fever, hyperglycaemia, and swallowing dysfunction in acute stroke (QASC): a cluster randomized trial. *The Lancet* https://doi.org/10.1016/s0140-6736(11)51485-2.

Moser, D., Kimble, L., and Alberts, M. (2007). Reducing delay in seeking treatment by patients with acute coronary syndrome and stroke: a scientific statement from the American Heart Association Council on Cardiovascular Nursing and Stroke Council. *Journal of Cardiovascular Nursing* 22: 326–343.

Mozaffarian, D. (2007). Acute myocardial infarction: a prediabetes risk equivalent? *The Lancet* **25**: 667–675.

Mulnier, H. (2012). Macrovascular disease and diabetes. *Journal of Diabetes Nursing* **16** (8): 307–313.

Nagel, G., Peter, R., Braig, S. et al. (2008). The impact of education on risk factors and the occurrence of multimorbidity in the EPIC-Heidelberg cohort. *BMC Public Health* **8** (384) https://doi.org/10.1186/1471-2458-8-384.

National Institute of Clinical Care Excellence (NICE) (2009). Guidelines for Managing Diabetes. www.nice.org.uk (accessed march 2012).

National Institute of Clinical Studies (NICS) (2005). *Evidence-Practice Gaps Report*, vol. **2**. Melbourne: NICS.

National Kidney Foundation (2018). Chronic Kideny Disease Classificatiion. http://www.kidney.org/professionals/guidelines/guidelines_commentries/chronic-kidney-disease-classification.

National Prescribing Service (NPS) (2012). Cardiovascular disease risk in type 2 diabetes. www.nps.org.au (accessed September 2012).

Nelson, M. and Woodward, M. (2019). Developing cardiovascular risk prediction models for *Australia. Medical Journal of Australia* **210** (4): 158–159.

Newton, P.J., Davidson, P.M., Reid, C.M. et al. (2016). Acute heart failure admissions in New South Wales and the Australian Capital Territory: the NSW HF Snapshot Study. *Medical Journal of Australia* **204** (3): 113–113.

Nishikawa, T., Edelstein, D., and Du, X. (2000). Normalising superoxide production blocks three pathways of hyperglycaemic damage. *Nature* **404**: 787–790.

Pfisterer, M. (2004). In elderly patients with chronic angina, drugs offer outcomes equal to invasive treatment. Circulation on line. http://www.medscape.com/viewarticle/488214 (accessed August 2007).

Piccone, J.E. (2012). Painless compliance. *Health Management Technology* **33** (9): 18.

Pittler, M., Guo, R., and Ernst, E. (2008). Hawthorn extract for treating chronic heart failure. *Cochrane Database of Systematic Reviews* (1): CD005312. https://doi.org/10.1002/14651858.CD005312.pub2.

Player, M., King, D., Mainous, A., and Geesey, M. (2007). Psychosocial factors and progression from prehypertension to hypertension or coronary heart disease. *Annals of Family Medicine* **5** (5): 403–411.

Ponikowski, P., Voors, A.A., Anker, S.D. et al. (2016). 2016 ESC Guidelines for the diagnosis and treatment of acute and chronic heart failure: The Task Force for the diagnosis and treatment of acute and chronic heart failure of the European Society of Cardiology (ESC). Developed with the special contribution of the Heart Failure Association (HFA) of the ESC. *European Journal of Heart Failure* **18** (8): 891–975.

Reddy, P. (2008). Diabetes and depression. Practical tools for the diabetes educator. Sanofi-Aventis Diabetes Partnership Seminar (12 April 2008). Novotel, Melbourne.

Ridker, P., Cook, N., and Lee, I. (2005). A randomized trial of low dose aspirin in the primary prevention of cardiovascular disease in women. *New England Journal of Medicine* **352**: 1293–1304.

Rosano, G., Vitale, C., and Seferovic, P. (2017). Heart failure in patients with diabetes. *Cardiac Failure Review* **3** (1): 52–55.

Rosenfeldt, F., Haas, S., and Krum, H. (2007). Coenzyme Q_{10} in the treatment of hypertension: a metaanalysis of the clinical trials. *Journal of Human Hypertension* **21**: 297–306.

Sanchis, J. (2007). Risk score useful in assessing chest pain with normal troponin levels. *American Journal of Cardiology* **99**: 797–801.

Schernthaner, G., Lotan, C., Baltadzhieva-Trendafilova, E. et al. (2018). Unrecognised cardiovascular disease in type 2 diabetes: is it time to act earlier? *Cardiovascular Diabetology* **17** (1): 145.

SIGN (2010). *Management of Diabetes: A National Clinical Guideline*. Edinburgh: SIGN.

Sindone, A. (2019). Fenofibrate and dylipidaemia – relevant, practical therapy. *Research Review* www.researchreview.com.au.

Singer, J., Palmas, W., Teresi, J. et al. (2012). Adiponectin and all-cause mortality in elderly people with type 2 diabetes. *Diabetes Care* https://doi.org/10.2337/dc11-2215.

Taylor, A., Price, K., Gill, T. et al. (2010). Morbidity – not just an older person's issue. Results from an Australian biomedical study. *BMC Public Health* **10**: 718.

United Kingdom Prospective Study (UKPDS) Group (1998). Effect of intensive blood glucose control with metformin on complications in overweight patients with type 2 diabetes. *Lancet* **352**: 854–865.

Vale, M., Jelinek, M., Best, J. et al. (2003). Coaching patients on achieving cardiovascular health (COACH): a multicenter randomized trial in patients with coronary heart disease. *Archives of Internal Medicine* **163**: 2775–2783.

Verdecchia, P., Angeli, F., Mazzotta, G., and Carofe, M. (2012). Ambulatory blood pressure monitoring: day-night dip and early-morning surge in blood pressure in hypertension. *Hypertension* **60**: 34–42.

Wang, H., Yuan, J., Zhang, B. et al. (2017). Phototherapy for treating foot ulcers in people with diabetes (review). *Cochrane database Systematic Reviews* (6): CD011979. https://doi.org/10.1002/1451858.CD011979.pub2.

Weber, C. and Schnell, O. (2009). The assessment of glycemic variability and its impact on diabetes-related complications: an overview. *Diabetes Technology & Therapeutics* **11** (10): 623–633.

Wells-Knecht, K., Zyzak, D., and Litchfield, J. (1995). Mechanism of autoxidative glycosylation: identification of glyoxal and arabinose as intermediates in the autooxidative modification of proteins by glucose. *Biochemistry* **34**: 3702–3709.

Wen, Y., Hung, L., Te, L. et al. (2012). Variability in hemoglobin A1c predicts all-cause mortality in patients with type 2 diabetes. *Journal of Diabetes and its Complications* **26** (4): 296–300.

White, W.B., Kupfer, S., Zannad, F. et al. (2016). Cardiovascular mortality in patients with type 2 diabetes and recent acute coronary syndromes from the EXAMINE trial. *Diabetes Care* **39** (7): 1267–1273.

Williams, J., Chimowitz, M., Cotsonis, G. et al. (2007). WASID investigators. Gender differences in outcomes among patients with symptomatic intracranial arterial stenosis. *Stroke* **38**: 2055–2062.

Wilmot, E., Edwardson, C., Achana, F. et al. (2012). Sedentary time in adults and the association with diabetes, cardiovascular disease and death: a systematic review and meta-analysis. *Diabetologia* https://doi.org/10.1007/s00125-012-2677-z.

Young, D., Furler, J., Vale, M. et al. (2007). Patient engagement and coaching for health: the PEACH study – a cluster randomised controlled trial using the telephone to coach people with type 2 diabetes to engage with their GPs to improve diabetes care. *BMC Family Practice* **8** (20): 8–13.

Zannad, F. (2008). Cardiovascular high risk patients – treat to protect, but whom? *Medscape Journal of Medicine* **10** (Suppl. 2): 1–11.

Zhang, Y., Hu, G., Yuan, Z., and Chen, L. (2012). Glycosylated haemoglobin in relation to cardiovascular outcomes and death in patients with type 2 diabetes: a systematic review and meta-analysis. *PLoS One* **7** (8): e42551.

Diabetes and eye disease

Antonetti, D., Barber, A., Bronson, S. et al. (2006). Diabetic retinopathy: seeing beyond glucose-induced microvascular disease. *Diabetes* **55** (9): 401–411.

Clemons, T., Milton, R., Klein, R. et al. (2005). Risk factors for the incidence of advance age-related macular degeneration in the Age-Related Eye Disease Study (AREDS). *AREDS report no. 19. Ophthalmology* **112**: 533–539.

Gupta, A., Gupta, V., Thapar, S., and Bhansali, A. (2004). Lipid-lowering drug atorastatin as an adjunct in the management of diabetic macular oedema. *American Journal of Ophthalmology* **137** (4): 675–682.

Khan, J., Shahid, H., and Thurlby, D. (2006). Age-related macular degeneration and sun exposure, iris colour, and skin sensitivity to sunlight. *British Journal of Ophthalmology* **90**: 29–32.

van Leeuwen, R., Boekhoorn, S., and Vingerling, J. (2005). Dietary intake of antioxidants and risk of age-related macular degeneration. *Journal American Medical Association* **294**: 3101–3107.

Lim, J. (2006). Risk factors for age-related macular degeneration. *eMedicine.* http://www.medscape.com/viewarticle/532642 1–5 (accessed November 2007).

Nurko, S. (2006). Anemia in chronic kidney disease: causes, diagnosis, treatment. *Cleveland Clinic Journal of Medicine* **73** (3): 289.

Ryan, C., Geckle, M., and Orchard, T. (2003). Cognitive efficiency declines over time in adults with type 1 diabetes: effect of micro- and macrovascular complications. *Diabetologia* **46** (7): 940–948. https://doi.org/10.1007/soo125–003-1128–2.

Seddon, J., Gensler, G., Milton, R. et al. (2004). Association between C-reactive protein and age-related macular degeneration. *Journal American Medical Association* **292**: 704–710.

Sen, K., Misra, A., Kumar, A., and Pandey, R. (2002). Simvastatin retards progression of retinopathy in diabetic patients with hypercholeserolaemia. *Diabetes Research and Clinical Practice* **56** (1): 1–11.

Stanway, L. (2012). Multi-ability alert dogs for people with diabetes and visual impairment. *Diabetes Voice* **57** (1): 39–42.

Diabetes and renal disease

American Society of Nephrology (ASN) (2012). Kidney disease recommendations. *Clinical Journal of the American Society Nephrology* http://www.asnonline.org/publications/kidneynews/.../2012/KN_2012_07_jul.pdf.

Bosman, D., Winkler, A., Marsden, J. et al. (2001). Anemia with erythropoietin deficiency occurs early in diabetic nephropathy. *Diabetes Care* **24** (3): 495–499.

Briguori, C. (2007). Renal insufficiency following contrast media administration trial (REMEDIAL): a randomized comparison of 3 preventative strategies. *Circulation* **115**: 1211–1217.

Cass, A., Cunningham, J., Arnold, P. et al. (2002). Delayed referral to a nephrologist: outcomes among patients who survive at least one year. *Medical Journal of Australia* **177** (3): 135–138.

Chan, M. (2001). Nutritional management in progressive renal failure. *Current Therapeutics* **42** (7): 23–27.

Chan, M. (2008). Nutrition, diabetes and chronic kidney disease. *Diabetes Management Journal* **25**: 6–7.

Chan, M. (2012). Nutrition, diabetes and chronic kidney disease. *Australian Diabetes Educator* **15** (3): 18–23.

Chobanian, A., Bakris, G., and Black, H. (2003). National Heart, Lung, and Blood Institute Joint National Committee on Prevention, Detection, Evaluation, and Treatment of High Blood Pressure National High Blood Pressure Education Program Coordinating Committee. The Seventh Report of the Joint National Committee on Prevention, Detection, Evaluation, and Treatment of High Blood Pressure: the JNC 7 report. *Journal of the American Medical Association* **289**: 2560–2572.

Choudhury, D. and Luna-Salazar, C. (2008). Preventive health care in chronic kidney disease and end stage renal failure. *Clinical Practice Nephrology* 4 (4): 3–16.

Churchill, D. (1996). Results and limitations of peritoneal dialysis. In: *Replacement of Renal Function by Dialysis* (eds. C. Jacobs, C. Kjellstrand, K. Koch and F. Winchester). Boston: Kluwer Academic Publishers.

Culleton, B. (2007). Frequent nocturnal hemodialysis may have better outcomes than conventional hemodialysis. *Journal of the American Medical Association* 298: 1291–1299.

DCCT (Diabetes Control and Complications Trial Research Group) (1993). The effect of intensive treatment of diabetes on the development and progression of long-term complications in insulin-dependent diabetes mellitus. *New England Journal of Medicine* 329: 977–986.

Duncan, H., Pittman, S., Govil, A. et al. (2007). Alternative medicine use in dialysis patients: potential for good and bad. *Nephrology and Clinical Practice* 105 (3): 108–113.

Dunning, T., MacGinley, R., and Ward, G. (2012). Is point of care testing for anaemia (Hb) and microalbumin feasible in people with type 2 diabetes attending diabetic outpatient clinics? *Renal Society of Australasia Journal* 8 (2): 76–81.

Dunning, T. and Martin, P. (2018). Palliative and end of life care of people with diabetes: Issues, challenges and strategies. *Diabetes Research and Clinical Practice* 143: 454–463.

Ernst, E. (1998). Harmless herbs? A review of the recent literature. *American Journal of Medicine* 104 (2): 170–178.

Gilbert, R., Tsalamandris, C., Allen, T. et al. (1998). Early nephropathy predicts vision-threatening retinal disease in patients with type I diabetes mellitus. *Journal of the American Society of Nephrology* 9: 85–89.

Hays, R., Kallich, J., Mapes, D. et al. (1994). Development of the kidney disease quality of life instrument (KDQOL-SF). *Quality of Life Research* 3: 329–338.

Hodeib, H., Hagras, M., Abelhai, D. et al. (2019). Galectin-3 as a prognostic biomarker for diabetic nephropathy. *Diabetes, Metabolic Syndrome and Obesity: Targets and Therapy* 12: 325–331.

HOPE (Heart Outcomes Prevention Evaluation Study Investigators) (2000). Effects of ramipril on cardiovascular and microvascular outcomes in people with diabetes mellitus: results of the HOPE study and MICRO-HOPE substudy. *Lancet* 355: 253–259.

Howes, L. (2001). Dosage alterations in the elderly: importance of mild renal impairment. *Current Therapeutics* 42 (7): 33–35.

Iliescu, E. (2006). Glycaemic control often poor among hemodialysis patients. *Diabetes Care* 29: 2247–2251.

Kalantar-Zadeh, K., Kuwae, N., and Wu, D. (2006). Association of body fat and its changes over time with quality of life and prospective mortality in hemodialysis patients. *American Journal Clinical Nursing* 83: 202–210.

Keane, W. (2001). Metabolic pathogenesis of cardiorenal disease. *American Journal of Kidney Disease* 38 (6): 1372–1375.

Kerr, P. (2008). Diabetic nephropathy: who to refer and when. *Diabetes Management Journal* 25: 4–5.

Ko, R. (1998). Adulterants in Asian patent medicines. *New England Journal of Medicine* 339: 847.

Kovesdy, C., Furth, S., Zoccali, C., and for the World Kidney Day Steering Committee (2017). Obesity and kidney disease: hidden consequences of the epidemic. *Journal Diabetes Nursing* 21 (2): 45–48.

Lehto, S., Ronnemaa, T., Pyorala, K., and Laakso, M. (1999). Poor glycaemic control predicts coronary heart disease events in patients with type 1 diabetes without nephropathy. *Arteriosclerosis Thrombosis Vascular Biology* 19: 1014–1019.

Levin, S., Coburn, J., Henderson, W. et al. (2000). Effect of intensive glycaemic control on microalbuminuria in type 2 diabetes. Veterans affairs cooperative study on glycaemic control and complications in type 2 diabetes. *Diabetes Care* 23 (910): 1478–1485.

Lopes, A., Elder, S., Ginsberg, N. et al. (2007). Lack of appetite in haemodialysis patients: associations with patient characteristics, indicators of nutritional status and outcomes in the international DOPPS. *Nephrology Dialysis Transplant* 22 (12): 3538–3546.

Meschi, M., Detrenis, S., Musini, S. et al. (2006). Facts and fallacies concerning the prevention of contrast medium-induced nephropathy. *Critical Care Medicine* 34 (8): 2060–2068.

Moustakas, J., Bennett, P., Nicholson, J., and Tranter, S. (2012). The needs of older people with advanced chronic kidney disease choosing supportive care: a review. *Renal Society of Australasia Journal* 8 (2): 70–75.

Myhre, M. (2000). Herbal remedies, nephropathies and renal disease. *Nephrology Nursing Journal* 27 (5): 473–480.

National Kidney Foundation (2002). Clinical practice guidelines for nutrition in chronic renal failure. Kidney outcome quality initiative. *American Journal of Kidney Disease* 35 (6 Supp. 2).

Oomichi, T., Emoto, M., Tabata, E. et al. (2007). Impact of glycemic control on survival of diabetic patients on chronic regular hemodialysis: a 7-year observational study. *Diabetes Care* 29: 1496–1500.

Ravid, M., Savin, H., and Jutrin, I. (1993). Long-term stabilising effect of angiotensin-converting enzyme on plasma creatinine and on proteinuria in normotensive type II diabetic patients. *Annals of Internal Medicine* 118: 577–581.

Ritz, E. (2001). Advances in nephrology: success and lessons learnt from diabetes. *Nephrology Dialysis Transplant* 16 (Suppl. 7): 46–50.

Rudnick, M., Kesselheim, A., and Goldfarb, S. (2006). Contrast-induced nephropathy: how it develops, how to prevent it. *Cleveland Clinic Journal of Medicine* 73 (1): 75–87.

Rutecki, G. and Whittier, F. (1993). Intraperitoneal insulin in diabetic patients on peritoneal dialysis. In: *Dialysis Therapy* (eds. A. Nissenson and R. Fine). Philadelphia: Hanley & Belfus.

Scales, C., Smith, A., Hanley, J. et al. (2012). Urologic disease in America project: prevalence of kidney stones in the United States. *European Urology* 62: 160–165.

Schetz, M., Vanhorebeck, I., Wouters, P. et al. (2008). Tight blood glucose control is renoprotective in critically ill patients. *Journal American Society of Nephrology* https://doi.org/10.1681/asn2006101091.

Terrill, B. (2002). *Renal Nursing: A Practical Approach*. Melbourne: Ausmed Publications.

Wu, M., Yu, C., and Yang, C. (1997). Poor pre-dialysis glycaemic control is a predictor of mortality in type II diabetic patients on maintenance haemodialysis. *Nephrology Dialysis Transplant* 12: 2105–2110.

Yu, M., Rees-Lyles, C., Bent-Shaw, L., and Young, B. (2012). Risk factor, age and sex differences in chronic kidney disease prevalence in a diabetic cohort: the pathways study. *Nephrology* 36 (3): 245–251.

Peripheral and autonomic neuropathy

Abusaisha, B., Constanzi, J., and Boulton, A. (1998). Acupuncture for treatment of chronic painful diabetic neuropathy: a long-term study. *Diabetes Research Clinical Practice* 39: 115–121.

Aly, N. and Weston, P. (2002). Autonomic neuropathy in older people with diabetes. *Journal of Diabetes Nursing* 6 (1): 10–14.

Apelqvist, J. and Larsson, J. (2000). What is the most effective way to reduce incidence of amputation in the diabetic foot? *Diabetes/Metabolism Research and Reviews* 16 (Suppl. 1): s75–s83.

Bakker, D. (2000). Hyperbaric oxygen therapy and the diabetic foot. *Diabetes/Metabolism Research and Reviews* 16 (Suppl. 1): s55–s58.

Bianchi, C., Penno, G., Pancani, F. et al. (2007). Nontraditional cardiovascular risk factors contribute to peripheral arterial disease in patients with type 2 diabetes. *Diabetes research and clinical practice* 78 (2): 246–253.

Boulton, A., Gries, F., and Jervell, J. (1998). Guidelines for the diagnosis and outpatient management of diabetic peripheral neuropathy. *Diabetes Medicine* 15: 508–514.

Brismar, K., Johansson, T., Lindström, B. et al. (2007). C-peptide replacement therapy and sensory nerve function in type 1 diabetic neuropathy. *Diabetes Care* 30 (1): 71–76.

Brod, M. (1998). Quality of life issues in patients with diabetes and lower limb extremity ulcers: patients and caregivers. *Quality Life Research* 7: 365–372.

DRS (1981). Photocoagulation treatment of proliferative diabetic retinopathy: clinical implications of DRS findings. DRS Report No. 8. *Ophthalmology* 88: 583–600.

Edmonds, M., Bates, M., Doxford, M. et al. (2000). New treatments in ulcer healing and wound infection. *Diabetes/Metabolism Research and Reviews* 16 (Suppl. 1): s51–s54.

EDTRS (1991). Early photocoagulation for diabetic retinopathy: EDTRS Report No. 9. *Ophthalmology* 98 (Suppl): 767–785.

Harding, K., Jones, V., and Price, P. (2000). Topical treatment: which dressing to choose. *Diabetes/Metabolism Research and Reviews* 16 (Suppl. 1): s47–s50.

Hotta, N. (2006). Epalrestat may delay progression and reduce symptoms of diabetic neuropathy. *Diabetes Care* 29: 1538–1544.

Karlson, B., Herlitz, J., and Hjalmarson, A. (1993). Prognosis of acute myocardial infarction in diabetic and nondiabetic patients. *Diabetic Medicine* 10: 449–454.

Lipsky, B. and Berendt, A. (2000). Principles and practice of antibiotic therapy of diabetic foot infections. *Diabetes/Metabolism Research and Reviews* 16 (Suppl. 1): s42–s46.

Litchy, W., Dyck, P., Tesfaye, S., and for the MBBQ Study Group (2002). Diabetic peripheral neuropathy (DPN) assessed by neurological examination and composite scores is improved with LY333531 treatment. *Diabetes* 45: A197.

Locke, D., Ill, G., and Camileri, M. (2000). Gastrointestinal symptoms among persons with diabetes in the community. *Archives of Internal Medicine* 160: 2808–2816.

Lowe, J. (2002). Hypertension in diabetes. *Australian Prescriber* 25 (1): 8–10.

Malmberg, K., Ryden, L., Efendic, S. et al. (1995). Randomised trial of insulin–glucose infusion followed by subcutaneous insulin treatment in diabetic patients with acute myocardial infarction (DIGAMI study): effects on mortality at 1 year. *Journal of the American College of Cardiology* 26: 57–65.

Papas, N., Boulton, A., Malik, R. et al. (2013). A simple new non-invasive sweat indicator test for the diagnosis of diabetic neuropathy. *Diabetic Medicine* 30: 525–534.

Pecorara, R. (1990). Pathways to diabetic limb amputation. *Diabetes Care* 13 (5): 513–530.

Sadiya, A. (2012). Nutritional therapy for the management of gastric paresis: a clinical review. *Diabetes, Metabolic Syndrome and Obesity Targets and Therapy* 5: 329–335.

Semla, T., Beizer, J., and Higbee, M. (eds.) (2002). *Geriatric Dosage Handbook*. Hudson, Ohio: Lexi-Company.

Spallone, V. and Menzinger, G. (1997). Autonomic neuropathy: clinical and instrumental findings. *Clinical Neuroscience* **4** (96): 346–358.

Standl, E. and Schnell, O. (2000). A new look at the heart in diabetes: from ailing to failing. *Diabetologia* **43**: 1455–1469.

Steinberg, F. (1991). Rehabilitation after amputation. *Diabetes Spectrum* **4** (1): 5–9.

Todd, M., Welsh, J., Key, M. et al. (2008). Survey of Doppler use in lymphoedema practitioners in the UK. *British Journal Community Nursing* **13** (4): S11–S12, S14, S16–17.

UKPDS Group (1998). Intensive blood glucose control with sulphonylureas or insulin compared with conventional treatment and risk of complications in patients with type 2 diabetes (UKPDS 33). *Lancet* **352**: 837–853.

Vinik, A., Park, T., Stansberry, K., and Henger, P. (2000). Diabetic neuropathy. *Diabetologia* **43**: 957–973.

Wegener, M., Borsch, G., Schaffsten, J. et al. (1990). Gastrointestional transit disorders in patients with insulin-treated diabetes. *Digestive Disorders* **8** (1): 23–26.

Zhang, W., Kamiya, H., and Ekberg, K. (2007). C-peptide improves neuropathy in type 1 diabetic BB/Wor-rats. *Diabetes Metabolism Reviews* **12**: 1471–1488.

Ziegler, D., Nowak, H., Kempler, P. et al. (2004). Treatment of symptomatic diabetic neuropathy with antioxidant alpha-lipoicacid: a meta-analysis. *Diabetic Medicine* **21**: 114–121.

Chapter 9

Management in Hospital, Surgery, and Investigations

Think beyond just, OK, what's their blood sugar?

(Dr. Tony Madsen, ED Physician, 2019)

Emergency department

Key points

- People with diabetes often present to the emergency department (ED) and often referred for investigations and/or admitted to hospital.
- Diabetes is the most common disease classification for people > age 65 who visit ED and they have longer stays in ED and require more interventions,
- Coordinating care, rapid assessment and identifying and managing the cause of the presentation, managing glycaemia and stabilisation are important care goals.
- Atypical presentations and 'silent' disease such as pain, urinary tract infections (UTI), and cardiac events can complicate assessment and diagnosis.

Rationale

People with diabetes present to ED with an acute/urgent condition such as hyperosmolar hyper-glycaemic states (HHS), diabetic ketoacidosis (DKA) or for nondiabetes-related reasons such as trauma. Nondiabetes-related presentation affects metabolic status, consequently diabetes must be considered when deciding care. Yet they are often treated differently, which can lead to more serious complications and influence diagnosis and treatment (Wells et al. 2018). Common reasons people with diabetes present to ED are chronic obstructive pulmonary disease (COPD), renal disease, cardiac disease, peripheral vascular disease, hypo- and hyperglycaemia, and fall-related injuries (Castillo 2019). Diabetes can be diagnosed in ED, e.g., T1DM presenting with DKA and T2DM presenting in an HHS.

For new presentations of diabetes, keeping the person safe and coordinating care are important to outcomes (Ford et al. 2014).

Care of People with Diabetes: A Manual for Healthcare Practice, Fifth Edition. Trisha Dunning and Alan Sinclair.
© 2020 John Wiley & Sons Ltd. Published 2020 by John Wiley & Sons Ltd.

Management strategies

Determine whether the person has T1DM or T2DM and their usual self-care and medicine regime, including self-prescribed and complementary medicines and the reasons for the presenting to ED. The assessment and any investigations will be informed by that information. Ford et al. (2014) indicate that investigations could include:

- Symptoms, e.g. nausea, vomiting, altered conscious state (Glasgow Coma Scale)
- Temperature, pulse, and respiration
- Various blood tests, including blood glucose and ketones, depending on the severity of the illness. If the person is critically ill, blood gases, cardiac enzymes, and other investigative procedures might be indicated.
- Screen for infection.
- General urinalysis, but urine ketones are not as accurate as blood ketones and may be misleading if the person is using sodium glucose cotransporter inhibitor-2 (SGLT-2) medicines, which can cause euglycaemic ketoacidosis (Chapter 5).
- Pregnancy test in women of childbearing age might be indicated.
- Drug and alcohol screen.
- Assess older people for geriatric syndromes and frailty.
- Consider mental health conditions.
- Various X-rays, MRIs, EEG may be warranted, such as for atypical chest pain.
- Perform an HbA1c if the blood glucose is >7.8 mmol/l (>140 mg/dl) when admitted to hospital.

Severe hypoglycaemia is a significant reason people with diabetes present to ED. These people might be treated with glucagon (if a dose was not already given) but the sometimes need IV glucose to restore the blood glucose to a safe level. Once they recover, their hypoglycaemia management plan and glucose-lowering medicines (GLM) doses and dose regimen might need to be reviewed (see Chapter 6). Likewise, their sick-day management plan and medicines might need to be reviewed if they present with HHS or DKA (Chapter 7). Counselling for repeat attendances for the same reason or if suicide ideation is indicated might be advisable (Chapter 15).

Indications for hospital admission depend on the individual, the presentation, and clinical judgement. Some reasons include (ADA 2019):

- Life-threatening acute metabolic decompensation – HHS, DKA, lactic acidosis (rare), and sometimes severe hypoglycaemia and neuroglycopenia.
- New diagnosis in children and adolescents and possibly older people.
- Frequent presentations for chronic complications and inadequate metabolic control, e.g. to assess and manage end-stage renal disease.
- New diagnosis of insulin-requiring diabetes in pregnancy if the blood glucose cannot be stabilised otherwise.
- Cancer and other associated conditions (Chapter 10).

Surgical procedures

Key points

- Organisations have policies in place that support clinicians to deliver quality care to people with diabetes during surgical procedures and diagnostic investigations.
- Surgery induces the counter-regulatory response that can increase the blood glucose six to eight times higher than normal in people with and without diabetes. Optimal control before, during, and after surgery reduces morbidity and mortality and length of stay.

- Preventing hyperglycaemia reduces the risk of adverse outcomes in people with diabetes.
- Morning procedures are desirable.
- Insulin should never be omitted in people with type 1 diabetes.
- Complications should be stabilised before, during, and after surgery.
- Cease oral glucose lowering medicines 24–36 hours before the procedure depending on the particular medicine and their duration of action; but note some experts recommend continuing oral agents until the day of surgery if the blood glucose is high.
- Ascertain whether the person is using any complementary therapies, especially herbal medicines, with a high risk of interacting with conventional medicines and/or causing bleeding. Provide advice about how to manage their CAM in the operative/investigative stages.
- Ascertain whether the person can following information about pre- and positive operative care and/or has support to do so after discharge.
- An insulin-glucose infusion is the most effective way to manage hyperglycaemia in the operative period.

Rationale

Diabetes is associated with an increased need for surgical procedures and invasive investigations and higher morbidity than nondiabetics. Anaesthesia and surgery are associated with a complex metabolic and neuroendocrine response that involves the release of counter-regulatory hormones and glucagon leading to insulin resistance, gluconeogenesis, hyperglycaemia, and neutrophil dysfunction, which impairs wound healing. The stress response also occurs in people without diabetes but is more pronounced and difficult to manage in people with diabetes due to the underlying metabolic abnormalities. Advances in diabetes management, surgical techniques, anaesthetic medicines, and intensive care medicine have significantly improved surgical outcomes for people with diabetes.

Minor surgery refers to day procedures and major surgery to procedures where the individual is admitted overnight or longer (Australian Diabetes Society (ADS) 2012).

The Joint Commission on Surgical Care Improvement Project (SCIP) (2012) included 'tight' diabetes control as an indicator for surgical improvement.

Introduction

People with diabetes undergo surgery for similar reasons to those without diabetes; however, because of the long-term complications of diabetes, they are more likely to require:

- Cardiac procedures such as:
  - angioplasty or stents
  - bypass surgery
- Ulcer debridement, amputations (toes, feet)
- Eye surgery such as cataract removal, repair retinal detachment, vitrectory
- Carpal tunnel decompression
- Bariatric surgery due to the increase in overweight and obesity
- Dental procedures

Surgical-induced stress results in endocrine, metabolic, and long-term effects that have implications for the management of people with diabetes undergoing surgery (see Table 9.1). Stress induces hyperglycaemia, which causes osmotic diuresis, increased hepatic glucose output, lipolysis, and insulin resistance. Unless these metabolic abnormalities are controlled, surgical stress increases the risk of DKA, HHS, and lactic acidosis (see Chapter 7), infection, impaired wound healing, and cerebral ischaemia. The risk of HHS is high in procedures such as cardiac bypass surgery and has a high mortality rate (Dagogo-Jack and Alberti 2002).

In addition, anaesthesia and surgical stress, as well as medicines, induce gastrointestinal instability that can compound gastric autonomic neuropathy and lead to nausea and vomiting and predispose the individual to dehydration and exacerbate fluid loss via osmotic diuresis and blood loss during surgery. As a result, electrolyte changes, particularly in potassium and magnesium, increase the risk of cardiac arrhythmias, ischaemic events, and acute renal failure (Dagogo-Jack and Alberti 2002). The risk is particularly high in people with chronic hyperglycaemia ($HbA_{1c} > 8\%$), existing diabetes complications, older people, and those who are obese, all of which are associated with increased risk of interoperative and postoperative complications (Dickerson et al. 2003; ADS 2012).

Obesity is associated with functional risks in addition to the metabolic consequences of surgery that need to be considered when positioning the patient. The respiratory system is affected and functional residual capacity and expiratory reserve volume may be reduced possibly due to excess weight on the chest wall and/or displacement of the diaphragm. Severe obesity can lead to hypoventilation and obstructive sleep apnoea. These factors predispose the individual to aspiration pneumonia. Various cardiac changes increase the risk of heart failure and inadequate tissue oxygenation. In addition, the risk of pressure ulcers is increased due to the weight, and activity level is often compromised, increasing the risk of venous stasis and emboli.

The need for nutritional support may be overlooked in obese individuals and protein deprivation can develop because protein and carbohydrate are used as the main energy sources during surgery rather than fat. In addition, energy expenditure is higher, which impacts on wound healing (Dickerson 2004; Mirtallo 2008). In addition people with sarcopenia and frailty may already have nutritional deficits and require frailty assessment prior to surgery (Eamer et al. 2017). Likewise, a comprehensive geriatric assessment can improve postoperative outcomes including length of stay (Harari et al. 2007).

Different types of surgery present specific risks, as do the person's age: the very young and older people are particularly at risk. The specific risks are summarised in Table 9.1. The blood

Table 9.1   Hormonal, metabolic, and long-term effects of surgery.

Hormonal	Metabolic	Long-term effects if optimal blood glucose control is not achieved
↑ Secretion of[a] epinephrine, norepinephrine, ACTH, cortisol and growth hormone ↓ secretion of insulin due to impaired beta cell responsiveness Insulin resistance	Catabolic state and ↑ metabolic rate Hyperglycaemia Insulin resistance ↓ Glucose utilisation and glycogen storage ↑ Gluconeogenesis ↓ Protein catabolism and reduced amino acid and protein synthesis in skeletal muscle ↑ Lipolysis and formation of ketone bodies ↓ Storage of fatty acids in the liver Osmotic diuresis with electrolyte loss and compromised circulating volume ↑ Risk of cerebrovascular accident, myocardial arrhythmias infarction electrolyte disorders ↑ Blood pressure and heart rate ↓ Peristalsis	Loss of lean body mass – impaired wound healing, ↓ resistance to infection Loss of adipose tissue Deficiency of essential amino acids, vitamins, minerals, and essential fatty acids Surgical complications Longer length of stay

[a] Norepinephrine is mostly augmented during surgery and epinephrine postoperatively. Stress stimulates glucagon secretion from the pancreatic alpha cells and together with growth hormone and cortisol, potentiates the effects of norepinephrine and epinephrine. Cortisol increases gluconeogenesis.

glucose must be controlled to prevent DKA and HHS, promote healing, and reduce the risk of infection postoperatively. The target blood glucose range in the perioperative period is 5–10 mmol/l (ADS 2012).

Hyperglycaemia inhibits white cell function and increases coagulability (Kirschner 1993). The magnitude of the metabolic/hormonal response depends on the severity and duration of the surgical procedure, metabolic control before, during, and after surgery, and the presence of complications such as sepsis, acidosis, hypotension, and hypovolaemia (Marks et al. 1998; ADS 2012). Significantly, metabolic disturbances can be present in euglycaemic states (De and Child 2001). Surgery is often performed as a day procedure, often without appropriate consideration of the effects of surgical and the related psychological stress on metabolic control. A multidisciplinary approach to planning is important.

People with diabetes are at risk of readmission (Morris and Richman 2017). These researchers found the average 30-day readmission risk in the US Veteran Affairs Study (n = 237 000) was 11%. Most readmissions occurred in the first postoperative week and then the rate declined. Admission risk depended on the type of procedure and the individual. Renal failure was the most significant risk factor. Wound complication was a common reason for readmission.

Surgery should be postponed if the HbA1c is >9% (75 mmol/mol), if it is safe to do so. The target blood glucose range is 5–10 mmol/l, but may be tighter is critical illness if hypoglycaemia can be avoided (ADA 2004).

Children with diabetes undergoing surgical procedures

Generally, children with type 1 and type 2 diabetes needing general anaesthesia should be admitted to hospital and must receive insulin to prevent ketosis even if they are fasting and should be managed with a glucose infusion to prevent hypoglycaemia if they need to fast for more than two hours (Betts et al. 2009). Blood glucose must be monitored hourly prior to and every 30–60 minutes during surgery to detect hypo- and hyperglycaemia. As in adults it is best to perform surgery when metabolic control is optimal and children should be first on the list if possible (Betts et al. 2009; ADS 2012). An IV insulin-glucose infusion should be commenced two hours prior to surgery.

Older people with diabetes and surgical procedures

The Geriatric Surgery Expert Panel of the American College of Surgeons recently released a comprehensive guideline for assessing older people prior to surgery (Chow et al. 2012). The recommendations are not specific to people with diabetes, but diabetes-related information could be incorporated into the guidelines. In addition to conducting a thorough history and physical assessment, the Expert Panel recommended assessing the individual's:

- Type of diabetes and diabetes management and blood glucose and HbA1c.
- Cognitive ability and capacity to understand the proposed surgery (give informed consent).
- Mental health: undertake a depression screen.
- Risk of developing delirium postoperatively.
- Alcohol, tobacco, and other substance use.
- Functional status.
- Falls history.
- Frailty status (see Chapter 12).
- Nutritional status.
- Medicine regimen to determine whether the regimen may need to be adjusted and to assess the level of polypharmacy and adherence to their medicine regimen. (Note information about insulin and other GLMs in this chapter.)
- Expectations of the surgery.
- Social and family support.

- Undertake appropriate investigations. These include renal function tests haemoglobin, and serum albumin, and in some cases, white cell count, platelet count, coagulation studies, electrolytes and blood glucose, and a urinalysis to detect UTI.

Tests of physical and cognitive function are discussed in Chapter 12. Interestingly, the guidelines do not mention CAM use, but as indicated, people with diabetes use CAM and many herbal medicines interact with conventional medicines and increase the risk of adverse events. It is also important to assess older people's self-care skills and available support at home.

Management

The aims of management include the following:

(1) Identify underlying problems that could compromise surgery and recovery by undertaking comprehensive presurgical assessment and manage them prior to surgery (ADS 2012; Dhatariya et al. 2012).
(2) Achieve normal metabolism by supplying sufficient insulin to counterbalance the increase in stress hormones during fasting, surgery, and postoperatively and avoid the need for prolonged fasting.
(3) Normalise metabolic control using regimens that minimise the possibility of errors and have the fewest adverse outcomes: target blood glucose range. 5–10 mmol/l and is best achieved with an insulin-glucose infusion (ADS 2012).
(4) Supply adequate carbohydrate to prevent catabolism, hypoglycaemia, and ketosis.
(5) Ensure that the patient undergoes surgery in the best possible physical condition.
(6) Prevent:
    - Hypoglycaemia, children <5 years are prone to hypoglycaemia during anaesthesia and surgery (Kirschner 1993). Undertake a hypoglycaemia risk assessment and mange risks (Chapter 6).
    - Hyperglycaemia predisposing the patient to dehydration, electrolyte imbalance, ketoacidosis, and hyperosmolar states.
    - Complications of surgery.
    - Electrolyte imbalance.
    - Worsening of preexisting diabetic complications.
    - Infection.
(7) Avoid undue psychological stress.
(8) Ensure safe discharge home or transfer to rehabilitation or other relevant services.

Preoperative care

Good preoperative care is important for both major and minor procedures. Preadmission clinics have an important role in identifying and managing preventable surgical risks. Sometimes people need to be admitted two to three days before major surgery to stabilise blood glucose levels and manage complications (see Table 9.2). Many procedures only require a day admission. In all cases, careful explanation about what is required and *written* instructions that are at a suitable language level and are culturally relevant are vital.

The individual's blood glucose profile needs to be reviewed and their diabetes regimen may need to be adjusted prior to surgery to achieve good metabolic control. Erratic control could indicate the presence of infection that should be treated prior to surgery. Alternatively, it could indicate brittle diabetes that might require investigation because of the risk of hypoglycaemia and delayed gastric emptying depending on the underlying cause (Chapter 10). If possible, schedule for a morning procedure to avoid the need for prolonged fasting and counter-regulatory hormone release that leads to hyperglycaemia.

Table 9.2 Common complications of diabetes that can affect surgery and postoperative recovery.

Complication	Possible consequences	Preoperative evaluation
Cardiovascular	Hypertension.	Careful history and examination
	Ischaemic heart disease.	ECG
	Cardiomyopathy.	Manage existing conditions such as heart failure.
	Myocardial infarction – can be 'silent' and in the presence of autonomic neuropathy cause sudden tachycardia, bradycardia, and/or postural hypotension.	Assess for silent cardiac disease autonomic neuropathy; indicators include: shortness of breath, palpitations, ankle oedema, tiredness, and atypical chest pain
	Cerebrovascular disease.	Assess resting heart rate.
	Increased resting heart rate is associated with increased risk of death in older people.	Ask about daytime sleepiness or assess formally, for example, using the Epworth Sleepiness Scale (ESS).
	Daytime sleepiness is associated with 4.5-fold increased risk of stroke and other vascular events.	
Neuropathy Autonomic Peripheral	Cardiac as above.	Lying and standing blood pressure is abnormal if decrease >30 mmHg.
	Patient unable to maintain body temperature during anaesthesia.	Heart rate response on deep breathing is abnormal if increase >10 beats/min.
	Pressure areas on feet and ulceration.	Foot assessment; assess for active and occult infection and signs of neuropathy.
	Foot infection.	
	Falls risk increases postoperatively.	
Renal	Nephropathy may affect medication excretion.	Urine culture to detect UTI, which should be treated with the relevant antibiotics.
	Urinary tract infection (UTI) may be silent and predispose to sepsis.	Microalbuminuria and creatinine clearance, eGFR.
	Acute renal failure and the need for dialysis.	Blood electrolytes, correct potassium >5 mmol/l before surgery.
	Risk of UTI increases if catheterisation is needed.	
Respiratory Airway	Obese people and smokers are prone to chest infections.	Counsel to stop smoking.
	Obesity may be associated with reduced respiratory reserve and displacement of the diaphragm.	Chest physiotherapy.
	Reduced tissue oxygenation.	Chest X-ray.
	Soft tissue, ligament, and joint thickening might involve the neck, making it difficult to extend the neck and intubate and might predispose the individual to neck injury and postoperative pain.	Blood gases.
		Nebulised oxygen pre- and postoperatively if indicated.
		See test for musculoskeletal disease (see page 341–342).
		Take extra care of the neck.
Gastrointestinal	Autonomic neuropathy can lead to gastric stasis delayed gastric emptying, gastric reflux, regurgitation, and aspiration on anaesthesia induction.	Assess history of heartburn or reflux and whether the person sleeps in an upright position.
	Ileus.	A H_2 antagonist and metoclopramide might be indicated preoperatively.
	May need to modify nutritional support if required postoperatively and given enterally.	Erratic food absorption can affect blood glucose levels.
Eyes	Cataracts, glaucoma, and retinopathy can be exacerbated by sudden rise in blood pressure.	Assess retinopathy stage.
Neutrophil dysfunction	Increased risk of infection.	Check for possible foci of infection: including feet, teeth, and gums, UTI.
	Inability to mount an appropriate response to infection.	Ensure optimal blood glucose control.
		Optimise vascular function.
Polypharmacy	Risk of medicine interactions with anaesthetic agents and postoperative medicines.	Medicine review
	Risk of lactic acidosis increases with metformin.	Ask about complementary medicines.
	Some medicines increase the risk of hyperglycaemia some hypoglycaemia.	Give the person clear, concise written instructions about how to manage their medicines preoperatively and postoperatively on discharge.
Musculoskeletal	Difficulties with intubation and tube placement.	Assess, for example, prayer sign, Dupuytren's contracture, trigger finger.
	Falls risk increases.	Check for foot abnormality, including Charcot foot.

(Continued)

Table 9.2   (Continued)

Complication	Possible consequences	Preoperative evaluation
Sarcopenia and frailty	Undernutrition can compromise would healing and contribute to hypoglycaemia. Loss of muscle mass (protein) and flexibility increases falls risk.	Undertake a nutrition review and frailty assessment, which could be part of a comprehensive geriatric assessment. Encourage early ambulation.
Obesity	Increased systemic vascular resistance can lead to reduced tissue oxygenation and increased risk of lactic acidosis in people on metformin, especially if renal function is compromised and those with surgical wound infections. Sleep apnoea and associated daytime sleepiness with associated risk of cardiovascular events. Difficulty intubating the person. Assumption that the person is well nourished when in fact nutritional deficiencies, especially protein, are common. High prevalence of hypertriglyceridaemia. Cardiovascular and respiratory effects, which affect postoperative nutrition support if it is required. Non-alcoholic fatty liver. Risk of pressure ulcers.	Assess nutritional status. Assess cardiovascular and respiratory status. Ask about daytime sleepiness or assess formally, for example, using the ESS. Check skin condition.

Many of the conditions described here may be documented in the person's medical record and they may undergo regular complication assessment but health status can change rapidly especially older people. Therefore, the current complication status should be assessed prior to surgery. Hyperglycaemia must be controlled.

Clinician actions

(1) Confirm time and date of the operation and inform the patient, verbally an in writing/electronically in a format and language they can understand. Some services send reminder prompts.

(2) Explain the procedure and postoperative care to the patient and/or family members if appropriate; for example, a child. Those patients on controlled GLMs may require insulin *during surgery and immediately postoperatively*. They should be aware of this possibility. Insulin during the operative period does not mean that diet- or tablet-controlled patients will remain on insulin when they recover from the procedure. People controlled by diet and exercise with good metabolic control (HbA1c, 6.5%) may not require an IV insulin infusion for minor procedures but one to two hourly blood glucose monitoring is necessary (ADS 2012). Diet-controlled people who become hyperglycaemic may require supplemental insulin peri- and/or postoperatively. If control is suboptimal, and for procedures longer than one hour, an IV insulin/dextrose infusion is advisable (Dagogo-Jack and Alberti 2002; Kwon et al. 2003). In fact, Kwon et al. (2003) suggested 'Perioperative glucose evaluation and insulin administration in patients with hyperglycaemia are important quality targets'. It should be noted that suboptimal control is common in diet-treated individuals.

(3) Ensure all documentation is completed:
- Consent form
- Medication chart
- Monitoring guidelines
- Chest X-ray and other X-rays
- Scans, MRI (magnetic resonance imaging)
- Electrocardiogram (ECG)

(4) GLMs: Sulphonylureas, metformin, repaglinide, acarbose, thiazolidinediones (TZDs) and the incretins can be continued until the day of surgery to prevent preoperative

hyperglycaemia (ADS 2012). Chlorpropamide should be given 36 hours preoperatively because it is long acting; however, it is rarely used nowadays and is no longer available in some countries, e.g. Australia because of the significant hypoglycaemia risk. Metformin is traditionally ceased 24 hours preoperatively, but there is little evidence that ceasing metformin or continuing metformin in the perioperatic period increases the risk of hyperglycaemia. Metformin is associated with a risk of lactic acidosis, although the risk is low; however, surgical procedures, hypotension secondary to blood loss, myocardial ischaemia, sepsis, and anaestheic agents can contribute to the development of lactic acidosis, especially in people with renal impairment (Chapter 7). It can be recommended after surgery if the serum creatinine is in a safe range. Thus, a careful clinical assessment of the risks and benefits of ceasing/continuing metformin in individual patients is essential insulin therapy must be initiated before the procedure in people with type 1 diabetes. SGLT-2 inhibitors should be stepped before major surgery because of the risk of euglycaemic ketoacidosis (Australian Department of Health 2018) (Chapter 5).

(5) Encourage patients who smoke to stop.

(6) Assess:
- Metabolic status: blood glucose control, ketones in blood and urine, hydration status, nutritional status, presence of anaemia, diabetic symptoms.
- Educational level and understanding of diabetes.
- Family support available postoperatively.
- Any known allergies or medicine reactions. This should include asking about complementary therapies, particularly herbal medicines, because some herbs predispose the person to haemorrhage and/or interact with anaesthetic agents and should be stopped at least seven days prior to surgery (see Chapter 19).
- Presence of diabetic complications and other comorbidities, for example, renal, hepatic, cardiac disease (ECG for people >50 years to detect the risk of silent infarction is performed in some units), presence of neuropathy. Patients with autonomic neuropathy pose special problems during anaesthesia: gastroparesis delays gastric emptying and the stomach can be full despite fasting and increases the possibility of regurgitation and inhalation of vomitus; or the vasoconstrictive response to reduced cardiac output may be absent and they may not recognise hypoglycaemia.
- Current medication regimen. Ask about self-prescribed medicines and CAM as well.
- Presence of infection; check feet and be aware of silent infections such as UTI.
- Self-care potential and available home support.

Note: Complications should be managed before the operation where possible (see Table 9.2).

Major procedures

Major surgery refers to procedures requiring anaesthesia and lasting longer than one hour (Dagogo-Jack and Alberti 2002).

Minor procedures

Minor surgery may be performed on an outpatient basis. The metabolic risks are still a consideration if the person is expected to fast for the procedure. Ensure the procedure is fully explained to the patient at the time the appointment is made. Give *written* instructions about how to manage insulin, oral agents, and other medications. Preoperative care is the same as for major surgery on the day of operation as regards:

- Managing diabetes medicines
- Complication screening and managing complications when they are present

Morning procedure is preferred.

Day of the operation

For both major and minor procedures, premedication and routine preparation for the scheduled operative procedure should be performed according to the treatment sheet and standard protocols.

Where insulin is required, for example, type 1 diabetes, major surgery, and poor control, an IV insulin infusion is the preferred method of delivering the insulin. The insulin dose should be balanced with adequate calories to prevent starvation ketosis, for example, saline/dextrose delivered at a rate that matches the insulin dose (Alberti and Gill 1997; Gill 1997); see Chapter 5. Fluid replacement should be adequate to maintain intravascular volume; normal saline/dextrose in water is the preferred solution for this purpose. Preoperative hyperglycaemia especially if polyuria is present can cause significant fluid deficits and intracellular dehydration. Clinical signs of dehydration are:

- Thirst and a dry mouth: water loss <5% of body weight
- Capillary refill >2 seconds (normal <2 seconds), reduced skin turgor, sunken eyes, reduced urine output, orthostatic hypotension, fainting on standing, low CVP/JVP: water loss 5–10% of body weight
- Unconscious or shock: water loss >10% of body weight (French 2000)

Morning procedure

(1) Ensure oral medications were ceased on the operative day or earlier in specific circumstances.
(2) Fast from 12 midnight.
(3) Ascertain insulin regimen: commence insulin infusion.
(4) Monitor blood glucose one to two-hourly. If the individual an insulin pump they should continue their usual basal rate (Joslin Diabetes Centre 2009; ADS 2012; ADA 2019).

Afternoon procedure

(1) Fast after an early light breakfast.
(2) Ensure oral medications are ceased.
(3) Ascertain insulin dose, usually one-half to one-third of usual dose (best given after IV dextrose has been commenced).
(4) It is preferable for IV therapy to be commenced in the ward to:
    - Prevent hyperglycaemia and dehydration.
    - Reduce the risk of hypoglycaemia. This will depend on the surgical and anaesthetic and usual hospital procedure. Some anaesthetists prefer to commence the infusion in theatre. It is preferable to insert the IV line in theatre in children unless blood glucose is <4 mmol/l (Werther 1994).
(5) Monitor blood glucose.

Practice points

- Sliding insulin scales are NOT appropriate to manage blood glucose postoperatively if they are used as the only method of managing uses blood glucose because they can lead to inadequate/inappropriate insulin administration and wide swings in the blood glucose levels.
- Supplemental insulin doses given in addition to the individual's medicine regimen is appropriate. Supplemental insulin is always short- or rapid-acting insulin and given before meals in addition to the insulin/GLM dose prescribed at that time.

- A daily review of the individual's blood glucose pattern and insulin requirements is essential to enable insulin doses to be calculated for the following day (ADS 2012).
- Persistent hyperglycaemia could indicate underlying infection or surgical or metabolic complications and severe pain.
- People using continuous blood glucose monitoring and an insulin pump may be able to manage their glycaemia for minor procedures with the support of a diabetes educator and/or endocrinologist.

The anaesthetist is usually responsible for intraoperative blood glucose monitoring. Interoperative blood glucose monitoring is essential to detect hypo-and hyperglycaemia. The anaesthetic masks the usual signs of hypoglycaemia. Precautions are needed to avoid regurgitation and aspiration, cardiac arrhythmias, and postural hypotension in young children and patients with autonomic neuropathy. Hypoglycaemia increases the risk of seizures. In all cases careful explanation about what to expect and how to prepare for the procedure to the patient and their family/carers is essential.

The National Health Service in the UK released guidelines for managing people with diabetes in the perioperative period in 2012 (Dhatariya et al. 2012). The guidelines describe seven stages of the surgical journey, including referrals from primary care, the surgical outpatient department, preoperative assessment, hospital admission, surgery, postoperative care, and discharge. The guidelines highlight the value of insulin infusions and blood glucose monitoring during the operative process as well as the importance of patient education. The guidelines raise a number of areas of controversy, such as whether high preoperative HbA1c is associated with worse outcomes, using oral GLMs in the perioperative period, and whether metformin is associated with adverse events when radio contrast media are needed for investigative purposes.

The guidelines highlight two key points:

(1) Managing elective surgery in adults with diabetes should involve minimal fasting time, e.g. only one missed meal, and suggest that modifying the individual's usual medicine regimen is preferable to intravenous insulin infusions. However, this particular recommendation is not consistent with other experts who recommend insulin infusions during surgery.
(2) A poor glycaemic control leads to worse outcomes and more adverse events and should be addressed before surgery.

Postoperative care

Immediate care

(1) Monitor and record vital signs. Pain is a vital sign.
(2) Monitor blood glucose (and ketones in type 1 diabetes) initially two-hourly.
(3) Observe dressings for signs of haemorrhage or excess discharge.
(4) Ensure drain tubes are patent and draining.
(5) Maintain an accurate fluid balance. Document all information relating to and output, especially:

Input	Output
IV fluid	Drainage from wound
Oral	Vomitus
Enteral nutrition (EN) and total parenteral nutrition (TPN)	Diarrhoea
	Urine

(6) Maintain care of IV insulin/glucose infusion.
(7) Ensure vomiting and pain are controlled.
(8) Ensure psychological needs are addressed, for example, change in body image.
(9) Ensure referral to appropriate allied health professional, for example, physiotherapist.
(10) Insulin therapy is continued for people on oral GLMs until they are eating a normal diet and blood glucose levels are stabilised. Plans for ceasing the insulin infusion and commencing GLM should be in place and usually commenced two hours before the infusion is stopped (Joslin Diabetes Centre 2009/ADS 2012).
(11) Provide pressure care, including high-risk neuropathic feet.

Ongoing Care

(1) Document all data accurately on the appropriate charts.
(2) Prevent complications:
- Infection – aseptic dressing technique including IV sites
- Venous thrombosis – anti-embolic stockings, physiotherapy, early ambulation, anticoagulants
- Hypo/hyperglycaemia
- Pressure ulcers
(3) Instruct patient and family/carers in wound care and medication management.
(4) Follow up with rehabilitation.

Antibiotics, heparin, and other medicines should be administered according to individual patient requirements and medical orders.

Clinical observation

People sometimes complain of a sore throat for 24 hours after a general anaesthetic. They need to be reassured that this is normal and resolves spontaneously but advised to seek medical advice if it persists.

Guidelines for informing people with diabetes about what they should do prior to surgical procedures

Examples of instructions for people undergoing outpatient procedures can be found in Example Instruction Sheets 2 (a) and (b) (see pages 298 and 299).

Note: These are *examples only* and protocols in the clinician's place of employment should be followed. Adjusting medications for investigations and day procedures is becoming more complex as the range of available insulin, oral agents, and other medicines increase, and multiple insulin injections, insulin pumps, and combining insulin and oral agents is common practice.

It is important to consider the individual's blood glucose pattern, the medication regimen they are on and the type of procedure they are having when advising them about preoperative medication self-care.

Where people are on basal bolus regimens and scheduled for a morning procedure, the bedtime insulin dose may need to be reduced and the morning dose omitted. If the procedure is scheduled for the afternoon the morning dose may be given and the lunchtime dose omitted.

When people are on a combination of insulin and oral GLMs, the oral GLMs are usually withheld on the day of the procedure and the morning dose of insulin may be withheld for morning procedures. A reduced dose of insulin will usually be given if the procedure is scheduled for the afternoon.

Practice point

Advice about medications should also include information about how to manage complementary medicines/therapies the person may be taking besides insulin and oral glucose-lowering medicines.

Morning procedure

(1) Insulin may or may not be withheld in the morning on the day of the procedure, depending on the type of diabetes and blood glucose range.
(2) Test blood glucose and ketones if type 1 before coming to hospital.
(3) Fast from 12 midnight.
(4) Some hospitals ask the individual to bring their insulin to hospital.
(5) Advise the patient to have someone available to drive him or her home after the procedure.
(6) Explain before discharge:
   (a) the risk of hypoglycaemia if not eating;
   (b) what to take for pain relief;
   (c) when to recommence OHAs/insulin;
   (d) what and when to eat;
   (e) any specific care, for example, wound dressings or care of a biopsy site.

Afternoon procedure
(7) Light breakfast (e.g. tea and toast).
(8) Fast after the breakfast. It may be necessary to explain what 'fasting' means.
(9) Test blood glucose and ketones in type 1 before coming to hospital.
(10) Give insulin dose according to blood glucose test as ordered by the doctor.
(11) Explain before discharge:
   (a) the risk of hypoglycaemia if not eating;
   (b) what to take for pain relief;
   (c) when to recommence OHAs/insulin;
   (d) what and when to eat;
   (e) any specific care, for example, wound dressings or care of a biopsy site.

In both cases:

(i) Test blood glucose at the end of the procedure and before discharge and administer OHA or insulin dose.
(ii) Ensure the patient has appropriate follow-up appointments with doctors and other relevant health professionals (e.g. diabetes educator and dietitian).
   (a) Ensure the patient has someone to accompany them home.
   (b) Allay concerns about the procedure.
   (c) Provide appropriate care according to the medical orders.
   (d) Inspect all wounds before discharge.
   (e) It is not advisable to drive, operate machinery or drink alcohol until the following day.

Clinical observations

It is important to ensure the patient and their family/carers understand what is meant by 'fasting' and 'light breakfast'. People have stated that they will 'come as fast as I can but I can only move slowly because of my hips'.

Insulin pump therapy in patients undergoing surgery

Insulin pumps or continuous subcutaneous insulin infusion (CSII) are becoming more common and sophisticated. The managing diabetes team in consultation with the individual, the anaesthetist and surgical team should determine the best way to manage the person's insulin needs during surgery. If the individual elects to continue using an insulin pump and/or continuous subcutaneous blood glucose monitoring, he or she should indicate their decision on the consent form.

If the person does continue pump therapy during surgery a clearly visible identification tag should state the person is wearing a pump and clinicians must take great care to ensure the devices are visible and do not become dislodged before, during and after surgery (ADS 2012).

The anaesthetist must have access to the pump during surgery and know how it operates and how to turn it off or disconnect it if necessary – for example, in persistent hypoglycaemia. Once euglycaemia is restored the pump therapy can be recommenced at a lower basal rate, which may be temporary. Alternatively, the pump can be recommenced at the same basal rate and the rate of the glucose infusion increased, or the pump can be left off and an IV insulin infusion commenced (Queensland Health 2012).

If the decision is to continue to administer insulin using the pump, then it is important to ensure the infusion site is secure and that the tubing cannot be inherently disconnected during transport to and from the operating room or surgery.

If the surgery is of short duration, the usual basal insulin rate can be continued and an IV infusion of 5% glucose administered according to the individual's caloric requirement (Betts et al. 2009). The usual morning insulin bolus is not given except to correct hyperglycaemia.

Blood glucose must be monitored at least hourly pre- and postoperatively and every 30 minutes during surgery. If needed, correction insulin doses can be administered via the pump. However, if hyperglycaemia occurs, it is important to ensure the pump is still functioning correctly, the infusion tubing is patent, and the needle has not been dislodged from the infusion site. If the pump is not functioning, an IV insulin-glucose infusion may be required to prevent ketosis and hyperglycaemia, which may compromise outcomes.

A bolus does of insulin is usually administered when the person is ready to eat postoperatively.

However, managing an insulin pump requires a great deal of knowledge and skill and should not be used if the surgical team does not have the necessary knowledge, skills, and experience. Nassar et al. (2012) demonstrated inconsistent documentation of pump use and blood glucose monitoring throughout the perioperative period in 35 patients with insulin pumps who had surgical procedures in the United States between 2006 and 2010. Likewise, it was not clear whether the pump was functioning during most procedures. The authors recommended guidelines be developed. Their recommendation is interesting, given at least three such guidelines exist (Betts et al. 2009 [ISPAD]; ADS 2012; Queensland Health 2012).

Emergency procedures

Approximately 5% of people with diabetes will need emergency surgery at some stage of their lives. These may be for general surgical emergencies such as appendicitis or diabetes-specific such as acute foot ulcer. Abdominal pain in the presence of DKA may not be an abdominal emergency. However, if the abdominal pain persists after the DKA is corrected, an abdominal emergency should be considered. Likewise, functional problems associated with gastroparesis, gastroenteropathy, and cyclical vomiting may be mistaken for a surgical emergency. Thus, even in an emergency situation it is important to undertake a thorough assessment and medical history.

The specific management will depend on the nature of the emergency. If possible, the metabolic status should be stabilised before surgery is commenced. Many patients requiring emergency surgery have suboptimal control. The minimum requirements are:

(1) Adequate hydration. IV access should be obtained and blood drawn for glucose, ketones, electrolytes, pH, and other tests as indicated by the presenting problem.
(2) If possible, surgery should be delayed until the underlying acid–base derangement is corrected if ketoacidosis (DKA), hyperosmolar, or lactic acidosis is present. Dehydration is often severe in hyperosmolar states, and the fluid volume needs to be replaced quickly, taking care not to cause fluid overload or cerebral oedema. If the patient presents with an abdominal emergency, ensure that it is not due to DKA before operating.

Specific treatment depends on the following:

• Nature of the emergency
• Time of last food intake and presence of autonomic neuropathy/gastric stasis
• Time and type of the last insulin dose
• Blood glucose level, which should be monitored hourly
• Presence of complications such as cardiac arrhythmias and renal disease

Postoperative care will depend on the reason for the emergency and will encompass the care outlined earlier in the chapter.

Bariatric surgery

Bariatric surgery, a solution to obesity when other methods fail, is becoming safer and more acceptable (see Chapter 14). A recent study demonstrated that laparoscopic adjustable gastric banding (LAGB) and conventional diabetes management had five times the diabetes remission rate than other methods in 60 obese people with type 2 diabetes (Dixon et al. 2008). Of those who had LAGB, 73% achieved diabetes remission, there was an average weight loss of 20%, and average BMI fell from 36.6 to 29.5, and 80% achieved normoglycaemia. A recent report of a 15-year follow-up study involving 3000 Australians who had laparoscopic and adjustable banding surgery lost an average of 26 kg and maintained the weight loss for >10 years (O'Brien et al. 2006). There were no deaths in the Australian cohort, but 1 in 20 people had the band removed in the follow-up period.

People who successfully lose weight after gastric banding are more likely to have improved insulin sensitivity, reduced fasting blood glucose and HbA1c, especially those with type 2 diabetes, and the lipid profile improves in people with type 2 diabetes and those with impaired glucose tolerance (Geloneze et al. 2001; O'Brien et al. 2006). However, the risks and benefits need to be carefully considered on an individual basis.

Diabetes Australia recommends bariatric surgery should be a last resort for very obese adults when lifestyle changes are unsuccessful.

Investigative procedures

Key points
• Careful preparation and explanation to the individual and their family/carers.
• Never omit insulin in type 1 diabetes.
• Radio-opaque contrast media may cause tubular necrosis in older people with diabetes, so fluid balance must be monitored carefully.
• Complementary therapies, especially herbs and topical essential oils, may need to be stopped temporarily.

Rationale

Metabolic stress occurs to a lesser degree during investigative procedures than during surgical procedures but still occurs and needs to be managed appropriately to limit adverse outcomes.

Clear written instructions about managing medications and any specific preparation required can improve the individual's understanding and compliance with instructions.

Management protocols for patients undergoing medical tests/procedures such as X-rays, gastroscopy, or laser therapy is not as intricate as those for ketoacidosis or major surgery. However, vigilant nursing care is equally important to prevent excursions in blood glucose levels and consequent metabolic effects, and psychological stress.

Note: Morning procedures are preferred.

The objectives of care

(1) It is important to prevent hyperglycaemia during surgical procedures to improve outcomes. Hyperglycaemia and insulin therapy can affect the uptake of the radio isotope fluorine-18-fludrodeoxyglucose in the area to be investigated using positron emission tomography (PET) scans.
(2) Ensure correct preparation for the test.
(3) Ensure the procedure has been explained to the individual and that they understand what they need to do and what the procedure involves.
(4) Provide verbal written instructions for the individual/family, especially if the procedure will be performed on an outpatient basis. The information should include what to do about *all* the medicines they are taking and how to recognise and manage hypoglycaemia should it occur whilst they are fasting. They should also warn the person that it may not be safe to drive home, depending on the procedure.

Usually, the doctor referring the person for a procedure should explain the procedure to the individual as part of the process for obtaining informed consent to undertake the procedure. All clinicians involved have a duty of care to ensure instructions have been given and were followed.

General management

(1) Be aware insulin pumps and continuous glucose monitoring devices should not be exposed to strong magnetic fields during X-rays, MRIs, and CT scans, although they are designed to withstand common electromagnetic interference (ADS 2012).
(2) Insulin/oral hypoglycaemic agents:
   • Insulin is *never omitted* in people with type 1 diabetes.
   • If the patient needs to fast, insulin doses should be adjusted accordingly.
   • OHAs are usually withheld on the morning of the test.
   • Ensure written medical instructions are available, including after the procedure.
(3) Aim for a morning procedure if fasting is required and avoid prolonged fasting that results in a catabolic state and counter-regulatory hormone release (see Chapters 1 and 7).
(4) Monitor blood glucose before and after the test and during the night (3 a.m.) if fasting and in hospital.
(5) Observe for signs of dehydration. Maintain fluid balance chart if these conditions are present:
   • Fasting is prolonged.
   • Bowel preparations are required – some may lead to a fluid deficit especially in the setting of hyperglycaemia.
   • An IV infusion is commenced.

- Dehydration in older people may predispose them to kidney damage if a radio-opaque contrast medium is used.
- An IV infusion may dilute some radio-opaque contrast media. The advice of the radiographer should be sought if IV therapy is necessary. Continue IV infusions and oral fluids after the procedure to wash out contrast medium.

(6) Control nausea and vomiting and pain, which can increase the blood glucose level.

(7) Ensure the patient can eat and drink normally after the procedure to avoid hypoglycaemia.

(8) Assess puncture sites (e.g. angiography) before discharge.

(9) Recommence medications as per the medical order.

(10) Counsel not to drive home if relevant.

Bowel procedures, for example, colonoscopy

(1) Iron, aspirin, and arthritis medications may need to be stopped one week before the procedure. Diabetes medications should be adjusted according to the procedures outlined for day procedures. Insulin doses may need to be reduced during the bowel preparation and people may only require long acting insulin. Oral medicines may not be absorbed because of the bowel preparation.

(2) The day before the colonoscopy only clear fluids are permitted and some form of bowel preparation is usually required to clean out the bowel and allow a better view of the mucosa. Bowel preparations should be diluted in water because cordial can contribute to diarrhoea. Older people are at risk of dehydration and should be carefully monitored. Modern preparations are not absorbed and do not usually lead to significant electrolyte disturbances.

(3) Fasting for at least six hours is usually necessary.

(4) If diabetes is unstable or the individual is hyperglycaemic and the procedure is urgent, admission to hospital and an IV insulin-glucose infusion during the procedure may be advisable (ADS 2012).

(5) Frequent blood glucose monitoring, e.g. at least two hourly, is important especially for people who have unstable or brittle diabetes.

Eye procedures

People with diabetes are more prone to visual impairment and blindness than the general population. The eye manifestations of diabetes can affect all ocular structures. The time of appearance, rate of progression, and severity of eye disease vary amongst individuals. However, most patients have some evidence of damage after 25 years of diabetes and vision is threatened in 10% of people with diabetes.

Retinopathy is symptomless and may remain undetected if an ophthalmologist or optician does not examine the eyes regularly. Retinal cameras are commonly used to assess the degree of retinopathy and do not require papillary dilation. Fluorescein angiography and retinal photography may aid in determining the severity of the disease. Management aims to conserve vision, and laser therapy is often effective in this respect.

Risk factors for eye disease include hypertension, pregnancy, nephropathy, hyperlipidaemia, and smoking (see Chapter 8).

Care during fluorescein angiography

Fluorescein angiography is usually an outpatient procedure. It provides useful information when unexplained vision loss occurs. A recent technique, ultrawide fluorescein angiography, provide more information than the usual process. The reasons for the test and the procedure should be carefully explained to the individual/family. They should be aware of the following:

- Transient nausea may occur.
- The skin and urine may become yellow for 12–24 hours.
- The dye is injected into a vein.
- Drinking adequate amounts of fluid will help flush the dye out of the system.

Care during laser therapy (photocoagulation)

Laser is an acronym for light amplification stimulated emission of radiation. There are many types of laser. The ones that are used to treat diabetic patients are the argon, krypton, and diode lasers. The lasers absorb light, which is converted into heat, which coagulates the tissue. Laser therapy is frequently used to treat diabetic retinopathy and glaucoma.

The goals of photocoagulation are to maintain vision:

- by allowing fluid exchange to occur and reducing fluid accumulation in the retina;
- by photocoagulating the retina, which is ischaemic, and thereby causing new vessels that are prone to haemorrhage, to regress.

Laser therapy is usually performed on an outpatient basis. Fasting is not required and medication adjustment is unnecessary.

Practice point

Laser therapy may not increase vision, but can prevent further loss of vision.

Clinician responsibilities

Ensure the purpose of laser therapy has been explained. Advise the person to ask their doctor whether it is still safe to drive after the treatment – not just immediately after but generally. The majority can still drive safely, but a driving assessment might be required:

(1) Before the procedure, the person should know that:
- The procedure is uncomfortable.
- The pupil of the eye will be dilated.
- Anaesthetic drops may be used.
- The laser beam causes bright flashes of light.
- Vision will be blurred for some time after the laser treatment.
- They should test their blood glucose before and after laser treatment.
- They should not drive home and may have tunnel vision after the procedure, which can limit the visual field. The possible effects on driving should be explained (see Chapter 10).
(2) After the procedure, the person should know that:
- Sunglasses will protect the eye and help reduce discomfort.
- Spots may be seen for 24–48 hours.
- There can be some discomfort for two to three weeks.
- Headache may develop after the procedure.
- Paracetamol may be taken to relieve pain.
- Activities that increase intraocular pressure, for example, lifting heavy objects, straining at stool, should be avoided for 24–36 hours.
- Night vision may be temporarily decreased.
- Lateral vision may be permanently diminished; this is known as *tunnel vision* and can have implications for peripheral vision and driving safety.

Practice point

Aspirin is best avoided because of its anticoagulant effect. If new vessels are present due to retinopathy, they can bleed and threaten sight.

Other eye procedures include cataract operations.

Practice point

Blurred vision does not necessarily indicate serious eye disease. It can occur during both hypo- and hyperglycaemia. Vision often also becomes worse when diabetic control is improved, for example, after commencement of insulin therapy. Although this is distressing for the patient, vision usually improves in six to eight weeks. Prescriptions for glasses obtained in these circumstances may be inappropriate. Glasses are best obtained when the eyes settle down.

The nursing care of people who are vision impaired is discussed in Chapter 14.

Care of when radio-contrast media are used

Radio-contrast media are eliminated through the kidneys and can cause contrast-induced nephropathy that can result in lactic acidosis in people taking metformin, especially if the radio-contrast media is injected IV (Klow et al. 2001; ADS 2012). Metformin-induced lactic acidosis following injection of radio-contrast media almost always occurs in people with preexisting renal impairment. Thus, the serum creatinine should be measured prior to the procedure and before metformin is recommenced after the procedure. Most radiological services recommend withholding metformin 24 hours prior and 48 hours after procedures requiring radio-contrast media.

Fasting is often required before the procedure and the patient can become dehydrated, especially if they are kept waiting for long periods, and kidney complications can occur. People most at risk:

- are over 50 years old;
- have established kidney disease;
- have had diabetes for more than 10 years;
- are hypertensive;
- have proteinuria;
- have an elevated serum creatinine, but note the limitations of serum creatinine discussed in Chapter 3.

Kidney problems caused by radio-contrast media may not produce symptoms. Reduced urine output following procedures requiring radio-contrast media may indicate kidney damage and should be investigated.

Management

(1) Ensure appropriate preparation has been carried out.
(2) Ensure the person is well hydrated before the procedure (intravenous therapy may be needed).

(3) Maintain an accurate fluid balance chart.
(4) Avoid delays in performing the procedure.
(5) Monitor urine output after the procedure.
(6) Assess serum creatinine and/or other kidney function tests after the procedure.
(7) Maintain good metabolic control.
(8) Encourage the person to drink water to help flush out the contrast media.

Complementary medicines and other therapies during surgery and investigative procedures

A version of the following information was published in the *Australian Diabetes Educator* 2008; see also Chapter 19. Of patients undergoing surgical and investigative procedures, 50% use complementary and alternative medicines (CAM). Women aged 40–60 years are high users and often use CAM on the advice of friends (Norred 2000; Tsen 2000). Thus, CAM use is an important consideration for people with diabetes having surgical and/or investigative procedures.

Significantly, despite the high rates of CAM usage, most conventional practitioners do not ask about CAM use (Braun 2006). CAM use can improve health outcomes of patients undergoing surgery. For example, essential-oil foot massage reduces stress and anxiety post CAGS (Stevenson 1994), essential oils lower MRI-associated claustrophobia and stress, acupuncture and peppermint or ginger tea reduce nausea, a range of strategies relieve pain and improve sleep, and CQ10 prior to cardiac surgery improves postoperative cardiac outcomes (Rosenfeldt 2005).

However, there are also risks, which need to be considered in the context of the particular surgery or investigation required and overall management plan. Bleeding is the most significant risk. Other risks include hypotension, hypertension, sedation, and cardiac effects such as arrhythmias, renal damage, and electrolyte disturbances (Norred 2000, 2002). It is well documented that many conventional medicines need to be adjusted or ceased prior to surgery. Less information about managing CAM in surgical settings is available, but a growing body of evidence suggests many CAM medicines may also need to be stopped or adjusted prior to surgery and some investigative procedures.

The following general information applies to people already using CAM medicines and those considering using them before or after surgery. Conventional practitioners may be able to provide general advice regarding CAM use, but people with diabetes should be advised to consult a qualified CAM medicine practitioner because many therapies should be used under qualified supervision and for specific advice. Self-prescribing is not recommended in the surgical period because of the complex metabolic and neuroendocrine response to surgery.

Preoperative phase

People need written information about how to manage CAM medicines and conventional medicines in the operative period as well as any special preparation needed for the surgery or investigation. Conventional health professionals can provide such information if they are qualified to do so or refer the person to a qualified CAM practitioner. Such information should be provided in an appropriate format relevant to the individual's health literacy level; see Chapter 16.

Great care is needed for major and high risk such as heart, orthopaedic, or neurosurgery, if the person has renal or liver disease, or is very young or elderly. The conventional medication list is unlikely to include CAM medicines or supplements, although it should; thus, health professionals should discuss CAM use with people during all structured medicine reviews and preoperative health assessments.

Some CAM medicines such as evening primrose oil, bilberry, cranberry, fish oils, ginger, Gingko, liquorice, guarana, willow bark, meadowsweet, and ginseng need to be stopped at least one week before surgery. St John's wort and supplements such as vitamin E should be stopped two weeks before surgery, primarily because of the risk of bleeding. In addition, medicines such as St John's wort, need to be stopped gradually (like conventional antidepressants). However, when CAM medicines are the main form of treatment, alternative management may be required to prevent the condition deteriorating and affecting the surgical outcome (e.g. glucose-lowering herbal medicines).

In addition to the bleeding risk, some commonly used CAM medicines may/can interact with some anaesthetic agents and prolong their sedative effects, some affect blood pressure and heart rate, others cause changes in the major electrolytes, potassium, calcium, and sodium levels in the blood. Grapefruit juice interferes with the action of some antibiotics such as cyclosporine, which may be needed pre- or postoperatively. These problems do not occur in everybody who uses CAM in the same way that not everybody experiences adverse events associated with conventional treatments. It is sometimes difficult to predict who will or will not have problems. Some hospitals have policies and guidelines about using CAM, and people who wish to continue using CAM in hospital should clarify such policies with the relevant hospital and surgeon before they are admitted. Most do not prescribe or supply CAM.

In addition to managing CAM and conventional medicines, achieving the best possible health status before surgery improves postoperative recovery. The preoperative assessment is an ideal time to revise the importance of eating a healthy balanced diet and exercise within the individual's capability, controlling blood glucose and lipids, which will support immune system functioning and enhance wound healing. Most people should continue their usual physical activity unless it is contraindicated to maintain strength and flexibility. Stress management strategies such as meditation, guided imagery, essential oils administered in a massage or via an inhalation, and music help reduce anxiety and fear about the surgery. Ginger capsules or tablets taken one hour before surgery reduces postoperative nausea (Gupta and Sharma 2001).

The preoperative assessment is also an ideal time to discuss postoperative recovery, including managing pain and promoting sleep. CAM may be a useful alternative to some conventional medicines provided a quality use of medicines (QUM) framework is adopted; see Chapter 5. For example, valerian, hops, and lavender in a vapourised essential oil blend, administered via massage or as herbal teas or medicines, promote restful sleep and have a lower side-effect profile than most conventional sedatives.

Postoperative phase

CAM users need information about whether and when it is safe to start using CAM again postoperatively, considering any new conventional medicines that were prescribed (e.g. anticoagulants), which could influence the choice and/or dose of CAM medicines. Likewise, some nonmedicine CAM therapies might need to be used with care, such as needle acupuncture and deep tissue massage, because they can cause bruising and/or bleeding.

A range of CAM strategies can be used to manage pain in the immediate postoperative phase as well as in the longer term. Most are less likely to cause constipation and drowsiness than pethidine and morphine-based medicines. Alternatively, if these medicines are the best method of managing pain, high-fibre CAM food/medicines such as aloe vera juice, probiotics, and psyllium can reduce constipation once oral feeding is permitted. Probiotics also increase bowel health and support natural bowel flora. Peppermint or ginger tea reduces mild-to-moderate nausea. Lymphatic drainage massage is very effective after some surgery to reduce swelling and relieve pain.

Some CAM products promote wound healing, for example, aloe vera, Medihoney, and calendula and could be used depending on the wound. Arnica ointment reduces bruising but should not be used on open wounds. Comfrey poultices are very effective at reducing local oedema and local pain but should not be used on open wounds or taken internally.

Implications for care

- CAM has both risks and benefits for people with diabetes undergoing surgery and investigative procedures.
- Not all the CAM therapies people use are medicines, and not all CAMs carry the same level of risk or confer equal benefits.

- Adopting an holistic QUM approach can optimise the benefits and reduce the risks. A key aspect of QUM is asking about and documenting CAM use.
- People with diabetes who use CAM need written advice about how to manage their CAM during surgery and investigations.
- People with diabetes and cardiac or renal disease and those on anticoagulants, older people, and children are at particular risk of adverse events if they use some CAM medicines.

References

Alberti, G. and Gill, G. (1997). The care of the diabetic patient during surgery. In: *International Textbook of Diabetes Mellitus*, 2e (eds. G. Alberti, R. DeFronzo and H. Keen), 1243–1253. Chichester: Wiley.

American Diabetes Association (ADS) (2019). Standards of medical care in diabetes. *Diabetes Care* https://care.diabetesjournals.org/content/42/Supplement_1/S61.

Australian Department of Health (2018). Sodium glucose co-transporter 2 safety advice: diabetic ketoacidosis and surgical procedures. www.tga.gov.au/alert/sodium-glucose-co-transporter-2-inhibitors.

Australian Diabetes Society (ADS) (2012). *Peri-operative Diabetes Management Guidelines*. Canberra: ADS.

Betts, P., Brink, S., Silink, M. et al. (2009). Management of children and adolescents with diabetes requiring surgery. *Paediatric Diabetes* 10 (Suppl 12): 169–179.

Braun, L. (2006). Use of complementary medicines by surgical patients. In: *Undetected and unsupervised. Proceedings of the Fourth Australasian Conference on Safety and Quality in Health Care*. Melbourne.

Castillo, E. (2019). Frequent ED visits common for older adults with diabetes. *Annals of Emergency Medicine* **2019** https://doi.org/10.1016/j.annemrgmed.2018.12/013.

Chow, W., Rosenthal, R., Merkow, R. et al. (2012). Optimal preoperative assessment of the geriatric surgical patient: a best practice guideline from the American college of surgeons national surgical quality improvement program and the American geriatrics society. *Journal of the American College of Surgeons* https://doi.org/10.1016/jamcollsurg.2012.06.017 (accessed December 2012).

Dagogo-Jack, S. and Alberti, G. (2002). Management of diabetes mellitus in surgical patients. *Diabetes Spectrum* **15**: 44–48.

De, P. and Child, D. (2001). Euglycaemic ketoacidosis – is it on the rise? *Practical Diabetes International* **18** (7): 239–240.

Dhatariya, L., Levy, N., Kilvert, A. et al. (2012). NHS Diabetes guideline for the perioperative management of the adult patient with diabetes. *Diabetic Medicine* **29**: 420–433.

Dickerson, L., Sack, Y., and Hueston, W. (2003). Glycaemic control in medical inpatients with type 2 diabetes receiving sliding scale insulin regimens versus routine diabetic medicines: a multicentre randomized control trial. *Annals of Family Medicine* **1**: 29–35.

Dickerson, R. (2004). Specialised nutrition support in the hospitalized obese patient. *Nutrition in Clinical Practice* **19**: 245–254.

Dixon, J., O'Brien, P., Playfair, J. et al. (2008). Adjustable gastric banding and conventional therapy for Type 2 diabetes: a randomized contolled trial. *Journal of the American Medical Association* **299** (3): 316–323.

Eamer, G., Gibson, J., Gillis, C. et al. (2017). Surgical frailty assessment: a missed opportunity. *BMC Anesthesiology* **17**: 99. https://doi.org/10.1186/s12871-017-0390-7.

Ford, W., Self, W., Slovis, C. et al. (2014). Diabetes in the emergency department and hospital: acute care of diabetes patients. *Current Emergency Medicines Reports* mar 1 **1** (1): 1–9. https://doi.org/10.1007/s40138-012-0007-x.

French, G. (2000). Clinical management of diabetes mellitus during anaesthesia and surgery. *Update in Anaesthesia* **11** (13): 1–6.

Geloneze, B., Tambascia, M., Pareja, J. et al. (2001). The insulin tolerance test in morbidly obese patients undergoing bariatric surgery. *Obesity Research* **9**: 763–769.

Gill, G. (1997). Surgery and diabetes. In: *Textbook of Diabetes* (eds. G. Williams and J. Pickup), 820–825. Oxford: Blackwell Science.

Gupta, Y. and Sharma, M. (2001). Reversal of pyrogallol-induced gastric emptying in rats by ginger (*Zingber officinalis*). *Experimental Clinical Pharmacology* **23** (9): 501–503.

Harari, D., Hopper, A., Dhesi, J. et al. (2007). Proactive care of older people undergoing surgery (POPS): designing, embedding, evaluating and funding a comprehensive geriatric assessment service for older elective surgical patients. *Age and Ageing* **36** (2): 190–196.

Joint Commission on Surgical Care Improvement (SCIP) (2012). Cardiac Surgery Patients With Controlled Postoperative Blood Glucose. https://www.jointcommission.org/assets/1/6/2w_SCIP-Inf-4.pdf.

Joslin Diabetes Centre (2009). *Guideline for Inpatient Management of Surgical and ICU Patients with Diabetes (Pre, Peri and Postoperative Care)*. Boston, USA: The Joslin Centre.

Kirschner, R. (1993). Diabetes in paediatric ambulatory surgical patients. *Journal of Post Anaesthesia Nursing* **8** (5): 322–326.

Klow, N., Draganov, B., and Os, I. (2001). Metformin and contrast media-increase risk of lactic acidosis? *Tidsskr Nor laegeforen* **121** (15): 1829.

Kwon, S., Thompson, R., Dellinger, P. et al. (2003). Importance of perioperative glycaemic control in general surgery: a report from the surgical care and outcomes assessment program. *Annals of Surgery* **257** (1): 8–14.

Madsen, T. (2019). Patients are treated differently in the ER. https://healthcare.utah.edu/the-scope/shows.php?shows=0_qw8dqn39.

Marks, J., Hirsch, J., and de Fronzo, R. (eds.) (1998). *Current Management of Diabetes Mellitus*, 247–254. St Louis: C.V. Mosby.

Mirtallo, J. (2008). Nutrition support for the obese surgical patient. *Medscape Pharmacist* http://www.medscap.com/viewarticle/566036 (accessed February 2008).

Morris, M. and Richman, J. (2017). What increases postoperative readmissions? *Annals of Surgery* **264**: 621–631.

Nassar, A., Boyle, M., Seifert, K. et al. (2012). Insulin pump therapy in patients with diabetes undergoing surgery. *Endocrinology Practice* **18** (1): 49–55.

Norred, C. (2000). Use of complementary and alternative medicines by surgical patients. *Journal of the American Association of Nurse Anaesthetists* **68** (1): 13–18.

Norred, C. (2002). Complementary and alternative medicine use by surgical patients. *AORN Journal* **76** (6): 1013–1021.

O'Brien, P., Dixon, J., and Laurie, C. (2006). Treatment of mild to moderate obesity with laparoscopic adjustable gastric banding or an intensive medical program: a randomized trial. *Annals of Internal Medicine* **144** (9): 625–633.

Queensland Health (2012). *Inpatient Guidelines: Insulin Infusion Pump Management*. Australia: Queensland Health.

Rosenfeldt, F. (2005). Coenzyme CQ-10 therapy before cardiac surgery improves mitochondrial function and *in vitro* contractility of myocardial tissue. *Journal of Thoracic and Cardiovascular Surgery* **129**: 25–32.

Stevenson, C. (1994). The psychophysiological effects of aromatherapy massage following cardiac surgery. *Complementary Therapies in Medicine* **2** (1): 27–35.

Tsen, I. (2000). Alternative medicine use in presurgical patients. *Anaesthesiology* **93** (1): 148–151.

Wells, K., Craven, P., Steenblik, J. et al. (2018). Prevalence and treatment of anxiety among emergency department patients with pain. *The American Journal of Emergency Medicine* **36** (7): 1315.

Werther, G. (1994). *Diabetes Mellitus and Surgery*. Melbourne: Royal Children's Hospital Melbourne www.rch.org.au/clinicalguide/cpg.cfm?doc_id=5190 (accessed February 2008).

Example Information 2(a): Instructions for people with diabetes on oral glucose-lowering medicines having procedures as outpatients under sedation of general anaesthesia

Person's Name: .... UR...

Time and Date of Appointment: ....

Where to go:...

IT IS IMPORTANT THAT YOU INFORM NURSING AND MEDICAL STAFF THAT YOU HAVE DIABETES

Morning

If your diabetes is controlled by diet and/or diabetes tablets and you are going to the operating theatre in the morning:

- Take nothing by mouth from midnight.
- Test your blood glucose and bring your blood glucose record to the hospital with you.
- Do not take your morning diabetes tablets.

Afternoon

If your diabetes is controlled by diet and/or diabetes tablets and you are going to the operating theatre in the afternoon:
- Have a light breakfast only (coffee/tea, two slices of toast with spread), and nothing by mouth after that
- Test your blood glucose and bring your blood glucose record to the hospital with you
- Omit your morning diabetes tablets unless your doctor tells you to take them.

If you have any questions:

Contact: ....   Telephone: ....

Note: The inappropriate paragraph can be deleted or, better still, separate forms can be produced for morning and afternoon procedures.

Example Instruction Sheet 2(b):   Instructions for people with diabetes on insulin having procedures as outpatients under sedation or general anaesthesia

Patient's Name: .... UR: ....

Time and Date of Appointment:...

where to go:.......................................

**IT IS IMPORTANT THAT YOU INFORM NURSING AND MEDICAL
STAFF THAT YOU HAVE DIABETES**

Morning

If your diabetes is controlled by insulin and you are going to the operating theatre in the morning:

- Take nothing by mouth from midnight.
- Test your blood glucose and bring your blood glucose record to the hospital with you.
- Omit your morning insulin. OR Take units of insulin.

Afternoon

If your diabetes is controlled by insulin and you are going to the operating theatre in the afternoon:

- Have a light breakfast only (coffee/tea, two slices of toast with spread), and nothing by mouth after that.
- Test your blood glucose and bring your blood glucose record to the hospital with you.
- Take .... units of insulin.

If you have any questions:

Contact: .... Telephone: ....

Note: The inappropriate paragraph can be deleted or, better still, separate forms can be produced for morning and afternoon procedures.

Chapter 10

Conditions Associated with Diabetes

Key points

- Some of the conditions described in this chapter are rare; others are more common.
- Many have common underlying contributory factors such as chronic inflammation.
- Many are overlooked in the focus on managing diabetes and achieving metabolic targets.
- Diabetes may be overlooked when managing conditions such as tuberculosis (TB) and HIV/AIDs.
- Most conditions could be identified as part of a comprehensive assessment that includes diabetes and preventative screening programmes.
- The concomitant presence of one or more of these conditions may influence diabetes management choices, health outcomes, diabetes self-care capability, and mental health.
- Concomitant diabetes can affect the life course and outcomes of concomitant conditions.

Introduction

This chapter outlines some conditions that are associated with diabetes. They are often managed in specialised services and some are very rare. A basic knowledge about these conditions can alert clinicians to the possibility that other conditions could be present, allow appropriate care plans to be formulated with the individual, and facilitate early referral for expert advice, which ultimately improves the health and well-being of the individual and often their families.

The conditions covered in this chapter are:

- Enteral and parenteral nutrition (see Chapter 4)
- Diabetes and cancer
- Smoking and alcohol addiction
- Brittle diabetes

Care of People with Diabetes: A Manual for Healthcare Practice, Fifth Edition. Trisha Dunning and Alan Sinclair.
© 2020 John Wiley & Sons Ltd. Published 2020 by John Wiley & Sons Ltd.

- Illegal drug use
- Oral health
- Liver disease
- Breast mastopathy
- Coeliac disease
- cystic fibrosis-related diabetes (CFRD)
- Incontinence
- Sleep disturbance
- Tuberculosis
- HIV/aids
- Hearing deficits
- Musculoskeletal disorders
- Corticosteroid and antipsychotic medications
- Diabetes and driving
- Fasting for religious observances

Other conditions that can co-occur with diabetes include thyroid disease, especially with T1DM, which is discussed in Chapters 1 and 13, sarcopenia and frailty, see Chapter 12 and schizophrenia and other mental health conditions, which are discussed in Chapter 15.

Enteral and parenteral nutrition

Practice points

- The guidelines, policies, and procedures of relevant health services and countries should be followed when caring for people with central lines, percutaneous endoscopic gastrostomy (PEG) tubes, and nasogastric tubes.
- Administering medicines can be challenging. It is important to know which medicines can be crushed, which ones are affected by some foods and when alternative dose forms are required.
- Enteral and parenteral nutrition is used to supply nutritional requirements in special circumstances such as malnourished patients admitted with a debilitating disease and where there is a risk of increasing the malnourishment, for example, fasting states and palliative care. It can be used temporarily or be required permanently. Malnourishment leads to increased mortality and morbidity, thus increasing length of stay in hospital, especially in older people (Chapters 4 and 12) (Middleton et al. 2001). Malnourishment can also affect medicine choices. Often the patient is extremely ill or has undergone major gastrointestinal, head or neck surgery, or has gastroparesis diabeticorum, a diabetes complication that leads to delayed gastric emptying and can result in hypoglycaemia due to delayed food absorption, bloating, and abdominal pain. Alternatively, hyperglycaemia can occur. Gastroparesis is very distressing for the individual.
- Malnourishment can be due to depression, recent significant loss/bereavement, isolation, food insecurity, swallowing difficulties, which have many causes, oral/periodontal conditions, reduced appetite, which can be a side effect of some medicines, e.g. Ramipril (an ACEI), eating disorders and drug and alcohol use. Age-related changes play a role, e.g. declining production of hydrochloric acid in the stomach declines with age, which affects absorption of vitamin $B_{12.}$ Reduced appetite is common in the last stages of life.

Malnutrition can lead to:

- Weight loss
- Loss of subcutaneous fat
- Loss of muscle mass
- Fluid accumulation, oedema
- Reduced grip strength (Hand et al. 2016)

Aims of enteral and parental nutrition

(1) Improve nutrition by supplying essential energy, protein, and nutrients.
(2) Reduce anxiety associated with the condition requiring enteral therapy and the procedure by involving the individual in management decisions, explaining the process and why enteral feeding is necessary. In some cases, family members/carers will need to be included in the education. Ample time should be allowed to enable people's concerns to be addressed.
(3) Prevent sepsis and other adverse events.
(4) Maintain an acceptable blood glucose range (4–8 mmol/l) except in frail older people when 6–8 mmol/l might be appropriate. Monitoring frequency depends on the individual and the reasons for using enteral feeding.
(5) Maintain normal urea, electrolytes, liver function tests, and blood gas levels.
(6) Supply adequate nutrition in terms of protein, fat, and carbohydrate to support normal body functions and promote growth and repair.
(7) Achieve positive nitrogen balance.
(8) Prevent complications of therapy.
(9) The long-term aim of enteral/parenteral feeding is the return of the patient to oral feeding. However, if life expectancy is reduced and/or in older people, it may be permanent (Chapters 4 and 12). In such cases, decisions about when to discontinue the feeding should be made proactively, documented in an advanced care plan (Dunning et al. 2018). Blood glucose monitoring and reviewing the diabetes management regimen, including medicines, is essential when oral feeding resumes (Australian Diabetes Society [ADS] 2012; American Diabetes Association 15 2019).

It may also be necessary to consider the balance of bacteria in the gut and the role these organisms play in altering dietary and metabolic processes. Specific 'good bacteria' appear to play a role in reducing systemic inflammatory processes. They also appear to play a role in fasting hyperglycaemia, obesity, steatosis, insulin resistance, and hyperinsulinaemia, as well as in the secretion of gastrointestinal hormones such as the incretins; see Chapter 1. Prebiotics and probiotics could be beneficial to the microbiota and overall health of malnourished people.

Complications of enteral nutrition

(1) Mechanical problems such as aspiration, poor gastric emptying, and reflux can occur, especially if the person has altered mental state and/or a suppressed gag reflex.
(2) Metabolic consequences include hyperglycaemia and hypernatraemia, depending on the feed used, the supplements added to the feed, and when a high feeding rate is used. Hyperglycaemia in people receiving enteral nutrition is associated with increased risk of cardiac complications, infection, sepsis, and acute renal failure. Significantly, people with mean blood glucose >9.1 mmol/l have a 10-fold greater risk of death than people with mean blood glucose 6.9 mmol/l, independent of age, gender, and presence of diabetes complications (ADS 2012). Feeding into the small bowel rather than the stomach minimises metabolic disturbance. People who cannot indicate that they are thirsty and who have altered mental status, particularly older people, are at risk of these metabolic consequences. Hypoglycaemia can occur if food is not absorbed, the calorie load is reduced, and if there are blockages in the feeding tubes.

(3) Medicine interactions can contribute to hyper or hypoglycaemia when feeds do not coincide with the action profile of prescribed glucose lowering medicines (GLMs); see Chapters 5–7.
(4) Gastrointestinal problems, commonly diarrhoea, which is usually osmotic in nature. Gastroparesis may be present.
(5) Enteral feeding is 'not normal' and can affect the person's dignity and self-concept.

Routes of administration

Enteral feeds

The enteral route supplies nutrients and fluids when the oral route is inadequate or obstructed. Feeds are administered via a nasogastric, duodenal, jejunal, or gastrostomy tube.

Enteral feeding is preferred over parenteral feeding when the gut function is normal and oral feeds do not meet the patient's nutritional requirements (McClave et al. 1999; ASPEN 2017). Nasogastric tubes may be used in the short term. Nasogastric feeds have a significant risk of pulmonary aspiration. The tubes are easily removed by confused patients and cause irritation to the nasal mucosa and external nares that can be uncomfortable and is an infection risk in immunocompromised patients and people with hyperglycaemia.

Duodenal and jejunal tubes do not carry the same risk of pulmonary aspiration but the feeds can contribute to gastric intolerance and bloating, especially in the presence of gastroparesis; see Chapter 8.

Gastroscopy tubes are used in the long term when the stomach is not affected by the primary disease, which may preclude their use in people with established autonomic neuropathy that involves the gastrointestinal tract. The tubes can be inserted through a surgical incision and the creation of a stoma. More commonly, percutaneous endoscopic techniques (PEG) are used (Thomas 2001). Inserting a PEG tube involves making an artificial tract between the stomach and the abdominal wall through which a tube is inserted. The tube can be a balloon tube or a button type that is more discrete and lies flat to the skin. An extension tube is inserted into the gastroscopy tube during feeding.

Gastrostomy (PEG) feeds

Feeds can usually be undertaken 12–24 hours after the tube is inserted but can be given as early as 4–6 hours after tube insertion in special circumstances. The initial feed may be water or dextrose saline, depending on the patient's condition.

Mode of administration

(1) Bolus instillation: may result in distension and delayed gastric emptying. Aspiration can occur. Diarrhoea may be a complication. *This method is not suitable for people with diabetes who have autonomic neuropathy, especially gastroparesis.*
(2) Continuous infusion: via gravity infusion or pump. This can lead to hyperinsulinaemia in T2DM because the infusion stimulates glucose-mediated insulin production. The effect on blood glucose can be minimised by using formulas with a low glycaemic index. Administering insulin via the IV route enables the caloric input to be balanced with the insulin requirements, but is not suitable for long-term use or in some clinical settings.

The strength of the feeds should be increased gradually to prevent a sudden overwhelming glucose load in the bloodstream. An IV insulin infusion is an ideal method to control blood glucose levels. Blood glucose monitoring is essential to gauge the impact of the feed on blood glucose and appropriately titrate medication doses.

The feeds usually contain protein, fat, and carbohydrate. The carbohydrate is in the form of dextrose, either 25% or 40%, and extra insulin may be needed to account for the glucose load. A balance must be achieved between caloric requirements and blood glucose levels. Patients who are managed using GLMs usually need insulin whilst they are on enteral feeding.

Parenteral feeds
Refers to administering nutrients and fluids by routes other than the alimentary canal, that is, intravenously via a peripheral or central line.

Mode of administration
Parenteral supplements are either partial or total:

(1) *Peripheral.* Used after gastrointestinal surgery and in malabsorption states. Peripheral access is usually reserved for people in whom central access is difficult or sometimes as a supplement to oral/enteral feeds. It is not suitable if a high dextrose supplement is needed because dextrose irritates the veins, causing considerable discomfort. It can cause significant tissue damage if extravasation occurs.
(2) *Central.* Supplies maximum nutrition in the form of protein, carbohydrate, fats, trace elements, vitamins, and electrolytes. For example, in patients with cancer or burns, larger volumes can be given than via the peripheral route. In addition, it provides long-term access because silastic catheters can be left in situ indefinitely. If patients are at risk of sepsis, the site of the central line is rotated weekly using strict aseptic technique. Central lines enable the person to remain mobile, which aids digestion and reduces the risk of pressure ulcers. Activity, itself is beneficial if it is possible and safe.

If insulin is required the dose regimen should be divided into basal, prandial, and correction doses, especially people with T1DM. For those on continuous feeds the insulin dose can be calculated as 1 unit of insulin for every 10–15 g carbohydrate per day. People on bolus enteral feeds can be administered rapid acting insulin can be given subcutaneously every four to six hours before the bolus fed.

People receiving continuous peripheral or central parental nutrition regular insulin can be added to the solution, especially if the person required >20% units of correction doses in 24 hours (Umpierrez 2009; ADA 2019).

Choice of formula

The particular formula selected depends on the person's nutritional requirements and absorptive capacity. It is usual to begin with half strength formula and gradually increase to full strength as tolerated. The aim is to supply adequate:

- Fluid
- Protein
- Carbohydrate
- Vitamins and minerals
- Essential fatty acids
- Sodium spread evenly over the 24 hours
- Preserve/enhance gut health

Generally, feeds low in carbohydrate/dextrose and high in monosaturated fatty acids are preferred for people with diabetes (ADS 2012). Nutritional requirements can vary from week-to-week; thus, careful monitoring is essential to ensure the formula is adjusted proactively and appropriately.

GLMs, insulin or other agents, are adjusted according to the emerging blood glucose pattern. The dose depends on the feeds used as well as other prescribed medicines, and the person's condition. Generally, the insulin/other GLM doses are calculated according to the caloric intake.

There is very little good quality research into the effects of glucose lowering medicines on blood glucose in people receiving enteral/parental nutrition.

Care of Nasogastric Tubes

(1) Explain purpose of tube and the insertion procedure to the individual and their family.
(2) Confirm the position of the tube with an X-ray, once it is inserted.
(3) Recheck position of the tube regularly to ensure it is in the stomach to prevent pulmonary aspiration and monitor for signs the tube could be dislodged.
(4) Change the position of the tube in the nose daily to avoid pressure areas.
(5) Flush regularly to ensure the tube remains patent.
(6) Check residual gastric volumes regularly to avoid gastric distension and reduce the possibility of aspiration, especially if gastroparesis is present.

Care of PEG tubes

The same care required for nasogastric tubes applies. Additional care:

(1) Monitor gastric aspirates at least daily.
(2) Elevate the head of the bed where there is a risk of pulmonary aspiration.
(3) Weigh the patient to ensure the desired weight outcome is achieved.
(4) Monitor nutritional status; see Chapter 4.
(5) Manage nausea and vomiting if they occur because they increase the risk of aspiration, represent fluid loss, and are uncomfortable for the patient. Record the amount and type of any vomitus. Antinausea medication may be required. Warm herbal teas such as chamomile, peppermint, or ginger may be helpful nonmedicine alternatives if oral intake is permitted.
(6) If the PEG tube blocks it can sometimes be cleared with a fizzy soft drink but local protocol should be followed because fizzy drinks can lead to electrolyte imbalances if they are used frequently.
(7) Ensure there is adequate fluid in the feeds to avoid dehydration and the consequent risk of hyperosmolar states; see Chapter 7 (Thomas 2001).

Care of IV and central lines

(1) Dress the insertion site regularly using strict aseptic technique according to usual protocols.
(2) Check position of the central line with a chest X-ray.
(3) Maintain strict aseptic technique.
(4) Maintain patency, usually by intermittently installing heparinised saline (weekly or when line is changed).
(5) Patients should be supine when the central catheter is disconnected and IV giving sets should be carefully primed to minimise the risk of air embolism.
(6) Check catheter for signs of occlusion (e.g. resistance to infusion or difficulty withdrawing a blood sample). Reposition the individual; if the occlusion is still present, consult the doctor.
(7) Observe exit site for any tenderness, redness or swelling. If bleeding occurs around the suture or exit site, apply pressure, and notify the doctor.
(8) Monitor the patient for signs of infection (e.g. fever). Note that elevated white cell count may not be a sign of infection in people with diabetes if hyperglycaemia is present.

General care

(1) Ensure the person is referred to a dietitian.
(2) Maintain an accurate fluid balance chart, including loss from stomas, drain tubes, vomitus, and diarrhoea.
(3) Monitor serum albumin, urea, and electrolytes to determine nutritional requirements, nitrogen balance, and energy requirements.
(4) Weigh regularly (weekly) at the same time, using the same scales with the person wearing similar clothing to ensure energy balance and sufficient calories are supplied. Excess calories lead to weight gain and hyperglycaemia. Insufficient calories lead to weight loss and increase the risk of hypoglycaemia.

(5) Monitor blood glucose regularly, four to six hourly, initially, but sometimes more frequently, e.g. in intensive care unit (ICU). If elevated, be aware of possibility of a hyperosmolar event or diabetic ketoacidosis (DKA) (see Chapter 7). If stable, less frequent monitoring might be appropriate.

(6) Record temperature, pulse, and respiration and report if elevated (>38 °C) or if any respiratory distress occurs.

(7) Check the label, including the date and appearance of all infusions before they are administered.

(8) Most medicines are given separately from the formula; check with the pharmacist which, if any, medicines can be added to the formula. Follow pump instructions and local guidelines carefully. Be very careful with medicines whose names look alike and sound alike.

Insulin therapy should include regular basal insulin (intermediate or long-acting) and prandial and correctional doses, if needed. Insulin is essential in people with T1DM (ADA 2019). If the blood glucose is unstable, an intravenous insulin infusion might be indicated (Umpierrez 2009; ADS 2012). Sliding-scale insulin/top-up doses increase the risk of hypoglycaemia and are not recommended (ADA 2019; American Geriatrics Society 2019). However, prandial correction doses might be needed; see Medicines, Chapter 5. Not all oral medicines can be crushed: it is essential to check before crushing *any* medicines for oral administration or given via enteral tubes.

(9) Skin fold thickness and mid-arm muscle circumference measurements can also help ascertain weight loss/gain/stability.

(10) Maintain skin care around tube insertion sites and stoma care for gastrostomy tubes to prevent infection.

Care when recommencing oral feeds

(1) Monitor blood glucose carefully. Long-acting insulin is often commenced when oral feeds are resumed so there is a risk of hypoglycaemia. Only rapid or short-acting insulin can be given intravenously.

(2) Monitor and control nausea or vomiting, and describe vomitus.

(3) Maintain accurate fluid balance chart, usually two-hourly subtotals.

Diabetes and cancer

Most cancer occurs in older people.

Diabetes, especially T2DM, has been linked to various forms of cancer, particularly cancer of the pancreas, kidney, liver, gallbladder, uterine corpus, colorectal cancer, and multiple myeloma. Endometrial cancer also appears to be associated with diabetes and obesity (Wideroff et al. 1997; National Cancer Institute, 2017). Diabetes may be an early sign of pancreatic cancer (Carreras-Torres et al. 2017). One study demonstrated a significant increased risk for all cancers at moderately elevated HbA1c levels (6–6.9%) with a small increased risk at high levels (>7%) (Travier et al. 2007). These findings support the hypothesis that abnormal glucose metabolism and the associated inflammatory response and obesity contribute to the increased risk of some cancers but may not explain the mechanism or causal relationship.

Other cancers such as lung cancer do not appear to be associated with an increased cancer risk in people with diabetes; the evidence for an association with kidney cancer and non-Hodgkin's lymphoma is inconclusive. Few researchers have explored the association between T1DM and cancer (Giovannuci et al. 2010). Interestingly, diabetes appears to be associated with lower risk of prostate cancer and the risk of pancreatic cancer appears to be restricted to people with diabetes that precedes the diagnosis of pancreatic cancer by at least five years.

Researchers also suggest that diabetes is an independent predictor of death from colon, pancreas, liver, bladder cancer and breast cancer in men and women (Coughlin et al. 2004). Verlato et al. (2003) reported increased risk of death from breast cancer in women with T2DM compared with people without diabetes and suggested controlling weight could reduce the mortality rate. Likewise, median survival time is shorter (Bloomgarden 2001).

Common risk factors for cancer and diabetes appear to be ageing, gender, obesity, physical inactivity, diet, excess alcohol consumption, and smoking. Ethnicity and genetics also appear to play a role but the relationship is not straightforward. Likewise, the interrelated effect of hyperinsulinaemia, hyperglycaemia, inflammation, and insulin-like growth factors (IGF) in carcinogenesis is unclear.

There is some evidence that some GLMs cause/contribute to cancer risk: for example, associations between cancer and thiazolidinediones, sulphonylureas, incretins, and insulin glargine have been reported. The findings may be confounded by factors such as the effects of other cancer risks and cancer not being a primary end point in many studies. More research is needed into these issues (Giovannuci et al. 2010).

However, pioglitazone appears to be associated with increased risk of bladder cancer. Rosiglitazone was not associated with increased risk (Tuccori et al. 2016). The finding suggests the cancer risk may apply to individual medicines, and not be a class effect.

Metformin appears to be associated with lower cancer risk. Recent research eepidemiological and basic research suggest metformin inhibits cell proliferation, reduces colony formation, and causes partial cell cycle arrest in cancer cells (Alimova et al. 2009). A number of ongoing clinical trials are underway to determine the antitumor activity of metformin (Zi et al. 2018).

Objectives of care

Many people with cancer survive, and some experts regard cancer survivors as having a chronic disease, Thus, the focus is on 'supportive care' and tailored care, managing residual pain and helping the person live with their cancer and often diabetes if it was diagnosed after the cancer diagnosis (Ahmedzai 2019). Supportive care refers to 'prevention and management of adverse effects of cancer and its treatment' (Ahmedzai 2019). Supportive care includes physical and psychosocial care as well as rehabilitation and survivorship (i.e. the care/life continuum (Multinational Association for Supportive Care in Cancer www.mascc.org). Supportive care should include diabetes management when relevant.

Primary prevention

People with chronic diseases such as diabetes often do not receive usual preventative health strategies such as cancer screening (Psarakis 2006). For example, Lipscombe et al. (2005) found that Canadian women with chronic diseases were 32% less likely to receive routine cancer screening even though their doctors regularly monitored them. The discrepancy in screening rates could not be explained by other variables. However, the current focus on individualised and person-centred care suggests general health advice and screening could, or even should, be encompassed in diabetes complication screening programmes.

Proactive cancer screening and prevention programmes are important and should be promoted to people with diabetes, for example, mammograms, breast self-examination, and prostate checks. The findings also highlight another indication for normoglycaemia, controlling lipids, and weight management. Preventative healthcare also needs to encompass smoking cessation, reducing alcohol intake, and appropriate exercise and diet. In addition to the specific management of the cancer indicated by the cancer type and prognosis, diabetes management aims are to:

(1) Optimise cancer management considering the end of life stages: stable, unstable, deteriorating and terminal (Palliative Care Outcomes Collaboration (PCOC)—CareSearch 2008; Dunning et al. 2011) to meet the needs of the individual.
(2) Achieve as good a lifestyle as possible for as long as possible by optimising comfort, safety, quality of life, and enabling the person to make necessary life decisions by controlling symptoms and providing support and psychological care to the individual and their families.

(3) Achieve an acceptable blood glucose range in order to avoid the distressing symptoms associated with hyperglycaemia and hypoglycaemia and the consequent effect on comfort, cognitive function, mood, and quality of life deepening on life expectancy (end of life phase), diabetes type and indications and contraindications for various GLM, Chapter 5 (Dunning et al. 2011; Savage et al. 2012; ADS 2012). Insulin may be required. The type of insulin and the dose and dose regimen depends on individual needs and the effects of other treatment such as medicines, feeding, and pain on blood glucose levels. Insulin analogues such as levemir and glargine may provide adequate control in a simple regimen; see Chapters 5 and 18. The short-acting glitinides may be a useful GLM option if vomiting is not an issue. Pioglitazone has been associated with a small but absolute risk of bladder cancer (Lewis et al. 2011) and should be avoided in people with or at risk of bladder cancer. Metformin may be contraindicated depending on the cancer and the status of the gastrointestinal tract. As with all care planning, the individual and their relevant carers should be involved in care decisions.

(4) Prevent/manage malnutrition, cachexia, dehydration, and hyperglycaemia, which affect healing and reduce resistance to infection and increase the risk of hypoglycaemia. Diet should be appropriate for the presenting cancer symptoms and in some cases is part of the treatment of some cancers. Sufficient protein and carbohydrate are needed for hormone synthesis and to maintain stores that are being depleted by the cancer. Small frequent feeds, enteral or total parenteral nutrition (TPN) feeds, may be needed. Enteral and TPN feeding can lead to hyperglycaemia and be exacerbated by corticosteroid medicines, stress, and infection. Short- or rapid-acting insulin may be needed, usually 1 unit of insulin to 10 g of carbohydrate initially, but higher doses may be needed. As indicated previously, selecting formulas developed for people with diabetes reduces the impact on blood glucose. High-fibre diets can cause diarrhoea, vomiting, and bloating if the cancer involves the bowel.

(5) Adequately control pain. Pain is due to various causes, including the investigative procedures and surgery and metastatic disease. Some 35% of people with cancer report pain early in the disease and 64% experience pain at the end of life (Van den Beuken et al. 2016). Pain has a negative effect on well-being and recovery. Comorbidities, including diabetes, are an important cause of pain, especially in older people.

(6) Control nausea and vomiting, which are common side effects of chemotherapeutic agents as well as some cancers and some diabetes complications. Preventative measures to avoid DKA and hyperosmolar states that can require admission to hospital, must be factored into the care plan (Chapter 7). Other causes include bowel obstruction, gastroparesis, infection, liver disease, medicine interactions, and increased intracranial pressure such as cerebral oedema and radiation therapy. Nausea and vomiting can affect hydration status and physical comfort.

(7) Prevent trauma.

(8) Monitor renal and hepatic function before, during, and after administering cytotoxic medicines and before using some GLMs such as metformin.

(9) Encourage exercise within the individual's capacity.

(10) Provide education and psychological support. Prepare for end-of-life care if the person has not already documented an advance care plan/directive; see Chapter 18. Limitation of medical treatment orders may also be documented to aid decision-making and reduce decisional uncertainty for clinicians and family (Chapter 18).

Clinician responsibilities

(1) Provide a safe environment.

(2) Consider the psychological aspects of having cancer and diabetes, such as fear of death, body image changes, denial, and grief and loss.

(3) Involve the individual and their relevant carers in management decisions, proactively plan for end-of-life care, including discussing documenting advanced care directives and plans, power of attorney, and making a will.

(4) Ensure appropriate diabetic education if diabetes develops as a consequence of the altered metabolism of cancer or medicines.

(5) Proactively attend to pressure areas, including the feet and around nasogastric tubes.

(6) Provide oral care, manage stomatitis and mucositis, and ensure a dental consultation occurs.

(7) Control nausea, vomiting, and pain, which contribute to fatigue and reduce quality of life.

(8) Manage radiotherapy. Fatigue often occurs as a consequence of radiotherapy; the rates vary between 14 and 90% of patients and can have a significant impact on quality of life and recovery (Jersczek-Fossa et al. 2002). Radiotherapy is usually localised to a specific site, and side effects are also usually localised but radiation-induced pneumonitis and fibrosis (late complication) can exacerbate fatigue and cause considerable discomfort, which compounds fatigue. The pattern of fatigue changes over the course of treatment and often declines on no-radiotherapy days. Ensuring the person understands and is given strategies to help them cope with fatigue is essential. Information should be oral and written. Stress management and relaxation techniques can be helpful, as can providing an environment conducive to rest and sleep.

(9) Monitor blood glucose levels as frequently as necessary.

(10) Accurately chart fluid balance, blood glucose, temperature, pulse, and respiration (TPS), weight.

(11) Ensure referral to the dietitian, psychologist, and diabetes nurse specialist/educator.

(12) Be aware of the possibility of hypoglycaemia if the person is not eating/fasting for a procedure, is vomiting or has a poor appetite. Hypoglycaemia is a significant risk when the appetite is poor and food intake is inadequate. QID insulin regimens using rapid-acting insulin such as Novorapid or Humalog and/or long-acting insulin analogues may reduce the hypoglycaemia risk. GLMs with long duration of action may need to be stopped because of the risk of hypoglycaemia. In addition, if hypoglycaemia does occur, it can be more profound and the energy reserves in the liver and muscles may be insufficient to respond to the counter-regulatory response to hypoglycaemia (Chapters 1 and 6). Short-acting sulphonylureas or insulin may be indicated in T2DM. Biguanides may be contraindicated if renal or hepatic failure is present because of the risk of lactic acidosis. Thiazolidinediones (TZDs) take some time to have an optimal effect, are difficult to adjust in the short term, and contribute to oedema, and can reduce haemoglobin and contribute to fatigue. TZD are contraindicated in people with heart failure and those at high risk of fractures (Chapter 5). TZD may be useful if prolonged low-dose steroids are required (Oyer et al. 2006). Incretin mimetics reduce postprandial hyperglycaemia, but research into their benefit in corticosteroid use is limited. In addition, they cause significant nausea, vomiting, and weight loss, which can exacerbate malnutrition and increase morbidity in people with cancer.

(13) Be aware of the possibility of hyperglycaemia as a result of medications such as corticosteroids and antipsychotics, pain, and stress.

(14) Monitor biochemistry results and report abnormal results.

(15) Provide appropriate care during investigative and surgical procedures; see Chapter 9.

(16) Consider the possibility that people with cancer often try complementary therapies in an attempt to cure or manage their cancer. It is important to ask about the use of complementary therapies and provide or refer the person for appropriate information about the risks and benefits of such therapies (see Chapter 18).

(17) Maintain skin integrity by appropriate skin care especially where corticosteroid medications are used. They cause the skin to become thin and fragile and it is easily damaged during shaving and routine nursing care, brittle hair, which can exacerbate the effects of chemotherapy, and bone loss. Corticosteroids are also associated with mood changes, which can cause distress to the patient and their relatives. Careful explanations and reassurance are required.

Clinical observations

(1) Narcotic pain medication can mask the signs of hypoglycaemia.

(2) Insulin/oral agents may need to be adjusted frequently to meet the changing metabolic needs and prevailing appetite and food intake. In the terminal stages of cancer, these medicines can be withheld, as long as the individual is comfortable and not subject to excursions in blood glucose that can lead to uncomfortable symptoms, dehydration, and pain.

(3) There is evidence that yoga, tai chi, and mindfulness increase well-being and reduce medicine side effects: however, people who use complementary and alternative medicine (CAM) and forgo conventional cancer treatments are twice as likely to die within five years than people who use conventional cancer treatments (National Cancer Institute 2017).

(4) People with diabetes in the end-of-life stages, and their family carers, want their blood glucose maintained in a range that avoids hypo- and hyperglycaemia to promote comfort and quality of life (Dunning et al. 2012; Savage et al. 2012).

Managing corticosteroids in people with cancer

People with cancer are often prescribed corticosteroids as a component of chemotherapy to prevent or manage nausea, reduce inflammation or following neurological procedures. These medicines cause postprandial hyperglycaemia by down-regulating GLUT-4 transporters in muscle, which impairs glucose entry into cells. They also promote gluconeogenesis. Thus, diabetes can be diagnosed after the cancer diagnosis.

Not all glucocorticoids have the same effect on blood glucose. The effect depends on the dose, duration of action, and duration of treatment. Morning prednisolone doses usually cause elevated blood glucose in the afternoon but the blood glucose usually drops overnight and is lower in the morning. Insulin is recommended to manage hyperglycaemia (ADS 2012; ADA 2019), using morning basal insulin or a premixed insulin at the midday meal because the blood glucose tends to rise towards the afternoon. People already using insulin are likely to require higher doses whilst they are receiving corticosteroid medicines. Generally, corticosteroid doses are reduced slowly and blood glucose monitored to adjust GLM doses.

Complementary medicines and therapies and cancer

Many people with cancer use a variety of complementary medicines and other therapies (CM). Estimates vary from 7% to 83%: mean 31%. High usage occurs in children, older people, those with specific cancers such as prostate and breast cancer (Wyatt et al. 1999; Kao and Devine 2000; Horneber et al. 2012; Cancer Council Australia 2018; Buckner et al. 2018). The type of CM therapies used varies amongst countries and ethnic and cultural groups.

There is evidence to support the effectiveness of some CM; others have not been assessed for efficacy or safety and some are ineffective and harmful (Cancer Council Australia 2018).

A common complaint from conventional practitioners is that people do not disclose their CM use. People who use CM do not disclose their CM use for a range of reasons: mostly because conventional practitioners do not ask about CM. Asking about CM is a core aspect of a holistic assessment. Characteristics of CM users with cancer include:

- Women
- Younger age
- Higher education
- Higher socioeconomic group

- Prior CM use
- Active coping and preventive healthcare behaviours, and a desire to do everything possible to maintain or improve health and quality of life, as well as take an active part in management decisions
- Participate in cancer support groups
- Have a close friend or relative with cancer who uses CM
- General and cancer-related health beliefs

Many conventional practitioners are concerned that CM holds out false hope of a cure, interferes with or delays conventional treatment, poses a risk of CAM medicine side effects and interactions, and is not always evidence-based. Many of these concerns are well-founded; see Chapter 19. Where CM is used, the selection and use of CM needs to be informed and integrated into the overall care plan to optimise the benefits of both CM and conventional management strategies.

Some benefits of CM use are longer survival time, reduced anxiety, and improved quality of life using mind–body medicine, music and art therapy, massage, aromatherapy, and support group programmes (Eremin and Walker 2009, Cancer Council Australia 2018), as well as reduction in chemotherapy-induced stomatitis (Oberbaum et al. 2001).

Here are seven useful CM strategies that can be alone or in combination (see, e.g. Mayo Clinic 2018b):

(1) Mind–body therapies include relaxation techniques, visualisation, meditation, massage, and creative therapies such as music, art, and writing (Mayo Clinic 2018b).
(2) Including prayer as a form of CAM greatly increases the percentages of people who say that they use CAM. Prayer is overwhelmingly perceived as being helpful (Chui et al. 2004).
(3) Gentle exercises such as some forms of tai chi and yoga, which combine meditative practices, and walking (Mayo Clinic 2018b). The latter can include pet therapy e.g. walking the dog. In Australia, women with breast cancer have participated in Dragon Boat racing.
(4) Essential oils can be used in psychological care as well as massage and education and some reduce stomatitis (Wilkinson 2008). The oils need to be chosen to suit the individual because some odours contribute to nausea or may provoke unpleasant memories. Alternatively, they can recall happy memories. 'Fragrant' oils are vastly different from essential oils chemically and should not be applied to the skin, used in baths, or taken orally but they have useful emotional effects when inhaled.
(5) Nutritional medicine that focuses on a healthy well-balanced diet, whole foods, low in fat and sugar, and using vitamin and mineral supplements, especially in immunocompromised patients if they are not contraindicated. Probiotics can help sustain normal gut flora. Soy products and vitamin D supplementation improve bone mineral density. However, megadoses of vitamins and mineral can interfere with chemotherapy. Other potentially dangerous supplements include calcium for bone disease for women with breast cancer, iron and vitamin C in those receiving blood transfusions, nutritionally inadequate diets and 'cleansing' enemas (Breast Cancer Network Australia, 2016).
(6) Acupressure and acupuncture to acupuncture point P6 reduce nausea. These are useful additions to conventional methods of controlling nausea (Mayo Clinic 2018b; Dibble et al. 2007).
(7) Herbal medicines such as milk thistle complement the action of chemotherapy agents and reduce the toxic effects on the liver in animal models (Abenavoli et al. 2010) and anti-inflammatory agents such as curcumin may have a role but more research is needed.

For information about advising people about the safe use of CM, see Chapter 19.

Management

Generally, a number of investigations are required to diagnose cancer, and the results often mean more tests are required before the individual receives a definitive diagnosis. Thus, a diagnosis of cancer is loaded with meaning, often interpreted as a 'death sentence' that induces significant distress to the individual and family, which needs to be factored into the diabetes care plan.

People with diabetes should be encouraged to participate in appropriate cancer screening programmes the same as those without diabetes, e.g. mammograms, bowel screens and prostate checks. Even though prostate cancer may not be associated with diabetes, if it occurs glycaemic control is likely to be affected, and it is a common and devastating cancer. A healthy well-balanced diet low in fat and alcohol and regular exercise are important preventative strategies as well as part of diabetes and cancer management plans.

Cancer management is the same for people with diabetes as for people without diabetes; however, some extra considerations apply. Cancer cells trap amino acids for their own use, limiting the protein available for normal body functions, which sets the scene for weight loss, especially where the appetite is poor, and the senses of smell and taste are diminished. Malabsorption, nausea and vomiting, and radiation treatment further exacerbate weight loss. Whilst weight loss may confer many health benefits, it is often excessive in cancer and causes malnutrition, which reduces immunity and affects normal cellular functioning and wound healing. Glucose enters cancer cells down a concentration gradient rather than through insulin-mediated entry and metabolism favours lactate production. Lactate is transported to the liver, increasing gluconeogenesis. Hypoalbuminaemia also occurs.

For the person with diabetes, lactate production can contribute to hyperglycaemia and reduce insulin production, with consequent effects on blood glucose control. Hyperglycaemia is associated with higher infection rates, and the risk is significantly increased in immunocompromised patients and those on corticosteroid medications. In addition, hyperglycaemia-associated symptoms cause discomfort (Dunning et al. 2011; Diabetes UK 2018; Savage et al. 2012).

Diabetes management should be considered in relation to the prognosis and cancer therapy. Preventing long-term complications of diabetes may be irrelevant if the prognosis is poor, but controlling hyperglycaemic symptoms and consequences has benefits for comfort, quality of life, and functioning during the dying process (Quinn et al. 2006; Dunning et al. 2012; Diabetes UK 2018).

However, many people have existing diabetes complications such as renal and cardiac disease that need to be managed to promote comfort and quality of life (see Chapter 18). For example, the chemotherapeutic agent cisplatin causes renal insufficiency and can exacerbate existing renal disease; cisplatin, paclitaxel, and vincristine might exacerbate neuropathy. Side effects from chemotherapeutic agents are usually permanent. Where the prognosis is good, improving the complication status as much as possible and controlling blood glucose and lipids may help minimise the impact of chemotherapy.

Specific treatment depends on the type of cancer the patient has, the prognosis and values, care goals, and preferences. Diagnosis of some types of cancer such as endocrine tumours can involve prolonged fasting and radiological imaging and/or other radiological procedures. The appropriate care should be given in these circumstances (see Chapter 9). Corticosteroid therapy is frequently used in cancer treatment and can precipitate diabetes in people without diabetes, especially if diabetes risk factors are present, and cause hyperglycaemia in people with diabetes. Corticosteroids may be required for a prolonged time or given in large doses for a short period. Therefore, blood glucose needs to be monitored regularly in patients on corticosteroid medications, which are discussed later in this chapter.

Smoking, alcohol, and illegal drug use

Substance use refers to intentionally using a pharmacological substance to achieve a desired recreational or therapeutic effect. The term *use* does not imply illegal use and is nonjudgmental. However, the term *substance abuse* is both negative and judgmental. Continued drug abuse can become an addiction. The American Psychiatric Association (DSM-V 2013) defined criteria for diagnosing psychiatric disease including drug abuse and drug addiction (see Table 10.1.)

Table 10.1   American Psychiatric Association criteria for drug abuse and drug addiction.

Criteria for drug abuse	Criteria for drug dependence/addiction
Recurrent drug use and not fulfilling important/usual life roles	Tolerance
	Withdrawal symptoms when not using
Using drugs in dangerous situations	Taking increasing amounts over time and for longer than intended (needing more drug to achieve an effect)
Encountering legal problems from using drugs	Wanting to or unsuccessfully trying to reduce use or quit
Continuing to use drugs despite encountering problems	Spending a considerable amount of time obtaining, using or recovering from drug use
	Usual activities are affected by drug use
	Continuing to use despite knowing it is harmful

Drug abuse is diagnosed when a person exhibits three of these criteria for 12 months.

Smoking

> Giving up smoking is the easiest thing in the world. I know because I've done it thousands of times.
>
> (Mark Twain)

The prevalence of smoking has decreased in many countries but smoking continues to be the most common underlying morbidity and mortality risk factor for many diseases (Australian Institute of Health and Welfare 2018). Smoking is hazardous to health, regardless of whether the individual has diabetes. In addition, constantly being in a smoke-filled environment is a hazard for non-smokers causing ~50 000 deaths annually in the United States (DHHS Surgeon General's Report 2006). Smoking during pregnancy has adverse effects on the foetus as well as the mother's health.

Smoking is a strong and independent risk factor for cardiovascular disease in a dose-dependent manner in the general population. Stopping smoking reduces the risk, but the degree of risk reduction depends on the duration of smoking (SIGN 2010). The evidence for an association between smoking and microvascular disease is unclear, although a Swedish study suggests people who smoke currently or up to five years before the study are at significant risk of chronic renal disease (Ejerblad et al. 2004). Smoking may be at risk factor of retinopathy in type 1 diabetes (Stratton et al. 2001 Mayo Clinic 2018a).

Smoking is also associated with respiratory diseases such as emphysema, chronic obstructive pulmonary disease (COPD), chronic bronchitis as well as oral, laryngeal, bladder and cervical cancers, and tooth and gum disease (Orisatoki 2013). In addition, environmental tobacco smoke or second-hand smoking can have the same or more adverse effects in non-smokers because there is three times the amount of tar and more than six times the amount of nicotine in second-hand smoke (Orisatoki 2013). Second-hand smoke can affect the foetus and children. For example, infant death and preterm birth as well as low birth weight is associated with maternal smoking, and there is a higher incidence of middle-ear infections, coughing, wheezing, and asthma in children (National Native Addictions Partnership Foundation 2006) and emotional and behavioural problems in children whose parents smoke (Weiser et al. 2010).

Nicotine is the primary alkaloid found in tobacco and is responsible for addiction to cigarettes. Tobacco also contains about 69 carcinogens in the tar, the particulate matter that remains when nicotine and water are removed, 11 of these substances are known carcinogens and a further 7 are probably carcinogens (Kroon 2007). Of these, polycyclic aromatic hydrocarbons (PAH) are the major lung carcinogens and are potent hepatic cytochrome P-450 inducers, particularly 1A1, 1A2, and possible 2E1. Thus, smoking and quitting can interact with commonly prescribed medicines and foods. Smoking status is an important aspect of routine medication reviews and when prescribing medicines.

Interactions that can occur between tobacco smoke and many commonly prescribed medicines include:

- Subcutaneous and inhaled insulin. Absorption of subcutaneous insulin may be reduced due to insulin resistance, which is associated with smoking. Inhaled insulin is rarely used, but when it is, smoking enhances absorption rates and peak action time is faster and insulin blood levels are higher than in nonsmokers.
- Propanolol and other beta-blocking agents.
- Heparin: reduced half-life and increased clearance.
- Hormone contraceptives particularly combination formulations.
- Inhaled corticosteroids, which may have reduced efficacy in people with asthma.
- Tricyclic antidepressants.
- Other medicines such as olanzapine, clozapine, benzodiazepines, and opoids (Zevin and Benowitz 1999).

Other medicines and foods can also be affected, leading to less than optional therapeutic effects and subtle malnutrition. Dose adjustments of many medicines may be required when people smoke and may need to be readjusted once they quit. The side effects of medicines may contribute to smoking withdrawal symptoms.

People most likely to smoke:

- Are members of some ethnic groups such as Indigenous Australian, African American, and Hispanic peoples.
- Have a mental health problem – 70% of people with a mental health problem smoke. In addition, people often commence smoking when they develop a mental health problem.
- Use illegal drugs and/or alcohol.

Quitting smoking reduces the risk of cardiovascular disease, respiratory disease, cancer, and a range of other diseases, and dying before age 50 by 50% in the following 15 years. The risk of developing many of these conditions is increased in the presence of obesity and uncontrolled diabetes. Smoking in middle and old age is significantly associated with a reduction in healthy life years (Ostbye and Taylor 2004; SIGN 2010). A meta-analysis of observational studies suggests smoking increases the risk of developing type 2 diabetes (Willi et al. 2007; Mayo Clinic 2018b). Willi et al. found smoking was independently associated with glucose intolerance, impaired fasting glucose and type 2 diabetes.

Quitting smoking is difficult and requires significant behaviour change on the part of the individual and support from their family, friends, and clinicians. The person must first recognise smoking is a problem. The desire to change may not be the same as wanting help to change. Almost 75% of smokers report they want to quit (Owen et al. 1992), but <7% remain smoke free after 12 months and the average smoker tries to quite six to nine times in their lifetime (American Cancer Society 2007). Smoking at night appears to be a predictor of nicotine dependence and is a significant predictor of relapsing within six months of trying to quit (Bover et al. 2008). In addition, smoking at night is associated with poor treatment outcomes (Foulds et al. 2006) and impacts on sleep quality, also important to health. Bover et al. (2008) suggested health professionals should specifically ask about night smoking when assessing readiness to quit.

Research suggests timing smoking cessation interventions to coincide with the individual's readiness to change is important to success. In addition, sociologists highlight the importance of life course transitions in behaviour change and suggest the longer people live, the more likely they are to make transitions in later life and the more likely such transitions are to be accompanied by changes in behaviour (George 1993). Thus, targeting smoking cessation interventions to coincide with life transitions may be more likely to succeed.

For example, Lang et al. (2007) suggested individuals retiring from work are more likely to stop smoking than those who remain at work after controlling for retiring due to ill health. They recommended interventions be developed for those making the transition to retirement and employers should incorporate smoking cessation programmes into their retirement plans. Health events, particularly those that are disabling or affect work and lifestyle, also affect smoking cessation rates (Falba 2005). These and other studies suggest several key transitions could be used to target smoking cessation in addition to regular prevention messages.

However, population health models and strategies as part of every country's public health framework that focuses on all the interrelated personal and social factors involved is essential. Significantly, health professionals should be appropriate role models and not smoke.

Nicotine addiction

Nicotine receptors, a_4b_2 nicotinic acetylcholine receptors (nAChRs), are located throughout the central nervous system. Nicotine binds to these receptors, and acts as an agonist prolonging activation of these receptors and facilitating the release of neurotransmitters such as acetylcholine, dopamine, serotonin, and beta-endorphins, which engenders pleasurable feelings, arousal, reduced anxiety and relaxation. Nicotine action mode reinforces dependence in a cyclical manner: smoking stimulates dopamine, the dopamine level falls as the nicotine level falls producing withdrawal symptoms. Smoking again suppresses the cravings by restimulating the nAChRs receptors.

The area of the brain concerned with addiction appears to be the insula, a small structure within the cerebral cortex. People with damage to the insula from trauma or stroke often suddenly stop smoking and remain non-smoking (Naqvi et al. 2007). Five milligrammes of nicotine per day is a large enough dose to cause addiction. Each cigarette contains between 0.13 and 2 mg of nicotine; thus, even light smokers can be addicted. Nicotine is present in the blood stream within 15 seconds of smoking a cigarette, which provides immediate gratification (Watkins et al. 2000). Chronic nicotine use desensitises the receptors, and increasing amounts of nicotine are required to achieve pleasurable effects.

Withdrawal symptoms usually occur within the first 24 hours and can be very stressful. Withdrawal symptoms include:

- Craving tobacco
- Difficulty concentrating, which affects work and usual daily activities and may be compounded by disturbed sleep and night smoking
- Headache
- Impaired motor performance
- Fatigue
- Irritability
- Anxiety and restlessness
- Sleep disturbances
- Nausea
- Hunger and weight gain

All of these symptoms can lead to inadequate diabetes self-care. For example, concern about putting on weight can be a significant barrier to quitting. Smoking cessation programmes need to help the individual manage their symptoms. In addition, smoking may increase addiction to cannabis if the individual also uses this drug.

Assisting the person to stop smoking

Brief advice from clinicians has a limited effect: only 2–3% quit per year (Lancaster and Stead 2004) but the effect size can be increased if other strategies such as referral to 'Quit' programmes, interested supportive follow-up, setting achievable goals with the individual and pharmacotherapy. The 5As approach can be helpful. It consists of the following:

Ask about smoking habits and systematically document the information at each visit. Provide brief advice to quit in a clear supportive, non-judgmental manner regularly.

Assess interest in quitting so that advice can be appropriately targeted to the stage of change and to opportunistically support attempts to quit. Assess whether the individual has tried to quit in the past and the factors that prevented them from quitting and those that helped, as well as the level of nicotine dependence: ~70–80% of smokers are dependent on nicotine and will experience withdrawal symptoms when they try to quit. Nicotine addiction is a chronic relapsing condition (Wise et al. 2007). Repeated efforts to quit can be demoralising and set up learned helplessness. Helping the individual manage the symptoms can support their attempt. Sometimes mental health problems become apparent when a person stops smoking; thus, mental health should be monitored.

Advise about the importance of quitting on a regular basis and provide new information as it arises. Advice can include information about smoking risks and quit programmes. Advice is more useful if it is tailored to the individual. In Australia, some health insurance funds offer member discounts to quit programmes, such as Allen Carr's Easy Way to Stop Smoking. This method consists of a combination of psychotherapy and hypnotherapy.

Assist those who indicate they want to quit by asking what assistance they feel would help them most, refer them for counselling, provide written information or recommend other therapies as indicated and follow up at the next visit. Relapsing after attempting to quit is common. Praise and support are essential, as are exploring the reasons for relapsing and discussing strategies for continuing the quit process. Motivational interviewing can be a useful technique.

Arrange a follow-up visit, preferably within the first week after the quit date (Torrijos and Glantz 2006). Some pharmaceutical companies offer support programmes through newsletters and Internet sites. Fu et al. (2006) showed 75% of relapsed smokers were interested in repeating the quit intervention (behavioural and medicines strategies) within 30 days of quitting, which highlights the importance of support and constant reminders. Advising and supporting partners may also be important.

Non-pharmacological strategies can be combined with the 5As. These include opportunistic and structured counselling that encourages the individual to think about the relevance of quitting to their life, helps them identify their personal health risks, and helps them determine the barriers and facilitators they are likely to encounter develop strategies to strengthen the facilitators and overcome the barriers.

Improving nutrition is important to health generally. Diets rich in tyrosine, tryptophane, and vitamins B_6, B_3, C, and magnesium, zinc, and iron may stimulate the dopamine pathway and help reduce the effects of nicotine withdrawal by increasing serotonin levels (Osiecki 2006). Improving nutrition can also reduce oxidative damage, which is increased in smokers and help reduce weight gain.

CAM strategies may help manage withdrawal symptoms. These include acupuncture and acupressure to specific pressure points to reduce the withdrawal symptoms (Mitchell 2008). People may be able to learn to self-stimulate relevant acupressure points. Treatment consists of biweekly session for two weeks and then weekly for two to six weeks. Herbal preparations include green tea and lemon balm tea capsules, which improve focus and concentration and reduce anxiety, without causing drowsiness; Ashwaganda capsules, an Ayurvedic medicine, increases energy levels and well-being, *Silymarin* (milk thistle) before meals may help manage blood glucose and support the liver, flower remedies, melatonin, and high-dose vitamin B. All of these interventions need to be combined with education, support, and counselling and be included in the management plan.

Self-help websites describe a time frame when symptoms resolve and people can expect to feel better, which gives them a goal to aim for. They also suggest some steps to stopping, which include:

- Make a firm decision to stop and ask for help without shame or guilt.
- Ask people who successfully quit how they did it.
- Quit with a friend to support each other.

- Wash your clothes and air out the house to get rid of the smell and if possible avoid smoke-filled environments.
- Write down the reasons you want to quit and the things that can help you succeed.
- Obtain information about all the quit options and decide which one/s is most likely to suit you.
- Set small achievable goals.

These strategies can be used in combination and included in other strategies. Recently, the Australian government has legislated for significant changes to labelling on tobacco packaging that included graphic pictures such as the effects of smoking on the mouth and gums, and advertising campaigns as well as regulating where people can smoke in public building and environments has had a significant impact on smoking in Australia.

Medicines to support smoking cessation

A number of medicines are available to assist smoking cessation, but they are not a substitute for counselling and support, which need to continue if medications are indicated. Commonly used medicines to help people quit smoking are shown in Table 10.2. A combination of dose forms can be used, for example, patches and gums, which can be used in combination. In addition, nicotine replacement therapy can be prescribed for pregnant and lactating women but nonmedicine options are preferred for pregnant women, people with cardiovascular disease, and young people aged 12–17 years (Tonstad et al. 2006).

Other medicines and an anti-nicotine vaccine are currently being developed to reduce the link between smoking and nicotine concentration in the brain to lower the related gratification. Transcranial magnetic stimulation (TMS) may be adapted in the future to specifically target the insula. Currently, TMS does not penetrate beyond peripheral tissues.

Many cultures smoke, chew, or sniff a range of smokeless tobacco products such as Gul, Gutcha, Iq'mik, Pan Masal (betal quid), and different snuff preparations. These chemical products often contain chemicals such as bicarbonate and other ingredients such as spices. The Third International Conference on Smokeless Tobacco held in 2002 concluded there is evidence that smokeless tobacco causes cancer in humans, especially in the oral cavity, and increases the risk of head and neck cancer. In addition, they lead to other noncancerous conditions, and some are as addictive, or more addictive, than nicotine (National Native Addictions Partnership Foundation 2006). The Third International Conference (2002) produced a number of fact sheets about these products that could be useful in cultures where smokeless tobacco products are used such as India and Native American Peoples.

In some countries, e-cigarette use (vaping) is promoted to reduce smoking rates; however, it only reduces cigarette smoking by 50% and needs to be used with behavioural therapy. Since e-cigarettes contain nicotine, over time some people become addicted to nicotine and commence cigarette smoking (Wilson et al. 2019). Likewise, nicotine has been linked to fatty deposits in the liver and change liver function in mice (Mangubat et al. 2019), which many have implications for people with existing liver disease.

Alcohol addiction

Alcohol is also an addictive substance associated with significant morbidity and mortality. Between 15% and 20% of primary care consultations relate to alcohol (Lee 2008). Short-term consequences include injury and domestic violence; longer-term effects include other risk-taking behaviours such as smoking, neglected self-care, driving whilst intoxicated, cognitive impairment, peripheral neuropathy, liver cirrhosis, and foetal damage in pregnant women. Hepatic encephalopathy (Gundling et al. 2013) and peripheral neuropathy are significant consequences of alcohol addiction.

Approximately 10% of Australians and 20% of Indigenous Australians drink more than the recommended level (National Health and Medical Research Council [NHMRC] 2007). Young people are also likely to consume higher than recommended amounts of alcohol. Recommendations

Table 10.2 Medicines available to assist people to stop smoking.

Medicine	Dose	Duration of treatment	Side effects and precautions
Nicotine formulations: Gum (Nicorette)	2–4 mg: 1 piece of gum 1–2 hourly	Up to 12 weeks	Sore mouth, hiccups, dyspepsia Caution: unstable angina, 2 weeks post MI, serious cardiac arrhythmias Acidic drinks and caffeine affect absorption
Lozenge	2–4 mg: 1 lozenge 1–2 hourly for 6 weeks then 1 every 2–4 hours in weeks 7–9 and 1 every 4–8 hours in weeks 10–12 (9–20/day according to need)	Up to 12 weeks	Caution: uncontrolled hypertension, recent MI, arrhythmias, gastric ulcers, diabetes
Transdermal patch (NicoDerm CQ, habitrol)	Available in 7, 14, and 21 mg doses. Patch applied every 16–24 hours	8–10 weeks	Localised skin reactions, headaches, disturbed sleep Caution: unstable angina, 2 weeks after MI, cardiac arrhythmias
Inhaled	168 cartridges; 10 mg nicotine/ cartridge but delivered dose is 4 mg; 1–2 doses/hour as required	Up to 8 weeks dose needs to be reduced in the last 4–6 weeks.	Nasal irritation Caution: unstable angina, 2 weeks after MI, cardiac arrhythmias Contraindicated if severe airways disease such as asthma and COPD is present
Nasal spray	100 mg nicotine/10 ml bottle, dose delivered per spray is 0.5 mg; one dose is 1 mg in each nostril (1 spray)	Up to 6 months	Nasal irritation May be contraindicated if severe airways disease such as asthma and COPD is present
Bupropion SR (Zyban)	Starting dose 150 mg/day for 3 days then 150 mg BD	Up to 24 weeks	Nausea, vomiting, constipation
Varenicline (Champix)	Starting dose 0.5 mg/day for 3 days then 0.5 mg BD for 3 days followed by 1 mg BD	Up to 24 weeks	Nausea, vomiting, constipation Mercola (2011) suggested Chantix can cause extreme mind-altering behaviours and movement disorders by releasing dopamine in the brain and blocking the pleasure centres in the brain and can lead to severe depression. Chantix may also have adverse cardiovascular effects. Mercola listed the following psychological side effects: depression, anger, hostility, suicidal ideation, mania, paranoia, agitation, anxiety, confusion and sleep disorders

MI = myocardial infarction.
They should be combined with other counselling and support strategies and good nutrition and be considered as part of the medication record and their benefits and risks reviewed regularly whilst they are being used. The prescribing information should be consulted for specific information about each medicine.

for alcohol intake were discussed in Chapter 1 and are defined in the NHMRC and other guidelines such as the American Diabetes Association (2019) guidelines: generally one drink per day or less for women and two drinks per day or less for men.

Excess alcohol >40 g/day increases the risk of liver disease, hypertension, and violent death (SIGN 2010). Likewise, drinking two to three units of alcohol/day may not result in hypoglycaemia, but alcohol consumption reduces hypoglycaemia awareness. In addition, both alcohol and hypoglycaemia affect cognitive function in an additive manner (SIGN 2010). Alcohol is associated with both benefits and risks for cardiovascular disease and psychological well-being. Alcohol in small doses may prevent cardiovascular disease and death in people with type 2 diabetes; however, the threshold for admission to hospital with an acute cardiac event occurs at a lower level of alcohol consumption: one glass of wine/day (SIGN 2010).

A diagnosis of alcohol dependence is made if three of the following factors are present:

- Alcohol tolerance;
- Withdrawal symptoms;
- Drinking more than the recommended level or for longer than planned;
- Previous unsuccessful attempts to reduce consumption or stop drinking;
- Spending a significant amount of time procuring or drinking alcohol;
- Neglecting social interactions and work responsibilities because of alcohol;
- Continuing to drink alcohol despite the actual and potential health risks.

The strategies outlined for helping people quit smoking can be adapted to help people reduce alcohol consumption to the recommended levels or stop drinking. Screening for alcohol dependence can be accomplished using the World Health Organization (WHO) Alcohol Use Disorders Identification Test (AUDIT) (Saunders et al. 1993). High AUDIT scores indicate the need for a comprehensive intervention and counselling. Support groups such as Alcoholics Anonymous have a well-recognised role in stopping drinking and preventing relapse. Anecdotally, Men's Sheds also play a supportive role in encouraging men to talk about their problems with peers, encouraging social interactions and hobbies and also have a positive impact on mental health and wellbeing.

Diabetes is difficult to manage because GLMs are often contraindicated because of the risk of lactic acidosis (metformin) and hypoglycaemia. Insulin is often indicated but adherence is often suboptimal and is compounded by erratic intake and malnutrition, which put the individual at risk of hypoglycaemia. Withdrawal processes for heavy drinkers need to be supervised and people require a significant amount of support.

Medicines to assist alcohol withdrawal include Acamprosate and Naltrexone, which are generally well tolerated and can be continued if the person drinks alcohol. They are effective at preventing relapse, delaying return to drinking and reducing drinking days. Disulfiram (Antabuse) causes acute illness if the person drinks alcohol whilst taking the medication. Supervision is required if Antabuse is used because life-threatening reactions can occur. It is not the ideal first-line treatment and probably should only be prescribed by doctors with experience using it or use it under the guidance of such experts (Shand et al. 2003).

Illegal drug use

The effect of marijuana, cocaine, and other illegal drugs on diabetes is unclear. These substances are associated with poor health outcomes and risk-taking behaviours in nondiabetics and people with diabetes. In addition, illegal drugs and the associated risks may compound or contribute to short- and long-term diabetes complications. The fact that they are illegal makes illegal drug use harder to detect. Generally, illegal drugs fall into three main categories:

- Uppers, for example, ecstasy, ice, crystal meth, cocaine, snow, speed
- Opiates, for example, morphine, heroin, smac.
- Hallucinogens, for example, marijuana (cannabis, pot, weed), LSD, solvents such as petrol, glue, and paint

Table 10.3 The effects of medicine or medicine combinations and duration of action.

Main class of illlegal drug	Duration of action	Possible effect on blood glucose[a]	Some commonly reported effects
Uppers	Usually 4–6 but up to 24 hours	Hyperglycaemia from missing injections/OHA increasing the risk of diabetic ketoacidosis (DKA)/hyperosmolar states (HHS) Hypoglycaemia due to inadequate intake, nausea, and vomiting	Increased energy Tachycardia Weakness and lethargy Heightened sensations Ecstasy can cause boundless energy and the user might not want to rest or eat Cocaine often reduces appetite Sleep disturbances and/or lethargy and prolonged sleep due to 'come down' as the effects of the drug wear off Dilated pupils Nausea and/or vomiting Weight loss Impaired memory and cognition These affect self-care and the ability to recognise hypoglycaemia
Opiates	4–24 hours	Hypo or hyperglycaemia due to inadequate self-care such as OHA/ insulin mismanagement and increased risk of DKA/HONK	Euphoria Hallucinations Relaxation Slurred speech Disinhibition Confusion and altered perception Diminished libido Constricted pupils Nausea/vomiting Pain relief (therapeutic use)
Hallucinogens	Often rapid onset, for example, Cannabis begins acting within 6–12 minute and may be stored in fat deposits for weeks	Hyperglycaemia due to increased intake and/or s forgetting to take OHA/insulin Increased possibility of DKA/HONK Hypoglycaemia with some drugs such as large doses of marijuana	Euphoria and disorientation Hallucinations Disinhibition Marijuana increases appetite Difficulty with coordination, making judgement Tiredness Can lead to psychiatric disorders including depression and paranoia

[a] Note the effects on blood glucose may not be a direct effect of the drug but a consequence of cognitive impairment, effects on judgement, hypoglycaemia symptoms not recognised or confused with the effect of the drug, and inadequate self-care (Glick 2003). Frequent blood glucose testing is recommended if a person with diabetes uses illegal drugs but the cognitive effects of the drugs often means they do not test.

Table 10.3 outlines the effects of these substances and their proposed impact on blood glucose. Note: medical cannabis in becoming accepted treatment for debilitating conditions such as epilepsy, schizophrenia and other psychotic disorders, type 2 diabetes, inflammatory bowel disease and some tumours when conventional medicine are ineffective(Alcohol and Drug Foundation 2019). Medical cannabis contains different cannabinoids from recreational cannabis and is less likely to cause 'highs'. It has more analgesic, anti-inflammatory, and anti-oxidant properties and reduces vomiting. The main pharmaceutical cannabis products are nabiximols (Sativex), synthetic cannabinoids such as Dronabinol. The products are available as a nasal or oral spray.

In addition, many herbs have psychogenic properties. They may be stimulants, sedative, cognitive enhancing, or analgesics as well as uppers, hallucinogens, or act in a similar way to opiates (Spinella 2005). Significantly, herbs may contain more than one chemical substance and are sometimes used to manufacture illegal drugs. Examples include but are not limited to:

- *Acorus calamus* (calamus). Ecstasy can be manufactured from calamus.
- *Salvia divinorum*. This is sometimes called sage or salvia. The leaves hold opioid-like compounds that induce hallucinations.
- Ephedra species. Pharmacological effects vary among the dozens of species.
- *Amantia muscaria*. These psychoactive mushrooms are sometimes called magic mushrooms, fly agaric, or fly amantia.
- A herbal mixture called hoasia, yaje, or daime. The names often indicate the country in which the mixture originates.

The effect of any drug depends on the dose and its pharmacokinetics and pharmacodynamics, bioavailability, and metabolism and elimination. Thus, the effect depends on the administration route, how the individual metabolises drugs, and is usually dose-dependent. Common routes of illegal drug administration are:

- Enteral:
  ○ oral
  ○ sublingual
  ○ rectal
- parenteral:
  ○ IV
- Subcutaneous, for example, 'skin popping' heroin
- Inhalation smoking, pipe, cigarettes, hookah

Effects on diabetes

Illegal drugs appear to have two inter-related consequences for people with diabetes: physical effects, although the pharmacological effects on blood glucose appear to be minor (Glick 2003), effect on cognitive processes, which disrupt problem-solving, decision-making, and self-care. Cognitive effects are significant and contribute to erratic blood glucose control. They are also associated with other general health risks such as sexually transmitted disease, malnutrition, and reduced immunity, which impact on diabetes-related well-being.

As well as contributing to the development of long-term diabetes complications through inadequate self-care and hyperglycaemia, addiction to some illegal drugs exacerbates existing diabetes complications. Illegal drugs exert significant haemodynamic and electrophysiological effects. The specific effects depend on the dose, the degree of addiction (see Table 10.3), and the drug formulation. Marijuana, the most commonly used illegal drug, is associated with cerebrovascular events and peripheral vascular events (Moussouttas 2004) and atrial fibrillation and increased cardiovascular morbidity (Korantzopoulos et al. 2008). Smoking exacerbates the vascular effects and nerve damage may be exacerbated by excessive alcohol use.

Cardiovascular effects include:

- Slight increase in blood pressure, especially in the supine position;
- Rapid tachycardia, most likely due to enhanced automaticity of the sinus node, which increases cardiac output and reduces oxygen carrying capacity due to increased carboxyhaemoglobin when smoking marijuana;
- Constriction of blood vessels increasing the risk of cardiovascular and cerebrovascular disease (e.g. cocaine);

- Reduced peripheral vascular resistance but the extent varies in different peripheral sites;
- Angina and acute coronary syndromes, especially in older people with postural or orthostatic hypotension.

Interactions with medicines

Information about interactions between illegal drugs, oral hypoglycaemic agents (OHAs), and insulin is unclear, but some drugs might affect GLM/insulin bioavailability. In addition, the different illegal drugs and the different dose forms (inhaled, smoked, intravenous, oral) are likely to have different pharmacodynamics and pharmacokinetics (Brown 1991). A significant problem is the fact that many such drugs are manufactured illegally and there are no quality control standard processes to ascertain purity, bioavailability, or the contents of the drug.

Management

Management is challenging and requires a great deal of tact and understanding. Referral to an appropriate 'drug and alcohol' service is advisable. Health professionals should be able to identify illegal drug use and refer early to reduce the likelihood of addiction developing (see Table 10.3). The effects of drug or drug combination and duration of action depends on a number of factors including the dose and frequency of use and individual factors. Long-term use can contribute to homelessness and psychiatric disorders: conversely, psychiatric disorders can trigger illegal drug use. Illegal drugs can interact with conventional and/or complementary medicines and sometimes alcohol. All can lead to addiction, which has social, professional, and financial implications and increases the risk of inadequate diabetes care, coma, and death.

Strategies include the following:

- Provide an environment where patients feel safe and able to discuss difficult issues.
- Take a thorough medical, work and social history, and monitoring changes.
- Assess whether there are any existing mental health problems and their relationship to illegal drug use.
- Assess diabetes status and self-care capacity and provide information about ways to enhance safety that are consistent with the advice of the specific drug service if they continue to use illegal drugs. Having appropriate information about how drugs work and their potential effects can help the individual develop strategies to reduce the risk of immediate and long-term adverse events if they continue to use drugs. Diabetes-specific advice might include:
  - Importance of frequent blood glucose testing.
  - Need to test for ketones if the blood glucose is high. This is especially true for individuals with type 1 diabetes.
  - Need to continue OHA/insulin. However, the doses may need to be adjusted according to blood glucose tests. Advice about how to make such adjustments may be needed.
  - Importance of maintaining adequate fluid and food intake to avoid dehydration.
  - Importance of being able to recognise and treat hypoglycaemia and strategies for distinguishing hypoglycaemia from the effects of the drug.
  - Importance of seeking medical advice early if they are unwell or develop an infection. For example, they might have intractable nausea and/or vomiting, depression, or have signs of infection at the IV drug injection site.
- Explain ways to reduce personal risk, such as:
  - Make sure they obtain drugs from a reputable source.
  - Use sterile techniques and do not share needles (e.g. risk of HIV and hepatitis C) or pipes/ hookahs (e.g. risk of TB, influenza).
  - Do not drive after using illegal drugs.
  - Practice safe sex.
  - Use with a trusted person who can support their self-care and seek medical care if an adverse event occurs and using in a safe environment.
  - Safely dispose of sharps.

Practice points

(1) Although the risk of psychiatric disorders is high, not all illegal drug users have psychiatric disorders and not all people with psychiatric conditions use illegal drugs.
(2) Co-occurring psychiatric disorders, substance addiction, and diabetes are highly challenging to manage, and there is very little evidence for the most effective strategies because such people are usually excluded from clinical trials (Wusthoff et al. 2012).
(3) Advice is easy to give but very difficult to follow because of the mental effects of most drugs on cognition, decision-making, and judgement, which affect self-care capacity.
(4) Larger doses of drugs are often needed to achieve the desired effect as addiction worsens.
(5) Coffee, tea, and chocolate are also stimulants.

Brittle or labile diabetes

Brittle diabetes means different things to different people.

Introduction

Brittle diabetes is difficult to define. Some experts consider it to be a psychological condition; others regard it as having a physical basis, it often has both physical and psychological components. Brittle diabetes is rare. The term usually refers to wide fluctuations in the blood glucose pattern despite optimal medical management. Vantyghem and Press (2006), National Institute of Health [NIH] 2017) suggested the term *brittle diabetes* should be reserved for people in whom 'instability, whatever its cause, results in disruption of life and often recurrent and/or prolonged hospitalisation'. Whichever definition is used, brittle diabetes is difficult to manage, affects quality of life and emotional well-being, and requires an holistic approach. Repeated admissions to hospital for bouts of DKA or severe hypoglycaemia often occur and could be an early indication of gastroparesis (Chapter 8).

Brittle diabetes affects 3/1000 people with type 1 diabetes, mostly young women (Vantyghem and Press 2006). The causes of brittle diabetes are multifactorial. Three forms of brittle diabetes are described:

(1) Recurrent diabetic DKA
(2) Predominant hypoglycaemic forms
(3) Mixed glucose instability

Causes of brittle diabetes

Physical causes of brittle diabetes include:

- Impaired insulin response. This could be due to rare conditions such as degradation of insulin at the injection site. In these cases, an insulin pump can improve insulin absorption. In other cases, insulin absorption from specific injection sites can be reduced or delayed. Changing sites may help (Garrett et al. 2019).
- Communication problems such as dyslexia can make education and therefore self-care difficult. People frequently hide their difficulty, and tactful questioning is needed to identify it.
- Drug addiction can be a factor.
- Gastroparesis leading to erratic food absorption is discussed in Chapter 8. Other gastrointestinal problems can also be present, such as coeliac disease and CFRD, which are discussed in this chapter, and should be excluded.
- Seizure disorders.
- Inappropriate management regimen.

- Presence of other disorders, for example 2–3% of people with T1DM have Hashimoto's thyroiditis. Coeliac disease is also common in people with T1DM.
- Eating disorders, either under- or overeating.
- Unrecognised hypoglycaemia and inappropriate insulin dose increases can lead to further hypoglycaemia, rebound hyperglycaemia, and DKA.

Psychological causes include:

- Anger and nonacceptance of diabetes can be factors.
- Difficult relationships can lead to using diabetes to 'escape' from the situation or to manipulate it, or gain attention.
- Sexual abuse can trigger brittle diabetes.

Role of the clinician

Support and patience are required to manage people with brittle diabetes. Nurses need to be aware that it exists and that it can have a physiological basis as well as an underlying psychological component.

Nurses can play a key role in organising case conferences, supporting diabetes education, and identifying barriers to learning, which might include inspecting injection sites and observing the person administering an injection and monitoring their blood glucose. Follow agreed management protocols and/or identify strategies to enhance management and ensure the person has follow-up appointments with appropriate health professionals on discharge. Regular blood glucose monitoring in hospital and continuous subcutaneous blood glucose monitoring can help identify excursions in blood glucose levels and identify unrecognised hypoglycaemia, which will assist with appropriate care planning.

Management

Management is protracted and requires a great deal of patience and support for the person with diabetes and their family. Taking a careful holistic history and a thorough physical assessment can identify physical causes. Processes used to quantify blood glucose variability include:

- Mean amplitude of largest glycaemic excursions (MAGE)
- Mean of daily differences (MODD)
- Lability index (LI)
- Low blood glucose index (LBGI)
- Clarke's score
- Hyposcore
- Continuous blood glucose monitoring
- A range of psychometric measures to exclude/detect psychological causes; see Chapter 15

A long-term management strategy is required that involves an agreed coordinated care plan that is communicated to all relevant health professionals and the patient and their family/carers. Managing the underlying organic problems where possible is important and optimising insulin therapy is essential. Continuous subcutaneous insulin therapy (insulin pump) might be indicated. In some cases an islet cell transplant can be considered provided the individual meets the criteria for transplantation: hypoglycaemic unawareness, BMI <25, normal renal function and no plans to become pregnant (Vantyghem and Press 2006; NIH 2017).

Regular case conferencing with the relevant health professionals is important. Liaison with a psychiatrist is desirable if the underlying cause is psychological, and may help the individual come to terms with their diabetes by going back to the time of diagnosis and exploring the issues in operation at the time. The focus should be taken off diabetic *control* and placed on quality of life, initially. If other issues are addressed metabolic control is easier to achieve. A basal bolus regimen using rapid-acting insulin can be commenced if it is not already being used.

Oral health and diabetes

Introduction

People with diabetes are at increased risk of periodontal disease (Khazaii and Kamareh 2018). Periodontal disease is a deep infection that affects bone and is caused by bacteria (plaque), which destroy the fibrosis attachment that anchors the teeth in the jaw (Southerland et al. 2006). Periodontal disease increases cardiovascular risk and may have a role in the pathogenesis of dementia (Chapter 12). Periodontal disease has been called the 'sixth diabetes complication' (Andersen et al. 2007).

Various causal processes are proposed, such as increased glucose levels in saliva that reduces the buffering power of saliva and saliva flow rates (Carramolino-Cuéllar et al. 2018). The pattern of dental decay and the decay rates vary between young and older people with diabetes and are influenced by individual susceptibility to periodontal disease, the degree of inflammation and destruction of bone, and environmental factors.

People with diabetes also have increased rates of oral candidiasis and a range of other oral cavity diseases, for example, lichen planus and painless swelling of the salivary glands (sialosis) that could be due to disordered fat metabolism and/or changed taste sensation (Lamey et al. 1992).

Symptoms of oral cavity disease

- Bleeding gums
- Swollen gums
- Halitosis
- Inflamed receding gums
- Pus around the gums
- Loose teeth
- Oral candidia
- Dental plaque, caries loose, worn or chipped teeth or ill-fitting dentures
- Painful abscesses, which are a late symptom and indicate permanent damage (Dunning 2009; Khazaii and Kamareh 2018)

Loss of or decay in teeth affects people's food intake and the type of food they eat. There is a propensity to choose low-fibre, low-protein foods, which represents a significant risk of hypoglycaemia and nutritional deficiencies, which, in turn, affect mental and physical functioning and quality of life; see Chapters 4, 15, and 12. Conversely, high sugar and fat food choices have a role in the development of tooth and gum disease, as well as diabetes.

Ageing also leads to submucosal changes and increasing prevalence of gum disease due to hyperglycaemia and the resultant dry mouth. Saliva production can be reduced (xerostomia) and is often exacerbated by medications that cause dry mouth (National Health Medical Research Council [NHMRC] 2013). The degree of metabolic control, duration, age, and dental hygiene influence the likelihood of gum disease occurring.

Younger people with diabetes are also at risk of tooth and gum disease, primarily as a result of inappropriate diet and inadequate dental care.

Causal mechanisms

- Accumulation of plaque on tooth surfaces and resultant gingivitis can contribute to inflammation and destruction of the bone that supports the teeth.
- Gingivitis can lead to periodontitis when bacteria or their products such as liposaccharides cause inflammation in the deeper connective tissues.
- The bacteria may cause an immune response with increased production of inflammatory cytokines and other proinflammatory markers, which reduce tissue repair (Khazaii and Kamareh 2018).

- Defective neutrophil function such as reduced chemotaxis and phagocytosis during hyperglycaemia can be present.
- Immune response can be depressed during hyperglycaemia.

Insulin resistance and deteriorating metabolic control can occur as a result of oral infection and may require adjustment to the GLM medicine regimen.

Management

- Regular oral health assessment should be part of everybody's healthcare. People with oral health problems who do not have a diagnosis of diabetes can be screened for risk diabetes risk, e.g. in dental clinics (Rogers et al. 2017).
- Consider the possibility of oral problems where signs of eating disorders, infection or deteriorating control are present in people with diabetes.
- Include dental assessment in the health history and assessment and annual complication screening programmes. Periodontal disease is associated with other inflammatory disease such as cardiovascular disease (Rogers et al. 2017).
- Provide opportunities for cleaning teeth during hospitalisation and in aged-care facilities.
- Clinicians have a responsibility to educate people with diabetes about preventative oral hygiene. This includes:
  - The need to have regular dental checks and education about ways to maintain oral health
  - Choosing a good toothbrush and toothpaste
  - Good blood glucose control
  - Eating a healthy well-balanced diet
  - Seeking dental advice early for any pain, bleeding, redness, and persistent bad breath so infection can be treated early
  - Using the correct method of brushing teeth, not gums, to reduce bleeding risk
- Refer for dental assessment if existing disease is identified.
- Check dentures regularly to ensure they fit.
- Educate dental practitioners about diabetes. Dental practitioners should also be aware of the possibility their patients could have undiagnosed diabetes and the risk of hypoglycaemia occurring during dental procedures in people with diabetes treated with insulin, and how to manage it; see Chapters 6 and 9.

Diabetes and liver disease

Introduction

Research suggests liver disease is an important cause of death in people with type 2 diabetes (Balkau et al. 1991; de Marco et al. 1999), and diabetes may be the most common cause of liver disease (US Organ Procurement and Transplantation Network and Scientific Registry of Transplant Recipients 2004; Tolman et al. 2007). Some studies show cirrhosis accounts for 4.4% of diabetes-related deaths (Balkau et al. 1991). Hepatic steatosis, like insulin resistance, might precede the onset of type 2 diabetes (Zarrinpar and Loomba 2012). Bile acids have an important role in glucose homeostasis and their effects are mediated by the farneold X receptor (FXR) and the cell receptor TGR5 (Zarrinpar and Loomba 2012).

A range of liver diseases occur in type 2 diabetes:

- Abnormal liver enzymes – elevated alanine transferase (ALT) is common in type 2 diabetes and may be associated with liver disease. Some studies show elevated ALT is associated with liver disease in up to 98% of cases, commonly fatty liver nonalcoholic fatty liver disease (NAFLD) and chronic hepatitis. Alkaline phosphatase (AST) may also be elevated.

- NAFLD is the most common liver disease in obese people with type 2 diabetes and affects other body systems, thus it is a multifactorial disease that increases the risk of cardiovascular and renal disease (Scheen 2018). NAFLD is defined as fatty liver disease with no alcohol intake or amounts <20 g/day (Caldwell et al. 1999; King 1996–2012). Insulin resistance is a significant contributing factor to NAFLD. It is estimated to occur in 34–74% of people with type 2 diabetes and up to ~100% of obese people with type 2 diabetes (Tolman et al. 2007). NAFLD is characterised by a range of liver diseases such as steatosis and nonalcoholic steato-hepatitis (NASH). NASH is a similar condition that consists of steatosis, inflammation, necrosis, and fibrosis and can lead to cirrhosis. Of people with NAFLD, 50% have concomitant NASH and 19% have cirrhosis at diagnosis. These conditions rarely produce symptoms in the early stages. The exact cause is unknown. The associated lipid pattern, elevated triglycerides, low HDL, high LDL, and high cholesterol also occur in type 2 diabetes. Insulin resistance contributes to lipolysis and elevated free fatty acids (FFA), which overload the hepatic mitochrondrial b-oxygenation system, and FFAs accumulate in the liver and affect normal liver function. NAFLD has been described as the hepatic manifestation of insulin resistance (Marchesini et al. 2003). Adipokines may play a role in the development of NASH. NAFLD is associated with increased risk of early morbidity and mortality and may have worse overall survival than people with alcoholic liver disease (Liu et al. 2018) In addition, moderate to severe sleep apnoea and hypoxia are common in people with NAFLD (Fuchs 2012).
- Cirrhosis is often due to alcohol addiction and is also associated with insulin resistance and reduced insulin secretion, which have implications for diabetes management. GLM therapy is limited by hepatic damage and the risk of hypoglycaemia. (Gundling et al. (2013) found the prevalence of diabetes in a cohort of people with cirrhosis ($n = 87$) was 30.5, and 31% of these were prescribed medicines that could have serious adverse effects. Most continued to drink alcohol and 41.4% did not adhere to their medicine regimen. Only 28.7% of those with diabetes achieved HbA1c < 6.5%; those who did achieve acceptable glycaemic control had lower risk of hepatic encephalopathy, hepatocellular carcinoma, arterial hypotension, and hypercholesterolaemia. However, hepatic encephalopathy was significantly more common in people with diabetes then nondiabetics. The safety and risk of aiming for HbA1c in people with cirrhosis needs to be considered because it affects liver glucose stores and the individual's ability to mount an effective counter-regulatory response (Chapters 1 and 6).
- Hepatocellular carcinoma appears to be associated with insulin resistance, increased lipolysis, accumulation of lipids in liver cells, oxidative stress leading to cell damage, fibrosis, and proliferation of procarcinogenic cells (El-Serag and Everhart 2002).
- Haemochromatosis is due to excess iron being deposited in many tissues, including the liver (next section) (Raju and Venkataramappa 2018).
- Acute liver failure can also occur, although the exact mechanism is unclear. Contributing factors include some medications and/or diabetes-related abnormalities.

Alcohol is also an addictive substance associated with significant morbidity and mortality. Between 15% and 20% of GP consultations relate to alcohol (Lee 2008). Short-term consequences include injury and domestic violence; longer-term effects include other risk-taking behaviours such as smoking, neglected self-care, driving whilst intoxicated, cognitive impairment, peripheral neuropathy, liver cirrhosis, and foetal damage in pregnant women. Hepatic encephalopathy (Gundling et al. 2013) and peripheral neuropathy are significant consequences of alcohol addiction.

- There is an association between the hepatitis C medication a-interferon and type 1 diabetes (Fabris et al. 2003).

Managing people with diabetes and liver disease

Managing people with diabetes and concomitant liver disease is complicated by changes in medicine metabolism, contraindication to medicines such as metformin, and increased risk of medicine interactions. Screening for liver disease consists of:

- Liver function tests
- Abdominal ultrasound
- Computerised tomography
- Magnetic resonance imaging
- Liver biopsy

Management is essentially the same as for any person with diabetes, but the exact strategy depends on the severity of the liver disease and the blood glucose and lipid pattern. Identifying the presence of liver disease appears to be important. Counselling to help people realise the severity and consequences of the problem is essential. It is important to consider concomitant comorbidities such as sleep apnoea, obesity, and cardiovascular disuse and manage these conditions.

Diet and exercise are important. Many people with liver disease are malnourished, which compromises their immune status and health outcomes. Nutrition and exercise are discussed in Chapter 4. Supplemental vitamins B_{12}, D, thiamine, and folic acid may be indicated. Alcohol and smoking should be avoided because of their toxic effects on the liver. Alcohol is a liver toxin and is high in calories. In addition, it contributes to vitamin deficiencies. Bile acid sequestrants such as colesevelum have been shown to improve glycaemic control. Likewise, enterohepatic bile acid recirculation can change after gastric bypass surgery and contribute to the improved glycaemic control noted after such surgery (Zarrinpar and Loomba 2012).

Recent research suggests that individual SGLT-2 inhibitors reduce liver fat and other biomarkers of liver disease such as ALT in people with NAFLD and T2DM. Dapagliflozin reduced all biomarkers of hepatocyte injury, including ALT, AST, GGT and fibroblast growth factor 21 (Eriksson et al. 2018). When dapagliflozin was combined with omega-3, liver fat was further reduced. Pioglitazone and liraglutide show some preliminary effects (Sumida and Yoneda 2018).

The usual contraindications to medicines should be considered. Liver failure, ascites, coagulopathy, and encephalopathy is associated with altered medicine metabolism. The risk of lactic acidosis with metformin needs to be considered. TZDs appear to improve ALT and liver histology (Harrison et al. 2005) but are associated with weight gain, see Chapter 5. ALT levels should be ascertained before commencing TZDs and monitored regularly. Insulin is frequently required. Lipid-lowering agents are usually also needed. The usual diabetes self-care and education is necessary; see Chapter 16 and consideration given to end of life care in end stage liver disease.

CAM medicines

CAM medicine use should be monitored. People often take CAM medicines 'to support liver function'. These include (*Silymarin marianum*) milk thistle, alpha-lipoic acid, vitamins E, C, and B, cysteine, and omega-3 fatty acids. However, some CAM medicines cause liver damage or worsen existing liver damage. Some interact with conventional medicines. The liver damage caused by CAM medicines is the same as other forms of liver damage due to conventional medicines (Chitturi and Farrell 2000).

People with the various forms of hepatitis and HIV infections, frequently use CAM. There is some preliminary evidence that one CAM medicine, Jianpi Wenshen Recipe, might help reduce the viral load of hepatitis B surface and e-antigen. Some studies show beneficial effects of a Chinese herbal medicine formula used with interferon on viral clearance, but the research methods are often flawed (Lipman 2007).

Prolonged ingestion or repeated exposure may play a role in the development of chronic damage with some medicines (e.g. Jin Bu Huan). The type of herbs likely to be used depends on geographical location, but migration and travel means they are often widespread. Significantly, many CAM medicines contain a mixture of herbs and sometimes supplements so it can be difficult to identify the specific liver toxin, which might actually be due to contaminants rather than the herb itself if CAM medicines are not obtained from a reputable source. CAM medicines should be taken under the direction of a qualified practitioner. Some commonly used CAM medicines that are reported to cause liver damage are shown in the following list (see also Chapter 19):

- Chaparral.
- Dai-saiko to.
- *Chelidonium majus* (greater celandine).
- *Lycopodium serratum* (Jin Bu Huan).
- *Ephedra* species such as Ma-Huang.
- Oral ingestion of essential oils containing pulegone such as pennyroyal. Pennyroyal is not usually used in aromatherapy.
- *Serenoa* species (saw palmetto) is often used to manage prostate disease.
- *Valerian officinalis.*

Monitoring the effect of smoking, including e-cigarettes on the liver, may also be important, especially in people with existing liver disease.

Haemochromatosis

Haemochromatosis is an inherited disease and occurs secondary to thalassaemia, some types of anaemia, and excess alcohol consumption. It is characterised by increased iron absorption and eventually iron overload in many body tissues. The onset of symptoms rarely occurs before age 40 because it takes time for the iron to accumulate and affect tissue and organ function (Raju and Venkataramappa 2018). The primary form is due to a mutation of HPE or non-HPE genes and is more common in Caucasians. Secondary haemachromotosis is due to alcohol, excessive iron or vitamin C intake, some oral contraceptives, and blood transfusion.

The excess iron is deposited in the liver, pancreas, heart, skin, joints, gonads, and the pituitary gland, causing tissue damage that disrupts the normal function of these organs and glands. The liver is usually the first organ to be affected. Approximately 50% of people with haemochromatosis have T1DM or T2DM because the iron overload in the pancreas, which damages beta cells and affects insulin release and insulin sensitivity.

Sixty-five percent of people with haemochromatosis have a family history of impaired glucose tolerance or a diagnosis of diabetes (Mendler et al. 1999). Men are 10 times more likely than women to develop haemochromatosis. This could be due, in part, to iron loss with menstruation in women. The peak incidence occurs in people 40–60 years old.

Other diabetic complications such as nephropathy, neuropathy, and peripheral vascular disease are often also present. Arthropathy occurs in two-thirds of people with acute crystal synovitis, which can make self-care tasks (e.g. insulin administration) difficult (Sherlock 1981).

Iron overload

Iron overload is associated with various metabolic conditions besides diabetes. Steatohepatitis is an iron overload condition distinct from haemochromatosis. It is characterised by hyperferritinaemia and transferrin saturation. Liver damage includes steatosis and nonalcoholic fatty liver disease (NASH). Type 2 diabetes is often associated with NASH (Mendler et al. 1999). Obesity and hyperlipidaemia that can lead to fibrosis and cirrhosis of the liver are common. The excess iron can increase the risk of cancer, and most probably stroke. Diagnosis is by MRI, liver biopsy, and blood glucose and lipid levels.

Symptoms include fatigue, weakness, weight loss, apathy, pain in arm, and leg muscles and leg cramps. Hyperpigmentation can occur and can resemble sunburn in the early stages.

Management

Management consists of:

- Early diagnosis to enable early treatment, which can prevent T2DM. This involves a careful family history.
- Hepatic iron index >0.9 μmol/year and abnormal liver function tests suggest primary haemochromotosis.
- Genetic testing and genetic counselling for first-degree relatives.
- Venesection to remove excess iron. Hypoglycaemia can occur after venesection and the nurse needs to be aware of the possibility and know how to prevent and manage hypoglycaemia. The patient should be informed of the possibility of hypoglycaemia and how to manage their diet and medications on venesection days to reduce the hypoglycaemia risk.
- Blood glucose can be easy to control or the patient might require large doses of insulin because of insulin resistance. Oral hypoglycaemic agents often do not lead to acceptable blood glucose control and insulin is needed.
- Blood glucose monitoring to enable changes to medication and diet to be made early.
- Regular blood tests to monitor ferritin, iron levels, and metabolic control.
- Counselling and medication to manage depression, if indicated.
- Care during tests and procedures such as liver biopsy (see Chapter 9).

Diabetic mastopathy

Diabetic mastopathy is rare, occurring in 0.6–13% of women, often women with long-standing type 1 diabetes around the time of the menopause (Khan et al. 2016). Most women with diabetic mastopathy also have microvascular disease and often other concomitant diseases such as auto-immune thyroid disease and cheiroarthropathy. There is relatively little information available about the causes of the disease, but it is possible that it occurs as a result of an immune reaction to deposits in the breast as a result of hyperglycaemia.

The breast masses are usually firm-to-hard, poorly defined, freely movable, not fixed to the skin, and can be mistaken for breast cancer. It is usually benign, but it is important to exclude cancer to allay fear and anxiety and avoid unnecessary biopsies and surgical intervention (Wilmshurst 2002).

Diagnosis

Investigations include:

- Mammogram or ultrasound.
- Fine-needle aspiration biopsy. This is often difficult to perform in people with diabetic mastopathy because the fibrous tissue is difficult to aspirate into the needle. Frequently, core or excision biopsy is required. The tissue is usually fibrous with lymphocyte infiltration but no glandular changes.

Management

(1) Counselling and reassurance is important.
(2) Regular annual follow-up is necessary with repeat mammogram and ultrasound on a regular basis.
(3) Single lesions can be removed. However, 63% of lesions are bilateral and often recur after excision.
(4) Supportive bras may help relieve breast discomfort.
(5) Regular breast self-examination and early help-seeking should be routine practice.

Diabetes and coeliac disease

Coeliac disease, also known as gluten-sensitive enteropathy, is a chronic autoimmune disorder where the lining of the small intestine is damaged as a consequence of sensitivity to gluten (Marsh 2011). Coeliac disease leads to malabsorption and sometimes involves many body systems. The link amongst the various disorders and coeliac disease is clear for some but not all disorders (Duggan 2004; Juvenile Diabetes Research Foundation [JDRF] 2008). Coeliac disease can be present with few clinical signs and occurs in 0.5–1.0% of the population (Fasano et al. 2003).

The causal association between type 1 diabetes and coeliac disease is currently under investigation and possibly involves similar human leukocyte antigen (HLA) genes, which are associated with other autoimmune disorders such as Addison's disease and thyroid disease. The impact of environmental factors on the genetic predisposition is unclear. Current studies investigating these issues include the Disease Autoimmunity Research (CEDAR) study and the Diabetes Autoimmunity Study in the Young (DAISY). People with type 2 diabetes may have gluten sensitivity but there is no known link between the two conditions because type 2 is not an auto-immune disease.

Coeliac disease is caused by a complex immunological response to gliadin, the main protein in wheat. Rye, barley, and oats have smaller quantities of gliadin. T cells associated with HLA-DQ2 or HLA-DQ-8 antigen become sensitised to gliadin and produce cytokines, which causes tissue damage such as villous atrophy in the mucosa and activates plasma cells to produce antibodies to gliadin. Not everybody with the particular HLA antigens develop coeliac disease, for unknown reasons. Interestingly, cigarette smoking reduces the risk of coeliac disease by 80% (Suman et al. 2003). Peak diagnostic times for coeliac disease occur at three to five years and during the forties, and affects more women than men (Green and Jabri 2003).

Untreated coeliac disease can affect growth and development in children and cause long-term health problems in children and adults such as osteoporosis, infertility, miscarriage, tooth decay and increased risk of gastrointestinal cancers. It can also affect glycaemic control and represents a hypoglycaemia risk (Mohn et al. 2001). Consequently, glucose-lowering medicine doses may need to be reduced.

Commonly associated diseases include:

- Liver disorders such as fatty liver, transaminitis, or hepatitis
- Dermatitis herpetiformis psoriasis
- Irritable bowel syndrome
- Anaemia, which is often a result of malabsorption of iron and/or folate and which responds to iron supplements
- Bone loss
- Various cancers
- IgA nephropathy
- Epilepsy
- Neuropathies
- Myelopathies
- Ataxias
- Male and female infertility

Type 1 diabetes is also associated with coeliac disease. The prevalence of coeliac disease in type 1 diabetes is 1.3–6.4% (Farrell and Kelly 2002; Buysschaert and Tomasi 2005) and the prevalence of type 1 diabetes in people with coelaic disease is 5% (Colin et al. 1994). There is limited information about whether a gluten-free diet relieves symptoms in people with type 1 diabetes and coeliac disease (Duggan 2004). Cavallo (2004) suggests that 1 in 20 people with type 1 have coeliac disease and 1 in 10 test positive for transglutaminase IgA antibodies.

Signs and symptoms

Common signs and symptoms include:

- Family history of coeliac disease
- Chronic tiredness, weakness, and lethargy
- Poor appetite
- Weight loss, failure to thrive
- Delayed growth in children
- Abdominal symptoms such as bloating, discomfort, malabsorption syndromes, pot belly, diarrhoea if most of the intestine is involved.
- Irritability and depression
- Discoloured tooth enamel
- Skin disorders such as psoriasis
- Unexplained hypo- or hyperglycaemia
- Elevated transglutaminase and endomysial antibody titres
- Anaemia
- Histological changes on endoscopy and duodenal biopsy such as flattened villi

Other less common signs and symptoms include easy bruising, mouth ulcers, muscle cramps if serum calcium levels are low, folate, and vitamin B_{12}, A, D, E, and K (fat-soluble vitamins) deficiencies, memory, and concentration deficits and bone/joint pain (Marsh 2011).

Diagnosis

Screening people with these symptoms and those with IgG antibodies and IgA deficiency may be useful because a gluten-free diet is likely to improve the symptoms and quality of life (Sjoberg et al. 1998; Green and Jabri 2003; Duggan 2004). Some experts suggest universal screening is not warranted and recommending a gluten-free diet when there are no symptoms may not be beneficial, may be socially restricting, and may reduce quality of life. However, Buysschaert and Tomasi (2005) advocated screening all people with type 1 diabetes and repeating the test every year for three years if the initial result is negative.

Likewise, the International Society for Paediatric and Adolescent Diabetes (ISPAD) recommends screening all children with type 1 diabetes at diagnosis and that screening be continued annually for the first five years after diagnosis and then every two years (Mahmud et al. 2018). In addition, screening should be undertaken if there are clinical signs and symptoms suggestive of coeliac disease, especially if the person has a first-degree relative with coeliac disease.

Diagnosis usually consists of the following steps:

(1) Screen blood tests to measure antibodies: anti-tissue transglutaminase (tTG), deaminated gliadin peptide (DGP), IGA, and IgG, which are sometimes used in place of anti-gliadin antibodies (AGA), and anti-endomyal antibodies (EMA). *Note:* These are screening tests rather than diagnostic tests because false positives can occur.
(2) Tissue is biopsied from different sections of the small intestine. Atrophied villi confirm the diagnosis. However, if the person has been on a gluten-free diet, that person must resume eating gluten-containing foods for at least six weeks before the biopsies are performed.
(3) Genetic testing is conducted by blood test or swab to detect HLA DQ2 or HA DQ8. However, genetic testing cannot be used alone because not everybody who carries these genes develops coeliac disease.

Management

Wheat, including spelt, kumut, saitan, rye, barley, and oats, must be eliminated from the diet, but the general principles of eating a healthy diet to manage blood glucose and lipids applies.

It is essential to ensure micronutrient intake is adequate to prevent anaemia and osteoporosis and other nutritional deficiencies such as vitamin B complex. Many gluten-free foods have a high GI and high fat content so referring the individual to a dietitian is essential. Grains such as buckwheat, chia, and millet are acceptable alternative grains. The range of gluten-free foods available on the market is increasing, which makes it easier for people to adhere to the strict gluten-free diet required to heal the intestine. Reading food labels to identify hidden gluten is essential.

Managing a gluten-free diet as well as balancing carbohydrate intake, insulin, and activity can be challenging and stressful. However, the long-term consequences in people with diabetes include chronic hypoglycaemia (see Chapter 6) that can cause neurological deficits. The individual should carry gluten-free hypoglycaemia treatment at all times but should ingest gluten-containing food if that is all that is available because the risks associated with moderate to severe hypoglycaemia are significant. If hypoglycaemia unawareness is present, the person might benefit from blood glucose awareness training (BGAT). Managing intercurrent illness and optimal health to reduce the incidence and physiological impact of these illnesses is important. Regular screening for depression and quality of life might be indicated.

Cystic fibrosis–related diabetes

Cystic fibrosis (CF) is the 'most common lethal autsomal recessive disease in Caucasians, with a worldwide prevalence of 1/2500 live births' (O'Riordan et al. 2009). Life expectancy for people with CF has improved over the past decade, thus complications, including CFRD, the most common comorbidity of CF, are beginning to emerge (Donoghue and Robinson, 2017). CFRD shares some characteristics in common with diabetes (Moran et al. 2010) but the pathophysiology of CFRD is not well understood. It is postulated that fatty infiltration in the pancreas leads to fibrosis and destruction of the beta cells that causes insulin deficiency (Moran et al. 2014). People with CFRD have shorter survival than those with CF not related to diabetes.

Identifying and treating people who develop CFRD early is important in order to maintain lung function and enhance survival. CFRD is more common in people with CF and liver disease. Recently, the Cystic Fibrosis Trust (CFT) (2004) in the United Kingdom recommended all people who develop CFRD be screened annually to detect diabetes and its complications. The SIGN (2010) guidelines recommend annual diabetes screening begins at age 10 and also recommends screening for associated conditions such as coeliac and thyroid disease. Both conditions can be present with few symptoms and can be missed during routine CF and CFRD care.

The prevalence of CFRD varies depending on the diagnostic criteria used. It can occur at any age but increases with age:

- 9% in 5–9 year olds
- 26% in 10–20 year olds
- 50% by age 30 (O'Riordan et al. 2009)

However, SIGN (2010) suggested 20% of people with CF are likely to develop diabetes by age 20 and the incidence of CFRD increases thereafter to 80% by age 35.

CFRD mostly occurs in people with serious CF mutations that are associated with pancreatic insufficiency. Chloride channels are abnormal in people with CF, which results in thick, viscous secretions obstructing the exocrine pancreas and fatty infiltration and progressive fibrosis that eventually affects the pancreatic alpha and beta cells. Thus, the beta cell destruction in CFRD is not usually an autoimmune process.

Diagnosis

Few people with CF have normal blood glucose levels all the time for a number of reasons; thus, diagnosing CFRD can be challenging and largely depends on detecting polyuria, polydipsia, and weight loss, but such symptoms only occur in about 33% of individuals with CFRD (Dyce and Wallymahmed 2012). The CFT (2004) and Moran et al. (2010) recommend oral glucose tolerance testing (OGTT). However, the results can be misleading if the test is not conducted under ideal testing conditions and if the OGTT is performed when the individual is unwell or when they are on high doses of corticosteroids, which also increase the risk of type 2 diabetes (Dunning 1996).

Variable intermittent post-prandial hyperglycaemia is the earliest sign, followed by impaired glucose tolerance, then diabetes without fasting hyperglycaemia and diabetes with fasting hyperglycaemia (O'Riordan et al. 2009). Significantly, a diagnosis of normal glucose tolerance on and OGTT does not exclude abnormal post-prandial blood glucose levels at home when the person is consuming their usual amount of carbohydrate as distinct from the 75 g used in an OGTT.

Some experts recommend the individual undertake regular blood glucose monitoring for a period of time to help diagnose the condition (CFT 2004). Blood glucose monitoring should be undertaken when corticosteroids are not being used for diagnostic purposes to make the blood glucose pattern easier to interpret. However, diabetes often presents when insulin resistance is increased, such as acute pulmonary infections and lung disease, which can cause hyperglycaemia especially when corticosteroid medicines are used to control the inflammatory response. Other insulin resistance-inducing factors include oral, intravenous, nasogastric, gastrostomy high carbohydrate supplements and feeds, and immunosuppressive therapy (e.g. after a transplant).

CF-specific factors that cause fluctuating blood glucose levels include:

- Respiratory infections and inflammation
- Increased energy expenditure
- Gastrointestinal abnormalities that affect food absorption, change intestinal motility, and liver disease
- Glucagon deficiency

HbA1c is currently being considered as a diagnostic test for diabetes but false negative results can occur in people with CF because of the increased red blood cell turnover. Fructosamine might be a useful alternative to monitoring diabetes control once the diagnosis is made.

Signs and symptoms

CFRD usually develops insidiously. Some signs and symptoms that should prompt investigation for CFRD include:

- Unexplained polyuria and/or polydipsia
- Inability to maintain or gain weight despite optimal nutrition
- Poor nutritional statues that affects growth
- Delayed puberty
- Unexplained decline in lung function and chest infections

Management

Several management guidelines are available in the United States, Australia, and the United Kingdom (e.g. Moran et al. 2014 and Middleton et al. 2014). Managing blood glucose is important but challenging. People might require insulin during exacerbations of CF that require corticosteroid treatment (see information in this chapter). A high-calorie, high-fat diet is recommended in CF (O'Riordan et al. 2009); thus, an appropriate insulin regimen is usually required. Insulin is the only glucose-lowering medicine recommended for CFRD (Moran et al. 1999) but the insulin regimen should be tailored to suit the individual.

The person needs to learn or have access to health professional support to increase insulin doses during acute illnesses, when the corticosteroid dose increases and when they are receiving parenteral supplements or feeds and in hospital. In these circumstances, the insulin dose may increase up to four times the usual insulin dose (Moran et al. 1999). The insulin dose must be reduced when these circumstances are managed to avoid hypoglycaemia.

Diabetes education and involving the individual in care decisions is essential, as is individualising the management plan to suit the individual. The plan should include plans for managing CFRD during period of wellness and plans for managing diabetes during exacerbations of CF, including adjusting glucose lowering medicines to manage blood glucose excursions, diabetes, and driving if they are insulin treated.

Incontinence

Incontinence is not a normal part of ageing. It can occur at any age. Untreated hyperglycaemia can lead to serious adverse events such as DKA and hyperglycaemic hyperosmolar states (HHS). Both states contribute to dehydration, confusion, falls and pain risk, and increased risk of death (Umpierrez 9). Polyuria and nocturia and can also indicate undiagnosed diabetes.

The damaging effects of hyperglycaemia on tissues and organs are well known in T1DM (DCCT 1991, 1993, 1997) and T2DM (UKPDS 1998). Glucose variability also damages tissues and organs (Krinsley 2008), including tissues and organs in the genitourinary and gastrointestinal tracts. Screening for and monitoring complication status includes renal function, neuropathic changes, and intercurrent infections and is central to diabetes care. However, incontinence is associated with diabetes and usual complication screening recommendations may not identify or misinterpret lower urinary tract symptoms such as urinary incontinence, urinary urgency, frequency, polyuria, and nocturia.

Definition and causes of incontinence

Urinary incontinence is defined as:

> Involuntary loss of urine in a place that is socially unacceptable that results in significant impacts on activities of daily living, quality of life and psychological aspects of culturally situated notions of health.
>
> (Zhang 2018)

Incontinence causes significant remediable distress and reduces quality of life (Felde et al. 2017). It increases the risk of falls, pressure ulcers, and polypharmacy, is a common reason older people are admitted to a residential aged care facility (RACF) (Wijk et al. 2018) and increased mortality (Zhang 2018). It is associated with dehydration and its consequences and may lead to or be caused by urinary tract infection (UTI).

Recurrent genitourinary infections in people with diabetes increase their risk of complicated pathogen-resistant UTIs, which often involve *E. coli*, *K. pneumoniae*, *Candida*, and *Enterococcus* (Gromiovits 2018). Complicated pathogen-resistant UTIs and include renal abscess, emphysematous pyelonephritis, fungal infections, and urolithiasis. In men it can be due to acute prostatitis and prostatic hypertrophy (Gromiovits 2018).

The aetiology of urinary incontinence is usually multifactorial in older people (Wagg et al. 2017), especially those with diabetes. The ability to remain continent of urine depends on:

- The bladder capacity to stretch and store urine until it is socially acceptable to void
- A competent sphincter mechanism
- A functional neurological system that co-ordinates urethral and bladder function and the shift from storage to voiding, when appropriate

Therefore, any condition that affects neural control of the bladder or damages anatomic structures that facilitate urethral closure can compromise continence. Neuromuscular damage to the pelvic floor during childbirth is the most common cause of stress incontinence in women (Salvatore et al. 2017). Women with stress incontinence can be treated with either surgery or conservative interventions. The latter include pelvic floor muscle training with or without biofeedback and electrical stimulation.

The most common causes of urinary incontinence in men are benign or malignant diseases of the prostate and their subsequent treatment (Salvatore et al. 2017). Pelvic floor muscle exercises and other conservative interventions are also helpful for men with post prostatectomy stress urinary incontinence.

Overactive bladder (OAB), a common cause of urinary incontinence, occurs in men and women. OAB refers to … *a symptom syndrome which is defined by the presence of urgency, with or without urge incontinence, but usually with frequency and nocturia in the absence of infection or other obvious aetiology* (Abrams et al. 2002). OAB usually causes urgency to urinate and/or urge incontinence (Abrams et al. 2002).

The causes of OAB are likely to be multifactorial but are not clearly defined. It is more common in people with cerebrovascular disease, Parkinson's disease, and people with spinal cord lesions above the lumbosacral level (Salvatore et al. 2017). Treating OAB-associated UI depends on diagnosing and treating the underlying causes and contributing factors. Other urinary symptoms include nocturnal enuresis, continuous incontinence, insensible incontinence, coital incontinence, functional incontinence, and multifactorial incontinence.

Diabetes and incontinence

Recent research suggests urologic complications are present in 75% of men and women with long-duration T1DM based on data collected from participants in the DCCT Epidemiology of Diabetes Interventions and Complications Cohort, at two time points: 2010 and 2011 ($n = 508$ women and 551 males) (Wessells et al. 2018). Sixty-five percent of women and 68% of males had at least one urologic symptom.

High HbA1c (>8.54%) was associated with increased risk of urologic complications in both genders (Wessells et al. 2018). Early studies did not identify a strong relationship between high HbA1c and the severity of urinary incontinence (Brown et al. 2006; Ebbesen et al. 2009), which is interesting, given the association between long-standing hyperglycaemia (HbA1c > 7%) and diabetes complications. HbA1c ≥ 7% is associated with inflammatory changes and tissue and organ damage that contribute to diabetes complications (Diabetes Control and Complications Trial [DCT] 1993, UKPDS 1998, ADA 2018).

Diabetes, age, and obesity (BMI > 30 kg/m^2) are independent risk factors for urinary incontinence in women with T1DM or T2DM (Sarma et al. 2009) but not men (Wessells et al. 2018). The association between diabetes and incontinence in men is less clear than in women. Significantly, diabetes is associated with earlier onset and increased severity of OAB, stress incontinence, impaired bladder contractility, and increased post-void residual urine, especially in women (Karoli et al. 2014).

Neuropathic and microvascular diabetes complications and benign prostate hyperplasia increases the risk of incontinence in men. Multimorbidity is common in diabetes and is associated with incontinence. A recent retrospective chart audit of people referred to a multidisciplinary continence clinic in Vancouver ($n = 225$) found 40% had Charlson Comorbidity Index >6 and were on >5 prescribed medicines and 52% were functionally dependent. The average age was 76: range 29–102 (Koo and Spencer 2018). It is not clear whether any participants had diabetes.

These long-term complications affect functional status, cognition, quality of life, dignity and autonomy, and reduce life expectancy. They have various effects on bladder and bowel function that predispose individuals, especially women, to UI and faecal incontinence (Ditah et al. 2014). Almost 50% of males and females with diabetes have some degree of bladder cystopathy: reduced bladder filling and sensation and poor contractility (Arrellano-Valdez et al. 2014). Consequently, they often have high residual urine volume post void, which increases their risk of UTI, especially if they are hyperglycaemic.

People with diabetes have more gastrointestinal symptoms than people without diabetes: 15.6% compared to 10%, respectively (Hillson 2018). Diarrhoea is a common symptom and has many causes. People with neuropathic gastrointestinal changes can have diarrhoea and/or constipation at differing times, which affects blood glucose and physical and psychological comfort (Du 2018). Colorectal cancer (Larsson 2005), coeliac, and pancreatic disease associated with diabetes and gastroenteritis can cause hyperglycaemia and polyuria (Clark et al. 1998). Many commonly used glucose-lowering medicines such as metformin, acarbose, and GLP-1 agonists can also cause/contribute to gastrointestinal issues (Hillson 2018).

Incontinence has a significant effect on personhood, self-concept, and dignity (Ostaszkiewicz et al. 2018). Continence assessment, management, and/or referral should be included in current diabetes guidelines and policies.

Sleep disturbance and diabetes

Chronic sleep deprivation increases the risk of obesity, insulin resistance, and diabetes (Shaw et al. 2008). Obstructive sleep apnoea (OSA) is the most common type; central sleep apnoea occurs when the brain signals to the muscles that control breathing are affected. Often, both types occur together. In addition, obese people and people with diabetes are more likely to develop OSA. Disturbed sleep results in daytime drowsiness. Shift workers are at increased risk of obesity and type 2 diabetes, possibly due to changes in insulin sensitivity and appetite regulation when meals are consumed in normal sleep time (at night).

Possible pathways linking OSA and diabetes include:

- Activation of the sympathetic nervous system resulting in hypoxia and repeated arousal from sleep.
- Hypoxia effects on insulin sensitivity.
- Systemic inflammatory effects. OSA engenders increased inflammatory markers such as CRB and IL6 independently of other causes of inflammation.
- Disruption of the hypothalamic–pituitary adrenal axis, which leads to elevated cortisol levels, which affect insulin secretion and glucose disposal.
- Suppressed slow-wave sleep. Slow-wave sleep is thought to be important to metabolic and emotional restoration. Lack of slow-wave sleep leads to insulin resistance independently of hypoxia and total sleep time.
- Fatigue from OSA and chronic sleep disturbance leads to less physical activity, which contributes to obesity and type 2 diabetes risk.
- Autonomic nerve dysfunction due to chronic hyperglycaemia, which affects sleep regulation and can contribute to OSA and/or reduce the person's response to hypoxia generated by existing OSA.
- OSA is independently associated with hypertension and exacerbated cardiovascular risk.

Sleep apnoea can develop at any age and occurs in both men and women, but it is more common in men, especially men over age 30 and high BMI. Quality slow-wave sleep is important to the way people process and store information they collect consciously and subconsciously during the day. Thus, sleep apnoea can affect memory.

Diagnosis

Common signs and symptoms include:

- Unrefreshing sleep especially if the person snores
- Insomnia
- Snoring, startling, and choking episodes during sleep
- Nocturia

- Night sweats
- Sexual dysfunction
- Cognitive impairment, difficulty concentrating, forgetfulness
- Depression
- Sleep-related driving incidents
- Systemic pulmonary hypertension
- Cardiac arrhythmias and angina at night (Young et al. 2002)

Physical examination should include neck circumference, which is often enlarged. In addition, microagnathia and enlarged tonsils might also be present. An oxygen desaturation index (ODI) >3–4% below baseline per hour of sleep represent severe OSA. Normal ODI is <5, and ODI >29 indicate severe OSA. The gold standard diagnostic test for OSA is polysomnography (PSG), which measures oral-nasal airflow, respiratory effort and oxyhaemoglobin desaturation, which is undertaken in sleep laboratories.

However, OSA can be measured at home using oximeters and noting symptoms of daytime drowsiness. In addition, valuable information can be obtained using the Insomnia Severity Index, the Epworth Sleepiness Scale, or the Berlin Questionnaire (Department of Veterans Affairs US 2012). Depression and OSA often coexist and may share some common aetiologies (Allen 2012). Thus, screening for and managing depression is also important.

Management

Management consists of weight loss and optimising blood glucose and lipid levels. This is essential because hyperglycaemia contributes to lethargy and sleepiness, exacerbates OSA, and increases the risk of death. It is important to avoid stimulant foods such as caffeine and spices at night and to limit alcohol. Likewise, avoiding sedatives is important.

Mouth appliances that opens the airways and continuous positive airway pressure (CPAP) improve sleep duration and quality (McDermott 2012). Screening people with OSA for metabolic derangements and asking about symptoms including snoring and daytime sleepiness is important. People who live with the individual can contribute important information.

Counselling about the risks associated with driving is essential. Significantly, partners should be involved unless the individual objects because they can often contribute important information to help clinicians support the couple and because sexual counselling might be beneficial.

Modern CPAP machines are not as noisy as the older models but they do emit an electric humming noise that can disturb partner's sleep.

Diabetes and tuberculosis

TB remains a major health issue. The link between diabetes and TB was documented in ancient Rome (Kapur et al. 2009), and the prevalence is increasing globally. Efforts to detect and manage diabetes may also help control TB (Viney 2017).

People with diabetes are three times more likely to develop TB (Jeon and Murray 2008), and people with TB have higher rates of TB treatment failure and death, even when TB treatment is appropriate (Dooley et al. 2009; Sullivan and Ben Amor 2012; WHO, 2017). People with diabetes have a two to three times higher risk of developing TB than people without diabetes; approximately 10% of TB cases are linked to diabetes. The link between diabetes and TB will become increasingly important because of the expected increase in obesity and diabetes in countries that have a high TB prevalence (e.g. Africa).

TB is often not diagnosed or diagnosed late in a large number of people with concomitant diabetes and TB (World Health Organization [WHO] 2011). Thus, everybody with TB should be regularly screened for diabetes and screening for diabetes in people with TB should be considered in high risk populations. It should be noted that such populations might exist in countries where TB has been eradicated, such as Australia and the United Kingdom, due to migration and refugees from TB-prevalent countries. In addition, many migrants and refugees are often also at high risk of diabetes. Although health checks are conducted before migrants and refugees enter Australia and other countries, diabetes and TB can be latent and become active at a later date.

Management

International Standards of TB care were published in 2014 and revised in 2017 (WHO 2017). Studies are currently in progress to determine whether diagnosing and treating diabetes early in people with TB can improve TB outcomes (Dooley et al. 2009). Early detection and management may improve outcomes. Blood glucose and lipids, blood pressure control, and complication screening should be individualised (see Chapter 1). Active TB should be treated and TB status monitored. Relevant family and community members should be educated about diabetes and infection control processes. Systematically documenting and sharing outcomes could contribute to the evidence base for managing these two conditions when they occur together.

Diabetes can adversely affect bacterial response to TB treatment and people are more likely to relapse and need retreatment, which increases the risk of drug-resistant TB developing (Mahishale et al. 2017). Ineffective treatment response and relapse are more likely in people with hyperglycaemia and high HbA1c and such people are more prone to infections.

Diabetes and HIV/AIDS

HIV/AIDs results in changes in glucose homeostasis possible through increased non-oxidative glucose disposal and increased glucose production in the liver (Spollett 2006). HIV is characterised by deficient immune status and is treated using combination therapy such as nucleoside reverse transcriptase inhibitors (NRTIs) and HIV-1 protease inhibitors (PI). The latter has been linked to hyperglycaemia, which resolves when the PI is discontinued or replaced with another class of medicine (Martinez et al. 1999). Other medicines, such as megestrol acetate, which is used as an appetite stimulant in people with AIDs-related cachexia, have glucocorticoid effects that predispose people with diabetes risk factors to hyperglycaemia and weight gain (Rathgaber et al. 1992). The benefits of these medicines for treating HIV most probably outweigh the risk of diabetes.

Management

There are generally three groups of people with HIV and diabetes:

- People with HIV and undiagnosed diabetes
- People who develop diabetes during treatment for HIV
- People who have diabetes and develop HIV

The optimal method of screening for diabetes in people with AIDs is still under debate and may differ amongst ethnic groups. Screening is recommended for people who have the classic risk factors for diabetes, especially women, because of the dual risk to the baby of HIV and diabetes-related foetal abnormalities including type 2 diabetes (Chapter 1) (Howard et al. 2005). However, there is some controversy over the best screening method to use. OGTT might detect diabetes more effectively than other methods in people with HIV (Spollett 2006). Some experts recommend performing fasting plasma glucose and a diabetes risk screen before commencing HIV treatment, especially with PIs are used because of the known hyperglycaemia risk associated with these medicines.

Choosing HIV medicines carefully and limiting the use of PIs where possible, especially in people at risk of diabetes or those who already have diabetes is a key strategy. However, the risk of developing/exacerbating diabetes needs to be considered in light of the benefits to be gained by reducing the HIV viral load and improving immune status.

Eating a healthy diet and exercising are key management strategies but need to be tailored to the individual's HIV status and capability. Nutrition supplements may be needed in HIV-related cachexia. GLMs might be indicated especially when PIs are used. Liver function should be tested before TZD are prescribed and during treatment with TZDs (Chapter 5). Before metformin is used the individual should screened for lactic acidosis and abnormal serum creatinine levels (Aberg et al. 2004). Lactic acidosis is a rare but serious side effect of metformin in certain circumstances (Chapter 5).

People receiving NRTI therapy, especially if the treatment lasts longer than six months, may be at higher risk of lactic acidosis. Stavudine, zidovudine, and didanosine are more likely to pre-cipitate lactic acidosis than other antiviral medicines. Although metformin is not contraindicated in people using antiviral medicines, clinicians must be aware of the possibility of lactic acidosis and educate the person accordingly. Insulin may be indicated for some people and the type of insulin and dose regimen needs to be individualised.

Diabetes complications need to be detected early and managed to improve outcomes. For example people with HIV and diabetes, especially those with a high viral load, prescribed the antiretroviral medicines Ziagen and the combination medicines Kivexa and Trizivir, have a high prevalence of albuminuria: twofold greater than for either disease alone (Kim 2011).

There is limited research on interactions between glucose-lowering medicines and antiretrovi-ral medicines, but such interactions are possible because both groups of medicines use similar metabolic pathways. Blood glucose monitoring is important to detect hypo- or hyperglycaemia, which could indicate an interaction. Significantly, safe disposal of sharps is paramount in people with diabetes and HIV.

Managing hyperglycaemia and its consequences is important to the individual's comfort and most likely outcomes. However, the added responsibility of managing diabetes as well as HIV may be overwhelming and compound/lead to depression. People with HIV and diabetes need tailored diabetes education that considers their HIV self-care, medication regimen, and other relevant personal information. People who are prescribed metformin need advice about recog-nising lactic acidosis (Chapter 7) and liver-related symptoms such as abdominal tenderness, ascites, and peripheral oedema (Aberg et al. 2004).

Although survival is improving for people with HIV and diabetes, end-of-life care should also be considered proactively and include diabetes management and management directions the individual chooses to document (Chapter 18).

Diabetes and hearing loss

The prevalence of hearing impairment is higher in people with diabetes compared with people without diabetes (Horikawa et al. 2012) and the association appears to be stronger in younger than older people (Bainbridge 2013). The prevalence of hearing loss appears to be approximately 30% higher in people with diabetes than in nondiabetics.

The pathophysiology of diabetes-related hearing loss is not clear but might be due to neuropathic changes in the vascular and/or neural systems in the inner ear. Autopsy evi-dence shows sclerosis of the internal auditory artery, thicker vessel walls in the stria vascu-laris and basilar membrane, demyelinisation of the cochlear nerve, atrophy of the spiral ganglion and loss of outer ear hair cells. However, age-related hearing changes need to be considered.

Causes of hearing loss

The causes of hearing loss are multifactorial:

- Older age is the most common cause of hearing loss. One in three people aged 65–74 have some degree of hearing loss, and after 75 the ratio increases to one in two people (Wilson et al. 1999). Genes and exposure to noise may play a role in aged-related hearing loss.

- Loud and continuous noise can damage hearing. People most at risk are those who work in loud workplaces, musicians, the military and people who constantly listen to loud music on smartphones or in nightclubs, for example. Wearing earplugs and limiting exposure to noise is important.
- Some medicines including antibiotics, chemotherapy medicines, aspirin, loop diuretics, and medicines used to treat malaria and erectile dysfunction; some 200 medicines are reported to trigger hearing loss.
- Some illnesses such as cardiovascular disease, hypertension, and diabetes, affect the blood supply to the inner ear and infections.
- Trauma that involves the eardrum, or skull. (WebMD 2013).

Sudden hearing loss >30 dB is uncommon and not particularly related to diabetes. It can occur over hours or days and often only affects one ear. The cause is often hard to identify. The degree of hearing loss is classified as mild, moderate, severe, or profound. As the hearing loss progresses, the ability to accurately understand conversational speech declines, and people become isolated and may become depressed. Progressive hearing loss associated with ageing often affects the high frequency sounds first. Therefore, in the early stages, high-pitched sounds such as women's voices and speech sound such as 'S' and 'F' become inaudible, whilst other lower pitched sounds may still be heard at relatively normal levels.

Other signs of hearing loss include:

- Difficulty understanding telephone conversations;
- Trouble hearing when there is background noise;
- Difficulty following conversations that involve several people speaking at once;
- Feeling people are mumbling;
- Misunderstanding what people say, which can lead to miscommunication and adverse events especially in healthcare settings;
- Needing to ask people to repeat themselves;
- Ringing, hissing, or other sounds in the ear;
- Other people complain about TVs, radios being too loud.

Diagnosis is through audiology testing.

Management

The earlier detection and management of hearing loss produces better outcomes. The earlier it is detected, the easier it is to treat. Unmanaged hearing loss has a negative impact on quality of life; appropriately managed hearing loss improves quality of life. However, hearing loss often occurs gradually and may go unnoticed by the individual concerned, although people around him/her may be aware of the changes. Diabetes-related hearing loss is typically high frequency sensorioneural hearing loss that can be managed using hearing aids. Ear infections that lead to temporary hearing loss can be treated with antibiotics; however, the specific treatment depends on the underlying cause, and frequent middle ear infections could permanently compromise hearing.

Clinicians need to be aware of the subtle changes in hearing and speak directly to the person whilst looking them in the face. Be sure you have the person's attention before you speak. Supplementing oral information with written information is helpful, provided it is at an appropriate literacy level and is culturally relevant. Given the prevalence of hearing loss and the effects on outcomes clinicians need to encourage people to have their hearing assessed and refer them to an audiologist or an ear specialist for assessment and appropriate management.

Group education programmes may be challenging for people with hearing loss but there is a range of options that can improve hearing and enable people with mild-to-moderate hearing loss to participate in groups. People with severe hearing loss would benefit more from individual education unless sessions are conducted with AUSLAN (Australian sign language) interpreters.

Learning AUSLAN takes time and it is recognised as a minority language. Learning sign language is rarely an option for older people with diabetes-related hearing loss.

In hospital settings, background noise may be distracting and consultations and beds should be placed in the quietest possible location with as few noise distractions as possible. A recent study also suggests much higher prevalence of hearing loss amongst hospital patients.

Diabetes, musculoskeletal disease, and osteoporosis

Musculoskeletal disorders associated with diabetes are often overlooked in usual diabetes care. Diabetes is associated with several specific musculoskeletal disorders and others occur concomitantly. Diabetes-related musculoskeletal disease reflects the multisystem effects of defects in glucose homeostasis. Potential causal mechanisms include (Brown et al. 2001; Smith et al. 2002):

- Nonenzymatic glycosylation of protein resulting in advanced glycated end products (age) and stiffened connective tissue
- Increased deposition of connective tissue as a result of myofibroblast proliferation
- Neuropathy
- Autoimmune diseases associated with type 1 diabetes
- Obesity-related changes and strain on joints
- Hyperinsulinaemia and associated hormonal abnormalities such as elevated growth hormone

Activities of daily living (ADL), quality of life, and driving safety are often associated with stress and lowered mood. Some cause chronic pain. Thus, they affect diabetes health outcomes. The prevalence of the following conditions tends to increase with long duration of diabetes, especially associated with chronic hyperglycaemia:

- Shoulder adhesive capsulitis is painful and limits movement.
- Shoulder–hand syndrome consists of painful shoulder capsulitis and swollen, tender hands.
- Cherioarthropathy (limited joint mobility) is specific to diabetes and causes stiffening of the small joints in the hands.
- Dupuytren's contracture is associated with vision-threatening retinopathy, increased risk of foot ulceration, and other musculoskeletal disorders in type 1 and type 2 diabetes.
- Carpal tunnel syndrome is also associated with hypothyroidism; the causal process is usually not due to inflammation.
- Hyperostosis and Forestier's disease is commonly occurs in obese middle-aged men with type 2 diabetes; the thoracic spine most commonly affected.
- Gout, pseudogout, and osteoarthritis. These health issues have a cyclical relationship with diabetes – they are both more likely to develop in a person with diabetes and more likely to contribute to a person subsequently developing diabetes (Hackethal 2014; Pan et al. 2016).
- Osteopenia, usually in type 1 diabetes, may be associated with retinopathy; bone density is usually normal or increased.
- Patient is unable to make the prayer sign – i.e. cannot press palms together when fingers are touching in the traditional prayer pose.
- Flexor tenosynovitis (trigger finger) occurs when a finger gets stuck in the bent position. It is more common in women than men.
- Diabetic foot diseases such as Charcot's foot; see Chapter 8.

Diagnosis is usually made on clinical grounds, but X-ray, MRI, and ultrasound may be required. Muscle biopsy or EMG testing may be useful. Improving metabolic control using an appropriate diet and exercise is essential. Strength and flexibility training programmes such as progressive weight training and some forms of gentle tai chi, physiotherapy massage, and appropriate pain management using nonmedicine options where possible are helpful.

Osteoporosis

Diabetes is associated with increased risk of fragility fractures: sixfold risk of hip fractures in T1DM and two- to threefold in T2DM. Poor glycaemic control increases the risk low trauma fractures in T1DM, but not T2DM (Vavanikunnel et al. 2019). The pathophysiology that contribute to skeletal fragility also differs between the two types. These include age at diabetes onset, insulin deficiency (T1DM) versus insulin resistance (T2DM) and the effects of some GLM medicines.T1DM diagnosed in adolescence and early adulthood have lower insulin levels and IGF-1 that may impair osteoclast function and lead to lower bone mass, smaller bones and changed bone microstructure (Vavanikunnel et al. 2019).

People with T2DM often have obesity-related insulin resistance and hyperinsulinaemia, normal to higher bone mass and preserved/increased trabecular bone volume with increased cortical porosity, particularly in people with fractures and microvascular disease. Complications, longstanding diabetes, glucose toxicity, chronic inflammation, and microvascular changes could play a critical role in bone ageing and progression to osteoporosis. These factors, combined with other comorbidities and medicine effects, can increase falls risk and fall-related injury such as fractures (Vavanikunnel et al. 2019).

Frailty status may play an important role in fragility fractures (Lee et al., 2017; Li 2019) (Chapter 12). There is a significant relationship between the frailty index (FI) and fragility fracture risk for every 0.1 increase in the FI and every 0.1 increase in risk of fragility fracture in people with diabetes and hip fracture and diabetes. Therefore, considering, managing, and monitoring frailty is an important aspect of care (Chapter 12).

Determinants of fracture risk include:

- Reduced bone mineral density (BMD) is usually measured using DEXA scan and reported as: normal, osteopenic, or osteoporotic, based on the T-score (ISCD Writing Group 2004). The fracture risk increases twofold for every one unit decrease in the T-score, and most occur in the osteoporotic range (Pasco et al. 2006).
- Advancing age.
- History of fragility fractures and falls.
- Frailty (Chen and Center 2015; Li 2019).

There are many fracture risk calculators. Absolute risk calculators generally include clinical risk factors as well as BMD; therefore, they and may quantify risk better and help decide optimal treatment (Chen and Center 2015). Fracture risk tools include The WHO Fracture Risk Assessment Tool (FRAX) www.shef.ac.uk/FRAX/tool.jsp) and the Garvan Fracture Risk Calculator (GFRC) (www.garvan.org.au/promotions,bone-fracture-risk/calculator).

The FRAX and T-score used together increase fracture risk prediction (Chen and Center 2015). However, the T-score has limitation is obese people and men, although these parameters are now included in the FRAX and it can be used in men and women. The GFRC is useful in both genders and has a similar prognostic performance to FRAX.

Management

The goal of management is to prevent fractures and other trauma. Optimal treatment is controversial (Ferrari et al. 2018). A healthy diet and exercise are important to support bone and gut health. Some people may require nutrition support (Chapters 4 and 12). Some evidence suggests long term treatment with denosumab is beneficial if people can tolerate the medicine and continue to respond to treatment. Response to treatment is defined as T-score >2.0–1.5 and reduced risk of fragility fractures.

Other treatment includes bisphosphonates and oestrogen receptor modulators (Ebeling and Ferrari 2019).

Some conditions such as carpel tunnel syndrome may require surgical management. The impact on quality of life, ADLs, and safety such as driving and falls risk must be regularly assessed, such as during annual complication screening programmes, any change in health status, and driving licence renewal assessment.

Corticosteroid medications and diabetes

> **Key points**
>
> - Corticosteroid medications predispose the person to insulin resistance, dose-related hyperglycaemia, and hyperinsulinaemia.
> - They increase blood glucose in people without diabetes, especially those at risk of diabetes.
> - They are used to control some disease processes or are given as hormone replacement therapy for some endocrine diseases; for example, pituitary tumours. In the latter case, corticosteroid doses are usually small or physiological levels and are less likely to cause hyperglycaemia.
> - Nondiabetics on high doses, long-term or intermittent corticosteroids should be monitored and should test their blood glucose. People with diabetes should test their diabetes and their medicines should be adjusted proactively.
> - Corticosteroids and atypical antipsychotic medicines can precipitate hyperosmolar states.

Introduction

Steroids are naturally occurring hormones produced by the adrenal glands under the control of the pituitary adrenocorticotropic hormone (ACTH). There are three major classes of steroid hormones:

(1) Glucocorticoids
(2) Mineralocorticoids
(3) Androgens and oestrogen

Corticosteroids and diabetes

Corticosteroid medicines are an essential part of the management of inflammatory disease processes, haematologic malignancies, allergic reactions, and shock. The long-term use, especially in high doses, predisposes the individual to steroid-induced diabetes or to hyperglycaemia in people with established diabetes. Corticosteroids have the propensity to cause insulin resistance, increased hepatic glucose output, reduced glucose transport, and to inhibit insulin secretion resulting in hyperglycaemia.

Effect on blood glucose
The effect on blood glucose depends to some extent on the biological action of the particular preparation used and the length of time it is required. Hyperglycaemia usually occurs with doses of prednisolone (or equivalent) >7.5 mg/day.

Specific short courses of corticosteroids usually only affect the blood glucose temporarily or not at all, but hyperglycaemia occurs if the dose is increased or the medication is needed intermittently or in the long term (Williams and Pickup 1992). If given for <1 week even large doses do not usually present problems, although impaired glucose tolerance can be present and can occur within 48 hours. IV steroids usually have a shorter duration of action than steroids given by other routes and do not increase the blood glucose if only one to two doses are given (Jackson and Bowman 1995).

Predisposing factors

People with existing risk factors for diabetes run the greatest risk of developing steroid-induced diabetes. These risks are described in Chapter 1. They include the following conditions:

* Old age
* Existing impaired glucose tolerance
* Current or previous gestational diabetes mellitus (GDM)
* Cardiac disease
* Psychosis

The presence of one or more of these risk factors may influence the decision to use steroids, the duration of the treatment, and the dose. In many cases steroids are the medicines of choice and management strategies should be implemented to minimise the impact on the blood glucose.

Corticosteroids and osteoporosis

Corticosteroids can also reduce bone formation and the viability of osteoblasts and osteocytes, reduce calcium absorption from the intestine, and increase renal calcium excretion predisposing the individual to osteoporosis and fractures (Romas 2008). These negative effects can be managed with supplemental oral calcium and vitamin D or calcitriol. In some cases, gonadal hormone production can be affected, which exacerbates the other bone effects. Changes are noted even at low doses of corticosteroids and fractures can occur soon after commencing these medicines, especially in high-risk individuals.

Risk factors include:

* Age
* Female gender
* Postmenopausal women who are at the highest risk
* Low bone mineral density

Bone mineral densitometry and dual energy X-ray absorptiometry of the lumbar spine and neck of the femur are warranted for all patients on corticosteroid therapy >3 months. Using a nonsteroid medicine if possible and using these medicines in the lowest possible dose for the shortest time helps reduce the risk of adverse effects. Oral bisphosphonates with vitamin D are important primary prevention medicines for people in the high-fracture-risk category.

Recent research suggests there is a significant inverse association between serum 25-dihydroxy vitamin D levels and the risk of developing type 2 diabetes (Chiu et al. 2004).

See Chapter 18 for information about corticosteroids and end-of-life care.

Management

Over 50% of people with type 2 diabetes treated with GLMs require insulin if they require corticosteroids, sometimes permanently (Williams and Pickup 1992). Shapiro (2007) suggested TZDs might be useful to overcome steroid-induced insulin resistance but recommended considering the individual characteristics before prescribing a TZD. However, TZD have a slow onset of action so they would not be beneficial when steroids are needed in the short term. When steroids are used in the long term, they exacerbate cardiovascular risk factors and lead to weight gain. In such cases, TZD may increase this because they also cause oedema and exacerbate heart failure.

Other GLM may be effective depending on the individual cautions and contraindication. The GLP-1 agents might be effective in some patients but more research is needed (van Raalte et al. 2009). The risk of lactic acidosis associated with metformin may preclude its use in many people with diabetes. Sulpuonylureas have a limited role in managing corticsteroid-induced hyperglycaemia (ADS 2012).

Therefore, insulin is often required. Dose flexibility is greater with insulin and the rapid onset of action and ease of dose titration are advantages. The insulin dose and dose regimen need to be individualised. Insulin regimens to manage steroid-induced hyperglycaemia include:

- Morning isophane insulin or morning premixed insulin
- Long-acting insulin in the morning, with or without rapid-acting insulin at mealtimes, which prevents new onset diabetes following immunosuppressive therapy following renal transplants

Insulin can be given by injection or insulin pump. In a small study (n = 10), people with type 1 diabetes on 80 mg prednisolone per day managed on insulin pumps required dose increases 30–100% (ADS 2012).

Managing corticosteroid use includes the following:

- Screen for the risk factors for diabetes before commencing corticosteroids.
- Where diabetes is present, GLM and/or insulin need to be reviewed and may require adjustment according to the blood glucose profile. In most cases, the postprandial blood glucose increases during the day but drops overnight and the fasting glucose may not be significantly elevated (Oyer et al. 2006).
- Select the optimal route of corticosteroid administration for the particular problem: oral, IV, inhaled, topical cream.
- Use the lowest effective corticosteroid dose for the shortest possible time.
- Monitor blood glucose four-hourly if the person has diabetes and at least weekly if they do not.
- Monitor for ketones, especially in type 1 diabetes because steroids predispose them to DKA.
- Explain to the patient the reasons for the blood glucose monitoring, especially if they do not have diabetes. Reassure them that steroids are the medicine of choice for their condition and that hyperglycaemia can be controlled.
- Steroids required on a temporary basis must be withdrawn gradually to allow the pituitary–adrenal axis to return to normal activity (Jackson and Bowman 1995).
- If GLM/insulin doses were commenced or increased they will need to be reduced as the steroid dose is reduced to avoid hypoglycaemia.
- Prolonged steroid use depresses the immune system. Aseptic technique is important if any invasive procedures are required, and the immune system should be supported with a healthy diet and regular activity within the individual's tolerance level.

Steroids can mask some of the signs and symptoms of infection, as can diabetes. Common infection sites should be closely monitored, such as injection sites, feet, mouth and gums, and the urinary tract:

- The skin can become thin and fragile and easily damaged if corticosteroids are required in the long term, predisposing the individual to bruising, skin tears, ulcers, and other trauma, especially older people. A protective skin care regimen is important.
- Protecting older people from falls that predispose them to trauma is essential where long-term corticosteroids are required because of the effects on bone and the increased risk of fractures if they fall.
- Alternate-day steroid regimens show greater effects on the blood glucose on the day steroid medications are taken. OHA/insulin regimes for steroid and nonsteroid days may be needed.
- Insulin is often required for people on GLMs if long-term steroids are required or if hyperglycaemia persists, despite compliance with their GLMs, and an appropriate diet.

- Where permanent steroid therapy is required, for example, after surgery for a pituitary tumour, the steroid dose usually needs to be increased during illness or surgery. Careful, *written* instructions detailing how to manage steroid dose reductions in these circumstances and close liaison with their endocrinologist is essential. OHAs/insulin will also need to be adjusted in these circumstances.
- Achieving acceptable growth and development in children on permanent steroids is important and should be closely monitored. Growth hormone may be required.
- Body changes can occur such as weight gain, moon face, thinning hair, and acne, which can affect body image.
- Steroids can cause mental changes ranging from mild changes to psychosis, which can affect the person's self-care. If psychosis occurs, it will need to be managed appropriately. The help of a psychiatrist may be necessary.

Antipsychotic medicines

Antipsychotic medicines more than double the risk of gestational diabetes in pregnant women using these medicines (Boden et al. 2012). The effect may be due to weight gain, insulin resistance and hyperlipidaemia. Significantly, infants of mothers taking Olanzapine and Clozapine are at double to risk of being born with larger than normal heads after adjusting for maternal risk factors. Thus, women using antipsychotic medicines should be closely monitored.

Some antipsychotic agents are also associated with prolonged QT intervals, which predisposes the individual to cardiac arrhythmias (O'Brien and Oyebode 2003). A number of different pharmacological mechanisms are proposed and vary amongst the different antipsychotic medicine groups. Prexisting cardiac disease and factors that predispose the individual to cardiac arrhythmias increase the risk.

There is considerable overlap between other cardiovascular risk factors, including excess alcohol consumption, smoking, lack of physical activity. In addition, antidepressants independently exacerbate dyslipidaemia, hyperglycaemia, and the metabolic syndrome.

Close monitoring of risk factors, especially in individuals at risk, is essential. Education about self-care and seeking medical advice is also important. It is important to choose the antipsychotic medicine with the least effect on blood glucose and cardiovascular functioning and use it at the lowest effective dose. However, managing the person's psychiatric diagnosis and enabling them to function as normally as possible is essential.

Diabetes and driving

Driving refers to driving any motorised vehicle (e.g. cars, trucks, farm equipment, motorised wheelchairs, motor bikes, and probably push bikes).

The Australian Diabetes Society (ADS) (2011) and the UK Government (2016) developed recommendations/standards that can help clinicians advise and assess people with diabetes' fitness to drive. The ADS recommends the blood glucose be 'above 5 to drive', the association amongst diabetes, diabetes complications, medications, coexisting comorbidities, intercurrent illness, alcohol intake, environmental conditions, and driving accidents is complex and multifactorial. Individual driving risk needs to be assessed and monitored regularly, for example, when a complication is diagnosed, when the medication regimen is modified, as the person grows older, and following a crash. In addition, the ability to operate other vehicles such as motorised wheelchairs and farm vehicles also needs to be considered.

Diabetes can have a significant impact on driving safety, yet many current diabetes management guidelines and diabetes complication screening programmes do not make provision for proactive structured assessment of driving ability, which usually only occurs when the driving licence needs to be renewed or following a serious hypoglycaemic event or traffic accident. Often licence renewal may not be required for several years and the health status can change significantly between renewal periods. Statistically young men and older people are most at risk of road crash but people need to be assessed on an individual basis. Diabetes-specific effects on driving are shown in Table 10.4.

Guidelines for assessing fitness to drive exist in most countries (e.g. the Australian AUSTROADS 2017 standards; US Department of Transportation 2013). Although the Australian standards are comprehensive, outline how health issues can impact on driving safety, and include standards for private and commercial licences. They do not stress the cumulative impact of comorbidities on driving safety, even where the standards are cross-referenced. Such guidelines recommend counselling people with diabetes about their rights and responsibilities with respect to driving and increasingly recognise that hyperglycaemia, as well as hypoglycaemia affects cognitive function.

Table 10.4 Possible pharmacological mechanisms of various antipsychotic medicines responsible for cardiovascular effects.

Antipsychotic medicine	Pharmacological mechanism likely to contribute to cardiovascular disease
Tricyclic antidepressants	Affect a broad range of receptor pathways that are implicated in therapeutic as well as adverse outcomes. For example, they inhibit central cholinergic neurotransmission, which affects autonomic functions such as tachycardia, which is accompanied by neuronal uptake of norepinepherine, which can exacerbate tachycardia. They can block alpha-adrenergic receptors, which can reduce systemic vascular resistance and cause hypotension or orthostatic hypotension. High doses increase sympathetic and reduce parasympathetic influences on heart rate variability. They inhibit sodium channel conduction, which delays phase 0 cardiac depolarisation, which can result in slower conduction within the His-Purkinje fibres and the ventricles, which prolongs the QRS complex (the deflections in an electrocardiogram (EKG) tracing that represent the ventricular activity of the heart).
Selective serotonin reuptake inhibitors	Cause cardiovascular effects mostly because of the release of excess serotonin within the central nervous system, which can cause mild systemic hypotension. Citalopram and Escitalopram can cause generalised seizures. The two medicines can lead to dose-dependent prolongation of the QT interval.
Monoamine oxidase inhibitors	Enhance the concentration of a broad range of central neurotransmitters including norepinephrine. Tachycardia and hypertension might occur as a consequence, particularly at high doses. The onset of cardiovascular effects might not occur for 12–24 hours after the medicine is taken because it takes time for the concentration of central neurotransmitters to accumulate. Consuming foods or medicines high in tyramine can precipitate severe hypertension; the so called 'cheese effect.' Cardiovascular effects may also be due to serotonin accumulation and include tachycardia and hypotension especially when Monoamine oxidase inhibitors are combined with serotonin reuptake inhibitors.
Serotonin and norepinephrine reuptake inhibitors	Venlafaxine, Reboxetine, and Duloxetine appear to stimulate cardiac sympathetic nerve activity, which cause mild tachycardia and systemic hypertension. If sympathetic activity is excessive, more serious tachyarrhythmias are possible especially if cardiomyopathy is present. Venlafaxine can block cardiac sodium conduction.
Lithium	Might be associated with several cardiac conduction defects such as complete heart block and impaired atrioventricular conduction and prolonged QTcB intervals. The onset of cardiotoxicty might be delayed after commencing lithium due to the delay in reaching equilibrium in cardiac tissue concentrations.

Prevalence of and risk factors for driving crashes

Evidence about driving crash rates in people with diabetes is confusing. Some old research suggests the traffic crash rate is similar between diabetics and nondiabetics (MacLeod 1999). Others report a lower mileage-adjusted crash rate per million miles driven in people with diabetes than in the general population (Eadington and Frier 1989). Older drivers generally appear to have a higher crash rate than any other age group except people <25 years (Guerrier et al. 1999; McGwin et al. 2000; Braver and Trempel 2004). Older women with heart disease, stroke, or arthritis are at high risk (McGwin et al. 2000). If they are in an accident, older people are more likely to suffer serious injury or die. The presence of diabetes was not reported in these studies. However, many older drivers voluntarily restrict their driving, such as not driving at night or in peak hour traffic (Penckofer et al. 2007).

Other modern risk factors for driving and other accidents include using mobile phones and other distractions whilst driving, especially if concentration is impaired by hypo- or hyperglycaemia, depression, alcohol, or other drugs or medicines such as sedatives. The prevalence of accidents relating to these issues is unknown.

Falls in older people, especially a fall in the previous year, increase crash risk (Margolis et al. 2002). Falls are more likely to occur when the following factors are present. Almost all of these apply to diabetes:

- Unstable balance
- Neurological problems
- Musculoskeletal problems
- Cardiovascular disease
- Vision deficits
- Cognitive impairment
- Insulin treatment
- Significant postural hypotension
- Female gender (Gregg et al. 2000)

Although insulin treatment is assumed to carry a higher crash risk, people managed by diet and exercise are also at significant risk (Sagberg 2006). Sagberg found a significant risk of road crashes and the presence of medical conditions, symptoms, and some medicines in drivers of all ages. In particular, Sagberg found significant associations amongst crash risk and diabetes, previous MI, wearing glasses whilst driving, myopia, difficulty getting to sleep, frequent tiredness, depression, and taking antidepressant medicines. Koepsell et al. (1994) also found increased crash risk when diabetes and heart disease were both present, people on insulin or OHA, and duration of diabetes >5 years. Experts suggest diabetes-related crashes involving insulin-treated people are often due to hypoglycaemia (Clark et al. 1980; Frier et al. 1980; Steel et al. 1981; Koepsell et al. 1994). However, McGwin et al. (1999) found no significant difference in crash rates according to diabetes treatment mode or in people with diabetes overall.

In some countries people on insulin are not permitted to drive articulated vehicles or other heavy vehicles such as passenger buses. However, there are no restrictions on driving other heavy vehicles such as tractors and farm vehicles in rural areas. Crashes involving these vehicles cause significant injury. Laberge-Nadeau et al. (2000) reported a higher crash rate associated with people with diabetes driving nonarticulated but not articulated trucks. In contrast, Laberge-Nadeau et al. (2000) found no significant differences in crash rates between people with diabetes and nondiabetics driving either type of truck. Interestingly, noninsulin users and those with no diabetes complications were more likely to be involved in a crash whilst driving trucks.

Cox et al. (2000) used driving simulators to determine the effect of hypoglycaemia on driving ability in young people with diabetes. No effect was detected at blood glucose 3.6 mmol/l but significantly more swerving, driving over the line or off the road, and compensatory slow driving occurred at 2.6 mmol/l. Fifty percent indicated they would not drive if their blood glucose were low. In a second simulator study, Cox et al. (2000) progressively lowered blood glucose to <2.8 mmol/l.

Most participants recognised they were hypoglycaemic but only a minority treated the hypoglycaemia or stopped driving despite impaired driving performance.

Lee et al. (2003) used a PC-simulator to assess older people's driving ability. Driving skill declined significantly with increasing age. Sommerfield et al. (2003) reported significant impairment in working memory, ability to make decisions under pressure, and less confidence driving at speed in a group of older people. It is not clear whether any of the participants in these studies had diabetes, but the findings mostly likely also apply to older people with diabetes.

However, driving simulators, particularly in research settings, may not be an appropriate way to assess actual driving behaviour because of distractions such as intravenous lines, wearing an electroencephalogram (EEG) cap, and being asked questions whilst driving, as occurred in Cox et al.'s study. In addition, a different set of skills is needed to drive in simulators from driving on the road. Simulators can cause stress and anxiety as well as being distracting, all of which affect driving skill and compound the effects of medical conditions. Some people may enjoy playing the game.

Driving can also be affected by weather and road conditions, level of vehicle maintenance, and the age and type of vehicle (Evans 2004). Some of these factors are significantly different from conditions operating when some older studies were undertaken. Likewise, many of the newer glucose-lowering agents and insulin analogues, and the trend towards using shorter acting OHA and insulin analogues have reduced the risk of hypoglycaemia.

Diabetes-related effects on driving

Diabetes-related factors that affect driving ability include:

- The duration of diabetes. Risk increases with increasing duration of diabetes largely because of the increasing risk of diabetes complications.
- Usual metabolic control. Hypoglycaemia is a recognised crash risk but hyperglycaemia also has short-term effects on driving ability and long-term consequences as a result of complications (see Table 10.5).
- Functional impairment and disability, for example, arthritis, and common diabetes complications; hypertension, stroke, and transient ischaemic attacks (TIA) are associated with functional decline (Stuck et al. 1999). Diabetes-related musculoskeletal disease can make it difficult to grip the steering wheel or feel the pedals and affect the degree of control over the vehicle and/or make turning to view traffic and road signs difficult and may compound the effects of arthritis and vision deficits.
- Impaired cognitive functioning due to age-related changes, hypo- or hyperglycaemia or other factors. Hyperglycaemia is linked to impaired cognitive functioning (Meneilly et al. 1993), slows recovery from injury following an accident (Scalea et al. 2007), and leads to tiredness and sleep disturbance, which affect concentration in the daytime.
- Long-term complications that cause functional and cognitive deficits such as cardiovascular disease, musculoskeletal problems, renal disease, retinopathy, and other vision deficits. Diabetic retinopathy is associated with a high rate of driving-related fear, Coyne et al. (2004). Autonomic neuropathy causing hypoglycaemic unawareness represents significant crash risk in insulin-treated people.
- Medicines likely to affect physical and/or mental functioning such as insulin and GLM, antihypertensive agents, sedatives, antidepressive agents, some herbal medicines, and illegal drugs. Polypharmacy is common in diabetes and medicine interactions and adverse events can occur that affect driving safety. Many people with diabetes use complementary medicines (CAM) and some CAM medicines can interact with conventional medicines (e.g. glucose-lowering herbal medicines).
- Self-care knowledge and behaviours, which encompasses diabetes-related and general self-care and safety considerations such as testing blood glucose before driving and not driving if it is low or goes low whilst driving.

Table 10.5 Diabetes-related complications that can affect driving ability and safety.

Complication	Effects	Possible consequences whilst driving
1. Short term		
Hypoglycaemia	Cognitive impairment Impaired decision making Vision changes Symptoms may be distracting Hypoglycaemic unawareness. If nocturnal, daytime lethargy Risk of falls Risk of coma	Can be distracting, for example, reaching for glucose to treat the 'hypo' May not be convenient to stop to treat the 'hypo' so mild hypoglycaemia progresses Impaired decision-making, not recognising the need to stop or treat the hypo Symptoms not recognised and episode not treated Inability to control the vehicle due to cognitive and functional changes Slow reaction time and erratic driving Difficulty reading road signs Loss of consciousness
Hyperglycaemia	Increased rate of intercurrent infection and if severe risk of ketoacidosis and hyperosmolar states Tiredness and lethargy Changed cognitive functioning Polyuria and polydipsia Vision changes Lowered mood Compromised self-care Risk of falls	Distractions, for example, need to pass urine Slowed reaction time Inability to control the vehicle Difficulty reading road signs Impaired decision-making Fall asleep whilst driving
2. Long term		
Microvascular disease:		

(a) Retinopathy	Vision impairment
	Visual field defects
	Self-care deficits
	Risk of falls
		Distractions.
		Slow reaction time as a consequence of the difficulty:
		   gauging distance
		   seeing oncoming vehicles
		   reading road signs
		   loss of peripheral vision
		Impact on night driving
		Wearing appropriate glasses for driving and ID necessary
		Effect of investigations such as retinal screening, angiograms and laser therapy

(b) Nephropathy	Changed medicine pharmacokinetics and pharmacodynamics Hypotension especially if on dialysis Increased hypo risk especially on dialysis days Discomfort Muscle weakness Lethargy Depression Risk of falls	Distractions Slow reaction time Inability to control the vehicle Difficulty reading road signs Impaired decision-making
Macrovascular disease:		
(a) Cardiac	Cardiac dysrhythmias Silent MI Disorientation and confusion Tiredness Lightheadedness Depression Risk of falls	Distractions MI during driving Sudden death whilst driving Impaired decision-making Daytime sleepiness

Table 10.5   (Continued)

Complication	Effects	Possible consequences whilst driving
(b) Cerebral	TIAs, stroke Not recognising 'hypos' Cognitive changes Risk of falls	Slow reaction time Impaired decision-making Reduces strength in affected limbs Difficulty operating pedals
(c) Peripheral	Intermittent claudication	More likely to use a car because of difficulty walking
Neuropathy:		
(a) Peripheral	Reduced sensation in feet and unstable gait Pain Risk of falls	Difficulty operating pedals Distraction
(b) Autonomic	Postural hypotension Hypoglycaemic unawareness Gastroparesis Incontinence Unstable blood glucose pattern Depression Silent MI Silent UTI Communication difficulties Lethargy Inadequate self-care Depression Suicide	Distractions Slow reaction time Inability to control the vehicle Erratic driving 'Hypo' not recognised and not treated May not be convenient to stop to treat a 'hypo' Difficulty reading road signs Impaired decision-making Sudden death
Musculoskeletal e.g.	Reduced fine motor skill affecting dexterity	Distractions
Carpal tunnel syndrome	Weakness Pain	Slow reaction time Difficulty controlling the vehicle
Dupuytren's contracture	Falls risk	Difficulty turning the head
Joint stiffness		

Sleep apnoea usually
   occurs as a
   consequence of
   obesity.
	Pain
	Day time lethargy
		Distraction
		Fall asleep whilst driving
		Difficulty fitting seat belts

Frequently more than one factor is present, therefore, the cumulative effect on driving ability needs to be considered. MI = myocardial infarction; 'Hypo' = hypoglycaemia.
Source: Reproduced with permission from Chapter 8 by Dunning in Odell (2009).

- Carrying hypoglycaemia treatment
- Not consuming alcohol or taking illegal drugs before driving
- Maintaining the vehicle in a roadworthy condition
- Considering environmental factors such as the weather when planning a trip
- Stopping regularly on long drives
- Wearing seat belts
- Obeying road rules
- Knowing what to do if an accident occurs

Hypoglycaemia effects on driving

Hypoglycaemia is the most significant side effect of insulin and most OHAs; see Chapter 5. Cox et al. (2000) undertook a simulator study and showed driving performance and decision-making were impaired during mild hypoglycaemia. Unless mild hypoglycaemia is treated, the blood glucose usually continues to fall. However, Marrero and Edelman (2000) suggested the blood glucose range at which driving is impaired and the specific driving actions that are impaired vary amongst individuals. Generally, judgement is impaired during moderate-to-severe hypoglycaemia.

Low blood glucose triggers a counter-regulatory response: at about 3.5–3.7 mmol/l adrenergic symptoms such as sweating and trembling appear. Fine motor skills, coordination, mental processing, concentration, and some memory functions are impaired <3.0 mmol/l (Heller and MacDonald 1996; Sommerfield et al. 2003) and affect driving safety. Sommerfield et al. (2003) suggested decision-making ability is affected when blood glucose <3.0 mmol/l. However, McAuley et al. (2001) found no significant effect on problem-solving ability but significant effects on attentional ability.

The Edinburgh Hypoglycaemia Scale is often used to grade hypoglycaemia severity in research projects and could help define driving risk National Health Service (NHS) 2018):

- Grade 1, mild: the person is aware of hypoglycaemia and responds and self-treats appropriately.
- Grade 2, moderate: the person cannot respond to hypoglycaemia and needs help. Oral treatment corrects the blood glucose level.
- Grade 3, severe: the person is semi- or unconscious and unable to self-treat. Glucagon or IV glucose may be required to correct the blood glucose.

Interpreting driving risk according to these grades suggests the person is at risk of an accident and should stop and treat hypoglycaemia immediately they recognise the symptoms. They are unlikely to manage alone and will be at greater risk if hypoglycaemia is moderate or severe. However, other factors that can affect judgement need to be considered. These include hypoglycaemic awareness, and alcohol and illegal drug use, which cloud judgement and may mask hypoglycaemic symptoms. If present, these factors significantly increase the risk of crash. Testing blood glucose before driving, not driving if the blood glucose is low and not drinking alcohol or using illegal drugs and driving reduce crash risk.

Most people recover from severe hypoglycaemia (Cryer 2007) without permanent effects on driving. The possibility of hypoglycaemia is increased with the trend towards stringent blood glucose targets, but the effects on driving crashes is unknown and the overall rate of severe hypoglycaemia is difficult to establish. Severe hypoglycaemia occurred in 0.4–2.3% of insulin-treated type 2 people per year compared with 0.4% on diet or sulphonylureas, in the UKPDS (1998).

In a later UKPDS substudy, Wright et al. (2006) reported hypoglycaemia grades 1 and 2 occurred in 0.8% in the diet group and 1.7% in the metformin group per year; and grades 2–4 in 0.1 and 0.3%, respectively, compared to 7.9%, and 1.2% in the sulphonylurea group. Hypoglycaemia increased significantly in the basal insulin group; 21.2% and 3.65; and 32%, and in those on basal bolus insulin, 5.5%. Hypoglycaemia frequency and severity in type 2 diabetes is lower than type 1 (Yki-Jarvinen et al. 1999).

The rate of GLM-induced hypoglycaemia may be lower than insulin-induced hypoglycaemia but when it does occur, it is often prolonged and can recur within 24 hours despite treatment, and carries a mortality rate of 4–10% (Shorr et al. 1997; Stahl and Berger 1999). In addition, 5% of survivors have permanent neurological damage (Salas and Caro 2002; Veitch and Clifton-Bligh 2004).

People on insulin have a higher crash risk than the general population but serious hypoglycaemia during driving is rare. Harsch et al. (2002) reported more hypoglycaemia in type 1 diabetes; the accident rate was 0.19–8.26, or 0.02–0.63 per 100 000 km per year per driver, depending on the intensity of the insulin regimen. Harsch et al. also found fewer events in those on basal bolus therapy and insulin pumps: 0.09–0.49 events per 100 000 km or 0.007–0.01 per driver per year. Likewise, Ziemer et al. (2007) found lower hypoglycaemia risk in people on basal bolus insulin regimens and no increase in driving risk.

Lower accident risk with basal bolus regimens might be due to the fact that rapid- or short-acting insulins have a shorter duration of action and smaller frequent doses significantly reduces the insulin depot. Long-acting insulin analogues also have a lower hypoglycaemic profile (see Chapter 5). Temporary driving restrictions usually apply if a person has severe hypoglycaemia. The licence may not be renewed until blood glucose is stabilised and is in a safe range. Loss of their driving licence can cause considerable hardship for the individual involved and sometimes their families and is a threat to independence and access to essential services including health professionals especially in outer suburban and rural areas.

If hypoglycaemic unawareness is a contributing factor, BGATT may help the individual learn to recognise impending hypoglycaemia and improve their safety and confidence. Cox et al. (2000) reported 6.8 crashes in a group of people participating in a BGATT programme per million miles driven versus 29.8 in the control group in a four-year observational study. BGATT did not improve the decision not to drive when blood glucose levels were low. In contrast, Broers et al. (2005) found a significant improvement in deciding not to drive during hypoglycaemia in BGATT participants. They also had a lower crash rate compared to controls: 0.6 versus 0.2 per patient per year. These findings of the BGATT programmes may be a useful addition to driver rehabilitation/safety programmes for people with severe hypoglycaemia.

Strategies to enhance driving safety

Clinicians could adopt a more proactive, holistic education and risk management approach to diabetes and driving safety:

- Conduct regular structured driving assessments as part of care planning, and annual complication screening, as well as during significant health and treatment changes. This would enable declining functional and cognitive ability and the potential effects on driving safety to be identified and remedial strategies implemented. If relevant, geriatric, mental health, and/or driving assessments should be sought. Such an approach would enable a gradual, planned transition to stopping driving to occur and reduce the physical and mental impact on the individual.
- Undertake opportunistic driving assessments instead of only at licence renewal time or when a severe hypoglycaemic event or a driving accident occurs. For example, during an emergency department/hospital presentation, when medicines are changed, and during the annual complication assessment, changes in mental and physical capabilities.
- Assess the individual's level of risk and counsel them and the family, appropriately about how to reduce their risk. Circumstances and the level of risk sometimes change rapidly; thus, forward planning for such contingencies is helpful, especially for older people. This could include developing a proactive driving/transport plan and recognising when to suggest the individual implements their plan. The driving plan could include making plans to cope during temporary incapacity, such as during acute illness, investigative procedures, or surgery, as well as a long-term plan to eventually stop driving.
- Be aware of the general and diabetes-related risk factors that contribute to unsafe driving and ensure they are considered when undertaking education, health assessments, and formulating management plans.
- Know the relevant driving legislation and where/how to access information for themselves and patients. When providing information, it needs to be relevant to the individual and in a format they are likely to use, for example, older people like and refer to written information, whereas Cox et al.'s (2000) simulator studies suggest computer programmes that involve 'playing a game' may be appropriate to younger people.
- Knowing the commonly used classes of medicines that can impair driving skills such as:
  - Anticonvulsants
  - Antihistamines
  - Antipsychotics
  - Benzodiazepines
  - OHA and insulin
  - Muscle relaxants

  - ○ Opioid analgesics
  - ○ Serotonin reuptake inhibitors
  - ○ Tricyclic and tetracyclic antidepressants
  - ○ Sympathomimetics (Drummer 2008)
- Consider driving safety when managing medicines including when undertaking medicines reviews, including home medicine reviews (HMRs) as a key aspect of safe prescribing and quality use of medicines (QUM). Ask about complementary therapy use, particularly herbal medicines and supplements.
- Ensure diabetes and other relevant education programmes encompass driving responsibilities and safety.

Information for people with diabetes to help them drive safely

The following information can be included in patient education programmes and supportive information such as handouts. It could also be used as a framework for assessing driving knowledge:

- Be aware of your responsibilities as a driver. Make sure you comply with legislation such as informing traffic authorities that you have diabetes, especially if you use insulin or glucose-lowering tablets.
- Regularly think about your driving ability, to help you decide your level of risk, and whether a formal driving assessment or attending a driving safety class would be useful. Advanced driving classes can be very helpful at improving driving safety for nondiabetics as well as people with diabetes and adapted for younger and older drivers in some countries. They can reduce the likelihood of an accident or improve the way you manage in high-risk driving situations. Formal driving assessment might be needed, for example, if you have a driving accident, a period of illness or your vision declines.
- Consider your own safety and that of your passengers, and other road users when you drive; for example, test your blood glucose before you drive if you are on insulin or diabetes tablets and do not drive if your blood glucose is low. Always carry glucose with you and wear a medical alert 'bracelet' containing relevant health information.
- Decide whether somebody should accompany you and/or whether you should inform relatives or friends where you are going.
- Discuss the factors likely to affect your driving safety with health professionals and your family on a regular basis, for example, when you have your annual diabetes complication check or winter influenza vaccinations. Make sure you have written advice about what to do when you are sick, have a hypo, need surgery, or an investigation such as an eye test. It may be advisable not to drive in these situations. Knowing beforehand will enable you to make other arrangements.
- Develop a formal driving/transportation plan to ensure you have strategies in place when you can no longer drive safely and ease the transition to not driving.
- Consider factors likely to affect driving safety before you drive. These include your health at the time and other factors such as the weather, distance to cover, road works, and the time of the day or night. Having a mobile phone enables you to call for help but should not be used whilst the vehicle is moving.
- Follow regulations such as wearing a seat belt, not speaking on a mobile phone whilst driving and not consuming alcohol or illegal drugs before or whilst driving. Make sure children and pets cannot move around in the car and place other objects such as groceries in the boot or secure them so they cannot move around and injure passengers if you have to stop suddenly.
- Stop regularly when driving long distances especially if you feel tired or have trouble concentrating. Test your blood glucose, walk around, have a powernap, and a drink and some food.
- If you feel unwell, stop and pull over immediately. Check your blood glucose and treat a hypo if your blood glucose is low. If you have chest discomfort, or feel dizzy or lightheaded call an ambulance.

- Make sure you know what to do if you have an accident.
- Be aware that motorised wheelchairs/vehicles, and farm machinery such as tractors can also cause traffic accidents and result in significant injury. Safe driving advice also applies to these vehicles, particularly farm machinery.

Diabetes and fasting for religious observances

Religious observances such as fasting are important to many people. Muslim and Buddhist rituals include fasting: Ramadan and Buddhist Lent (Vassa), respectively. Some Christians also fast, usually for a shorter time. Fasting can affect blood glucose and put the individual at risk of an adverse event. Exception from fasting for people with diabetes is permitted in many countries, but many people want to observe their religious conventions.

Ramadan is known as partial feasting because people are not permitted food or fluids from sunrise to sunset for a month each year. Alcohol is not permitted during Ramadan (Al Maatouq 2012; Assoug et al. 2015). Vassa is observed for three months in the rainy season. Fasting occurs from noon to midnight followed by a 12-hour period when the fast is broken (Latt and Kaira 2012). Glycaemia may improve, worsen or stay the same during religious fasting periods. People most at risk of adverse effects are older people, those with illnesses, children, and pregnant women (Assoug et al. 2015).

Potential effects of fasting:

- Severe hypoglycaemia in people with type 2 diabetes requiring hospital treatment increases during Ramadan (Chapter 6) (Salti et al. 2004; Assoug et al. 2015) and occurs in ~ 20% of people on sulphonylureas (Al Maatouq 2012). Hypoglycaemia symptoms may go unnoticed (e.g. when meditating during Vassa or praying). Likewise, hypoglycaemia can impair the meditation.
- Symptomatic hyperglycaemia can occur if people stop taking their GLM or reduce the dose inappropriately during fasting. Salti et al. (2004) reported a fivefold increase in hyperglycaemia during Ramadan. Excessive food intake during the nonfasting hours contributes to hyperglycaemia. Hyperglycaemia can cause polyuria, polydipdia, and lethargy, which contribute to dehydration. Ensuring the person sick-day-care plan encompasses fasting could be useful.
- Dehydration and volume depletion may be exacerbated in hot climates due to insensible fluid loss. Dehydration can lead to hyperosmolar states (HHS) orthostatic hypotension that can lead to syncope, falls, and injuries. The risk of postural hypotension is higher in people who have autonomic neuropathy. Older people may also be at increased risk because they may not experience thirst (Chapter 7).
- There is increased risk of cardiovascular events, including associated with hypoglycaemia. Undertaking a hypoglycaemia risk assessment could be useful in counselling individuals and families how to manage diabetes during Ramadan (see Chapter 6):
  ○ Cognitive changes due to hyper- and hypoglycaemia can affect decision-making.
  ○ Overeating can occur after the fasting period.

Education and counselling

Advice needs to be tailored to the individual and the way the manage Ramadan/Vassa and could include:

- Understand the risks associated with fasting.
- Know how to determine the individual's risk level from hypo-and hyperglycaemia (see Chapters 6, 7, and 12).
- Know how to adjust the medicine regimen for periods of fasting and nonfasting.
- Recognize the importance of monitoring blood glucose to determine the blood glucose patterns and using the information to manage the food and medicine regimen.

- Know when to test ketones, especially people with type 1 diabetes.
- Review hypoglycaemia and hyperglycaemia management if necessary and include specific information about when to break the fast for safety reasons. Al Maatouq (2012) recommends breaking the fast if the blood glucose is <3.9 mmol/l early in the fast because the blood glucose is likely to continue to fall, or if it is <3.3 mmol/l during the fast. These levels may be too low for some people at particular risk of hypoglycaemia, such as older people and children. No specific levels were recommended for hyperglycaemia.
- Know when to seek advice.
- Avoid calorie-rich foods during non-fasting periods.

Practice points

- Reflect on how having diabetes and two other concomitant diseases would affect your mental health, work, and social functioning and other aspects of your everyday life.
- What education, care and advice would you expect your healthcare providers to provide?
- How would you manage all the self-care tasks involved including medicines management if various health professionals gave you different information/advice?

References

Abenavoli, L., Capasso, R., Milic, N., and Capasso, F. (2010). Milk thistle in liver diseases: past, present, future. *Phytotherapy Research* 24 (10): 1423–1432.

Abrams, P., Cardozo, L., Fall, M. et al. (2002). The standardisation of terminology of lower tract function: report from the standardisation sub-committee of the international continence society. *Neurourology and Urodynamics* 21: 167–1678.

Aberg, J., Gallant, J., Anderson, J. et al. (2004). Primary care guidelines for the management of persons infected with human immunodeficiency virus: recommendations of the HIV Medicine Association of the Infectious Diseases Society of America. *Clinics of Infectious Diseases* 39: 609–629.

Ahmedzai, S. (2019). Challenges, opportunities and the role of palliative medicine in cancer. Research review www.researchreview.com.au.

Alcohol and Drug Foundation (2019). Medicinal cannabis. https://adf.org.au/drug-facts/medical-cannabis.

Allen, R. (2012). Home sleep studies. *Australian Prescriber* 25: 62–64.

Alimova, T., Liu, B., Fan, Z. et al. (2009). Metformin inhibits breast cancer cell growth, colony formation, and induces cell cycle arrest in vitro. *Cell Cycle* 8 (6): 909–915.

Al Maatouq, M. (2012). Pharmacological approaches to the management of type 2 diabetes in fasting adults during Ramadan. *Diabetes Metabolic Syndrome and Obesity: Targets and Therapy* 20 (25): 109–119.

American Cancer Society (2007). *Cancer Facts and Figures*. Atlanta, GA: American Cancer Society.

American Diabetes Association (ADA) (2018). Standards of Medical Care. https://professional.diabetes.org/content-page/standards-medical-care-diabetes.

American Diabetes Association 15 (2019). Diabetes care in hospital; standards of medical care in diabetes – 2019. *Diabetes Care* 42 (Suppl.10): S173–S181.

America Geriatircs Society (2019). Updated AGS Beers Criteria® for Potentially Inappropriate Medication Use in Older Adults. *Journal of the American Geriatric Society* 67: 674–694. https://doi.org/10.1111/jgs.15767.

American Psychiatric Association (APA) (2013). *Diagnostic and Statistical Manual of Mental Disorders (5) Text Revision (DSM-V)*. Washington DC: APA https://www.psychiatry.org/psychiatrists/practice/dsm/about-dsm.

American Society of Parenteral and Enteral Nutrition (ASPEN) (2017). Parenteral Nutrition Resources. http://www.nutritioncare.org/PNResources/.

Andersen, C., Flyvbjerg, K., and Holmstrup, P. (2007). Periodontitis is associated with aggravation of prediabetes in Zuker rats. *Journal of Periodontology* 78 (3): 559–565.

Arrellano-Valdez, T., Urrutia-Osorio, M., and Soto-Vega, E. (2014). A comprehensive review of urologic complications in patients with diabetes. *Springer Plus* https://doi.org/10.1185/2193-1801-3-549.

Australian Diabetes Society (2011). Diabetes and Driving. https://diabetessociety.com.au/downloads/Driving%20and%20Diabetes%20Booklet.pdf.

Australian Diabetes Society (2012). *Guidelines for Routine Glucose Control in Hospital Australian Diabetes Society, ADS, Canberra*. Australian Diabetes Society https://diabetessociety.com.au/documents/adsguidelinesfor routineglucosecontrolinhospitalfinal2012_000.pdf.

Australian Institute of Health and Welfare (2018). About Smoking. www.aihw.gov.au/reports-statistics/behaviours-risk-factors/smoking/about.

AUSTROADS (2017). Assessing Fitness to Drive. https://austroads.com.au/drivers-and-vehicles/assessing-fitness-to-drive.

Azzoug, S., Mahgoun, S., and Chentil, F. (2015). Diabetes mellitus and Ramadan in elderly patients. *Journal of the Pakistan Medical Association* http://jpma.org.pk/supplement_details.php?article_id=185.

Bainbridge, K. (2013). Diabetes and hearing impairment: an epidemiological perspective. In: *American-Speech-Language-Hearing Association*. American Speech-Language-Hearing Association https://www.asha.org/Articles/Diabetes-and-Hearing-Impairment-An-Epidemiological-Perspective.

Balkau, B., Eschwege, E., Ducimetiere, P. et al. (1991). The high risk of death by alcohol-related diseases in subjects diagnosed as diabetic and impaired glucose tolerant: the Paris prospective study after 15 years follow-up. *Journal of Clinical Epidemiology* **44**: 465–474.

Bloomgarden, Z. (2001). Diabetes and cancer. *Diabetes Care* **24**: 780–781.

Bodén, R., Lundgren, M., Brandt, L. et al. (2012). Antipsychotics during pregnancy: relation to fetal and maternal metabolic effects. *Archives of General Psychiatry* **69** (7): 715–721.

Bover, M., Foulds, J., Steinberg, M. et al. (2008). Waking at night to smoke as a marker for tobacco dependence: patient characteristics and relationship to treatment outcome. *International Journal of Clinical Practice* **62** (2): 182–190.

Braver, E. and Trempel, R. (2004). Are older drivers actually at higher risk of involvement in collisions resulting in deaths or non-fatal injuries among their passengers and other road users? *Injury Prevention* **10**: 27–32.

Breast Cancer Network Australia (2016). Healthy eating and breast cancer. https://www.bcna.org.au/media/2132/bcna-healthy-eating-booklet.pdf.

Broers, S., van Vliet, K., le Cessie, S. et al. (2005). Blood glucose awareness training in Dutch type 1 diabetes patients: one year follow up. *Netherlands Journal of Medicine* **63**: 164–169.

Brown, L. (1991). Clinical aspects of drug abuse in diabetes. *Diabetes Spectrum* **4** (1): 45–47.

Brown, D., McRae, F., and Shaw, K. (2001). Musculoskeletal disease in diabetes. *Practical Diabetes International* **18** (2): 62–64.

Buckner, C., Lafrenie, R., Dénommée, J. et al. (2018). Complementary and alternative medicine use in patients before and after a cancer diagnosis. *Current Oncology* **25** (4): e275–e281. https://doi.org/10.3747/co.25.3884.

Buysschaert, M. and Tomasi, J. (2005). Prospective screening for biopsy proven celiac disease, autoimmunity and malabsorption markers in Belgian subjects with type 1 diabetes. *Diabetic Medicine* **22**: 889–892.

Cancer Council of Australia (2018). Complementary and alternative therapies. https://www.cancer.org.au/about-cancer/treatment/complementary-therapies-and-cancer.html.

Caldwell, S., Oelsner, D., Iezzoni, J. et al. (1999). Cryptogenic cirrhosis: clinical characterisation and risk factors for underlying disease. *Hepatology* **29**: 664–669.

Carramolino-Cuéllar, E., Lauritano, D., Silvestre, F.-J. et al. (2018). Salivary flow and xerostomia in patients with type 2 diabetes. *Journal of Oral Pathology and Medicine* **47**: 526–530. https://doi.org/10.1111/jop.12712.

Carreras-Torres, R., Johansson, M., Gaborieau, V. et al. (2017). The role of obesity, type 2 diabetes, and metabolic factors in pancreatic cancer: A Mendelian randomization study. *Journal of the National Cancer Institute* **109** (9): djx012.

Cavallo, J. (2004). Celiac disease: Sometimes silent, often misleading, always serious. *JDRF (Juvenile Diabetes Research Foundation) Countdown* Summer.

Chen, W. and Center, J. (2015). Absolute fracture risk. What does it mean for your patient? *Endocrinology Today* **4** (5): 3134.

Chitturi, S. and Farrell, G. (2000). Herbal hepatotoxicity: an expanding but poorly defined problem. *Journal of Gastroenterology and Hepatology* **15**: 1093–1099.

Chiu, K., Chu, A., Go, V. et al. (2004). Hypovitaminosis D is associated with insulin resistance and β cell dysfunction. *The American Journal of Clinical Nutrition* **79** (5): 820–825.

Clark, B., Ward, J., and Enoch, B. (1980). Hypoglycaemia in insulin dependent diabetic drivers. *British Medical Journal* **281**: 586.

Clark, D., Stump, T., and Wolinsky, F. (1998). Predictors of onset of and recovery from mobility difficulty among adults aged 51–61 years. *American Journal of Epidemiology* **148** (1): 63–71.

Colin, P., Reunala, T., and Pukkala, E. (1994). Coeliac disease – associated disorders and survival. *Gut* **35**: 1215–1218.

Coughlin, S., Calle, E., Teras, L. et al. (2004). Diabetes mellitus as a predictor of cancer morality in a large cohort of US adults. *American Journal of Epidemiology* **159**: 1160–1167.

Cox, D., Gonder-Frederick, L., Kovatchev, B. et al. (2000). Progressive hypoglycaemia's impact of driving similation performance: occurrence, awareness and correction. *Diabetes Care* **23**: 163–170.

Coyne, K., Margolis, M., Kennedy-Martin, T. et al. (2004). The impact of diabetic retinopathy: perspectives from patient focus groups. *Family Practice* **21**: 447–453.

Cryer, P. (2007). Hypoglycaemia, functional brain failure and brain death. *Journal of Clinical Investigation* **117**: 868–870.

Cystic Fibrosis Trust (2004). *Guidelines for the management of cystic fibrosis-related diabetes*. Bromley, Kent, UK: Cystic Fibrosis Trust.

Department of Health and Human Services (DHHS) (2006). The Health Consequences of Involuntary Exposure to Tobacco Smoke: A Report of the Surgeon General – Executive Summary. Department of Health and Human Services (DHSS, Public Health Service, Center for Disease Control, Center for Chronic Disease Prevention and Health Promotion, Office of Smoking and Health, USA.

Department of Veteran's Affairs USA (2012). https://www.myhealth.va.gov.

De Marco, R., Locatelli, F., Zoppini, G. et al. (1999). Cause-specific mortality in type 2 diabetes: the Verona diabetes study. *Diabetes Care* **22**: 756–761.

Diabetes UK (2018). Hyperglycaemia symptoms. https://www.diabetes.org.uk/guide-to-diabetes/complications/hypos/having-a-hypo.

Diabetes Control and Complication Trial Research Group (DCCT) (1991). Epidemiology of severe hypoglycaemia in the diabetes control and complications trial. *American Journal of Medicine* **90**: 450–459.

Diabetes Control and Complication Trial Research Group (DCCT) (1997). Hypoglycaemia in the diabetes control and complications trial. *Diabetes* **46**: 271–286.

Diabetes Control and Complications Trial Research Group (DCCT) (1993). The effect of intensive treatment of diabetes on the development and progression of long-term complications in insulin dependent diabetes mellitus. *The New England Journal of Medicine* **329** (14): 977–986.

Dibble, S., Luce, J., and Cooper, B. (2007). Acupressure for chemotherapy-induced nausea and vomiting: a randomized clinical trial. *Oncology Nursing Forum* **34**: 813–820.

Ditah, I., Devaki, P., Luma, H.N. et al. (2014). Prevalence, trends, and risk factors for fecal incontinence in United States adults, 2005–2010. *Clinical Gastroenterology and Hepatology* **12** (4): 636–643.

Donaghue, K. and Robinson, P. (2017). Cystic fibrosis and diabetes mellitus. https://uptodat.com/contents/cysticpfibrosis-related-diabetes-mellitus.

Dooley, K., Tang, T., Golub, J. et al. (2009). Impact of diabetes mellitus on treatment outcomes of patients with active tuberculosis. *American Journal of Tropical Medicine and Hygiene* **80**: 634–639.

Drummer, O. (2008). The role of drugs in road safety. *Australian Prescriber* **31** (2): 33–35.

Du, Y. (2018). Gastrointestinal symptoms in diabetes, prevalence, assessment, pathogenesis and management. *Diabetes Care* **41**: 627–637.

Duggan, J. (2004). Coeliac disease: the great imitator. *eMedical Journal of Australia* **180** (10): 524–526. http://www.mja.com.au/public/issues/180_10_170504/dug10818_fm.html (accessed November 2007).

Dunning, T. (1996). Corticosteroids medications and diabetes mellitus. *Practical Diabetes International* **13**: 186–188.

Dunning, T. (2009). Periodontal disease 0 the overlooked diabetes complication. *Nephrology Nursing Journal* **36**: 171–181.

Dunning, T., Savage, S., Duggan, N., and Martin, P. (2011). Guidelines for Managing Diabetes at the End of Life. Centre for Nursing and Allied Health Research, Deakin University and Barwon Health http://clearinghouse.adma.org.au/browse-resources/guideline/guidelines-for-managing-diabetes-at-the-end-of-life/details.html.

Dunning, T., Savage, S., Duggan, N., and Martin, P. (2012). Diabetes and end of life: ethical and methodological issues in gathering evidence to guide care. *Scandinavian Journal of Caring Sciences* https://doi.org/10.1111/j.1471-6712.2012.01016.x.

Dunning, T., Martin, P., Orellana, L., and Orford, N. (2018). *Planning Palliative and end of life care: a suite of Information for older people with diabetes, families and health professionals*. Centre for Quality and Patient Safety Research. Geelong, Victoria: Deakin University Barwon Health Partnership.

Dyce, P. and Wallymahmed, M. (2012). Evaluating screening for long-term complications of cystic fibrosis-related diabetes. *Journal of Diabetes Nursing* **16** (6): 240–246.

Eadington, D. and Frier, B. (1989). Type 1 diabetes driving experience: an eight-year cohort study. *Diabetic Medicine* **6**: 137–141.

Ebbesen, M.H., Hannestad, Y.S., Midthjell, K., and Hunskaar, S. (2009). Diabetes-related risk factors did not explain the increased risk for urinary incontinence among women with diabetes. The Norwegian HUNT/EPINCONT study. *BMC Urology* **9** (1): 11. http://doi.org/10.1186/1471-2490-9-11.

Ebeling, P. and Ferrari, S. (2019). Long-term osteoporosis management requires lmh term thinking. Break-out session. International Osteoporosis Foundation regional 7th Asia-Pacific Osteoporosis Conference, Sydney (January 2019).

Ejerblad, E., Fored, C., Lindblad, P. et al. (2004). Association between smoking and chronic renal failure in a nationwide population-based case-control study. *Journal of the American Society of Nephrology* **15** (18): 2178–2185.

El-Serag, H. and Everhart, J. (2002). Diabetes increases the risky of acute liver failure. *Gastroenterology* **122**: 1822–1828.

Eremin, O. and Walker, M. (2009). Immuno-modulatory effects of relaxation training and guided imagery in women with locally advanced breast cancer undergoing multimodality therapy: a randomised controlled trial. *Breast* **18** (1): 17–25.

Eriksson, J.W., Lundkvist, P., Jansson, P.A. et al. (2018). Effects of dapagliflozin and n-3 carboxylic acids on non-alcoholic fatty liver disease in people with type 2 diabetes: a double-blind randomised placebo-controlled study. *Diabetologia* **61** (9): 1923–1934.

Evans, L. (2004). Overview of traffic fatalities. In: *Traffic Safety* (ed. L. Evans), 57–58. Bloomfield Hills, MI: Science Serving Society.

Fabris, P., Floreani, A., Tositti, G. et al. (2003). Type 1 diabetes mellitus in patients with chronic hepatitis C before and after interferon therapy. *Alimentary Pharmacology Therapy* **18**: 549–558.

Falba, T. (2005). Health events and the smoking cessation of middle-aged Americans. *Journal of Behavioural Medicine* **28**: 21–33.

Farrell, R. and Kelly, C. (2002). Celiac sprue. *New England Journal of Medicine* **346**: 180–188.

Fasano, A., Berti, I., and Gerarduzzi, T. (2003). Prevalence of celiac disease in at-risk and not-at-risk groups in the United States. *Archives of Internal Medicine* **163**: 286–292.

Felde, G., Ebbesen, M.H., and Hunskaar, S. (2017). Anxiety and depression associated with urinary incontinence. A 10-year follow-up study from the Norwegian HUNT study (EPINCONT). *Neurourology and Urodynamics* **36**: 322–328.

Ferrari, S., Napoli, N., and Schwartz, A. (2018). Diabetes and Fracture Risk. *Primer on the Metabolic Bone Diseases and Disorders of Mineral Metabolism*: 487–491.

Foulds, J., Gandhi, K., and Steinberg, M. (2006). Factors associated with quitting smoking at a tobacco dependence treatment clinic. *American Journal of Health Behaviour* **30**: 400–412.

Frier, B., Mathews, D., Steel, J., and Duncan, L. (1980). Driving and insulin-dependent diabetes. *Lancet* **8180**: 1232–1234.

Fu, S., Partin, M., and Snyder, A. (2006). Promoting repeat tobacco dependence treatment: are relapsed smokers interested? *American Journal of Managed Care* **12**: 235–243.

Fuchs, M. (2012). Non-alcoholic fatty liver disease: the bile acid-activated Farnesoid X receptor as an emerging treatment target. *Journal of Lipids* https://doi.org/10.1155/2012/934396.

Garrett, C.J., Choudhary, P., Amiel, S.A. et al. (2019). Recurrent diabetic diabetic ketoacidosis and a brief history of brittle diabetes research: contemporary and past evidence in diabetic diabetic ketoacidosis research including mortality, mental health and prevention. *Diabetic Medicine* Online first: https://doi.org/10.1111/dme.14109.

George, L. (1993). Sociological-perspectives on life transitions. *Annual Review of Sociology* **19**: 353–373.

Giovannuci, E., Harlan, D., Archer, M. et al. (2010). Diabetes and cancer: a consensus report. *Diabetes Care* **33** (7): 1674–1685.

Glick, D. (2003). *Legal and illegal drugs: what every person with diabetes should know before they party*. Diabetes and Health http://www.diabeteshealth.com/read/2003/11/0i/3163.html (accessed August 2008).

Gregg, E., Pereira, M., and Caspersen, C. (2000). Physical activity, falls, and fractures among older adults: a review of the epidemiologic evidence. *Journal of the American Geriatrics Society* **48**: 883–893.

Green, P. and Jabri, B. (2003). Coeliac disease. *Lancet* **362**: 383–391.

Gundling, F., Seidl, H., Haler, B. et al. (2013). Clinical manifestations and treatment options in patients with cirrhosis and diabetes mellitus. *Digestion* **87** (2): 75–84.

Gromiovits, K. (2018). An introduction to decreasing urologic complications related to uncontrolled diabetes. *Urologic Nursing* **38** (6): 289–302.

Guerrier, H., Manivannan, P., and Nair, N. (1999). The role of working memory, field dependence, visual search, and reaction time in left turn performance of older female drivers. *Applied Ergonomics* **30**: 109–119.

Hand, R., Murphy, W., Field, L. et al. (2016). Validation of the academy/ASPN malnutrition clinical characteristics. *Journal of Academic Nutrition Diet* **116**: 856–864.

Harsch, I., Stocker, S., Radespiel-Troger, M. et al. (2002). Traffic hypoglycaemias and accidents in patients with diabetes mellitus treated with different antidiabetic regimens. *Journal of Internal Medicine* **252**: 352–360.

Heller, S. and Macdonald, I. (1996). The measurement of cognitive function during acute hypoglycaemia: experimental limitations and their effect on study of hypoglycaemic unawareness. *Diabetic Medicine* **13**: 607–615.

Hillson, R. (2018). Diarrhoea in diabetes. *Practical Diabetes* **36** (6): 195–196.

Horneber, M., Bueschel, G., Dennert, G. et al. (2012). How many cancer patients use complementary and alternative medicine: a systematic review and metaanalysis. *Integrative Cancer Therapies* **11** (3): 187–203.

Horikawa, C., Kodama, S., Tanaka, S. et al. (2012). Diabetes and risk of hearing impairment in adults: a meta-analysis. *Journal of Clinical Endocrinology and Metabolism* 2012-2119v1 98/1/51.

Howard, A., Floris-Moore, A., Amsten, J. et al. (2005). Disorders of glucose metabolism in HIV infected women. *Clinics of Infectious Diseases* **40**: 1492–1499.

ISCD Writing Group (2004). Diagnosis of osteoporosis in men, premenopausal women and children. *Journal of Clinical Densitometry* 7: 17–26.

Jackson, R. and Bowman, R. (1995). Corticosteroids. *Medical Journal of Australia* 162: 663–665.

Jeon, C. and Murray, M. (2008). Diabetes mellitus increases the risk of active tuberculosis: a systematic review of 13 observational studies. *PLoS Medicine* 5 (8): e181. https://doi.org/10.1371/journal.pmed.00501.

Jereczek-Fossa, B.A., Marsiglia, H.R., and Orecchia, R. (2002). Radiotherapy-related fatigue. *Critical reviews in oncology/hematology* 41 (3): 317–325.

Juvenile Diabetes Research Foundation (JDRF) (2008). Type 1 diabetes and celiac disease. http://www.jdrf.org.au/living_w_diabetes/newsitem.asp?newsid=166 (accessed January 2008).

Kapur, A., Harries, A.D., Lönnroth, K. et al. (2009). Diabetes and tuberculosis–Old associates posing a renewed public health challenge. *Eureopean Endocrinology* 5: 10–12.

Kao, G. and Devine, P. (2000). Use of complementary health practices by prostate carcinoma patients undergoing radiotherapy. *Cancer* 88 (3): 615–619.

Karoli, R. et al. (2014). A study of bladder dysfunction in women with type 2 diabetes. *Indian Endocrinology and Metabolism* 18: 552–557.

Khan, F., Naab, T., and Cook-Sampson, E. (2016). Diabetic mastopathy, a rare fibrioinflammatory breast disease. *American Journal of Clinical Pathology* 146 (suppl_1): 264. https://doi.org/10.1093/ajcp/aqw159.035.

Khazaii, R. and Kamareh, S. (2018). Relationship between diabetes and periodontal disease: a review literature. *Annals of dental Specialty* 6 (1): 57–60.

Kim, P. (2011). Increased prevalence of albuminuria in HIV-infected adults with diabetes. *PLoS One* 6 (9): e24610. https://doi.org/10.1037/journal.pone.0024610.

King, M. (1996–2012). themedicalchemistrypage.org.LLC/info@themedicalchemistrypage.org (accessed November 2012).

Koo, R. and Spencer, M. (2018). Continence promotion and successful aging: the role of the multidisciplinary continence clinic. *Geriatrics* 3: 91. https://doi.org/10.3390/geriatrics3040091.

Koepsell, T., Wolf, E., McCloskey, L. et al. (1994). Medical conditions and motor vehicle collision injuries in older adults. *Journal of American Geriatrics Society* 42 (7): 695–700.

Korantzopoulos, P., Liu, T., Papaioannides, D. et al. (2008). Atrial fibrillation and marijuana smoking. *International Journal of Clinical Practice* 62 (2): 308–313.

Krinsley, J. (2008). Glycaemic variability: a strong predictor of mortality in critically ill patients. *Critical Care Medicine* 36 (11): 3008–3303.

Kroon, L. (2007). Drug interactions with smoking. *American Journal of Health-System Pharmacy* 64 (18): 1917–1921.

Lancaster, T. and Stead, L. (2004). Physician advice for smoking cessation. *Cochrane Database of Systematic Reviews, Issue* 4: CD000165.

Laberge-Nadeau, C., Dionne, G., and Ekoe, M. (2000). Impact of diabetes on crash risks of truck-permit holders and commercial drivers. *Diabetes Care* 23 (5): 612–617.

Lang, I., Rice, N., Wallace, R. et al. (2007). Smoking cessation and transition into retirement: analysis from the English longitudinal study. *Age and Aging* 36 (6): 638–643.

Lamey, P., Darwazeh, A., and Frier, B. (1992). Oral disorders associated with diabetes mellitus. *Diabetic Medicine* 9 (5): 410–416.

Larsson, S. (2005). Diabetes mellitus and risk of colorectal cancer: a metanalysis. *Journal of the National Cancer Institute* 97: 1675–1687.

Latt, T. and Kaira, S. (2012). Managing diabetes during fasting – A focus on Buddhist lent. *Diabetes Voice* 57 (4): 42–45.

Lee, N. (2008). Alcohol intervention: what works? *Australian Family Physician* 37 (1/2): 16–19.

Lee, H., Lee, A., Cameron, D., and Li-Tsang, C. (2003). Using a driving simulator to identify older drivers at inflated risk of motor vehicle crashes. *Journal of Safety Research* 34 (4): 453–459.

Lee, R., Sloan, R., Pieper, C. et al. (2017). Clinical fractures among older men with diabetes are mediated by diabetes complications. *Journal of Clinical Endocrinology and Metabolism* 103 (1): 281–287.

Lewis, J., Ferrara, A., Peng, T. et al. (2011). Risk of bladder cancer among diabeteic patients treated with pioglitazone. *Diabetes Care* 34: 916–922.

Li, G. (2019). Interaction between frailty, fractures provides insight for 'diabetes bone paradox'. *Diabetes Care* https://doi.org/10.2337/dc16-1965.

Liu, A., Galoosian, A., Kaswala, D. et al. (2018). Nonalcoholic Fatty Liver Disease: Epidemiology, Liver Transplantation Trends and Outcomes, and Risk of Recurrent Disease in the Graft. *Journal of Clinical and Translational Hepatology* 6 (4): 420–424. https://doi.org/10.14218/JCTH.2018.00010.

Lipman, T. (2007). The role of herbs and probiotics in GI wellness for older adults. *Geriatrics and Aging* 10 (3): 182–191.

Lipscombe, L., Hux, J., and Booth, G. (2005). Reduced screening mammography among women with chronic medical diseases. *Archives of Internal Medicine* 165: 2090–2095.

MacLeod, K. (1999). Diabetes and driving: toward equitable evidence-based decision-making. *Diabetes Medicine* 16: 282–290.

Mahishale, V., Avuthu, S., Patil, B. et al. (2017). Effect of poor glycaemic control in newly diagnosed patients with smear positive pulmonary tuberculosis an type 2 diabetes mellitus. *Iranian Journal Medical Sciences* **42** (2): 144–151.

Mahmud, F.H., Elbarbary, N.S., Fröhlich-Reiterer, E. et al. (2018). ISPAD Clinical Practice Consensus Guidelines 2018: Other complications and associated conditions in children and adolescents with type 1 diabetes. *Pediatric Diabetes* **19**: 275–286.

Mangubat, N., Lutfy, K., Lee, M. et al. (2019). Effect of nicotine in mice. *The Journal of Endocrinology*: 317–326. https://doi.org/10.1530/JOE=11-1350.

Marchesini, G., Bugianesi, E., Forlani, G. et al. (2003). Nonalcoholic fatty liver, steatohepatitis and the metabolic syndrome. *Hepatology* **37**: 917–923.

Margolis, K., Kerani, R., McGovern, T. et al. (2002). Study of osteoporotic fractures research, risk factors for motor vehicle crashes in older women. *Journals of Gerontology, Series A. Biological Sciences and Medical Sciences* **57**: M186–M191.

Marrero, D. and Edelman, S. (2000). Hypoglycaemia and driving performance: a flashing yellow light? *Diabetes Care* **23** (2): 146–147.

Marsh, K. (2011). Coeliac disease and type I diabetes. *The Australian Diabetes Educator* **14** (3): 18–21.

Martinez, E., Conget, I., Lozano, L. et al. (1999). Reversion of metabolic abnormalities after switching from HIV-1 protease inhibitors to nevirapine. *AIDS* **13**: 805–810.

Mayo Clinic (2018a). Smoking and diabetes risk. https://www.mayoclinic.org/diseases-conditions/…2-diabetes/…/diabetes/faq-20058540.

Mayo Clinic (2018b). Alternative cancer treatments: 10 options to consider. https://www.mayoclinic.org/diseases-conditions/cancer/in-depth/cancer-treatment/art-20047246.

McAuley, K.A., Williams, S.M., Mann, J.I. et al. (2001). Diagnosing insulin resistance in the general population. *Diabetes Care* **24** (3): 460–464.

McClave, S., Snider, H., and Spain, D. (1999). Use of residual volume as a marker for enteral feeding intolerance: prospective blinded comparison with physical examination and radiographic findings. *Journal of Parenteral and Enteral Nutrition* **16**: 64s–70s.

McDermott, R. (2012). Sleep disturbance as an independent risk factor for diabetes. *Diabetes Management Journal* **39**: 4–5.

McGwin, G., Sims, R., Pulley, L., and Roseman, J. (1999). Diabetes and automobile crashes in the elderly: a population-based case control study. *Diabetes Care* **22**: 220–227.

McGwin, G., Sims, R., Pulley, L., and Roseman, M. (2000). Relations among chronic medical conditions, medications, and automobile crashes in the elderly. *American Journal of Epidemiology* **152** (5): 424–431.

Mendler, M.H., Turlin, B., Moirrand, R. et al. (1999). Insulin resistance-associated iron overload. *Gastroenterology* **117**: 1155–1163.

Meneilly, S., Cheung, E., Tessier, D. et al. (1993). The effect of improved glycemic control on cognitive functions in the elderly patient with diabetes. *Journal of Gerontology* **48** (4): M117–M121.

Mercola.com (2011). Drug used to help people stop smoking may cause suicide. http://articles.mercola.com/sites/articles/archive2011/06/13/drug-used-to-help-people (accessed December 2012).

Middleton, P., Wagenaar, M., Matson, A. et al. (2014). Australian standards of care for cystic fibrosis-related diabetes. *Respirology* 2014 **19**: 185.

Middleton, M., Nazarenko, G., Nivison-Smith, I., and Smerdley, P. (2001). Prevalence of malnutrition and 12-month incidence of mortality in two Sydney teaching hospitals. *Medical Journal of Australia* **31**: 455–461.

Mitchell, D. (2008). Pushing the pin on smoking. *Journal of Complementary Medicine* **7** (2): 55–63.

Mohn, A., Cerruto, M., Lafusco, D. et al. (2001). Coeliac disease in children and adolescents with type I diabetes: importance of hyperglycaemia. *Journal of Paediatric Gastroenterology and Nutrition* **32**: 37–40.

Moran, A., Hardin, D., Rodman, D. et al. (1999). Diagnosis, screening and management of cystic fibrosis related diabetes mellitus: a consensus conference report. *Diabetes Research and Clinical Practice* **45**: 61–73.

Moran, A., Becker, D., and Castella, S. (2010). Epidemiology, pathophysiology and prognostic implications of cystic fibrosis-related diabetes. *Diabetes Care* **3**: 2677–2685.

Moran, A., Pillay, K., Becker, D. et al. (2014). ISPAD clinical practice consensus guidelines. Management of cystic fibrosis-related diabetes in children and adolescents. *Pediatric Diabetes* **15** (Suppl 20): 65.

Moussouttas, M. (2004). Cannabis use and cerebrovascular disease. *The Neurologist* **10**: 47–53.

Naqvi, N., Rudrauf, D., Damasio, H., and Bechara, A. (2007). Damage to the insula disrupts addiction to cigarette smoking. *Science* **315** (5811): 531–534.

National Cancer Institute (2017). Forgoing conventional cancer treatment for alternative medicine. https://www.cancer.gov/news-events/cancer…/alternative-medicine-cancer-survival.

National Health and Medical Research Council (NHMRC) (2007). Draft Australian Drinking Guidelines for Low Risk Drinking. www.nhmrc.gov.au/consult (accessed November 2007).

National Health Medical Research Council (NHMRC) (2013). *Dietary Guidelines for Older Australians*. Canberra: Commonwealth of Australia https://www.nhmrc.gov.au/about-us/publications/australian-dietary-guidelines.

National Institute of Health (2017). Brittle diabetes. https://rarediseases.info.nih.gov/diseases/11900/brittle-diabetes.

National Health Service (NHS) (2018). *The Hospital Management of Hypoglycaemia in Adults with Diabetes Mellitus*, 3e, 11. Edinburgh Hypoglycaemia Scale: Joint British Diabetes Societies on Inpatient Care https://www.diabetes.org.uk/professionals/position-statements-reports/specialist-care-for-children-and-adults-and-complications/the-hospital-management-of-hypoglycaemia-in-adults-with-diabetes-mellitus (accessed September 2019).

National Native Addictions Partnership Foundation (2006). Keeping the sacred in tobacco: a toolkit for tobacco cessation. http://www.nnapf.org/tobacco-sacred (accessed November 2012).

Oberbaum, M., Yaniv, I., and Beg, G. (2001). Treating chemotherapy-induced stomatitis with Traumeel. *Cancer* **92** (3): 684–690.

O'Brien, P. and Oyebode, F. (2003). Psychotropic medication and the heart. *Advances in Psychiatric Treatment* **9**: 414–423. https://doi.org/10.1192/apt.9.6.414.

O'Riordan, S., Robinson, P., Donaghue, K., and Moran, A. (2009). Management of cystic fibrosis-related diabetes in children and adolescents. ISPAD clinic practice compendium. *Paediatric Diabetes* **10** (Suppl 12): 43.

Orisatoki, R. (2013). The public health implications of the use and misuse of tobacco among aboriginals in Canada. *Clinical Journal of Health Science* **5** (1): 28–34.

Osiecki, H. (2006). *The Physician's Handbook of Clinical Nutrition*. Eagle Farm, Australia: Bio Concepts Publishing.

Ostbye, T. and Taylor, D. (2004). The effect of smoking on years of healthy life (YHL) lost among middle-aged and older Americans. *Health Services Research* **39**: 531–532.

Ostaszkiewicz, J., Tomlinson, E., and Hutchinson, A. (2018). 'Dignity': a central construct in nursing home staff understandings of quality continence care. *Journal of Clinical Nursing* **27**: 2425–2437. https://doi.org/10.1111/jocn.14293.

Owen, N., Wakefield, M., Roberts, L., and Esterman, A. (1992). Stages of readiness to quit smoking; population prevalence and correlates. *Health Psychology* **11**: 413–417.

Oyer, D., Shah, A., and Bettenhausen, S. (2006). How to manage steroid diabetes in the patient with cancer. *Supportive Oncology* **4** (9): 479–483.

Palliative Care Outcomes Collaboration (PCOC)—CareSearch (2008). www.caresearch.com.au/caresearch/tabid/99/Default.aspx (accessed February 2013).

Pasco, J., Seeman, E., Henry, M. et al. (2006). The population burden of fractures originates in women with osteopenia, not osteoporosis. *Osteoporosis International* **17**: 1404–1409.

Penckofer, S., Ferrans, C., Velsor-Fredrich, B., and Savoy, S. (2007). The psychological impact of living with diabetes: Women's day-to-day experiences. *The Diabetes Educator* **33** (4): 680–690.

Psarakis, H. (2006). Clinical challenges in caring for patients with diabetes and cancer. *Diabetes Spectrum* **19**: 157–162.

Quinn, K., Hudson, P., and Dunning, T. (2006). Diabetes management in patients receiving palliative care. *Journal of Pain and Symptom Management* **32** (3): 275–286.

Rathgaber, H., Sullivan, C., and McCabe, K. (1992). Diabetes mellitus induced by megestrol acetate in patients with AIDS and cachexia. *Annals of Internal Medicine* **116**: 53–54.

Rogers, M., Pawlak, J., Law, S. et al. (2017). Embracing change in dental practice to deliver better health outcomes: a type 3 diabetes screening in oral health pilot program. *Dentistry* **7**: 454. https://doi.org/10.4172/2161-1122.

Romas, E. (2008). Corticosteroid-induced osteoporosis and fractures. *Australian Prescriber* **21** (2): 45–49.

Raju, K. and Venkataramappa, M. (2018). Primary hemochromatosis presenting as type 2 diabetes mellitus: a case report with review of literature. *International Journal of Applied and Basic Medical Research* **8** (1): 57–60.

Sagberg, F. (2006). Driver health and crash involvement: a case control study. *Accident Analysis and Prevention* **38** (1): 28–34.

Salas, M. and Caro, J. (2002). Are hypoglycaemia and other adverse effects similar among sulphonylureas? *Adverse Drug Reactions Toxicology Review* **21**: 205–217.

Salti, I., Benard, E., and Detournay, B. (2004). EPIDIAR study. A population-based study of diabetes and its characteristics during the fasting month of Ramadan in 13 countries: results of the epidemiology of diabetes and Ramadan 1422/2001 study. *Diabetes Care* **27**: 2306–2311.

Salvatore, C., Rademakers, K., DeLancey, J. et al. (2017). Pathophysiology of urinary incontinence, faecal incontinence and pelvic organ prolapse. In: *Incontinence*, 6e (eds. P. Abrams, L. Cardozo, A. Wagg and A. Wein), 361–496. Anheim, The Netherlands: ICS-ICUD.

Sarma, A.V., Brown, J., Nyberg, L. et al. (2009). Urinary incontinence among women with type 1 diabetes – how common is it? *The Journal of Urology* **181** (3): 1224–1230.

Saunders, J., Aasland, O., and Babor, T. (1993). Development of Alcohol Use Disorders Identification Test (AUDIT). WHO collaborative project on early detection of persons with harmful alcohol consumption. Part 2. *Addiction* **88**: 791–804.

Savage, S., Dunning, T., Duggan, N., and Martin, P. (2012). The experiences and care preferences of people with diabetes at the end of life. *Journal of Hospice and Palliative Nursing* **14**: 293–323.

Scalea, T., Bochicchio, G., and Bochicchio, K. (2007). Tight glycaemic control in critically injured trauma patients. *Annals of Surgery* **246**: 605–610.

Scheen, A. (2018). Effect of sodium glucose cotransporter type 2 inhibitors on liver fat in patients with type 2 diabetes: hepatic beyond cardiovascular and renal protection? *Annals of Translational Medicine* **6** (Suppl 1): S68. https://doi.org/10.21037/atm.2018.10.39.

Shand, F., Gates, J., Fawcett, J., and Mattick, R. (2003). *Guidelines for the Treatment of Alcohol Problems*. Sydney: National Drug and Alcohol Research Center.

Shapiro, K. (2007). What is the role of rosiglitazone in steroid-induced diabetes? *Medscape* (March 6) http://www. medscape.com/viewarticle/552606 (accessed October 2012).

Shaw, J., Punjabi, M., Wilding, J. et al. (2008). Sleep-disordered breathing and type 2 diabetes a report from the international diabetes federation taskforce on epidemiology and prevention. *Diabetes Research and Clinical Practice* **81**: 2–12.

Sherlock, S. (1981). *Diseases of the Liver and Biliary System*. Oxford: Blackwell Science.

Shorr, R., Ray, W., Daugherty, J., and Griffin, M. (1997). Incidence and risk factors for serious hypoglycaemia in older persons using insulin or sulphonylureas. *Archives of Internal Medicine* **157**: 1681–1685.

SIGN (Scottish Intercollegiate Guidelines Network) (2010). *A National Clinical Guideline*. Edinburgh: SIGN.

Sjoberg, K., Eriksson, K., and Bredberg, A. (1998). Screening for celiac disease in adult insulin-dependent diabetes mellitus. *Journal of Internal Medicine* **243**: 133–140.

Smith, L., Burnet, S. and McNeil, J. (2002) Musculoskeletal Manifestations of Diabetes Mellitus. www.bjsm.bmj (accessed March 2008).

Spinella, M. (2005). *Concise Handbook of Psychoactive Herbs*. Oxford: Haworth Herbal Press.

Spollett, G. (2006). Hyperglycaemia in HIV/AIDS. http://spectrum.diabetesjournals.org/content /18/3/163 (accessed October 2012).

Sommerfield, A., Deary, I., McAuley, V., and Frier, B. (2003). Short-term delayed, and working memory are impaired during hypoglycaemia in individuals with type 1 diabetes. *Diabetes Care* **26**: 390–396.

Southerland, J., Taylor, G., Moss, K. et al. (2006). Commonality in chronic inflammatory diseases: periodontitis, diabetes, and coronary artery disease. *Periodontology* **40**: 130–143.

Stahl, M. and Berger, W. (1999). High incidence of severe hypoglycaemia leading to hospital admission in type 2 diabetic patients treated with long-acting sulphonylureas versus short-acting sulphonylureas. *Diabetic Medicine* **16**: 586–590.

Steel, J., Frier, B., Young, R., and Duncan, L. (1981). Driving and insulin dependent diabetics. *Lancet* **2** (8242): 354–356.

Stratton, I., Kohner, E., Aldington, S. et al. (2001). Risk factors for incidence and progression of retinopathy in type 2 diabetes over 6 years from diagnosis. *Diabetologia* **44** (2): 156–163.

Stuck, A., Walthert, J., Nikolaus, T. et al. (1999). Risk factors for functional status decline in community-living elderly people: a systematic review. *Social Science and Medicine* **48**: 445–469.

Sullivan, T. and Ben Amor, V. (2012). The co-management of tuberculosis and diabetes: challenges and opportunities in the developing world. *PLoS Medicine* **9** (7): e10011269. https://doi.org/10.1371/journal. pmed.1001260.

Suman, S., Williams, E., and Thomas, P. (2003). Is the risk of adult celiac disease causally related to cigarette exposure? *European Journal of Gastroenterology and Hepatology* **15**: 995–1000.

Sumida, Y. and Yoneda, M. (2018). Current and future pharmacological therapies for NAFLD/NASH. *Journal of Gastroenterology* **53**: 362–376.

Third International Conference on Smokeless Tobacco (2002). Smokeless tobacco fact sheets. Stockholm (22–25 September).

Thomas, B. (2001). *A Manual of Dietetic Practice*. Oxford: Blackwell Science.

Tolman, K., Fonseca, V., Dalpiaz, A., and Tan, M. (2007). Spectrum of liver disease in type 2 diabetes and management of patients with diabetes and liver diseases. *Diabetes Care* **30**: 734–743.

Tonstad, S., Tonnesesn, P., and Hajek, P. (2006). Effect of maintenance therapy with varenicine. *Journal of the American Medical Association* **296**: 64–71.

Torrijos, R. and Glantz, S. (2006). The US public health service treating tobacco use and dependence clinical practice guidelines as a legal standard of care. *BMC Journal of Tobacco Control* **15** (6): PMC2563672.

Travier, N., Jeffreys, M., Brewer, N. et al. (2007). Association between glycosylated hemoglobin and cancer risk: a New Zealand linkage study. *Annals of Oncology* **18** (8): 1414–1419.

Tuccori, M., Filio, K., Yin, H. et al. (2016). Poiglitazone use and risk of bladder cancer: a population based cohort study. *British Medical Journal* **352**: 11541. https://doi.org/10.101136/bmj.11541.

UK Government (2016). Assessing fitness to drive: a guide for medical professionals - GOV.UK www.gov.uk › ... › Driving and medical conditions.

UKPDS (United Kingdom Prospective Diabetes Study) (1998). Intensive blood glucose control with sulphonylureas or insulin compared with conventional treatment and risk of complications in patients with type 2 diabetes (UKPDS 33). *Lancet* **352**: 837–853.

Umpierrez, G. (2009). Basal versus sliding scale regular insulin in hospitalized patients with hyperglycaemia during enteral nutrition therapy. *Diabetes Care* **32**: 751–753.

US Department of Transportation Federal Highway Safety Information (2013). http://safety.fhwa.dot.gov.older_ users (accessed March 2013).

US Organ Procurement and Transplantation Network and Scientific Registry of Transplant Recipients (2004). Annual Report. http://www.optn.org/AR2005/904a_rec-dgn_li.htm (accessed January 2007).

Van den Beuken, H., van Everdingen, M. et al. (2016). Update on prevalence of pain in patients with cancer; systematic review and metanalysis. *Journal of Pain and Symptom Management* **51**: 1070–1090.

van Raalte, D., Ouwens, D., and Diamant, M. (2009). Novel insights into glucocorticoid-mediateddiabetogenic effects: towards expansionof therapeutic options? *European Journal of Clinical Investigation* **39**: 81–93.

Vantyghem, M. and Press, M. (2006). Management strategies for brittle diabetes. *Annals of Endocrinology* **67** (4): 287–296.

Vavanikunnel, J., Charlier, S., Becker, C. et al. (2019). Association between glycaemic control and risk of fracture in diabetic patients: a nested case-control study. *The Journal of Clinical Endocrinology and Metabolism* https://doi.org/10.1210/jc.2018-01879.

Veitch, P. and Clifton-Bligh, R. (2004). Octreotide treatment for sulfonylurea- induced hypoglycaemia. *Medical Journal of Australia* **180** (10): 540–541.

Verlato, G., Zoppini, G., Bonora, E., and Muggeo, M. (2003). Mortality from site specific malignancies in type 2 diabetes patients from Verona. *Diabetes Care* **26**: 1047–1051.

Viney, K. (2017). Diabetes and tuberculosis: what we know, why we care and what can be done. *Australian Diabetes Educator* **20** (2): 39–44.

Wagg, A.S., (Chair), Kung Chen, L. et al. (2017). Incontinence in frail older persons. In: *Incontinence*, 6e (eds. P. Abrams, L. Cardozo, A. Wagg and A. Wein), 1309–1442. Anheim, The Netherlands: ICS-ICUD.

Watkins, S., Koob, G., and Markou, A. (2000). Neural mechanisms underlying nicotine addiction: acute positive reinforcement and withdrawal. *Nicotine and Tobacco Research* **2** (1): 19–37.

WebMD (2013). Hearing Loss. http://www.wedmed.com/a-to-z-guides/hearing-loss-causes-symptoms-treatment (accessed January 2013).

Weiser, M., Zarka, S., Webeloff, N. et al. (2010). Cognitive test scores in male adolescent cigarette smokers compared to non-smokers: a population-based study. *Addiction* **105** (2): 358–363.

Wessells, H., Braffett, B., Holt, S. et al. (2018). The DCCT edict study. *Diabetes Care* https://doi.org/10.2337/dc18-0255.

Wideroff, L., Gridley, G., Mellemkjaer, L. et al. (1997). Cancer incidence in a population-based cohort of patients hospitalised with diabetes mellitus in Denmark. *Journal of the National Cancer Institute* **89** (18): 1360–1365.

Wijk, H., Corazzini, K., Lindstrom, I. et al. (2018). Person centred incontinence care in residential care facilities for older adults with cognitive decline. *Journal of Gerontological Nursing* **44** (11): 10–19.

Wilkinson, J. (2008). "Good gargling": Evaluation of the use of an essential oil mouthwash in the management of radiation-induced mucositis of the oropharyngeal area. In: *Proceedings of the 3rd International Congress on Complementary Medicine*, 26. Sydney, March 2008.

Willi, C., Bodenmann, P., Ghali, W. et al. (2007). Active smoking and the risk of type 2 diabetes: a systematic review and meta-analysis. *Journal of the American Medical Association* **298**: 2654–2664.

Williams, G. and Pickup, J. (1992). *Handbook of Diabetes*. Oxford: Blackwell Science.

Wilmshurst, E. (2002). Facts about diabetic breast disease all women should know. *Diabetes Conquest, Autumn* **13**.

Wilson, D., Walsh, P., Sanchez, L. et al. (1999). The epidemiology of hearing impairment in an Australian adult population. *International Journal of Epidemiology* **28** (2): 247–252.

Wilson, S., Pavlos, T., McNeil, A. et al. (2019). Perceptions of e-cigarettes and other nicotine products in a UK population smaple. *Addiction Journal* https://doi.org/10.1111/add.14502 m.

Wise, R., Sims, T., and Taylor, R. (2007). Smoking cessation – a practical guide for the primary care physician. *Primary Care Reports* **13** (4): 49–60.

World Health Organization (2017). International standards of TB care. https://erj.ersjournals.com/content/erj/51/3/1800098.full-text.pdf.

World Health Organization (WHO) (2011). *Tuberculosis and Diabetes: Collaborative Framework for Care and Control of Tuberculosis and Diabetes*. WHO http://www.who.int/tb (accessed November 2012).

Wright, A., Cull, C., Macleod, K. et al. (2006). For the UKPDS group hypoglycemia in type 2 diabetic patients randomized to and maintained on monotherapy with diet, sulfonylurea, metformin, or insulin for 6 years from diagnosis: UKPDS73. *The Journal of Diabetic Complications* **20**: 395–401.

Wusthoff, T., Smee, C., Merchant, N. et al. (2012). Prediction of neurodevelopmental outcome after hypoxic-ischemic encephalopathy treated with hypothermia by diffusion tensor imaging analyzed using tract-based spatial statistics. *Pediatric Research* **72**: 63–69.

Wyatt, G., Friedman, L., Given, C., and Beckrow, K. (1999). Complementary therapy use among older cancer therapy patients. *Cancer Practice* **7** (3): 136–144.

Yki-Jarvinen, H., Ryysy, L., Nikkila, K. et al. (1999). Comparison of bedtime insulin regimens in patients with type 2 diabetes mellitus. A randomised, controlled trial. *Archives of Internal Medicine* **130**: 399–396.

Young, T., Shahar, E., Nieto, F.J. et al. (2002). Predictors of sleep-disordered breathing in community-dwelling adults: the Sleep Heart Health Study. *Archives of internal medicine* **162** (8): 893–900.

Zarrinpar, A. and Loomba, R. (2012). Review article: the emerging interplay among the gastrointestinal tract, bile acids and incretins in the pathogenesis of diabetes and non-alcoholic fatty liver disease. *Alimentary Pharmacology and Therapeutics* **36**: 909–921.

Zevin, S. and Benowitz, N.L. (1999). Drug interactions with tobacco smoking. *Clinical Pharmacokinetics* **36** (6): 425–438.

Zhang, N. (2018). An evolutionary concept analysis of urinary incontinence. *Urologic Nursing* **38** (6): 289–295.

Zi, F., Zi, H., Li, Y. et al. (2018). Metformin and cancer: An existing drug for cancer prevention and therapy (Review). *Oncology Letters* **15**: 683–690. https://doi.org/10.3892/ol.2017.7412.

Ziemer, D.C., Barnes, C.S., Tsui, C.W. et al. (2007). Hypoglycemia Is Not Associated with Intensification of Diabetes Therapy. *Diabetes*: 56.

Chapter 11

Sexual and Reproductive Health

Key points

- Sexuality is a broad multifactorial concept that encompasses gender, sexual orientation, personhood, and is a key aspect of quality of life (Bauer et al. 2014).
- Sexual dysfunction is common in the general population. People with diabetes are at increased risk.
- The presence of a sexual problem and diabetes does not mean one led to the other: other causative factors need to be discussed.
- Physical, psychological, environmental, and social factors that affect sexual health should be considered.
- The needs and perceptions of each partner are important.
- Addressing sexual health and sex education should be part of preventative, holistic diabetes care.
- The sexual health needs of older people are often overlooked and not addressed, especially in aged-care homes.
- There is a fine line between taking a sexual history and voyeurism.
- The focus should be on what is normal and achievable for the individual/couple rather than dysfunction or 'performance'.
- Health professionals need to be comfortable with their own sexuality to advise other effectively.

Rationale

People with diabetes expect clinicians to be knowledgeable about the impact of diabetes on their sexual well-being. Sexuality is an integral component of health and sexual problems affect all aspects of health and well-being. Sexual dysfunction in men with diabetes is well documented, but sexual dysfunction amongst women with diabetes is still not well understood. The sexual response is an interaction between two (usually) people. Sexual dysfunction is also likely to involve both partners in the relationship (Masters and Johnson 1970). All clinicians are ideally

Care of People with Diabetes: A Manual for Healthcare Practice, Fifth Edition. Trisha Dunning and Alan Sinclair.
© 2020 John Wiley & Sons Ltd. Published 2020 by John Wiley & Sons Ltd.

placed to be able to emphasise the need for primary prevention and early identification of sexual difficulties and to dispel common sex myths. Yet, research suggests clinicians are reluctant to acknowledge sexual health needs (Poynten et al. 2013).

Significantly, the incidence of sexually transmitted infections (STIs) is increasing, including in Australia, the United States, Canada, and the United Kingdom across all age groups including in older people (Poynten et al. 2013; Kirby Institute 2016). People with HIV infections are ageing due to increasing lifespan and contracting HIV in older age (Poynten et al. 2013). STIs include chlamydia, gonorrhoea, syphilis (especially in men), Hepatitis B and C.
Several factors increase the risk of STIs (Bateson et al. 2012; WHO 2019):

- Increased numbers of new partners due to longer life and divorce rates
- Reduced use of condoms
- Lower rates of STI testing
- Uptake of medicines to treat erectile dysfunction (ED)
- Ease of travel to foreign countries
- Relationships that begin through internet dating

Sexual health

Sexual health is a core aspect of an individual's general health and well-being and is the result of an integration of many components into a unified complex system – endocrine hormonal regulators, and the vascular, nervous, and psychological systems. Diabetes can profoundly affect the individual's sexual identity and the physical ability to engage in sexual activity. Maximising sexual health should be an integral part of an holistic personalised management plan for people with diabetes.

Management should include education about screening for where relevant and managing diabetes-related complications and issues such as safe sex, contraception, STIs, and the importance of planning pregnancies (Chapter 14). Thus, a life continuum approach to sexual health is recommended.

Contraception

Female contraception is described in Chapter 14. Contraception options for men include:

- Condoms.
- Withdrawing before ejaculating. This is not recommended and has a high failure rate for pregnancies and sexual satisfaction.
- Billings method. This is a process of charting vaginal mucous conditions, and so it requires cooperation from female partners.
- Vasectomy.
- Male contraceptive agents are still under study, and include hormone contraceptives to stop sperm development, nonhormone contraception to prevent sperm entering the vagina, and methods to change the way the epididymis functions and sperm matures in the epididymis (National Health Service 2019).

Sexual issues are highly sensitive and must be approached with tact and consideration of the person's culture, sexual beliefs, and their privacy and confidentiality. Thus, although partners can often provide important information about their partner's sexual functioning, they should not be included in the consultation unless the individual agrees. The World Health Organization (WHO) (2010) stressed the importance of sexuality as an integral component of health and defined sexual health as:

A state of physical, emotional, mental and social wellbeing in relation to sexuality; it is not merely the absence of disease, dysfunction or infirmity. Sexual health requires a positive, respectful approach to sexuality and sexual relationships and the possibility of having pleasurable and safe sexual experiences, free of coercion, discrimination and violence. For sexual health to be attained and maintained, the sexual rights of all persons must be respected, protected and fulfilled.

(WHO 2010)

By the WHO definition, the majority of the general populations, including people with diabetes, may not achieve ideal sexual health!

Masters and Johnson first described the human sexual response in Masters and Johnson 1970. They described four phases: arousal, plateau, orgasm, and resolution (Masters and Johnson 1970). These phases blend into each other and sexual difficulties can occur in one or all of them. Kaplan (1979) described a biphasic response that involved parasympathetic nerve activity – vasocongestion, vaginal lubrication, and erection; and sympathetic nerve activity – reflex muscle contraction, orgasm, and ejaculation. Kaplan's description makes it easier to understand how diabetes can affect physical sex given that autonomic neuropathy causes nerve damage, which is a component of ED; see Chapter 8.

Sex counsellors continue to utilise many of the sexual counselling techniques developed by Masters and Johnson. Sexual difficulties do not occur in isolation from other aspects of an individual's life and relationships and a thorough assessment and history is necessary to identify the underlying inter-related causal factors. Masters and Johnson found that age and chronic disease processes do not affect female sexual responsiveness as severely as they affect male sexuality and stated the sexual response is more varied in women than in men. However, other studies suggest diabetes has a pervasively negative effect on women with type 2 diabetes' sexual health and well-being, which begins after the diagnosis of diabetes (Albright 2012).

Sexual development

Sexual development occurs across the lifespan:

- Chromosomal sex is determined at fertilisation.
- 3–5 years – diffuse sexual pleasure, fantasies, and sex play. Often form a close relationship with a parent of the opposite sex.
- 5–8 years – interest in sexual differences; sex play is common.
- 8–9 years – begin to evaluate attractiveness and are curious about sex.
- 10–12 years – preoccupation with changing body and puberty. Adolescents are often sexually active by this age; thus, sex education should start early and information provided in accordance to the child's capacity to understand and using appropriate language.
- 13–20 years – puberty, development of self-image and sexual identity.
- Late 30s–early 40s – peak sexual responsiveness.
- Menopause – variable onset and highly individual effect on sexuality.
- Old age – sexuality still matters, although older people often need to contend with physical difficulties, ageist attitudes/stereotyping, and limited opportunity.

Effective sex and diabetes education should be part of the diabetes management plan so that sexual health issues can be identified early and optimal sexual functioning maintained. Health professionals and people with diabetes often have limited information about the impact diabetes can have on their sexual health. Sex education, good metabolic control, early identification, and management of sexual problems are important but often neglected aspects of the diabetes care plan and should be included in annual complication screening programmes. When a sexual problem is identified, the focus is often on dysfunction and performance, rather than on what is normal or achievable, which can have a negative psychological impact on sexuality. Changing the focus to what can be achieved and focusing on feelings, intimacy, love, and warmth have a big impact on general and sexual well-being.

Sexual problems

Sexual satisfaction is a combination of physical and emotional factors. Sexual problems can be:

- Primary – usually defined as never having an orgasm.
- Secondary – difficulties occur after a period of normal sexual functioning. Most sexual difficulties fit into this category.
- Situational – where the situation itself inhibits sexual activity; other sexual problems may also be involved.

Possible causes of sexual difficulties and dysfunction

Sexual difficulties usually involve two people. The problem may be shared or each person may have individual issues that need to be considered. Interpersonal factors, the relationship, and environmental and disease factors need to be explored with the individuals and couple involved.

(1) Individual factors
  - Ignorance and misinformation, which are common, despite today's sexually permissive society and the surfeit of explicit sex in movies, books, and television programmes and advertisements (sell it with sex). A great deal of readily available literature in magazines and on television overemphasises performance, which can set up unreal expectations.
  - Guilt, shame, and fear, which may be fear of getting pregnant, contracting a STI, not pleasing their partner, or being rejected by them.
  - Gender insecurity/uncertainty and sexual preference.
  - Nonsexual concerns, such as worry about finances, children, and job.
  - Past sexual abuse.
  - Physical condition; for example, presence of diabetes especially diabetes complications such as autonomic neuropathy, and vascular disease.
  - Age-related changes and the menopause in women.
(2) Interpersonal factors
  - Sexual relationships are one of the most complex undertakings people ever make; yet most people prepare for sexual relationships and their sexual health casually and in an uninformed way.
  - Communication problems – the most common sexual difficulty.
  - Lack of trust.
  - Different sexual preferences and desires, for example, frequency of intercourse.
  - Relationship difficulties that can include difficulties associated with incompatibility, alcohol and violence, or be related to disease process, including diabetes.
  - Changes in lifestyle, for example, having children, retrenchment, retirement, and illness, including diabetes.
(3) Chronic disease sequelae
  - (a) Psychological.
    - Depression, anger, guilt, anxiety, fear, feelings of helplessness, changed body image and self-identification as a victim. Lowered self-image and self-esteem may or may not accompany the disease. Loss of libido is one of the classic signs of depression.
  - (b) Physical changes, for example, arthritis and diabetic neuropathy.
    - Pain, debilitation associated with changed mobility, for example, arthritis, bad odour associated with infections and candidia, cardiac and respiratory problems and sleep apnoea, and snoring. Some people worry about resuming sexual activity after a myocardial infarction (MI) or having a heart attack during sexual activity. Education can help allay such fears.

- Disease processes and hormonal imbalance, including diabetes, as well as other endocrine and reproductive conditions.
- Medications, for example, antihypertensive and antidepressive agents.

(c) Diabetes-related.
- Hypoglycaemia during intercourse can be frightening and off-putting, especially for the partner, and inhibit spontaneity and enjoyment in future encounters.
- Tiredness and decreased mood and decreased arousal and libido are associated with hyperglycaemia.
- Mood disorders such as depression and other psychological problems may be present, but mood can change with hypo- and hyperglycaemia and can cause temporary sexual problems.
- Autonomic neuropathy leading to ED in men and possibly decreased vaginal lubrication in older women. Vaginal dryness is also associated with normal ageing and not being aroused and may cause painful intercourse. Vaginal dryness has not been definitively linked to diabetes as a cause.
- Men with diabetes are likely to have low testosterone levels and low libido, especially if they have poor glycaemic control. Low testosterone is associated with increased risk of death. Testosterone supplementation improves glycaemic control (HbA1c), lipids, and well being (Heufelder et al. 2009).

(d) Infections such as vaginal/penile thrush.

(e) Musculoskeletal diseases that limit mobility and dexterity; these may cause pain; see Chapter 10.

(4) Environmental factors.
- Lack of privacy.
- Limited opportunity, for example, older people generally and especially those who live in aged-care facilities.
- Uncomfortable, noisy surroundings.
- Drugs and alcohol.
- Health professional and population ageist attitudes concerning older people's sexual needs.

Sexuality and older people

Older people are capable of having fulfilling sexual relationships but often lack the opportunity or are constrained by environmental factors, ageist attitudes, sexual stereotypes, and disease processes (see Chapter 12). Sensory impairment can change the individual's response to sexual stimulation and the multiplicity of medications required by many older people can inhibit sexual functioning. Touch is important throughout life, and caring touch as distinct from providing nursing care is often lacking. Touch can provide a great deal of sexual pleasure when intercourse is not possible. Many older people are deprived of touch when a partner dies or when they are separated in aged-care facilities.

There is increasing emphasis on considering older people's sexual health needs across the lifespan, including in aged-care facilities. In Australia, the Charter of Aged Care Rights (which replaced the Charter of Care Residents' Rights and Responsibilities) includes residents' right to privacy and control over their relationships, but the charter can be challenging to implement (see Australian Government Department of Health 2019). Some aged-care homes have developed policies to promote sexual health that consider privacy, staff, and other residents' safety, education for staff and families, the needs of people with dementia, and transgender people.

Like all care, decisions should be based on a comprehensive assessment: sexual health should be part of that assessment and part of the personalised care plan developed with the individual. The *Global Guideline for Managing Older People with Type 2 Diabetes* (International Diabetes Federation 2013) is one of the few diabetes guidelines that includes sexual health and well-being and does not just focus on diabetes-related complications (ED).

Women

The biological effect of diabetes on male sexual functioning has been well documented. The effects of diabetes on sexual function in women are poorly understood, and the evidence for any effect is less conclusive than the evidence for the effects on male sexual functioning (Leedom et al. 1991). Physicians regularly ask men about their sexual functioning but not women (Albright 2012; Copeland et al. 2012).

Women with diabetes are twice as likely to report low sexual satisfaction than women without diabetes (Copeland et al. 2012). In a study ($n = 2000$), women on insulin were more likely to report difficulty with vaginal lubrication and 80% reported difficulty achieving orgasm. Not surprisingly, women with diabetes complications such as peripheral neuropathy, renal dysfunction, and cardiovascular disease were more likely to report less sexual activity and less satisfaction than controls. However, a number of factors besides diabetes contribute to sexual dissatisfaction, as indicated in the previous section.

Women who have difficulty accepting that they have diabetes report higher levels of sexual dysfunction than those who accept their diabetes. Type 2 diabetes has a pervasively negative effect on women's sexuality (Schriener-Engel et al. 1991). There appears to be little or no effect in women with type 1 diabetes but they often have concerns about pregnancy, childbirth, and hypoglycaemia during sex in the younger years (Dunning 1994). There is a positive association between the degree of sexual dysfunction and the severity of depression that illustrates the connection between physical and psychological factors and the need for an holistic approach.

Fluctuating blood glucose levels can have a negative transient effect on desire and sexual responsiveness and women often report slow arousal, decreased libido, and inadequate lubrication during hyperglycaemia. Desire can fluctuate with stages of the menstrual cycle but this also occurs in women without diabetes. Polycystic ovarian disease and its effects could have adverse psychological effects, which, in turn, affect sexual health (see Chapter 14). Obesity can contribute to physical difficulties during sexual intercourse.

The developmental stage of the individual should also be considered when assessing sexual health and planning sex education and counselling.

- Children and adolescents – diabetes can affect normal growth and development if it is not well controlled and menarche and puberty can be delayed. This could impact negatively on body image and the development of sexual identity and self-esteem eating disorders. Insulin manipulation to manage weight can compound the problem.
- Young adulthood – attracting a partner, successful pregnancy, and birth can be areas of fear and concern that affect sexual health (Dunning 1994). Hyperglycaemia can occur during menstruation and contribute to tiredness, decreased arousal and libido. Vaginal thrush is common and causes itch and discomfort during sexual intercourse. It may be associated with taking oral contraceptives or antibiotics for intercurrent illness. Thrush and balanitis can inhibit male sexual activity. Brittle diabetes (Chapter 14) may also inhibit sexual functioning and health.
- Older age group – hormonal changes due to menopause and associated fatigue and depression inhibit sexual enjoyment. Often, a long-term partner's life courses are different and can affect their sexual relationship. There are fewer partners and opportunities for sexual activity for older women especially those in care facilities.

Specific problems should be investigated, depending on their presentation. Diabetes management should be revised to achieve good glycaemic control and a medicines review may be indicated. Preventative sexual health care such as breast self-examination, mammograms, and cervical (pap) smears should be part of the care plan. Contraception is discussed in Chapter 14.

Men

Diabetes has physical effects that cause ED. Other ED causes include:

- Andropause, which leads to a normal, gradual reduction in male hormones such as testosterone and sex hormone binding globulin (SHBG) akin to the menopause in women. Andropause can result in depression, low libido, ED, and irritability. Men with diabetes tend to experience andropause earlier and the symptoms are more pronounced then men without diabetes (Andropause Report 2013).
- Vascular damage, both systemic atherosclerosis and microvascular disease.
- Neurological diseases such as spinal cord damage, multiple sclerosis, and diabetic neuropathy.
- Psychological causes such as performance anxiety, depression, and mood changes may be associated with hypo- or hyperglycaemia.
- Endocrine diseases that result in lowered sex hormones: testosterone, SHBG, prolactin, follicle-stimulating hormone (FSH), and luteinizing hormone (LH). Hypogonadism can occur in chronic disease.
- Obesity can contribute to physical difficulties during sexual intercourse.
- Surgery and trauma to genitalia or its nerve and vascular supply.
- Anatomical abnormalities, for example, Peyronie's contracture, which is often associated with Dupuyten's contracture and other glycosylation diseases including diabetes; see Chapter 10.
- Medicines such as thiazide diuretics, beta blockers, lipid lowering agents, antidepressants, SSRI, smoking, alcohol, and illicit drug use.
- Normal ageing.

ED is defined as the inability to achieve or maintain an erection sufficient for satisfactory sexual performance – penetration and ejaculation. It is common in men with diabetes especially if other diabetic complications are present. It occurs in 50% of men 10 years after the diagnosis of diabetes especially those who smoke. ED is gradual, insidious, and progressive (Krane 1991). ED may be a predictor of cardiovascular risk and there is a higher incidence of undiagnosed coronary disease in men with ED. Elevated blood fats and hypertension and antihypertensive agents also play a part in the development of ED. Lowered sperm counts are associated with obesity, smoking, and poor diet.

ED significantly reduces the man's quality of life, especially in the emotional domain, and has a negative effect on self-esteem. However, ED also has a significant effect on the man's partner. Partners play a key supportive role in the man's treatment and treatment success (Dean et al. 2008). When sexual functioning improves, improvement in mental and social status follows. Other sexual issues for men are fatigue, fear of performance failure, and concern about not satisfying their partners, but most men do not involve their partners when they seek advice about ED (Dean et al. 2008).

Aboriginal and Torres Strait Islander men have higher incidence of ED; ~10% in men younger than 35 years and 28% in men 55–74 years. Those with a chronic disease or living in remote areas are more likely to have moderate to severe ED and a similar low level of help-seeking as nonindigenous men. Barriers to help-seeking in indigenous men are shame, cultural inappropriate services, and lack of awareness (Adams et al. 2013). It is not clear whether similar issues apply to other indigenous peoples. Sexual health assessment, education and management programmes need to be culturally sensitive and should be developed by/with relevant indigenous people.

Investigation and management

A thorough history and physical examination are required. Some of the questions that need to be asked are very personal, which may be difficult and stressful. Thus, time, privacy, and tact are essential. The assessment includes diabetic complication status and blood glucose and lipid control, identifying the cause, and determining the extent of the dysfunction (e.g. using rigiscan and snap gauge to determine whether nocturnal erections occur), and sleep apnoea studies. There is an association between poor sleep, sleep apnoea, and ED. Doppler studies are carried out to determine local blood flow.

Testosterone, FSH, LH, SHBG, and prolactin levels are measured to identify central causes of hypogonadism. Blood might be collected between 8 and 11 A.M. when serum testosterone is highest. The value for 'low' testosterone is controversial (Lue et al. 2017). Symptoms of hypogonadism are more common in men with total testosterone levels <320 ng/ml and free testosterone <64 ng/ml (Lue et al. 2017). Low testosterone should be confirmed with repeat testing rather than relying on a single test result.

Management consists of the following:

- Good metabolic control to prevent ED and improve andropause symptoms. If the testosterone is low, supplementation might improve symptoms. Testerosterone can be given by injection, patch, topical gel, and implants.
- Early intervention if ED occurs.
- Assess fitness for sex and modifying risk factors, for example, managing cardiovascular health, losing weight, managing pain, smoking cessation, and reducing alcohol intake.
- Ensure appropriate diet and exercise programme. Tai chi and strength training can improve flexibility and strength and general well-being in older men.
- Sex education should include setting realistic expectations and planning for regular sexual health checks, for example, prostate disease.
- Diabetes education.
- Counselling should include partners and inform them about treatment options to help the couple find fulfilling sexual alternatives if the man cannot achieve erections.

Men are often reluctant to seek help, especially for sexual difficulties. Programmes such as Men's Sheds in Australia have had a positive effect on mental health and well-being as well as helping men develop life skills in a peer education environment. It is not clear whether men discuss sexual health in men's sheds but diabetes educators have been invited to discuss diabetes in these sheds.

Medication management for ED

Oral Medicines
Medication management includes oral phosphodiesterase type 5 (PDE-5) inhibitors such as Sildenafil (Viagra) and Vardenafil (Levitra), which are vasodilators that enhance the natural sexual response. They can cause visual disturbances ('blue vision'), transient hypotension, and can unmask cardiac ischaemia. PDE-5 medicines are contraindicated if nitrate medications are used and when cardiovascular disease is present. Cimetidine and Ketoconozale can increase Viagra levels and Rifampicin decreases them. Other oral medicines are still under study.

Urethral and injected medicines
Urethrally introduced medicines such as MUSE have a success rate between 30% and 50% of men. Side effects include urethral pain and burning in 7–10% of men who use this medicine. Intracavernosal therapy or penile injections such the vasoconstrictor agents papaverine, alprostadil (Caverject), VIP, and the vasodilator phentalamine. Men and/or their partners need to learn the technique of penile injections, which should be done under supervision. A rare but serious side effect is priapism, which requires urgent treatment to reverse the effects of the vasoconstriction. Other side effects include the formation of scar tissue, bruising, and rarely infection at injection sites. Caverject sometimes causes pain in high doses.

Nonpharmacological therapy – penile prosthetics

Nonpharmacological therapy includes external vacuum pumps. Vacuum devices are a simple, effective method of achieving an erection. A man suffering from ED invented a device called

ErecAid® in the 1960s. It consists of a clear plastic cylinder, which has either a manual pump or batteries and a special tension ring. The penis is placed into the cylinder and the man or his partner holds the device firmly against the body to form an airtight seal and then pumps the air out of the cylinder, which creates a vacuum and causes the penis to become erect. The special tension ring is inserted over the device around the base of the penis to maintain the erection, and the device is removed. The whole process takes about 2 minutes and the erection is maintained for about 30 minutes (longer than natural erections). The ring *must* be removed after intercourse.

Vacuum pumps have very few side effects. Sometimes, small red dots called petechiae and bruising can occur on the penis but these are not harmful. They are more likely to occur if the individual is on anticoagulant medicines. The temperature in the penis drops 1–2°, which is caused by the tension ring. The device can be difficult to use, so learning how to use it is important. It can reduce sexual spontaneity, so it is very important that the man discusses sexual issues and their management options with his partner.

Hormone replacement therapy

Hormone replacement therapy (testosterone) might be indicated in 3–4% of men, but is contraindicated in men with liver disease, cardiovascular disease, renal disease, and prostate cancer. These contraindications probably apply to many men with diabetes. See subheading men.

Complementary and alternative medicines for sexual problems (CAM)

Men with sexual health problems commonly use CAM especially if they receive conflicting advice and worry a lot about the problem (Trutnovsky et al. 2001). CAM can be used to improve general health and well-being and manage stress that can have benefits for sexual health; see Chapter 19. Eating a healthy diet, regular exercise, and adequate rest and sleep are important to sexual health. Often CAM practitioners recommend supplements such as flaxseed oil, vitamins E, and C and zinc. However, rigorous evidence for a beneficial effect for most herbal medicines is lacking, and some are harmful. CAM therapies appear to target three main sexual health issues: improving sexual 'stamina', aphrodisiacs, and overcoming erection problems.

Commonly used CAM medicines to improve libido and erections include the following. They are often used in combination:

- L-arginine and *Gingko biloba*
- Horney goat weed
- Passion treatment
- Damiana
- Yohimbe
- Asian Ginseng
- Goji berries, which are sometimes referred to as 'natural viagra.' They are also sold covered in chocolate.

Many so-called aphrodisiacs carry significant health risks (often for animals as well as men) and are not recommended. These include powdered rhino horn, crushed pearls, Spanish fly, and animal testicles.

The risks and benefits of these medicines are not known and they may interact with conventional medicines, including those used to manage sexual problems. Therefore, it is important to ask men and women with sexual health problems about CAM use. The US FDA warned about two unapproved dietary supplements sold online to treat ED: 'Blue Steel' and 'Hero', which contain active ingredients with similar actions to sildenafil. These products could interact with conventional nitrate medicines and cause hypotension. People might unwittingly seek such alternatives if conventional ED medicines are contraindicated or if they do not feel comfortable discussing sexual health with their health professionals.

Involving partners in ED management

Partners may be able to contribute important information about the man's general health and sexual history but should only be involved if they are willing and the man agrees. The man, and ideally his partner, needs to be involved in selecting the best management option. Partner's attitudes affect the man's uptake of and adherence to ED treatment and long-term management is more successful if the partner is involved (Fisher et al. 2005). The Index of Sexual Life (ISL) (Chevret et al. 2004) is a validated tool developed to assess women's sexual desire and satisfaction when their partner has ED.

Chevret et al. (2004) and Fisher et al. (2005) found partners of men with ED had significantly reduced sexual drive, orgasm, satisfaction, and frequency of sex compared with partners of men who did not have ED, and prior to the onset of ED. In addition, partners of men with ED are more likely to have sexual dysfunction or avoid sexual activity. A number of studies demonstrate significant improvements in sexual function, satisfaction, and quality of life for both partners following treatment, especially with PDE-5 medicines (Fisher et al. 2005) but 10–45% discontinue treatment (Madduri 2001).

Clinical observations

- Improving sexual functioning can lead to positive changes in the relationship; it can also result in conflict and disharmony, especially if both partners are not involved in management decisions.
- Women have reported acute cystitis when their partners begin using Viagra due to the increased sexual activity, so-called 'honeymoon cystitis'.
- Sex education is part of the management for both men and women, and needs to include:
- Focus on what is achievable and not on improving 'performance'.
- Revision of diabetes knowledge and self-care and the importance of blood glucose and lipid control.
- Knowledge about sex and sexuality and 'normal' sexual functioning.

Sexual counselling

Good communication and trust is essential to sexual relationships. It is also essential to sexual counselling. Health professionals need knowledge of the human sexual response, normal ageing, and the potential effects of diabetes on sexual health, to counsel effectively. Questions about sexual health can be included when taking a nursing history. Including sexual questions in the nursing history can be simple and identify sexual problems that require specific questions to obtain a more detailed history or referral to a sex specialist. Respect and regard for the person and empathetic understanding and privacy are essential (Ross and Channon-Little 1991). The main areas to be covered when taking a sexual history are:

(1) Social aspects
  - Childhood experiences
  - Marital status
  - Family relationships
  - Number and sex of any children
  - Interests, activities
  - Job demands/unemployment
  - Religious and cultural beliefs
(2) Sexual aspects
  - Sexual knowledge, education, fears, fantasies
  - Previous sexual experiences

- Contraception method
- Current problems:
  - Whose problem does the person believe it to be?
  - Description of the problem in the person's own words.
  - Is the partner aware of the problem?
  - Does the problem follow a period of poor diabetic control or illness?
  - Have there been any previous sexual problems?
  - What were those problems?
  - How were they resolved?

(3) Psychological aspects
- Acceptance of diabetes by self and partner
- Body-image concepts
- Presence of depression or other psychological problem

(4) Diabetes knowledge
- Self-care skills
- Knowledge of effects of poor diabetic control

In addition, questions to assess the level of communication amongst partners could include:

- Have you discussed your issues with your partner? Be specific about the problem after the individual explains what the problem is, and address each problem separately if there is more than one problem.
- Do you know what your partner thinks about the problem?
- Is your partner supportive of you seeking treatment to improve the problem?
- Does your partner have any question or concern about the treatment?
- Do you think your partner would come with you to discuss ways to improve your sex life?
- Does your partner have any concerns about his/her sexual function or general health?
- Is there anything else you would like to tell me to help me understand the problem?

The ISI questionnaire could also be useful to understand the woman's perspective.

Measuring sexual health

General measures of well-being and psychological are useful indicators of mood and the effects of diabetes on these parameters; see Chapter 15. Following are examples of some of the many tools available. Some are old, but most are valid and reliable:

- Derogatis Sexual Function Inventory (DSFI)
- Sexual Concerns Checklist (SCC)
- Sexual Interest Questionnaire (SIQ)
- Harvard Sex Questionnaire
- Sexual Anxiety Scale (SAS)
- Body Attitude Scale (BAS)

Interpersonal relationships can also be measured if indicated using tools such as:

- Marital Satisfaction Inventory
- Index of Marital Satisfaction
- Caring Relationship Inventory
- Sexual Communication Inventory

Specific training in sexual counselling might be required to use these tools and interpret the findings and to use the information to help the individual. Some of the tools could be administered in stage one or two of the PLISSIT Model (next section) and forwarded to a sexual health counsellor with a referral for specific sexual counselling.

The WHO produced a manual: *Measuring Sexual Health: Conceptual and Practical Considerations and Related Indicators* (2010) that contains 17 global indicators governments can use to legislating for sexual health, equality, and safety. There are a number of tools clinicians can use as part of sexual counselling, with the PLISSIT model and as part of diabetes complication screening programmes.

The PLISSIT model

PLISSIT is an acronym for Permission–Limited Information–Specific Suggestions–Intensive Therapy. The model uses four phases to address sexual problems and moves from simple to complex issues. It can be used in a variety of settings and adapted to the individual's needs (Anon 1975). It is an old model but it is still effective and follows education theory; thus, the framework can be used to investigate other health issues.

(1) Permission-giving
  • Being open and nonjudgemental allows the person to discuss their problem by:
    ○ offering reassurance;
    ○ accepting the person's concerns;
    ○ Being open and non-judgemental;
    ○ establishing acceptable terminology;
    ○ being truly present in the consultation (Dunning 2013).

Questions about the person's sexuality can be asked or the nurse can respond to sexual questions the person asks. These actions establish that it is appropriate and acceptable to discuss sexual issues.

(2) Provide limited information
  • This involves giving limited information and general suggestions that might include practising safe sex, contraceptive advice, diabetes, and sex education and giving accurate, limited information.
  • This could include some reference information for home reading.
(3) Specific suggestions
  • These are usually made by a qualified sex therapist and often include sensate focus exercises and the squeeze technique for premature ejaculation.
  • Involve the partner.
  • Provide sex education.
(4) Intensive therapy

Therapy at this stage requires referral to a sex psychologist/psychiatrist. Techniques include a range of counselling techniques, behavioural therapy, and a range of other therapies.

Practice points

(1) The nurse must have adequate knowledge to undertake steps 3 and 4 in the PLISSIT model and know when and how to refer the person appropriately.
(2) Examples of information to give in stage 1 include information about the differences between men and women (e.g. women take longer to become aroused than men and need sufficient quality foreplay to be able to achieve orgasm), the effects of medications, smoking, alcohol, and diabetes on sexual responsiveness.

Role of the clinician

Clinicians have an important role in the early identification of sexual problems and helping the individual or couple develop a health plan that includes sexual health. Some STIs must be reported to government health authorities in some countries. Some specific nursing actions include the following:

- Be aware of the possibility that a sex problem may exist and allow people to discuss their concerns.
- Debunk sexual myths; for example, old people who have sex are 'dirty old men/women'.
- Identify sexual problems and address them or refer appropriately.
- Provide relevant care and information during investigative procedures and surgery.
- Provide medication advice and management.
- Provide advice about safe sex and contraception. People can be referred to family planning clinics, sexual health clinics, or clinics that manage STI if relevant. There is a great deal of useful information on the internet, but people need to be careful about the sites they access and the information provided. One useful booklet that can be downloaded free is *A Couple's Guide for the Treatment of Erectile Dysfunction* (Endocare 2004) available at www. osbonerecaid.com.
- Provide advice about monitoring quality sexual health.
- Provide information about self-care and when it is safe to resume sex after hospitalisation, such as after a myocardial infarct or cardiac surgery.
- In care homes for older people and rehabilitation settings, providing an appropriate environment and opportunities for couples to enjoy a sexual relationship might be possible.

References

Adams, M., Collins, V., Dunne, M. et al. (2013). Male reproductive health disorders among aboriginal and Torres Strait islander men: a hidden problem? *Medical Journal of Australia* **198** (1): 33–38.

Albright, A. (2012). *Women, Sex and Diabetes*. Diabetes Health Centre http://diabetes.webmed.com/features/women-sex-and-diabetes (accessed December 2012).

Andropause Report (2013). All About Diabetes, *Testosterone Replacement and Andropause*. http://andropausereport.com/all-about-diabetes-testosterone-replacement-and-andropause (accessed January 2012).

Anon (1975). *The Behavioural Treatment of Sexual Problems*. Honolulu: Enabling Systems.

Australian Government Department of Health (2019). Charter of Aged Care Rights. https://agedcare.health.gov.au/quality/single-charter-of-aged-care-rights.

Bateson, O., Weisberg, E., McCaffery, K. et al. (2012). When online becomes offline: attitudes to safer sex practice in older and younger women using an Australian internet dating service. *Sex Health* **9** (2): 152–159.

Bauer, M., Featherstonehaugh, D., Tarzia, L. et al. (2014). Supporting residents' expression of sexuality: the initial construction of a sexuality assessment tool for residential aged care facilities. *BMC Geriatrics* **14** (82) https://www.biomedcentral.com/1471-2318/14/82.

Chevret, M., Jaudinot, E., and Sullivan, K. (2004). Impact of erectile dysfunction (ED) on sexual life of female partners: assessment with the index of sexual life (ISL) questionnaire. *Journal of Sex and Marital Therapy* **30**: 157–172.

Copeland, K., Brown, J., Creasman, J. et al. (2012). Diabetes mellitus and sexual function in middle-aged and older women. *Obstetrics & Gynecology* **120** (2): 331–340.

Dean, J., Rubio-Aurioles, E., McCabe, M. et al. (2008). Integrating partners into erectile dysfunction treatment: improving the sexual experience for the couple. *International Journal of Clinical Practice* **62** (1): 127–133.

Dunning, P. (1994). Having diabetes: young adult's perspectives. *The Diabetes Educator* **21** (1): 58–65.

Dunning, T. (ed.) (2013). The teacher: moving from good to exceptional. In: *Diabetes Education: Art, Science and Evidence*, 62–77. Chichester, UK: Wiley Blackwell.

Endocare (2004). *A Couple's Guide for the Treatment of Erectile Dysfunction*. www.osbonerecaid.com.

Fisher, W., Rosen, R., and Mollen, M. (2005). Improving the sexual quality of life of couples affected by erectile dysfunction: a double blind, randomized, placebo controlled trial of vardenafil. *Journal of Sex Medicine* **2**: 699–708.

Heufelder, A.E., Saad, F., Bunck, M.C., and Gooren, L. (2009). Fifty-two-week treatment with diet and exercise plus transdermal testosterone reverses the metabolic syndrome and improves glycemic control in men with newly diagnosed type 2 diabetes and subnormal plasma testosterone. *Journal of Andrology* **30** (6): 726–733.

International Diabetes Federation (2013). Global guideline for managing older people with type 2 diabetes. www.idf.org.

Kaplan, H. (1979). *Making Sense of Sex*. New York: Simon & Schuster.

Kirby Institute (2016). HIV, viral hepatitis and sexually transmissible infections in Australia. Annual Surveillance Report. https://kirby.unsw.edu.au/report/annual-surveillance-report-hiv-viral-hepatitis-stis-2016.

Krane, R. (1991). Commentary on erectile dysfunction. *Diabetes Spectrum* **4** (1): 29–30.

Leedom, L., Feldman, M., Procci, W., and Zeidler, A. (1991). Severity of sexual dysfunction and depression in diabetic women. *Journal of Diabetic Complications* **5** (1): 38–41.

Lue, T., Brant, W., Shindel, A., and Bella, A. (2017). Sexual dysfunction in diabetes NCIB Bookshelf. https://www.ncbi.nlm.nih.gov/books/NBK279101.

Madduri, S. (2001). After 2 years, did Viagra live up to its expectations? *Missouri Medicine* **98**: 243–245.

Masters, W. and Johnson, V. (1970). *Human Sexual Inadequacy*. Boston: Little Brown Company.

National Health Service (2019). The pill for men. https://www.nhsinform.scot/healthy-living/contraception/the-pill/the-pill-for-men.

Poynten, Grulich, A., and Templeton, D. (2013). Sexually transmitted infections in older populations. *Current Opinion in Infectious Diseases* **26** (1): 80–85.

Ross, M. and Channon-Little, L. (1991). *Discussing Sexuality. A Guide for Health Practitioners*. Sydney: MacLennan & Pretty.

Schriener-Engel, P., Schiavi, P., Vietorisz, D., and Smith, H. (1991). The differential impact of diabetes type on female sexuality. *Diabetes Spectrum* **4** (1): 16–20.

Trutnovsky, G., Law, C., Simpson, J., and Mindel, A. (2001). Use of complementary therapies in a sexual health clinic setting. *International Journal of STD and AIDS* **12** (5): 307–309.

World Health Organization (WHO) (2010). *Measuring Sexual Health: Conceptual and Practical Considerations and Related Indicators*. Geneva: WHO.

World Health Organization (WHO) (2019). Sexually transmitted infections (STIs) https://www.who.int/gho/sti/en.

Chapter 12
Diabetes and Older People

It is important to keep in front of people's minds that old age is not a burden. In fact, it is a celebration of continuing life, of living to be 100.

(Honourable Ken Wyatt Australian Minister for Senior Australians and Aged Care 2019)

Key points

- 'Ageing' is a social construct describing transitions through different stages throughout the lifespan.
- An holistic proactive and integrated approach is needed to achieve effective diabetes management, manage age- and diabetes-related health risks, and ensure management strategies are appropriate for older people with diabetes.
- Increasing age is associated with insulin resistance that predisposes older people to diabetes.
- Diabetes is common in people over age 65. Most have type 2 diabetes, but type 1 and latent autoimmune diabetes in adults (LADA) also occur in older people.
- Older people rarely present with the textbook symptoms of hyperglycaemia; the onset of diabetes is often insidious and the nonspecific symptoms are often mistaken for advancing age or other conditions.
- Long-term complications are often present at diagnosis and often coexist with other functional changes and comorbidities. Frailty is a significant comorbidity. Screening for geriatric syndromes and determining when palliative care with usual care is indicated.
- There is high prevalence of diabetes in care homes: policies should be in place to screen for undiagnosed diabetes, manage those with diagnosed diabetes, and educate staff.
- The individual should be encouraged to maintain independent self-care within their capabilities for as long as possible, but carer assistance is often needed, especially during illnesses and in aged-care homes.
- There is limited evidence for metabolic targets in older people. Targets must be appropriate to the individual and limit the risk of adverse events such as hypoglycaemia, hyperglycaemia, cognitive changes, and falls.
- Pharmacovigilance is essential because age-related changes affect medicine absorption, distribution, metabolism, and elimination, leading to serious adverse events.

Care of People with Diabetes: A Manual for Healthcare Practice, Fifth Edition. Trisha Dunning and Alan Sinclair.
© 2020 John Wiley & Sons Ltd. Published 2020 by John Wiley & Sons Ltd.

- Being hospitalised leads to a decline in physical and cognitive functioning in older people. Older people are relatively immobile in bed or a chair for 95% of their time in hospital. Immobility is linked to venous stasis, reduced muscle mass and strength, and is a key reason for delayed discharge or admission to a care home.
- Where relevant, family carers' well-being should be considered.
- Despite the growing body of knowledge concerning care of older people with diabetes some challenges remain (Sinclair et al. 2015).

Rationale

By 2015, two billion people globally will be >age 60; >25% will have diabetes and obesity, 50% will have prediabetes (ADA 2019). People over age 65 are usually regarded as old. However, older people generally and those with diabetes are highly individual: they are not a heterogeneous group. Some are healthy and active; others are frail and have multiple health problems. Thus, care needs can differ amongst older individuals of the same age and within the individual at different times. Clinically relevant categories of older people that can help determine care needs are:

- Healthy older people who are independent and self-caring
- Older people who manage most activities of daily living (ADL) independently but require some assistance
- Frail older people whose care needs to be considered on an individual basis depending on their functional (physical and mental) status and available support
- Older people at the end of life (IDF 2013)

Managing diabetes in/with older people is a complex and increasingly important aspect of health care as the global population ages and because the incidence and prevalence of diabetes increases with increasing age. Diabetes manifests differently in older people, and their health-care needs are different from younger people. Likewise, diabetes and its complications are likely to adversely affect many ADL, including socialising and driving as well as physical and mental functioning, all of which affect self-care ability, independence, and psychological well-being.

Evidence suggests that older people with diabetes use more primary care services than older people without diabetes and frequently require hospital care and/or care in aged care homes (Sinclair 2011). Optimal holistic care could reduce the high cost of care and help older people with diabetes live more fulfilling lives.

Introduction

The *ageing process* refers to a progressive deterioration of bodily functions over the lifespan whose characteristics are destructive, progressive, intrinsically determined, and universal. Ageing occurs at different rates amongst individuals and amongst individual organs and tissues in the body. There are many theories, but no consensus, about what causes ageing. The two major schools of thought are: (i) ageing is programmed; and (ii) ageing is random, each school of thought is accompanied by specific theories (see Table 12.1).

These theories raise the question: Can ageing be cured, or should it be managed better to maintain wellness for longer with a short decline to death because ageing is a natural process?

Although ageing theories might still be debated, ancient wisdom has been substantiated by a great deal of modern research (Miller 2019). In fact, the core advice is unchanged:

- Eat a healthy diet.
- Be active every day.

Table 12.1   Theories of ageing.

Programmed theories	Damage theories
Ageing is a designed process (built in obsolescence)	Ageing is due to accumulated molecular damage especially to DNA and proteins that causes cell, organ, and system dysfunction.
Disposable soma Organisms exist to reproduce and then die.	Systematic damage theories: Immune system failure Failure of neuroendocrine regulation Failure to adapt
Antagonistic pleiotropy Genes that are essential and advantageous in young people cause damage in older people. Developmental programming Ageing is regulated by genes and damage only begins to occur after development is complete. Neuroendocrine programming Biological clock is regulated by the hypothalamus. Hormone production eventually diminishes and causes changes associated with ageing. Rate of living (live fast, die young). Every person has a fixed metabolic potential that can be affected by lifestyle, also known as metabolic burnout. Genetic programming. Ageing is preprogrammed in genes that might affect germ cell function, cell division, and cell death.	Cellular damage theories caused by free radical damage by reactive oxygen species (ROS), hyperglycaemia causing advanced glycated end products (AGE) and AGE binding to AGE receptors (RAGE). This results in oxidative and inflammatory effects, which are accelerated in diabetes, and/or chronic inflammation caused by inflammatory cytokines and eicosanoids With infection, these can induce oxidant-generating enzymes such as NADPH oxidase and nitric oxide synthase that produce ROS and reactive nitrogen species (RNS) that react with each other to form more potent reactive species that damage DNA and contribute to diseases such as cancer by activating oncogenes and/or suppressing tumour suppressor proteins.
	Damage to cell membranes
	Somatic mutations
	Failure of repair processes

Note: Currently there is no general agreement about the causes of ageing, but most experts favour cellular damage theories. These seem to apply to uncontrolled diabetes where similar theories are proposed for the development of diabetes complications. See Chapter 8.

- Learn something new every day.
- Contribute to society.

Strategies to maintain wellness include:

- Counsel and support the individual to reduce risk factors that accelerate ageing such as smoking, obesity, hypertension, and diabetes.
- Improve micronutrient deficiencies and use antioxidant supplements based on the Ames hypothesis that an adaptive triage process occurs in the body when micronutrients are scarce that favours short-term survival over long-term and health-energy pathways are favoured over DNA repair (Ames 2006).
- Anti-ageing strategies include the following:
  - Ensure optimal nutrition that includes adequate calories essential amino acids, fats and micronutrients.
  - Include anti-ageing nutrient supplements to reduce inflammation and oxidative stress such as superoxide dismutase (SOD), coQ10, ginkgo, ginseng, brahmi.
  - Consider hormones such as melatonin.
  - Include medicines to improve insulin sensitivity, vasodilators, and mind stimulants.
  - Keep physically active.
  - Keep mentally active, e.g. brain training.
- Under research: gene therapy, therapeutic cloning, cell therapy, nanotechnology (Grossman 2005).

Advancing age is associated with glucose intolerance, changes in renal function which alter medicine pharmacodynamics and pharmacokinetics, reduced sense of smell, hearing, sight, mobility, reduced muscle mass, and changed cognitive functioning, all of which increase the individual's vulnerability to ill health. Significantly, chronological age is not the most important factor to consider when deciding management options. The functional status and biological age are more important determinants of care. Some of the particular problems encountered in older people are shown in Table 12.2. It is important to realise that older people in hospital or living in aged-care facilities do not represent the majority of older individuals living in the community (Australian Institute of Health and Welfare [AIHW] 2002).

Table 12.2   Particular care issues encountered in older people with diabetes and the resultant risks associated with the issue. Individuals are likely to have more than one of these conditions and or other geriatric syndromes. Most of these conditions affect activities of daily living (ADL) and extended ADL. They represent a cumulative health burden and almost all represent a falls risk and many contribute to or complicate delirium and depression and increase the risk of driving accidents and death.

Health issue	Associated risk
The type of diabetes the person has, T1DM or T2DM, is not always clearly document or accessible in health records, especially in aged-care facilities.	• Inappropriate management of T1DM, leading to diabetic ketoacidosis (DKA). • Missed diagnosis of T1DM in older people.
Hyperglycaemia leading to:	• Overtreatment or complex medicine regimes and polypharmacy • Incontinence • Constipation • Postural hypotension • Dehydration and electrolyte imbalance • Polyuria and nocturia, which may present as urinary incontinence • Hyperosmolar hyperglycaemic states (HHS) and diabetic ketoacidosis (DKA) • Impaired cognition • Thrombosis • Infection, e.g. UTI, foot infections, pneumonia, periodontal disease • Impaired wound healing • Postural hypotension • Decreased pain threshold • Exacerbated neuropathic pain • Lowered mood, lethargy, compromised self-care • Driving deficits • Falls
Chewing problems and swallowing difficulties, low appetite	• Undernutrition • Difficulty swallowing oral medicines – the dose form may need to be changed. • Hypoglycaemia and its risks, such as falls and cardiovascular events • Gagging and choking
Nutritional deficiencies:	• Impaired immune response • Infection risk • Decreased plasma protein and anaemia • Compromised fluid intake, dehydration, and electrolyte changes, contributing to confusion, delirium, and falls • Impaired wound healing: • Higher fat intake • Sarcopenia and frailty, muscle wasting, and reduced strength in the lower limbs, which affect ADLs • Increased risk of systemic diseases such as cancer and cardiovascular diseases • Driving deficits • Inappropriate fluid and nutrition replacement at end of life that increases risks • Energy deficits • Increased morbidity and mortality • Falls

Table 12.2   (Continued)

Health issue	Associated risk
Cerebral insufficiency	• Stroke • Nonrecognition of hypoglycaemia (hypoglycaemic unawareness (Chapter 6) • Trauma • Impaired cognition • TIAs being confused with hypoglycaemia • Increased prevalence of vascular dementia (VD), Alzheimer's disease (AD), and other dementias • Falls • Driving deficits
Cardiac insufficiency	• Myocardial infarction, often with atypical pain • Confusion • Poor wound healing • Poor peripheral circulation affects uptake of subcutaneous medicines such as insulin and glucagon and affects medicine distribution to peripheral tissues. • Foot ulcers • Driving deficits • Falls
Autonomic neuropathy	• Postural hypotension • Gustatory sweating • Urinary tract infections and incontinence • Unrecognised hypoglycaemia • Silent myocardial infarction • Decreased/delayed food and medicine absorption and glycaemic variability if the gastrointestinal tract is affected • Poor nutrition • Infections, pain • Decreased motor skills • Erectile dysfunction • Driving deficits • Falls
Peripheral insufficiency	• Trauma • Foot/leg ulcers that can become infected and painful • Claudication • Falls
Peripheral neuropathy	• Unstable gait • Foot ulcers • Pain • Depression • Driving deficits • Falls
Other neuropathies such as Bell's palsy	• Reduced self-care • Loss of independence • Body image changes
Vision	• Self-care deficits, e.g. blood glucose monitoring, managing medicines, shopping • Reading • Falls risk • Driving
Sarcopenia and frailty	• Reduced physical reserve. • People over age 60 have three times the risk of frailty. • T2DM has been describe as a 'frail phenotype'. • People are often malnourished and have low cholesterol and serum albumin, weight loss, and low HbA1c. They are at high risk of falls and trauma. • Frailty predicts death.

(Continued)

Table 12.2   (Continued)

Health issue	Associated risk
Changed colour perception (red, blue, green, violet)	• Depression • Loss of independence • Social isolation • Education difficulties with types of materials used and, differentiating medications • Driving deficits
Skin atrophy	• Can be due to incontinence and can lead to pressure ulcers, skin tears • Infection • Progression of acute wounds to chronic wounds • Stress and depression • Oedema
Communication problems	• Misunderstanding • Confusion • Inaccurate self-care • Stress • Social isolation
Stress and depression	• Inadequate self-care • Hypertension • Hyperglycaemia • Hypoglycaemia • Impacts on wound healing • Driving deficits • Suicide risk • Falls
Renal disease associated with diabetes and normal age-related renal changes	• Decreased medicine clearance and prolonged activity • End-stage renal disease requiring dialysis • Difficulty interpreting investigative blood tests • Malnutrition • Reduced choice of GLM • Dehydration • Hyperosmolar coma • Lactic acidosis • Driving deficits • Falls
Failure to recognise thirst (normal ageing process)	• Dehydration • Hyperglycaemia • Confusion and delirium • Driving deficits • Falls
Cognitive impairment and dementia	• Self-care deficits, including managing medicines • Education difficulties • Reduced quality of life • Incontinence • Falls • Driving deficits
Musculoskeletal disorders such as Dupytren's contracture, cherioarthropathy, flexor tenosynovitis, carpal tunnel syndrome Osteoporosis (Chapter 10)	• Difficulty performing ADL • Pain and discomfort • Driving deficits • Falls

The Victoria Department of Health and Human Services (2013) identified nine guidelines for maintaining functional status:

(1) Optimise nutrition.
(2) Increase functional mobility including in hospital and aged-care homes.
(3) Preserve skin integrity.
(4) Reduce incontinence.
(5) Avoid and reduce the incidence of falls.
(6) Detect and manage cognitive changes (which can be associated with hyper- and hypoglycaemia), delirium. and dementia.
(7) Reduce medicine-related risks and maximising the benefits.
(8) Support and maintain self-care.
(9) Detect and manage depression.

It is essential that relevant services are available and that they function optimally and the health and well-being of carers is addressed. Integrated multidisciplinary health professional care is essential and that carers receive appropriate education and support to deliver quality care to older people with diabetes. Clinicians need to understand that atypical presentation of many illnesses is common in older people, including presentation of diabetes, hypo- and hyperglycaemia, and infections. Guidelines such as ADA (2019), ADS (2012), IDF (2013), Dunning et al. (2013), and position statements (Sinclair et al. 2012) make similar but stronger recommendations about individualising target ranges to avoid hypoglycaemia and significant hyperglycaemia.

Many illnesses present with atypical symptoms, which can delay appropriate diagnosis and management and result in death or significant morbidities and geriatric syndromes:

- Hypoglycaemia can present as a 'behaviour problem' because neuroglycopenic symptoms are more common in older people.
- Failure to thrive.
- Immobility.
- Postural instability.
- Incontinence.
- Confusion and delirium.
- Depression.
- Fatigue and lethargy.
- Weight loss.
- Undetected/untreated hyperglycaemia and LADA (Chapter 1) can be present in older people without diabetes and can be triggered by an intercurrent illness, a diabetes complication or emotional stress, and present as:
  ○ Constipation
  ○ Dehydration
  ○ Postural hypotension
  ○ Confusion
  ○ Polyuria or urinary incontinence
  ○ Infections such as urinary and upper respiratory tract infections (UTIs and URTIs)

Older people with diabetes usually have multiple health problems, some of which are the result of diabetes-related complications and are present at diagnosis in >20% of people (Kilvert and Fox 2017). Thus, actively and regularly screening older people for diabetes and its complications in hospital and aged-care facilities is warranted. Bayliss et al. (2007) found an average of 8.7 chronic diseases present per person in a cross-sectional survey of people aged >65 years. Compared with people without diabetes, older people have a 9% mortality rate, 40% more lower-leg complications (claudication, cellulitis), double the risk of cardiovascular disease including heart failure, double the risk of end-stage renal disease, and are 60% more likely to have vision problems (Kirkman et al. 2012). They are also at greater risk of falling, especially in hospital and aged-care facilities.

Managing diabetes, its complications, and other comorbid diseases requires multiple medicines, and often several doses per medicine per day. Many commonly used laboratory tests have lower specificity and sensitivity in older people, which can further complicate the clinical picture and clinical decision-making. For example, serum creatinine may not detect renal impairment especially in normal weight or underweight individuals (Giannelli et al. 2007; Howes 2001) and contraindicated medicines may not be stopped.

Fasting blood glucose may not be an appropriate screening test for older people, even though blood glucose levels increase with age. Loss of the first-phase insulin response means older people with normal fasting glucose can have high post prandial blood glucose levels that require treatment (Abdo and Flack 2012). Likewise, HbA1c <7% (53 mmol/mol) increases the risk of hypoglycaemia and its consequences. HbA1c > 10% (86 mmol/mol) has significant physiological effects as well as effects on neutrophil function and wound healing (Shekelle and Vijan 2007). Thus, the risks and benefits for the individual need to be considered when interpreting clinical assessments and laboratory data.

Evidence for ideal HbA1c target ranges in older people is limited, apart from the UKPDS (1998), which focused on preventing long-term complications rather than safety and maximising function. The Australian Diabetes Educators Association (ADEA) (2003) proposed targets based on a systematic review; however, the ADEA targets were not intended for older people in aged care facilities. Brown et al. (2003) and ADA (2019) recommend HbA1c < 7% (53 mmol/mol) for most older people; and <8% (84 mmol/mol) in frail older people because preventing the short-term consequences of hypo- and hyperglycaemia and their associated symptoms and risks to safety and quality of life (QoL), might be more important than preventing long-term complications.

Most diabetes-related guidelines published in the last four years recommend HbA1c 7–7.5% (53–58 mmol/mol) in general, but stress the need to individualise glycaemic targets, and recommend HbA1c ~8% in frail older people (Sinclair et al. 2012, Australian Diabetes Society (ADS) 2012; Dunning et al. 2013, ADA 2019). However, management also depends on the individual's functional status, risk profile, QoL, and life expectancy.

Interestingly, despite the association amongst obesity, morbidity, and mortality (Hu et al. 2004; Chen et al. 2008; Masters et al. 2013), being overweight is associated with longer life expectancy in men and women >80 years and underweight is associated with shorter life expectancy, even when other comorbidities are present (Takata et al. 2007). Weight loss is associated with total mortality in older people, independently of low body weight (Keller et al. 2004). These findings suggest recommending older overweight people lose weight may actually put them at risk.

Determining functional status

Functional ability refers to an individual's ability to perform ADL. There are two main types of ADL: physical activities of daily living (PADL) that encompasses essential daily activities such as bathing and dressing; and instrumental activities of daily living (IADL), which enable the individual to live independently in society and are more complex (Kock and Garratt 2001). IADL assessment must be based on activities relevant to the individual and take account of their physical surroundings, culture, and interests. For example, assessing an older person when they are in hospital and their blood glucose levels are in the optimal range may not accurately reflect their ADL and adverse event risk level at home (Dunning and Alford 1993). Significantly, older people with diabetes have more functional impairment than age- and gender-matched controls in the same community (Sinclair et al. 2008) as well as cognitive impairment that affects self-care capacity.

Older people in hospital and care facilities are a vulnerable group, and the latter often receive suboptimal care (Kirkland 2003). Sinclair et al. (1997) and Sinclair et al. (2015) found 40% of residents in aged-care facilities were on long-acting sulphonylureas: fewer than 1 in 10 had any regular diabetes follow-up, they had more hospital admissions than people without diabetes, stayed in hospital longer and had more complications. In addition, staff and resident knowledge about diabetes was deficient. Likewise, functional decline occurs in 30–50% of older people during hospitalisation and ~30% >70 years return home with ADL deficits (Royal Melbourne Hospital 2002). Functional decline is associated with long duration of hospitalisation and manifests gradually as malnutrition, reduced mobility, compromised skin integrity, incontinence, falls, delirium, depression, geriatric syndromes, and inadequate self-care. That is, gradual reduction of physical and mental reserves.

The degree of disability is likely to change over time, sometimes rapidly, and during illness, and affect the amount of assistance the individual needs, either on a temporary basis or in the longer term. Changing circumstances often have financial implications for the individual and the health system. Table 12.3 suggests some issues to explore to help decide the level of assistance needed and appropriate management. In addition, relevant assessment tools, geomaps, and ecomaps can provide a great deal of information about the individual's social network (social reserves) and relationships; see Chapter 2.

Annual diabetes complication screening/comprehensive health assessments should encompass screening for hypo- and hyperglycaemia risk, depression, comorbidities, falls risk, incontinence, pain and memory deficits, degree of frailty, functional status including driving ability, a structured

Table 12.3 Key issues that need to be considered when assessing functional ability in older people with diabetes.

Issues	Implications
What is the person's explanatory model for diabetes, and what are their values, goals, and preferences?	These are essential aspects of the person's story and affect care decisions.
What activities are limited and to what degree?	A precise description of the disability is important in order to plan appropriate medical and nursing care and evaluate outcomes.
Which disease processes are causing the disability?	Attributing disability to 'old age' is not an appropriate diagnosis. Common causes of disability include arthritis, cardiovascular disease, respiratory disease, frailty, stroke, and vision impairment. One or more of these comorbidities often coexist with diabetes. Polypharmacy is likely. In some cases, the medicine of choice for some comorbidities increases blood glucose levels. Medicine interactions are possible, and the person might be using self-prescribed and complementary medicines. What is their life expectancy?
What is the person's mental state? Various assessment tools are used to assess mental status, for example the Mini-Mental; however, their limitations need to be considered.	Evidence of memory loss, disorientation, confused behaviour and personality change may indicate diseases of the brain, dementia states or metabolic changes such as high or low blood glucose levels that impair mental processing. Consideration should also be given to the presence of anxiety, depression, and the individual's general mental approach to life (positive or pessimistic) and hearing deficits.
What is the person's social situation? See Figure 2.1.	Disability implies dependence on others. It is important to identify the services and people likely to be able to support the individual if they do require help. In addition, it is important to ensure the person who takes on the care is supported and their personal health and well-being considered preventing stress, sleep disturbance, and ill health in the carer, especially if they are also old.

Note: Repeat measures may be needed, especially during acute illnesses when the physical and mental condition can change rapidly. These issues should be considered as part of the standard diabetes complication screening process. (Dunning and Manias 2005]).

medicines review and general health needs such as vaccinations and cancer screening programmes. Many annual review programmes currently do not encompass all these issues. Ideally, a comprehensive assessment should be undertaken at every change in health status, hospital, aged-care home admission, or adverse event.

Determining the frailty level helps identify older people likely to suffer adverse health effects (Kulminski et al. 2007; Abdelhafiz and Sinclair 2015). Frailty is a consequence of declining physical reserve and altered functioning in multiple physiological systems, which make the individual vulnerable to physical and mental stressors (Bortz 2002; Fried et al. 2004; Abdelhafiz and Sinclair 2015). It is common, occurring in 20% of people >age 70 and 50% aged 80 and older (English and Padden-Jones 2010). Frailty is complex and not fully explained. Several definitions of frailty exist including the following:

> The frailty state can be described using a cumulative index of health and well-being deficiencies that is assessable for each individual … the fraction of deficits in a list of items that measure health and well-being [constitutes the frailty index (FI)]
>
> (Kulminski et al. 2007)

It is a distinctive state of health where body systems progressively decline and is related to ageing (Smith and Kydd 2017). Some experts suggest the degree of frailty could be a measure of healthy/ unhealthy ageing. The British Geriatric Society (2014) recommended older people should have a frailty assessment at all health-care consultations to help consider the benefits and risks of management options and the individual's safety. Frailty is often the result of sarcopenia, which is associated with loss of muscle mass and reducing muscle strength, which affects factors such as hand grip strength and balance and walking speed (Choi 2016). Not all frail older people are thin, although ageing is associated with loss of muscle mass and increase in visceral fat. The recent concept of sarcopenic obesity emerged and highlights the role of reducing muscle mass and strength in cardio-metabolic mortality, given that sarcopenia is associated with insulin resistance (Choi 2016).

A number of methods of estimating frailty are used. The most useful enable clinicians to use health information already collected to predict whether older people are at risk of adverse health outcomes and proactively plan preventative care. Various anthropometric measures are used in research. Biochemical estimates include low serum albumin and low cholesterol (Mehta et al. 2011).

There are more than 25 tools for measuring frailty: each has advantages and disadvantages and has varying degrees of complexity (Cruz-Jentoft et al. 2018). These tools include:

- Rockwood Accumulative Index
- Frail Scale
- Fried Phenotype
- Comprehensive Geriatric Assessment
- Jen Frailty Index SARC F
- TUG – timed up and go and chair stand
- Grip strength
- Gait speed

Clinically useful measures are hand-grip strength and Short Physical Performance Battery (SPPB); usual gait speed is part of the SPPB, and TUG indicates the time needed to accomplish a series of critical functional tasks.

Geriatric syndromes

The term *geriatric syndromes* refers to commonly occurring comorbidities in older people that make managing diabetes and the associated syndromes complex and challenging. They often include or coexist with frailty. The American Geriatrics Society (2013) described six commonly occurring geriatric syndromes:

- Polypharmacy; see Chapter 5.
- Depression; see Chapter 15 and this chapter.
- Cognitive impairment.
- Urinary incontinence.
- Injurious falls.
- Pain.

Other authors include delirium, renal disease, cardiovascular disease, infections, and frailty. As indicated, all of the coexisting comorbidities need to be identified and adequately treated as part of integrated, individualised care – not as silo conditions.

Cognitive functioning and dementia

Glucose is the main metabolic fuel for the brain; it uses 25% of total body glucose utilisation, and stable blood glucose levels are critical for normal brain function. Type 2 diabetes doubles the risk of dementia in older age and is associated with lower brain volume, decline in executive function, processing speed, verbal fluency and memory (Callisaya et al. 2018). Dementia is a growing health problem, yet the diagnosis is often missed or delayed (Bradford et al. 2009). Factors that contribute to missed/delayed diagnosis include dementia severity, degree of impairment, and frequency of interaction with primary care providers. Other significant reasons include attitudes towards dementia, person clinician communication, education deficits, and resource constraints (Bradford et al. 2009).

Huang et al. (2018) suggested adolescent boys who find it difficult to understand how basic machines work and girls who find it difficult to remember words are at increased risk of dementia: a 17% risk at age 70 for boys and girls with lower memory for words were at increased risk of neurodegenerative disease. The mechanisms may be unclear but the study highlights that risk in early life affect the life course. Thus, it is important to preserve cognitive reserve and attend to modifiable risk factors, including education, social support, high insensitivity progressive resistance training, stimulating activities, and engagement as part of a healthy lifestyle.

Nonpathological age-related cognitive changes are a normal part of ageing; however, pronounced, severe cognitive changes may reflect pathological changes such as Alzheimer's disease (AD). However, normal age-related cognitive changes can impair usual functioning such as managing finances, diabetes self-management including medicine self-management, remembering information and medical appointments (Vance 2012). Some researchers suggest cognitive reserve acts as a neurological reservoir that can sustain cognitive functioning during illness, substance abuse, depression, and underlying metabolic abnormalities associated with diabetes (Carmichael et al. 2010).

Cognitive reserve refers to the neuronal connections that organise, store, and transmit information. The strength of the neuronal connections affects the brain's ability to cope with damage before cognitive function is disrupted (Vance et al. 2012). Neuronal connections need to be used to remain efficient. Some experts recommend various 'brain training' activities to maintain/enhance neuronal reserve; however, cognitive reserve is difficult to measure and different factors affect cognitive reserve. Table 12.4 depicts some of the positive and negative factors that affect cognitive reserve.

Cognitive decline in older people with diabetes is multifactorial due to advancing age and vascular dementia (VD) but not other forms of dementia (Allen et al. 2004), hyperglycaemia (Morley and Flood 1990), hypoglycaemia, and increasing duration of diabetes. Large community studies suggest older people with diabetes have worse cognitive functioning than those without diabetes (Croxson 2000; Gregg et al. 2000; Logroscino et al. 2004), and the decline is more rapid in those with diabetes (Biessels et al. 2006). The Framingham Study suggests hypertension and diabetes are independent risk factors for poor performance on memory and visual organisation tests (Elias et al. 2005). Asimakopoulou et al. (2002) demonstrated minimal effects on verbal and logical memory when blood glucose control is optimal.

Table 12.4   Positive and negative factors that affect cognitive reserve.

Factors that contribute to positive neuroplasticity and enhance cognitive reserve	Factors that contribute to negative neuroplasticity and reduce cognitive reserve
Mental stimulation and cognitive-enhancing activates (use it or lose it)	Low education and health literacy level. Low health literacy predicts mortality (Bostock and Steptoe 2012) and compromises participation in activities that enhance cognition
Positive thinking, spirituality, and resilience	Mood disorders, including depression, which are associated with negative thinking and compromised resilience
Healthy diet	Inadequate nutrition (similarly muscle reserve protects older people from sarcopenia)
Optimal health status	Health status, e.g. cardiovascular risk factors, are associated with faster cognitive decline in older people (Dregan et al. 2012), and there is an association between higher Framingham risk score and worse cognitive functioning (Kaffashian et al. 2011).
Regular physical activity	Inactivity
Using few medicines and avoiding medicines and addictive substances that affect cognition	Some prescribed medicines as well as alcohol and drug abuse and smoking
Social engagement and stimulation	Social isolation
Regular dental care	Recent research suggests gum disease is associated with Alzheimer's disease (AD) due to *Porphyromonas gingivalis*, a bacteria involved in gum disease. It has been found in the cerebral cortex and other parts of the brain in people with Alzheimer's, including in amyloid and tau (MacKenzie 2019).

Note: Good cognitive reserve protects against age-related cognitive changes. The theory supports the need for and importance of proactive, lifelong optimal health-related self-care and regular comprehensive physical, spiritual, and mental assessments.

Older people with dementia have more hospital admissions, comorbidities, and mortality than those without dementia (Zuliani 2012). People with dementia in Zuliani's study (50 000 admissions and data collected over six years) had high rates of cardiovascular disease, pneumonia, and hip fractures. Dementia was associated with secondary diagnoses such as delirium, immobility, dehydration, and pressure ulcers. These findings might be expected, but they could also suggest some admissions could be prevented by optimal assessment and proactive, preventative care planning (Sinclair et al. 2014).

During acute illnesses, it is important to differentiate cognitive changes associated with hypoglycaemia, hyperglycaemia, and hyperosmolar states, delirium, MI, and other more permanent causes. Delirium is often missed and is associated with:

- Prolonged hospitalisation, poor outcomes, and admission to aged-care facilities
- Functional decline
- Increased use of chemical and other restraints that increase the risk of falls and may increase delirium
- Presence of infection, which can precipitate hyperosmolar states
- Multiple comorbidities (geriatric syndromes)
- Severe illness
- Dehydration, which can precipitate hyperosmolar states and may lead to a diagnosis of diabetes in undiagnosed at risk individuals (Chapter 7)
- Alcohol abuse
- Falls and fractures
- Prescribed psychotropic medications

Delirium, but not the severity, can be distinguished from nonreversible cognitive impairment using the Confusion Assessment Method (CAM) (Waszynski 2004); also see Table 12.5. The CAM

Table 12.5 Some of the presenting feature of dementia, delirium, and depression.

Parameter	Dementia	Delirium	Depression
Onset	Usually slow and progressive, occurring over years.	Usually occurs over hours or days.	May be sudden and often occurs during significant life transitions, such as death of a loved one and admission into an aged-care home. Changes persist for at least two weeks.
Course	Symptoms are irreversible and gradually progress over time.	The course is usually short, and cognitive changes may fluctuate over the day and may be worse at night. Once the underlying cause/s is/are identified and treated, symptoms usually abate to the individual's predelirium state.	Usually worse in the morning but could be seasonal (see Chapter 15). Usually improves with treatment (nonmedicine options and medicines as a last resort).
Duration	Depends on the type of dementia present; time varies from months to several years.	Usually less than four weeks.	Time varies from weeks to years.
Cognition	Person is generally alert.	Cognition varies from lethargic to hyperactive.	Normal, but person may be apathetic.
(1) Alertness	Usually normal in the early stages.	Depends on the degree of delirium.	Depends on interest and severity of the depression.
(2) Attention span	Individuals often have difficulty finding words and remembering and recalling people, and events.	Individuals have difficulty organising thoughts.	
(3) Thinking		Several types of delirium are described:	Thinking is usually intact but can be disordered.
	Difficulty learning new information.	• Hyperactive (agitation, restlessness, hallucinations).	
	Person may wander, become agitated, especially in the afternoon (Sundowner's syndrome) or withdrawn and may have coexisting depression.	• Hypoactive (person may be sleepy, difficult to rouse).	Person may show disinterest in activities and usual activities.
		• Mixed (combination of hyper- and hypoactive symptoms).	Individual may be withdrawn.
	Multiple cognitive deficits may be present.		Appetite often changes.
Mood	May be associated with depression.	Mood changes: may be angry, afraid, tearful.	
Commonly used screening and diagnostic tools[a]	• Mini-Mental Status Exam (Folstein). • Clock Drawing Test. • Mini-Co Dementia Screen. • Cohen-Mansfield Agitation Inventory (CMAI) if behavioural issues are present.	• Confusion Assessment Method (CAM). • IWATCH DEATH (Infections, **W**ithdrawal, **A**cute metabolic, **T**oxins, drugs **C**NS pathology, **H**ypoxia, **D**eficiencies, **E**ndocrine, **A**cute vascular, **T**rauma, **H**eavy metals.	• Geriatric Depression Scale (GDS) and the GDS Short Form. • Cornell Scale for Depression. • Patient Health Questionnaire (PHQ) and PHQ-2. • Whooley Depression Screen. • SIG ECAPS (DSM-1 V criteria.
Laboratory investigations	TSH, electrolytes, Ca. Blood glucose and ketones. PET scan to identify changes in relevant parts of the brain associated with memory, executive function.	Na, K+, Na, Ca, urea and electrolytes, creatinine, liver function tests, Hb, white cell count (which can be elevated in hyperglycaemia without indicating infection) Blood glucose and ketones. Oxygen saturation, blood gases, urinalysis, and culture. Alcohol/drug screen. Chest X-ray.	TSH, vitamin B_{12}, folate, ferritin, iron, K+, Hb, ESR, albumin, full blood count

[a] See Chapter 15 for commonly used diabetes-specific tools to identify diabetes-related distress.

has concurrent validity with the Mini-Mental State Examination (MMSE) but has not been tested in clinical settings and is associated with a 10% false-positive rate. The key aspects of the CAM are shown in the following list. A diagnosis of delirium is made if 1 and 2 and either 3 or 4 are present:

(1) Acute onset and fluctuating course during the day;
(2) Inattention such as being easily distracted and finding it difficult to recall what was said last;
(3) Disorganised thinking and unpredictable switching from topic-to-topic;
(4) Altered consciousness (Inouye et al. 1990; Waszynski 2004).

Recognising cognitive decline

The following strategies can slow cognitive decline and enhance mental health:

- Use appropriate, inclusive respectful language when discussing dementia and in conversations with individual's with dementia and their families (Dementia Australia 2018).
- Determine and monitor cognitive status as part of diabetes complication screening programmes, e.g. language, planning, problem-solving. Incorporate ADL assessment such as Barthel Index and the 'Get up and Go' test; and cognitive assessment such as MMSE, the Clock test and screen for depression using tools such as the Geriatric Depression Score (Sinclair 2011).
- Regularly screen for diabetes-related complications that can impair cognitive function such as cardiovascular disease (American Diabetes Association 2013).
- Establish individuals' risk of low cognitive reserve, delirium and depression, and the presence of geriatric syndromes.
- Make an accurate diagnosis, which might require referral to a geriatrician and/or psychiatrist. Make an accurate diagnosis includes differentiating between the '3Ds' dementia, delirium, and depression. Be aware that hypoglycaemic symptoms in older people are predominantly neurological and can be mistaken for delirium.
- Develop an appropriate care plan to manage the condition, which might include behavioural or psychosocial interventions and 'brain training'. Involve older people in group diabetes education programmes and diabetes self-care activities to the level of their ability, which can improve glycaemic control (Beverly et al. 2012). In aged-care homes, consider how the environment could affect mental health and well-being positively or negatively, including disrupting sleep.
- Manage diabetes by individualising management targets and medicine use and avoiding polypharmacy when possible.
- Undertake a comprehensive medicine review and, where possible, stop medicines that affect cognitive functioning. These include medicines prescribed to manage 'behaviours of concern' and sliding scales of insulin (American Geriatrics Society 2019). Consider medicine contraindications and interactions and ask about herbal medicine use.
- Manage pain.

Practice point

Poor blood glucose control is associated with reduced cognitive functioning and problem-solving and planning skills. Cognition sometimes improves when the blood glucose pattern improves (Gradman et al. 1993). Screening for cognitive impairment can be incorporated into the diabetes management plan using screening tools such as the MMSE and the results used to plan diabetes education strategies (Sinclair 1995).

Dehydration

Fluid balance disturbances are common in older people, largely as a result of changes in body water composition, declining renal function, and reduced thirst perception. Dehydration is common in community dwelling older people (Warren et al. 1994) occurring in ~6.7% of those >65 years in hospital and is the principal diagnosis in 1.4% (Warren et al. 1994). Dehydration is present in 50% of residents in aged-care facilities with a febrile illness who are often referred to hospital due to dehydration (Bourdel-Marchasson et al. 2004). Dehydration should be preventable in hospital and aged-care facilities. Management guidelines should encompass strategies to do so considering the following information.

Dehydration is associated with hyperglycaemia and diabetic ketoacidosis (DKA) and hyperosmolar hyperglycaemic states (HHS) (see Chapter 7), poor mental functioning, thromboembolism, infections, renal calculi, falls, and constipation, and it causes up to 50% mortality if it is not adequately managed (Wilson and Morley 2003; Faes et al. 2007). Early diagnosis is difficult because of the atypical presentation in older people and because there is no absolute definition of dehydration (Weinberg et al. 1995). A commonly used definition is:

> … a clinically relevant decrease of an individual's optimal Total Body Water (TBW) amount and may occur with or without loss of electrolytes. (Faes et al. 2007)

Thus, the degree of dehydration depends on the relative rather than the actual total intracellular and extracellular water loss. People with low body weight show signs of dehydration after losing small amounts of water. Significantly, ~25% of older people drink <1 l of fluid per day, especially those over 85 (Volkert et al. 2005). Risk factors for dehydration include:

- Age over 85 years
- Female
- Having ≥ chronic diseases
- Using ≥5 medicines
- Medicine-related factors such as high protein oral or enteral feeds, laxatives, antidepressants, and diuretics
- Fasting for surgery or investigative procedures
- Hyperglycaemia and the associated fluid loss such as urinary incontinence, diarrhoea, vomiting
- Being confined to bed/chair
- Poor mobility including manual dexterity
- Poor eye–hand coordination
- Communication difficulties
- Inability to feed themselves
- Social isolation
- Hot weather
- Having AD and other cognitive disturbances (Lavizzo-Mourey et al. 1988)

The diagnosis is made on clinical signs such as recent weight loss >3% body weight, presence of an intercurrent illness, dry mucous membranes, coated tongue, sunken eyes, confusion, hypotension, muscle weakness in the upper body, and falls. Laboratory investigations such as serum osmolality, creatinine, blood urea nitrogen (BUN), BUN/creatinine ratio, and electrolytes as well as urine pH and output are useful. Three forms of dehydration occur:

(1) Hypertonic: sodium >150 mmol/l or serum osmolality >300 mosmol/l.
(2) Isotonic dehydration occurs when water and electrolyte loss are balanced, for example, diarrhoea and vomiting.
(3) Hypotonic dehydration results when electrolyte loss is greater than water loss, e.g. overuse of diuretics.

The prevalence of the isotonic and hypotonic dehydration has not been studied systematically and may be underrecognised. Having a high level of suspicion and care strategies to ensure optimal fluid intake such as prompting older people to drink are important preventative measures. Specific treatment depends on the clinical assessment and may include IV fluid replacement, preventing venous stasis, pressure ulcers, and falls, as well as managing the underlying cause and uncontrolled hyperglycaemia. Care must be taken not to overhydrate the individual and cause cerebral oedema or water intoxication.

Depression and older people with diabetes

Given the increasing prevalence of diabetes in older people, the fact that depression is a risk factor for diabetes, and the twofold increased risk of depression in people with diabetes (Bogner et al. 2007), it is likely that many older people have undetected diabetes as well as undetected depression, which is a concern given that depression in older people is treatable in 65–75% of people (Ragan and Kane 2010). Undiagnosed depression contributes to physical and mental functional impairment and is a known risk factor for suicide (Cahoon 2012). Older people with depression require higher levels of informal care, even after adjusting for other comorbidities, and place a significant burden on family caregivers (Langa 2004). Managing depression reduces depression-related caregiver burden (Martire 2010).

Depression frequently precedes and may be the factor that leads to admission to an aged care facility. Depression may be due to grief over loss of functional and self-care ability and independence (Fleming 2002) and is significantly correlated with QoL (Goldney et al. 2004). Depression is often associated with diabetes-related complications such as cardiovascular disease (Fenton and Stover 2006; Cahoon 2012), diabetes (Verma et al. 2010), chronic pain, and unhealthy diet. Depression is more likely to be recurrent in older people (Cluning 2001) and leads to inadequate self-care, unstable blood glucose patterns, and affects cognitive functioning. Comorbidities need to comprehensively evaluated because when one comorbidity worsens, others also worsen, and if all comorbidities are not detected, then treatment could be ineffective (Cahoon 2012). Treating depression in older people reduces mortality by 50% (Bogner et al. 2007).

Commonly used depression screening tools are shown in Table 12.5. Some clinical indicators of depression in older people are:

- Constantly talking about physical symptoms and believing they have a serious illness (Cluning 2001)
- Grief over loss and lost opportunities, abilities, and self-determination
- Withdrawing from communal activities
- Experiencing chronic pain
- Having had a stroke or cardiovascular event
- Not receiving any visitors at least once a week in hospital and aged-care facilities
- Difficulty establishing relationships with staff and other aged-care residents in the first four weeks after admission

Depression management is discussed in Chapter 15. When possible, nonpharmacological options should be used first.

Dementia

The prevalence of dementia increases with age and ranges from 63% to 81% (Zimmerman et al. 2007). Approximately one in four Australians over age 85 have dementia (Gray et al. 2002). There are two main forms of dementia: AD accounting for 70% of known dementias and VD accounting for the remaining 20%. Both AD and VD are present in ~20% of people, especially those with diabetes (Stewart and Liolitsa 1999). The association between diabetes and dementia may be due to:

- Cardiovascular disease: Transient ischemic attacks (TIAs) and stroke can cause multifocal brain damage.
- Hypoglycaemia, especially if it is frequent and recurrent, may cause permanent neuronal destruction.
- Persistent hyperglycaemia increases protein glycosylation and contributes to the development of advanced contributes to advanced glycated end products (AGE) (see Chapter 8) found in AD plaques (Phillips and Popplewell 2002).

Nay and Garrat (1999) outlined three main stages of AD. The first is characterised by absent-mindedness, emotional instability, and poor concentration. These symptoms can include spatial disorientation, disturbed perception, changes in personal appearance and hygiene, a tendency to blame others for a range of occurrences, and an inability to successfully perform ADLs. Depression is often present in the early stages because the person is aware that something is 'not quite right' and they realise 'things are slipping away' from them (Katona 1994).

Stage two lasts up to 12 years. The person may withdraw, and behaviour is often variable, including anger, transient crying, poor sleep patterns, disorientation, and profound short-term memory loss. Gait often changes, people have difficulty recognising their own face in a mirror, and continence issues emerge, as well as other behaviours such as exhibitionism. The person cannot live safely by themselves in the community.

Stage three is often the shortest, lasting up to two years. Profound physical and cognitive decline occurs, finally resulting in stupor and coma. Depression, delirium, and dementia can occur concomitantly and have cumulative and compounding effects on physical and mental functioning. It can be difficult to differentiate amongst the three states: Table 12.5 compares some of the features to help differentiate amongst them to ensure treatment is timely and appropriate; refer to Table 12.5, which outlines some differences amongst dementia, delirium, and depression.

Caring for older people with diabetes

Age, life expectancy, other health problems, and the person's social situation should be considered when planning care. Achieving near-normal blood glucose levels and preventing long-term complications may not be priority management aims. It is important to control uncomfortable symptoms (polyuria, polydipsia, lethargy), maintain QoL and wellbeing and minimise the risk of hypoglycaemia and the attendant risk of falling.

Suboptimal metabolic control is associated with urinary incontinence, leg/foot ulcers, infections, nutritional deficiencies, exacerbates neuropathic pain, affects communication and cause confusion and aggression (Kirkland 2003). Strategies and care priorities need to be implemented using a stepwise approach and nonpharmacological measures where possible. Planning should include planning for end of life care (Chapter 18). The individual should be involved in planning their care, whenever possible.

Management aims

Caring for older people is complicated and diabetes adds to the complexity. Various models of care exist biased on the chronic disease model and the governments of some countries are introducing policies and service models to cope with the ageing population and the increasing prevalence of diabetes, for example, supporting people to remain living at home for longer (e.g. Department of Health 2003; Department of Health and Aging (DOHA) 2012; Victoria Department of Health and Human Services 2013).

Other strategies include geriatric evaluation units (GEM) in hospitals, which provide comprehensive assessment and plan care with the individual and their families/carers to support community-dwelling older people remain independent and self-caring for as long as possible. Older people managed in GEM units spend less time in hospital, are discharged taking fewer medicines, and have better outcomes (Verschoor 2012).

The Eden Alternative (https://www.edenalt.org), an innovative to residential aged care, has a philosophical approach that changes the focus in aged-care facilities from medical to creating environments that address common problems people living in aged-care facilities face loneliness, boredom, and helplessness. The Eden Alternative and its derivatives encourage contact with children, companion pets, hobbies, and indoor and outdoor gardens. Benefits include fewer infection and lower medicine use.

The main aims of care are to:

- Provide appropriate care for the diabetes type: T1DM and T2DM.
- Optimise nutrition.
- Prevent hypo- and hyperglycaemia by individualising blood glucose and other target ranges to suit the individual's health and functional status and safety.
- Undertake a structured medication management programme using a quality use of medicine framework, considering the Beers Criteria (American Geriatrics Society 2019) and deprescribing where possible to limit polypharmacy.
- Proactively screen for and prevent and/or manage diabetic complications, comorbidities, depression, and maintain independent self-care as long as possible.
- Undertake general preventative health measure such as vaccinations and health checks, for example, mammograms, prostate checks. Flu vaccine prevents respiratory illnesses, pneumonia, hospital admissions and death in older people (Gross et al. 1995). However, in years without influenza, booster vaccinations may not confer added benefits if routing trivalent vaccination does not produce seroprotection (Gaughran et al. 2007). Research suggests people with chronic diseases are less likely to receive preventative care despite attending health professionals frequently (Lipscombe et al. 2005).
- Manage coexisting illnesses to improve physical and mental functional ability and improve QoL.
- Maintain or enhance a positive attitude (cognitive reserve).
- Maintain a safe environment to limit adverse events such as falls.
- Regularly assess driving safety and help the individual develop and maintain a transportation plan to make the transition to stop driving. Be aware that operating motorised wheelchairs, Go-Fors, and farm machinery may also constitute a driving risk.
- Develop an end-of-life care plan to ensure a comfortable and peaceful death when the time comes.
- Undertake regular diabetes complication screening that includes geriatric syndromes, medicines, and mental health. Such screens may need to be undertaken at any change in physical and mental health status, not just annually.
- Proactively document and communicate an advance care plan, especially before admission to a care home (Chapter 18).

Factors that affect management decisions

- The individual's values, care preferences and life expectancy.
- Age, but age alone may not give an accurate picture of an individual's ability to cope with self-care tasks and ADL. Functional level should be assessed using appropriate tools in an appropriate familiar setting.
- Current diabetes control and complication status, including the presence of liver and kidney disease.
- Presence and severity of comorbidities.
- Life expectancy.

- Mental and physical capacity to self-care.
- Nutritional status. Inadequate nutrition predisposes the person to hypoglycaemia, falls, decreased immunity, delayed wound healing and infections, and other diseases.
- Learning capacity, which is influenced by the individual's learning style, sight, hearing and cognitive ability, interest in the topic, and the way the information is worded (language and designed) as well as the way it is used in conversations with the individual/families, see Chapter 16. Many people, not only older people, do not understand most health information.
- Social support from family and the community. Include strategies to reduce social isolation and loneliness. Pets often play a very important role in the health and well-being of older people and have been shown to prevent suicide (Cohen-Mansfield et al. 2015).
- Financial status and access to services.
- Advanced care plan (Chapter 18).
- Access to care, including using relevant technologies and 'gerontologies' to support independence matched to the person's needs and capabilities (Novak et al. 2009, Haufe et al. 2019) (Chapter 1).

Nutritional management

Older people are often malnourished. Malnourishment is associated with adverse outcomes, and weight change in older people is associated with longer length of stay in hospital and increased mortality (Middleton et al. 2001) and is particularly concerning in frail older people (Devitt 2011). The causes of poor nutrition are shown in Table 12.6. Sometimes it is difficult to distinguish between the effects of malnutrition and disease processes, which are

Table 12.6 Risk factors for inadequate nutrition and malnutrition in older people are mulitfactorial and encompass the factors shown in the table.

Risk factor	Potential outcome
Living in an aged-care home; forced food choices and mealtimes	Loss of control over environment, not eating or reduced eating, unhealthy gut microbiota, depression
	Not being able to reach food and/or feed themselves
	Not being exposed to sunlight, leading to vitamin D deficiency Nutritional deficiencies Weight loss, sarcopenia, and frailty
Diminished hunger sensation, anorexia, dysphagia, mouth pathology	Reduced intake Nutritional deficiencies Weight loss, sarcopenia, and frailty
Malabsorption	Bacterial infections, coeliac disease, medicines, disease processes, and diabetes complications such as gastric autonomic neuropathy, effects on the gut microbiota
Neurological deficits	Stroke, dementia, neuropathy
Medicines	Digitalis, alcohol, sedatives, and metformin, known to affect the absorption of vitamin B_{12}
Sensory deficits	Impaired sight and/or hearing, taste, and smell, communication difficulties
Dentition and swallowing difficulties	Ill-fitting dentures, caries, missing teeth, gum disease, malnutrition Nutritional deficiencies Weight loss, sarcopenia, and frailty
Social circumstances	Isolation, poverty, inability to shop or prepare food, depression, malnutrition
Medical problems	Chronic disease, pneumonia, heart failure, chronic infection, thyroid disease, malnutrition, low immunity

closely related (World Health Organization 1999). Significantly, undernutrition is often underrecognised and underdiagnosed.

It is important to take a broad approach to nutritional assessment and management in older people with diabetes rather than the usual focus on reducing dietary fat and sugar. Energy requirements usually reduce in older people, but they require nutrient-rich foods to ensure essential nutrients are included in the diet. Generally, caloric requirements reduce by 20–30%. Caloric requirements should be individualised according to age, gender, body size and composition, activity, and medicine regimen.

Older people need to be encouraged to:

- Incorporate omega-3 foods into the diet.
- Eat a variety of nutritious foods in at least three meals every day.
- Eat plenty of cereals, wholegrain bread, and pasta, especially those with a low Glycaemic Index; 50–60% of total intake.
- Have adequate protein intake, consisting of at least 15% of the total intake and not <0.8 g/kg/day Protein requirements increase during wound healing and stress conditions such as infections and might decrease in end-stage renal disease.
- Eat plenty of fruits and vegetables to reduce the risk of cardiovascular and degenerative diseases and supply essential vitamins and minerals, such as calcium.
- Have an adequate fluid intake, including water (about 1500 ml/day) to reduce the likelihood of dehydration, especially in hot weather, unless fluid restriction is indicated.
- Drink alcohol in moderation. Because of the reduced muscle mass, the volume in which alcohol is distributed is reduced; therefore, the concentration of circulating alcohol is higher, putting the person at risk of cognitive impairment, hypoglycaemia, and falls. However, moderate consumption of alcohol might have health benefits.
- Use low-salt food and only add small amounts of salt to food to help prevent hypertension (National Health and Medical Research Council 1999).

Practice points

(1) Many older people are malnourished even though they appear overweight. Malnutrition is common: 15% of homebound community dwelling, 35–65% of hospitalised people, and 50% of residential aged care residents (Szony 2004). Malnutrition is associated with longer length of stay in hospital, is a strong predictor of readmission, and is associated with pressure ulcers, delirium, and depression.

(2) There is limited data about the nutritional needs of very old people.

(3) People over the age of 70 have special nutritional needs (Drewnowski and Warren-Mears 2001), especially if they have diabetes.

(4) Enteral feeding and supplements are often required but can affect blood glucose levels unless the formula is carefully selected and the risks and benefits of enteral feeding are carefully considered.

Malnourishment can occur whilst older people are in hospital (McWhirter and Pennington 1994). In care facilities, rates between 36% and 43% are reported (Friedman and Kalant 1998).

Factors that increase risk

Concomitant diseases that increase the risk of malnutrition in older people with diabetes include:

- Psychiatric disorders including depression, see Chapter 15.
- Parkinson's disease.

- Chronic obstructive pulmonary disease.
- Polypharmacy, which is common in diabetes.
- Renal failure.
- Neurological dysfunction.
- Dental problems and chewing and swallowing difficulties. The latter also increases the likelihood that nasogastric or enteral feeding will be needed as well as the risk of coughing and choking during feeding and increases the risk of chest infections. Swallowing difficulties affect ~10% of hospitalised older people (Hudson et al. 2000).
- Disabled house-bound individuals.
- People with cancer or HIV/AIDS.
- At the end stages of life.

Addressing nutritional deficits

Specific nutritional deficits include vitamin D and calcium, which increases the risk of osteoporosis and fractures. Low intake of vitamin K-rich vegetables affects the stability of the INR in people on anticoagulant therapy (Franco et al. 2004). Factors that help maintain optimal nutrition for people over 80 living in the community are supportive family and friends, having a microwave oven, transportation, and proximity to a grocery store (Callan and Wells 2003). The Australian Nutrition Screening Initiative was developed to highlight the importance of identifying older people at risk of malnutrition. The tool can help nurses decide when a comprehensive nutritional assessment is required and refer the individual to a dietitian.

The Hydration Assessment checklist detects hydration problems in older people (Zembrzuski 1997), and the Mini Nutritional assessment (MNA) detects actual and potential malnourishment in people over 65 (Reilly 1996) and may predict mortality in older people (Persson et al. 2002). Other nutrition assessment tools are listed in Chapter 4.

Biochemical assessments include plasma proteins, recognising the concentration can be influenced by non-nutritional factors such as liver disease, some cancers, sepsis, and inflammatory bowel disease. Protein intake can be calculated using the BUN with the serum creatinine. If the creatinine is low, protein intake is low. If both the creatinine and BUN are low, a state of tissue catabolism such as that associated with hyperglycaemia, exists. Low serum albumin indicates chronic protein deficiency. However, albumin has a long half-life (~20 days), thus, it is not an accurate indicator of temporary protein lack (Baines and Roberts 2001). Specific tests for deficiencies such as zinc and vitamins may be indicated. Indicators of malnutrition include:

- Significant weight change: 10% of body weight in six months. Weight loss in older people often means loss of muscle mass, which affects strength and functional ability.
- Body Mass Index <22 or >27.
- Mid-arm circumference <10th percentile. Mid-arm circumference is often easier to measure in older people, especially frail older people and those in aged-care homes.
- Triceps skin fold <10th or >90th percentile.
- Serum:
  - prealbumin <16 mg/dl
  - transferrin <200 mg/dl
  - albumin <3.5 g/dl
  - cholesterol <160 mg/dl (Mooradian et al. 1999)

Nutritional supplements are a simple way of increasing the energy and nutrient content of the diet of older people. Even when the daily intake of vitamins and minerals is adequate these nutrients may not be bioavailable and supplements may be needed (Truswell 2003). For example, omega-3 supplementation may be beneficial to lower triglycerides of people with heart disease if the reference daily intake (RDI) cannot be consumed by eating oily fish. The American Heart

Foundation (AHA) (Orford et al. 2002) recommended doctors supervise omega-3 supplementation in older people. Omega-3 supplements may cause gastrointestinal disturbances and hyperglycaemia and may interact with warfarin and cause bleeding.

Nutrition in dementia

Inadequate nutritional intake is common in people with dementia who accept or refuse meals erratically and may be anorexic. When a person refuses meals, they can be encouraged to consume fluids and light foods such as hot chocolate, milkshakes, ice cream, fruit, yoghurt, and custard. Repeating favourite foods can sometimes help. For example, if the person likes breakfast foods, breakfast can be repeated at dinnertime. Nutritional supplements may also be useful; for example, 60 ml Two-Cal® administered with normal prescribed medications four times a day will increase protein intake. Having food available to enable them to 'graze' might be possible if food hygiene and infection control issues are considered.

Enteral therapy

An increasing number of older people, particularly those living in aged-care facilities, require enteral feeding. Usually, glucose-lowering medicines (GLMs)/insulin should be administered and blood glucose tests performed before administering the enteral feed but other medications may need to be administered separately from feeds to ensure they are absorbed. Nasogastric tubes are usually used when temporary enteral feeds are needed. Gastroscopy, jejunostomy, or percutaneous endoscopic gastrostomy (PEG) tubes are usually preferred when enteral feeding is required long term. Enteral therapy enables fluid and macronutrients to be provided to meet the individual's metabolic and nutritional requirements (see also Chapter 10).

Feeds are administered slowly initially to prevent refeeding syndrome and to limit the metabolic and haemodynamic effects. For example, electrolyte shifts can precipitate congestive cardiac failure, cardiac arrhythmias, and neuromuscular and respiratory dysfunction (Crook et al. 2001). The formula used depends on the indication, such as the need to reduce CO_2 production in respiratory disease when CO_2 excretion is compromised. There are no specific guidelines for people with diabetes at risk of malnutrition who require nutritional support. General dietary recommendations for people with diabetes may not be appropriate for older malnourished people with diabetes (Elias et al. 2005). Formulas with less impact on blood glucose are available for people with diabetes. Types of formulas include:

- Standard, which are often used when commencing enteral feeding. These are high in carbohydrate and low in fat and fibre and can cause hyperglycaemia because of their rapid transit time and nutrient absorption and lead to post prandial hyperglycaemia due to impaired muscle and splanchic glucose uptake (Basu et al. 2001).
- Hypercaloric, used if fluid intake needs to be restricted, for example, end-stage renal disease.
- Fibre to reduce constipation.
- A range of specialty formulas exists for renal, hepatic, respiratory disease, wound management, and cancer. Specialty formulas for people with diabetes include Nutrison low energy for diabetes, Nutrison diabetes, Resource diabetes, and Glucerna, which are all generally low GI. These formulas used as enteral feeds or supplements have less effect on blood glucose than standard feeds (Elias et al. 2005). Glucerna has less effect on blood glucose than Enrich, Ensure HN, and Compleat Modified (Peters and Davidson 1992). Diabetes-specific formulas contain fructose, fibre mono-unsaturated fatty acids, protein, and antioxidants. High-GI foods can precipitate osmotic diarrhoea, dehydration, and hyperosmolar states. If high-GI foods are indicated, they should be commenced slowly and increased slowly and oral hypoglycaemic agents/insulin adjusted according to the blood glucose pattern. Blood glucose should be monitored regularly.

- Elemental and subelemental formulas are easily digested and may be suitable for people with autonomic gastroparesis.
- Modular formulas, which contain a single nutrient, enable feeds to be tailored to the individual.

The effects on the individual need to be considered when commencing enteral feeding: these include isolation, depression, and reduced QoL. In addition, enteral feeds may not prevent malnutrition, even when they are carefully tailored. They may delay wound healing if they lead to hyperglycaemia, pressure sores and infection can develop around the tube insertion site, and the nasogastric tubes can become dislodged and cause aspiration pneumonia and are associated with increased risk of mortality. They can be a burden on carers, and incorrect administration of medicines through enteral feeding methods occurs in home, aged-care, and hospital settings, such as crushing enteric-coated long-acting medicines.

Guidelines for administering GLMs with enteral feeds

The policies and guidelines of the relevant facility should be followed. General recommendations can be found in (Department of Health and Aging *Guidelines for Medicine Management in Residential Aged care facilities* (DOHA) 2012).

(1) Liquid dose forms are the preferred formulations. If there are no contraindications to crushing tablets or opening capsules, they should be crushed to a fine powder and mixed with 10–15 ml of water.
(2) The feed should be stopped 30 minutes before the scheduled medication administration time and flushed with 30 ml water before administering the medicines when medicines need to be administered on an empty stomach and recommenced 30 minutes after all the medicine is administered.
(3) If medicine/enteral formula incompatibilities are possible; alternative medicines or formulas should be prescribed if possible. If it is not possible, the feed should be stopped two hours before medicine administered as a single daily dose and recommenced two hours after the medicine is administered. If more frequent doses are prescribed one hour should be allowed before and after the medicine/s are administered. However, this method does *not* guarantee complete bioavailability of the medicines but no incompatibility between commonly used diabetes medicines and enteral feeds were identified.
(4) Medicines should be remixed before they are administered using a syringe clearly labelled for oral dosing to avoid the possibility of a wrong route medication error. Allow the medicines to flow in by gravity. If the mixture does not flow easily, the plunger can be depressed very gently. Medicines should not be pushed through enteral tubes because they can obstruct the tube.

Different medicines should never be mixed together in a syringe

The syringe should be flushed with 5 ml of water between medicines when several medicines need to be administered at the same time. The tube should be flushed with 30 ml of water and clamped after all the medicines are administered. The feeding can then be recommenced. A feeding record should be maintained and the amount of water used to flush the tubing should be documented, especially when the person has oedema or renal disease. Medicines should be documented on the medication record.

It is advisable to consult a pharmacist before crushing medicines or opening capsules and administering them through enteral feeding tubes. Some medicines are more toxic if they are crushed, others have reduced efficacy, and the possibility of medicine interactions increases (Simpson 2005). If possible, liquid formulations should be used for enteral administration. Other dose formulations such as topical applications, intranasal sprays, patches, suppositories or injections should be used if applicable. Many lipid-lowering agents and antihypertensive medicines should not be crushed.

The Product Information sheets and quality medicine handbooks detail specific information about administering medicines in relation to food, solubility, and information about administering via enteral routes. For example, some medicines are absorbed.

Practice points

(1) Insulin should not be stopped in people with T1DM except in specific circumstances, e.g. fasting for a procedure and at the terminal stage of life.

(2) During acute illness, surgical procedures and trauma blood glucose levels can be controlled more effectively with and insulin infusion.

(3) Insulin may be preferable and reduce the risk of adverse medicine events if enteral feeding is required temporarily and in the long term.

(4) GLM may be contradicted in some disease states, see Chapter 5.

(5) Diabetes medication management must relate to enteral therapy routines and not usual medication/meal administration times. For example, if the individual is scheduled for an enteral feed five times a day, for example, at 6 A.M., 10 A.M., 2 P.M., 6 P.M., and 10 P.M., the diabetes medicines must be administered and blood glucose tested considering these feed times. Thus, many diabetes medications need to be administered at 6 a.m. with the first feed and not at 8 A.M. when breakfast is served. Capillary blood glucose testing should be performed before an enteral feed and/or two hours after the feed to determine postprandial glucose clearance.

There is no specific information about compatibility between various enteral feeds and many medicines. Therefore, patients should be monitored according to the indication for the medicine and the enteral feed to ensure management aims are met. Enteral feeding may not be a contraindication to medicines, but administering some medicines via enteral tubes can alter their bioavailability. For example, crushing may increase the absorption and affect the action profile of some medicines and increase the possibility of adverse events (Engle and Hannawa 1999; Gilbar 1999; Young 2004).

Education approaches

Diabetes education is discussed in detail in Chapter 16. Factors that affect learning in older people include the environment, the time the education is delivered, the duration of the session, the type of education materials used and the person's physical and mental state (Table 12.6). Where appropriate, people should have their glasses (spectacles) and hearing aid with them during diabetes education sessions (Jennings 1997; Rosenstock 2001).

Spouses and/or carers should be included in diabetes education sessions when appropriate, especially when cognition is impaired for whatever reason. Support groups have long-term benefits for knowledge retention, psychosocial functioning and improved metabolic control, and improve socialisation (Gilden et al. 1992). In the absence of dementia, the factor most likely to affect an older person's ability to learn, retain, and recall new information and skills and problem-solve depends on whether they are actively involved in their community. For example, an older person who participates in social activities is more likely to want to learn about their diabetes management than socially isolated older people.

Many diabetes education programmers are not age-specific and often occur in groups, which makes it difficult for hearing and vision impaired people to participate. Computer-generated learning packages are also difficult to see, access and use for some older people. In addition, many older people have low literacy skills. Small font sizes and/or text printed on shiny or coloured paper with insufficient contrast between the text and the background also compromise comprehension. Despite these limitations, older people like to receive written information and are likely to refer to it and use it in their diabetes care.

Participating in education programmes can provide mental stimulus and help preserve mental functioning as well as reduce hospital admissions and improve QoL. Memory, learning, information retrieval, and cognitive deficits have been demonstrated in people with type 2 diabetes, particularly when metabolic control is poor (Gilden et al. 1992). Several factors affect memory and learning besides cognitive function and vision changes. These include:

- Degree of wellness.
- Physical, psychological, and biological capacity.
- Social situation and available support.
- Degree of adjustment to being older and age-related changes, for example, wearing glasses.
- Sensory loss, tiredness, and incontinence can be barriers to effective education.
- Interest in the topic.
- Educator's style and skill. Diabetes education strategies must include methods of increasing concentration and enhancing attention, especially when vision and hearing are impaired. Incorporating relaxation techniques and other complementary therapies into the education session can relieve stress and enhance learning; see Chapter 18.
- The environment in which the education occurs.

When recommending self-care equipment to older people, consider factors such as whether they can hold it easily, and that numbers on meters and insulin devices are large and clear enough to see. Memory prompts and cues can be helpful for some people.

Many staff education programmer concerning care of older people do not address significant care issues, e.g. atypical symptoms.

Self-care

Self-care is important, and independent self-care should be maintained as long as possible. Older people may need help with some self-care tasks but not others. Health professionals need to realise that diabetes self-care is relentless and demanding. Self-care can be an added burden to carers who may be old and have illnesses themselves. Self-care capacity should be assessed regularly as part of the annual complication assessment, following a hospital admission, and when medicine or medicine doses change. Barriers to self-care include declining physical and mental functioning, depression, intercurrent illness, comorbidities, and the effects of medications. Specific factors associated with inadequate self-care include:

- Geriatric syndromes and frailty
- Lower levels of physical functioning
- Inadequate knowledge about the medical condition/s
- Limited participation in social activities
- Depression
- Financial constraints
- Male gender
- Low perceptions of health status
- High number of concomitant conditions (Bayliss et al. 2007)

Potential barriers include high levels of morbidity, cumulative effects of comorbidities, inadequate health professional/patient communication, and health professional clinical inertia. In addition, self-perception, the desire to remain independent, health beliefs and attitudes play a role. For example, in general, older people are reluctant to use walking aids. However, sudden changes in walking ability and positive cultural views about ageing make a difference to their willingness to accept a walking aid (Gooberman-Hill and Ebrahim 2007).

The person's home blood glucose testing record might provide important clues to self-care. For example, if it is smeared with blood, it might indicate visual, eye–hand coordination, or manual dexterity deficits. Food- and blood-stained record books and blood glucose meters might indicate testing from contaminated fingers. If these deficits are suspected, the issue needs to be approached with tact and in a nonjudgemental manner. Record books can be used proactively and constructively to help people understand the effects of food, activity, medicines and stress on their blood glucose, help them find solutions to problems and involve them in planning their care.

Wetzels et al. (2007) undertook a systematic review of the relevant literature that showed using a previsit record book in combination with an education session or consultation led to more questions and more self-reported health care.

Some older people find the print too small in commercial blood glucose record books and prefer to use 'exercise books'. Paper-based patient-held records are still popular with many people, despite modern meters that automatically record blood glucose results and have the capacity to download the results directly onto computers (Davis 2003).

Factors that can affect metabolic control

'Barriers to good control are often in the minds of physicians rather than the capacity of the elderly person with diabetes' (Halter 2001). A current term is *clinical inertia*. For example, some GPs are reluctant to commence insulin in older people when metabolic control deteriorates, even when the individual and their family/carers are willing. It is important to consider the clinicians' influence on an individual's health care, especially when the individual is old. Clinicians often judge older people in general by the older people they manage in aged-care facilities, who may not accurately represent the majority of self-caring elderly people living in the community. Some of the factors that can affect diabetes control in the elderly are shown in Table 12.7.

Table 12.7   Factors that can affect diabetes control and management in older people.

Clinicians	Attitudes and beliefs
	Inadequate knowledge about diabetes and/or about teaching and learning and communication skills
	Inappropriate advice, education materials
	Ageist attitudes and limited services and diabetes management choices
	Clinical inertia
	Constraints on time and services
Altered senses	Communication difficulties
	Diminished vision, hearing, and smell, altered taste, decreased proprioception
	Not understanding instructions Communication capacity
Cognitive status	Diminished cognition affects learning, memory, and recall
	May be temporarily affected by hypo- or hyperglycaemia
Food difficulties	Purchasing, preparing, and consuming food, understanding nutritional requirements, poor appetite, early satiety, gastrointestinal problems
	Disease processes
	Dental and oral problems
Disease processes/effects	Tremor, arthritis, poor dentition, gastrointestinal abnormalities, altered thirst sensation, altered renal and hepatic function, infection (acute and chronic)
Mobility	Limited ability to exercise
	Self-imposed driving restrictions or withdrawal of driving licence
Medicines	Alcohol, medications such as glucocorticoids, interactions, self-prescribed medications
Complementary therapies	Hypo- or hyperglycaemia, medicine/herb interactions, herb/herb interactions
Malabsorption	Owing to diabetes medications, disease processes, medicine interactions, diabetes complications
Psychological issues	Bereavement, depression, cognitive deficits
Social factors	Social isolation, living alone or in care facilities, family expectations
Financial status	Purchasing recommended foods, monitoring equipment, diabetes complication screening, podiatry services

Access and equity to diabetes services

Older people are often unable to attend mainstream diabetes services, especially where they are fragmented and essential services are offered on different days. Appointments scheduled to allow a 'one-stop' approach to diabetes management enhance attendance rates. People are often required to attend different sites to have their eyes, kidneys, and feet checked for diabetic complications. Therefore, integrated care and careful transition care, discharge planning, and involving the GPs is essential. In Australia, the GP incentive schemes and integrated care planning and assessment strategies and the National Service Framework in the United Kingdom have significantly improved diabetes care in general practice.

Infections

The presence of infection can significantly affect the health status of older people. Any sudden increase in blood glucose that cannot be accounted for by dietary changes, inactivity, medicines, or stress should be investigated. The temperature should be recorded. Foot inspection is important to exclude occult infection. Reduced mobility and sitting with feet in the dependent position can cause lower leg oedema, which puts pressure on fragile, less flexible older skin, causing small ruptures, weeping, and increasing the risk of infection and chronic ulcers. Mental stress associated with nonhealing wounds delays wound healing.

Urinary tract infections are common in older people. A urine dipstick test for white cells and nitrate should be performed. There is growing evidence that consuming cranberry formulations on a daily basis can prevent UTI in older people with diabetes. Cranberry formulations can interact with warfarin, so caution is needed in people on these medicines. As indicated, annual influenza vaccination should be part of the individual's routine health management plan.

An holistic approach to healing is needed that includes proactive screening for occult infections, optimal nutrition, education, and strategies that encompass physical, spiritual, and mental health. A single point-of-care coordination is desirable but the expertise of several health professional groups may be needed. For example, podiatrist, orthotist, endocrinologist, diabetes educator, dietitian, vascular surgeon, orthopaedic specialist, infectious diseases physician, and a wound consultant might all be required to manage an infected foot.

Quality of life

Quality of life refers to an individual's enjoyment of life and might or might not include prolonging life see Chapter 15. QoL issues specific to the individual are more likely to accurately gauge life enjoyment than objective QoL tools even those well validated and frequently used tools. Such tools are essential if the objective is to compare individuals. However, they may be less relevant if the objective is to sequentially monitor individual QoL. For example, pets enhance QoL and are treasured companions for many older people, yet pets are not mentioned on any QoL tools. Older people identify QoL as being more important than length of life (Medical Research Council 1994).

Many factors affect QoL in addition to personal QoL factors, these include:

- General health and medical issues such as diabetes type, treatment regimen, level of metabolic control and presence of complications. The greater the severity and effects of diabetes-related complications the greater the effect on QoL. Sexual health is often overlooked in older people. It is an important aspect of QoL often compromised by medical conditions, medications, the effects of age, and health professional and societal attitudes.
- Management strategies – the level of glycaemic control rarely relates to the level of well-being (Testa et al. 1998) but diabetes symptoms of hypo or hyperglycaemia are more directly related to QoL. Maaravi et al. (2000) identified nutritional status as a major determinant of QoL in a community dwelling people over 70 years. There are conflicting about the effects of the different types of diabetes treatment on the QoL of older people. QoL is lower in people

treated with insulin (Petterson et al. 1998; Rutherford et al. 2004; Speight et al. 2011). In contrast, Reza et al. (2002) reported better mental health, social functioning, and vitality and less carer strain associated with insulin.

- Cognitive functioning is affected by acute and chronic blood glucose fluctuations. The associated neuropsychological changes can reduce QoL of both the person with diabetes and their family.
- Health, diabetes, cultural, and general attitudes and beliefs, which influence factors such as self-efficacy and locus of control. Strategies that focus on understanding the individual's beliefs and attitudes, and encompass empowerment theories improve an individual's sense of well-being and involvement in their care.
- Demographic factors such as gender, education level ethnicity, age, and social support. Men report better QoL than women and young people better than older people. Higher education is associated with a higher QoL. Individuals with good support generally have a better QoL and reduced risk of depression.

Various tools to measure QoL and other related factors are shown in Chapter 15.

Safety

In many respects, diabetes management in older people encompasses managing risks, regardless of whether the individual lives in the community, in a care facility, or is being cared for in acute, ambulatory, or primary care settings. Safety is multifactorial and risks are often cumulative as can be seen from Table 12.2. Many safety programmes focus on falls, but driving and other safety issues also need to be addressed.

Falls are the sixth leading cause of death in older people with and without diabetes, but having diabetes significantly increases the risk. People who fall do so repeatedly, and falls are a common cause of placement in an aged-care home. Falls are a result of a combination of accumulated effects of disease processes, impairment, and medications (Quayle 2001). It can be seen from Table 12.2 that a significant number of diabetes-related problems significantly increase the likelihood that an older person with diabetes will fall.

General factors that increase the risk of falling include:

- Fell in the last year;
- Have difficulty with mobility and/or sensory deficits;
- Are on four or more medications, particularly oral GLMs, insulin, and antihypotensive and antidepressive agents;
- Have an acute illness;
- Were recently discharged from hospital;
- Have reduced strength and require a walking stick or frame;
- Wear inappropriate footwear;
- Live where there are environmental hazards;
- Have balance problems;
- Have diabetes complications such as autonomic neuropathy and vision loss;
- Are sedated, especially in an unfamiliar environment such as hospital or aged care facilities where the person can become disorientated and fall going to the toilet at night.

Diabetes is associated with a twofold increased risk of older people falling (Sinclair 2006) and older women are at increased risk of sustaining a fracture if they fall (Gregg et al. 2002). Ninety percent of those who fall are likely to fracture a hip, shoulder, or foot (Schwartz et al. 2001). Women with diabetes aged 70–79 are more likely to fall if their HbA1c is ≤6.8% and they are on insulin (Schwartz et al. 2003), which suggests hypoglycaemia may be implicated in many falls in older women with diabetes. Significantly, the presence of diabetes predicts failure to recover from mobility deficits, which increases the likelihood the individual will require supported care (Clark et al. 1998).

Some diabetes-specific factors related to falls are shown in Table 12.2. Others include:

- Insulin treatment leading to hypoglycaemia. Sulphonylureas, particularly long-acting agents, also cause hypoglycaemia but less frequently than insulin. The association between hypogly-caemia and GLM might be partly due to reduced renal clearance of active GLM metabolites of long-acting agents. Falls are associated with high levels of cystatin-c, an indicator of kidney function (Schwartz et al. 2008).
- Postural and postprandial hypotension. Hypertension is also associated with haemodialysis on dialysis days. See Chapter 10 and cardiovascular disease, and Chapter 8.
- Postural instability, gait, and balance problems. These are due to a wide range of health problems including erratic blood glucose pattern, muscle wasting and reduced lower limb strength, musculoskeletal problems, low vision and environmental factors.
- Weight loss and nutritional deficiencies.
- Neurological problems may slow recognition of and response to falls risk situations.
- Cardiovascular disease: About 77% of presentations to emergency department due to unexplained falls have their basis in cardiovascular disease (van der Velde et al. 2007). Poon and Braun (2005) suggested orthostatic hypotension might be contributory factor in up to 32% of falls associated with cardiovascular disease. Postprandial hypotension is also a falls risk. Postprandial hypotension is described as a blood pressure fall of 20 mmHg, an hour after eating. In aged-care facilities postprandial hypotension is associated with an increased incidence of falls, syncope, stroke, and new coronary events (Aronow and Ahn 1997).
- Withdrawing medicines that contribute to orthostatic hypotension reduces the falls rate. Tilt table tests might be useful to detect hypotension (van der Velde et al. 2007). However, this equipment is unlikely to be readily available in most clinical situations.
- Cognitive impairment might be due to hyper- or hypoglycaemia, hypotension, neurological problems, vascular disease, depression, dementia or a number of other causes.

Interestingly, Oates et al. (2007) showed older people, >80 years (n = 4071 from 10 US veteran's affairs sites) had lower five-year survival rates if they had low blood pressure than those with higher blood pressure, which suggests current blood pressure targets might be harmful in very old people, particularly given the associated falls risk. Research in other populations also demonstrated better outcomes in older people with higher than recommended target blood pressure levels (Vidan et al. 2010). However, blood pressure targets need to be considered in light of hypertension-associated risks such as stroke and cardiovascular events. All of these factors support the need for individualised, structured medicines reviews that are undertaken in the context of cumulative risk and QoL.

However, there is some evidence to support the following:

- Exercise and/physical therapy with vitamin D supplementation in community-dwelling older people (Moyer 2012) is beneficial.
- Tai chi improves balance and stability (Li 2012).
- LIFE programme (Lifestyle integrated Functional Exercise improve functional capacity (Clemson et al. 2012).
- Yoga (Patel et al. 2012) could improve well-being, but studies are small with different methodologies and yoga styles.
- In hospital:
  - Bedside handover
  - Hourly rounding
  - Ensuring the individual can reach walking aids and call bells and the environment is free from obstacles
  - Clinician rosters to ensure adequate staffing is maintained (Digby 2012).

Multifactorial strategies are usually needed to prevent and manage falls. Interestingly, a meta-analysis of the literature about hospital falls prevention programmes demonstrated falls reduction of 30–49% but few studies used sound methodologies or represent strong evidence for their benefit (Coussement et al. 2008). After adjusting for falls risk, Coussement et al. 2008 suggested current falls prevention programmes may only be useful in long-stay care units. They suggested more research into primary falls prevention in hospitals is needed in which the number of fallers, the effect of the setting in which the fall occurred, and individual falls risk are examined to determine the effect of the separate components of falls reduction programmes. A recent literature undertaken by the author and one of her PhD students suggests Coussement et al.'s suggestions have not been implemented. That is, it is difficult to combine data because of methodological differences and deficits.

Pharmacovigilance

Medications are discussed in detail in Chapter 5. Medication-related problems are 'common and costly and often preventable in older people:' adverse medicine events occur in 42% of older people living in aged-care facilities, most during prescribing and monitoring (American Geriatrics Society 2013). Age-related medicine pharmacokinetic and pharmacodynamic changes, nutritional status, cardiovascular status, and risk of polypharmacy and its consequences must be considered when deciding whether to use a medicine, which medicine, dose, and dose interval, to use; see the *Australian Medicines Handbook (AMH)* (Pharmaceutical Society of Australia, Australasian College of General Practitioners, and Australasian Society of Clinical and Experimental Pharmacologists and Toxicologists 2010) and the AMH *Aged Care Companion* (2018; also updated online yearly).

Inappropriate high-risk medicines should be avoided and nonmedicine options used where possible, such as the quality use of medicines (QUM) (Victoria Department of Health and Human Services 2019). The American Geriatrics Society (2019) Beers Criteria was developed for use to guide medicine use for people >65 years in all care settings in the United States, but it is used in many countries. The Beers Criteria were designed to enhance clinical judgement and highlight the need to seek safer alternative medicines and 'less-is-more'. The criteria encompass most classes of medicines, describes the rationale for the recommendation, the recommendation, and the quality of the evidence. The criteria strongly recommend avoiding sliding scales of insulin and long-acting sulphonylureas in older people with diabetes.

The Australian National prescribing Service (NPS 2004) developed a range of education programmes and multimedia campaigns to enhance medicine self-management in older people such as Medimate and other programmes such as home medicine reviews.

As indicated in Chapter 5, declining renal function is a normal consequence of ageing; consequently, long-acting medicines may be contraindicated if they have a prolonged half-life. Liver damage and inadequate or erratic food intake or food low in carbohydrate increases the risk of hypoglycaemia in insulin-treated individuals and with some CLMs. When swallowing difficulties are present medication dose forms may need to be reviewed. Suggested strategies to improved medicine safety when swallowing difficulties are present include the following:

- Identify medications that cannot be crushed and discuss these with the individual's doctor (hospital or GP) and pharmacist to determine whether the medicines are still required. If so, decide whether a nonmedicine option could be used or whether there is an alternative dose form.
- Place a medication alert and a swallowing alert in the person's medical record.
- Communicate the alerts to the relevant carers and health professional carers, especially when transferring amongst services.
- Provide education for people with diabetes, their carers, and health professionals.
- Regularly review medications.

Practice point

The medicine dose forms that cannot be crushed are enteric coated, extended release, sublingual, medicines that irritate the oral mucous membranes, have a bitter taste, contain incipients and dyes that could stain the teeth, when specific protection is required when handling the medicine (Mitchell 2011).

Antipsychotic medicines should be used with caution in older people with dementia because they are associated with increased risk stroke and a moderately increased risk of MI when corrected for age, gender and cardiovascular risk (Parlente 2012).

Some medicines affect nutritional status by altering appetite, taste, or sense of smell and affect food appreciation. Medicines such as antidepressants, sulphonylureas, and glucocorticoids contribute to weight gain. Others, such as anticholinergic medicines, lead to dry mouth and difficulty in swallowing. Some medicines impair absorption of vitamins and minerals, for example, antacids reduce iron and iron tablet absorption whereas vitamin C enhances iron absorption. There is increasing evidence that people with diabetic renal disease are at earlier risk of renal-associated anaemia, but the exact mechanism and role of nutrition in this process is not known.

Phenytoin is sometimes used to manage painful diabetic peripheral neuropathy as well as seizures. It can inhibit absorption of vitamin D and folic acid. Some foods modify the absorption of some medicines, which explains why the timing medication doses in relation to food is important, especially in enteral feeding regimens.

Exercise/Activity

Regular exercise has physical and mental benefits for people with and without diabetes of all ages. Exercise helps reduce the risk of developing diabetes and cardiovascular disease as well as improving mental wellbeing. Any movement of the body or limbs helps reduce cardiovascular fatalities by up to 50% and the chance of a second myocardial infarct by 25% as well as reducing hypertension and stroke risk.

However, exercise is difficult for many older people because of the decline in muscle mass and general mobility, strength, and energy. These factors increase the risk of falls, injury, and fractures. Thus, exercise needs to be planned and individualised considering safety. At least 30 minutes of aerobic exercise per day and strength-training exercises help maintain muscle mass and energy. In addition, adequate nutrition, especially protein, is important to preserving muscle mass and mobility, reduce falls, and improve well-being (Stressman et al. 2002; Vaitkevicius et al. 2002). It is not appropriate to merely recommend an older person to begin an exercise programme without assessing his/her physical status first. Assessment can be incorporated in usual care:

- Assess vascular status and detecting cardiac. Well older people in the community may require a graded exercise test. Blood pressure, lipid profile and assessment for autonomic neuropathy, which could lead to silent MI is advisable (Flood and Constance 2002).
- Examine the feet to detect peripheral neuropathy and any other foot pathology that could increase the risk of foot injury during exercise.
- Check eyes to detect the presence and status of retinopathy.
- Observe gait and balance.
- Measure blood glucose pattern and do not encourage activity if the blood glucose is <6 mmol/l or >10 mmol/l.
- Self-care knowledge. Be aware of the signs of hypoglycaemia, such as sweating, faintness, weakness, and dizziness, that can be missed or attributed to the effect of the exercise, especially if hypoglycaemic unawareness is present, or could have other causes such as angina, or silent MI. Important information includes:
  - Know that some physical activity can lower blood glucose for up to 48 hours; therefore, an adequate high GI intake is required when aerobic activities are planned and activity levels increased gradually.

○ Wear appropriate clothing and footwear that does not restrict blood flow and breathing or put the feet at risk.
○ Warm up and cool before and after exercise.
○ Know how to incorporate exercise/activity into the usual daily routine.
○ Consider personal safety and be aware of risks such as being attacked when out walking or risk of falling on poorly maintained footpaths.

The Society of Geriatric Cardiology recommends that older people participate in physical activity programmes that include aerobic and strength-training activities, such as tai chi, which reduces blood pressure, blood glucose, and lipids, and improves balance and well-being (Lan et al. 1998; Tsai et al. 2003). Resistance training reduces bone loss, improves strength, and makes routine activities such as carrying groceries and gardening easier (Meuleman et al. 2000; Simkin 2004). Walking 30 minutes/day or for 10 minutes three times per day is ideal. Swimming has the benefit of being non-weight-bearing and might be easier for overweight people to manage. A great deal of incidental activity occurs during usual activities, such as playing with grandchildren, housework, and gardening.

Hypoglycaemia

Hypoglycaemia is the most important side effect of insulin and some GLMs; see Chapters 5 and 6. Hypoglycaemia occurring in older people can be difficult to recognise. Usually the counter-regulatory response is triggered when the blood glucose drops below ~3.5–3.7 mmol/l, which triggers adrenergic symptoms such as sweating and trembling. Fine motor coordination, the speed of mental processing, concentration, and some memory functions are when blood glucose is <3 mmol/l (Sommerfield et al. 2003). The effects on decision-making are unclear. Some researchers suggest attentional ability is compromised but problem-solving ability remains intact (McAulay et al. 2001). Prolonged hypoglycaemia can result in neurological damage or death, but these are rare (Cryer 2007).

The usual hypoglycaemia signs and symptoms can be masked or absent in older people, and hypoglycaemia can present as chronic confusion, and not be recognised. The presentation of hypoglycaemia may resemble a cerebrovascular accident or mental confusion leading to an incorrect diagnosis of impaired mental function and delayed treatment or failure to treat the hypoglycaemia. The need to consider hypoglycaemia in older people with diabetes presenting to emergency departments has improved with education and since the introduction of capillary blood glucose testing on all unconscious patients presenting to emergency departments.

Hypoglycaemia caused by GLMs, especially long acting agents, is often profound and prolonged and can become chronic or fatal. If it is prolonged it can cause brain damage or provoke an MI (Tiengo 1999).

It is important to monitor the blood glucose of older peoples and residents presenting with these risk factors and to be aware that usually more than one risk factor is operating. The more risk factors present the greater the likelihood of hypoglycaemia occurring. Hypoglycaemia risk assessment tool is shown in Chapter 6.

The method of treating hypoglycaemia must reflect the individual's functional level and the severity of the hypoglycaemia; see Chapter 6.

Practice points

- Hypoglycaemia leading to unconsciousness is rare in older people. However, such an event is very stressful and can precipitate an MI. An ECG should be performed.
- In cold weather, prolonged hypoglycaemia can lead to hypothermia, which has a poor outcome.

Regular vaccinations against influenza and pneumonia are recommended for older people. A recent report recommended vaccinating infants as young as six months if they are in contact with frail elderly grandparents/relatives to reduce the spread of infection (Jackson and Janoff 2008). Interestingly, researchers found that although people's immune response depends on the vaccination they received, the side of their brain that is most active also had an effect on the degree of the response (Davidson et al. 2003).

Davidson et al. (2003), found people aged 57–60 with left-sided brain activity in the prefrontal cortex developed stronger immunity. The prefrontal cortex is associated with a positive outlook on life. Whilst the study is small, it demonstrates the effect of psychological parameters on physical status. Another earlier study (Graham et al. 2006), demonstrated that chronic stress reduces immune function in older people and impaired antibody responses to influenza vaccinations. These findings also apply to older carers. These studies suggest that chronically stressed older people, including carers, may be vulnerable to infection and because they are not able to mount an adequate immune response. Therefore, infection control procedures and appropriate preventative measure must be in place.

Overall care strategies

- Careful assessment of the individual from an holistic approach that incorporates physical, psychological, social, spiritual, and relationship functioning. The latter includes relationships with health professionals.
- Strategies need to be in place to assess and minimise the risk of falling. These include providing a safe environment, orientating the person to the ward, considering protective measures to avoid pressure ulcers such as hip protectors, careful discharge planning, and early referral to the social worker, domiciliary or aged-care team for home assessment.
- Time meals, PEG, and enteral feeds and medication rounds to reduce the risk of hypoglycaemia.
- Adequate preparation of the patient for surgical and investigative procedures, see Chapter 9.
- Remind the person to drink, especially in hot weather.
- Monitor blood glucose and take steps to correct persistent levels outside the target range.
- Provide clear, careful explanations when relevant and check that the person understands what is required of them. Written information enhances verbal information.
- Identify stress and depression and ensure appropriate assessment and management occurs.
- Identify the barriers to self-care and recognise and change those things that can be changed and those that cannot.
- Bed rest may be required initially, but it should not be prolonged because of the loss of muscle mass especially in the lower limbs, venous stasis, skin tears, pressure ulcers and falls risk. Thus, it is important to ensure timely assessment when an older person presents to the emergency department and to consult an aged care expert early in the admission to ensure appropriate management and reduce the likelihood of repeated presentations.

WHO (1983) emphasised the importance of helping older people live safe, dignified lives in society with their families and friends if possible and recognised the important role carers play in supporting older people in the community. Carers should be included in assessment and health planning and outcome monitoring processes where appropriate. Carers become concerned when they are not consulted when their older relative is hospitalised from an aged-care facility (Hong et al. 2004). Written action plans can support carers to manage older people at home but need to be relevant to the carer and the older person and revised regularly, bearing in mind the burden of care.

Having such strategies in place for respite and end-of-life care can relieve the burden of care and improve outcomes for carers and older people (Berthold et al. 1991). Carers presenting with health problems have the following possible challenges:

- They have long-standing health problems.
- They experienced health problems in the previous year.

- They are concerned about their health.
- A high level of frustration is common.
- Personal tasks such as bathing and dressing the older person fall on the carer, which can be distressing for both parties. Many older people do not want physical help from their family and friends (Connell 1991), even when they need it. Providing support when it is not wanted, even if it is needed, can result in negative outcomes and be perceived as interference. Carers often tread the fine line between support and 'interference' on a daily basis.
- They have difficulty communicating with the older person (Toraski 2004).
- There is inadequate respite care/support services in place.
- Carers can feel depressed and burnt out (Toraski 2004).

An education programme for caregivers that includes information about how to manage their relative's behaviour can foster closer relationships between the carer and their relative, as well as fewer incidents of acute confusion and faecal incontinence during hospital admissions and fewer depressive symptoms (Hong et al. 2004).

References

Abdelhafiz, A. and Sinclair, A. (2015). low hbA1c and increased mortality risk – is frailty a confounding factor? *Ageing and Disease* **6** (4): 262–270.

Abdo, S. and Flack, J. (2012). Diabetes as the years progress: how does management differ? *Endocrinology Today* **2**: 6–14.

Allen, K.V., Frier, B.M., and Strachan, M.W. (2004). The relationship between type 2 diabetes and cognitive dysfunction: longitudinal studies and their methodological limitations. *European Journal of Pharmacology* **490**: 169–175.

Australian Diabetes Educators Association (2003). *Guidelines for the management and care of diabetes in the elderly*. Weston, A.C.T.: *Australian Diabetes Educators Association*.

America Diabetes Association (2019). Older adults: standards of medical care in diabetes. *Diabetes Care* **42** (Suppl. 1): S139–S2147.

American Diabetes Association (2013). *Clinical Guidelines – Diabetes in Older People*. http://www.ndei.org/ADA-2013-Guideline-Diabetes-Older-Adults.aspx (accessed January 2013).

American Geriatrics Society Expert Panel on Care of Older Adults with Diabetes Mellitus, Moreno, G., Mangione, C.M. et al. (2013). Guidelines abstracted from the American Geriatrics Society Guidelines for Improving the Care of Older Adults with Diabetes Mellitus: 2013 update. *Journal of the American Geriatrics Society* **61** (11): 2020–2026. https://doi.org/10.1111/jgs.12514.

American Geriatrics Society (2019). Updated Beers Criteria for potentially inappropriate use in older adults. *Journal of the American Geriatrics Society* **67** (4): 674–694. https://www.ncbi.nlm.nih.gov/pubmed/30693946.

Ames, B. (2006). Low micronutrient intake may accelerate degenerative diseases of aging through allocation of scarce micronutrients by triage. *Proceedings of National Academy of Science USA* **103** (47): 17589–17594.

Aronow, W. and Ahn, C. (1997). Association of post prandial hypotension with incidence of falls, syncope, coronary events, stroke, and total mortality at 29 months follow-up in 499 older nursing home residents. *Journal of the American Geriatrics Society* **45**: 1051–1053.

Asimakopoulou, K.G., Hampson, S.E., and Morrish, N.J. (2002). Neuropsychological functioning in older people with type 2 diabetes: the effect of controlling for confounding factors. *Diabetic Medicine* **19** (4): 311–316.

Australian Diabetes Society (ADS) (2012). *Guidelines for Routine Glucose Control in Hospital*. Canberra: ADS.

Australian Institute of Health and Welfare (2002). Older Australia at a glance. https://www.aihw.gov.au/getmedia/ce13dbbe-542c-4957-849c-15109e6a69e7/oag04.pdf.aspx?inline=true.

Australian Medicines Handbook (AMH) (2018). *Aged Care Companion*, 3e. Melbourne: AMH.

Baines, S. and Roberts, D. (2001). Undernutrition in the community. *Australian Prescriber* **24** (5): 113–115.

Basu, A., Basu, R., Sha, P. et al. (2001). Type 2 diabetes impairs splanchnic uptake of glucose but does not alter intestinal glucose absorption during enteral glucose feeding. *Diabetes* **50**: 1351–1362.

Bayliss, E., Ellis, J., and Steiner, J. (2007). Barriers to self-management and quality of life outcomes in seniors with multimorbidities. *Annals of Family Medicine* **5** (5): 395–402.

Berthold, H., Landahl, S., and Svanborg, A. (1991). Intermittent care and caregivers at home. *Ageing* **3** (1): 51–56.

Beverly, E., Fitzgerald, S., Sitnikov, L. et al. (2012). Do older adults aged 60 to 70 years benefit from diabetes behavioural interventions? *Diabetes Care* **36** (6): 1501–1506.

Biessels, G., Staekenborg, S., Brunner, E. et al. (2006). Risk of dementia in diabetes mellitus: a systematic review. *The Lancet Neurology* **5** (1): 64–74.

Bogner, H., Morales, K., Post, E., and Bruce, M. (2007). Diabetes, depression, and death: a randomized controlled trial of a depression treatment program for older adults based in primary care (PROSPECT). *Diabetes Care* 30: 3005–3010.

Bortz, W. (2002). A conceptual framework of frailty: a review. *Journal of Gerontology* 75 (5): 283–288.

Bostock, S. and Steptoe, A. (2012). Association between low functional health literacy and mortality in older adults: longitudinal cohort study. *British Medical Journal* 3: 344. https://doi.org/10.1136/bmj.e1602.

Bourdel-Marchasson, I., Proux, S., Dehail, P. et al. (2004). One-year incidence of hyperosmolar states and prognosis in a geriatric acute care unit. *Gerontology* 50 (3): 171–176.

Bradford, A., Kunik, M.E., Schulz, P. et al. (2009). Missed and delayed diagnosis of dementia in primary care: prevalence and contributing factors. *Alzheimer Disease and Associated Disorders* 23 (4): 306.

Brown, A., Mangione, C., Saliba, D., and Sarkisian, A. (2003). California Healthcare Foundation/American Geriatrics Society Panel on Improving Care for Elders with Diabetes. Guidelines for improving the care of the older person with diabetes mellitus. *Journal of the American Geriatric Society* 55 Suppl Guidelines: S265–S280.

Cahoon, C. (2012). Depression in older adults. *American Journal of Nursing* 112 (11): 22–30.

Callan, B. and Wells, T. (2003). Views of community-dwelling old-old people on barriers and aids to nutritional health. *Journal of Nursing Scholarship* 35 (3): 257–262.

Callisaya, M., Beare, R., Moran, C. et al. (2018). Type 2 diabetes mellitus, brain atrophy and cognitive decline in older people: a longitudinal study. *Diabetalogia* https://doi.org/10.1007/s00125-018-4778-9.

Carmichael, O., Schwarz, C., and Drucker, D. (2010). Alzheimer's Disease Neuroimaging Initiative. Longitudinal changes in white matter disease and cognition in the first year of the Alzheimer's disease neuroimaging initiative. *Archives of Neurology* 67 (11): 1370–1378.

Chen, X., Beydoun, M.A., and Wang, Y. (2008). Is sleep duration associated with childhood obesity? A systematic review and meta-analysis. *Obesity* 16 (2): 265–274.

Choi, K. (2016). Sarcopenia and sarcopenic obesity. *Korean Journal of Internal Medicine* 31 (6): 1054–1060.

Clark, D.O., Stump, T.E., and Wollnsky, F.D. (1998). Predictors of onset of and recovery from mobility difficulty among adults aged 51–61 years. *American Journal of Epidemiology* 148 (1): 63–71.

Clemson, L., Fiatarone Singh, M., Bundy, A. et al. (2012). Integration of balance and strength training into daily life activity to reduce rate of falls in older people (the LIFE study): randomized panel trial. *British Medical Journal* 340 (c2244): 1042–1043.

Cluning, T. (2001). *Aging at Home: Practical Approaches to Community Care*. Melbourne: Ausmed Publications.

Cohen-Mansfield, J., Dakheel-Ali, M., Marx, M.S. et al. (2015). Which unmet needs contribute to behavior problems in persons with advanced dementia? *Psychiatry Research* 228: 59–64.

Connell, C.M. (1991). Psychosocial contexts of diabetes and older adulthood: Reciprocal effects. *The Diabetes Educator* 17 (5): 364–371.

Coussement, J., De Paepe, L., Schwendimann, R. et al. (2008). Interventions for preventing falls in acute- and chronic-care hospitals: a systematic review and meta-analysis. *Journal American Geriatric Society* 56: 29–36.

Croxon, S. (2000). Diabetes in United Kingdom care homes. *Practical Diabetes International* 17 (3): 1868–1869.

Cruz-Jentoft, A., Bahat, G., Bauer, J. et al. (2018). Saceopenia: revised European consensus on definition and diagnosis. *Age and Ageing* 48: 1–16. https://doi.org/10.1093/ageing/ary169.

Cryer, P. (2007). Hypoglycaemia, functional brain failure, and brain death. *Journal of Clinical Investigation* 117: 868–870.

Davidson, R., Kabat-Zinn, J., Schumacher, J. et al. (2003). Alterations in brain and immune function produced by mindfulness meditation. *Psychosomatic Medicine* 65 (4): 564–570.

Davis, T. (2003). Patient-managed records: Their use in diabetes care. *Diabetes Management Journal* 5 (18): 4–7.

Dementia Australia (2018). Dementia language guidelines. dementia.org.au.

Department of Health (2003). *Care Homes for Older People: National Minimal Standards. Care Standards Act 2001*. London: HMSO.

Department of Health and Aging (DOHA) (2012). *Guidelines for Medicine Management in Residential Aged Care Facilities*. Canberra: DOHA.

Devitt, H. (2011). Exploring nutrition for older people with diabetes. *Australian Diabetes Educator* 14 (2): 16–19.

Digby, R. (2012). Focus on falls prevention. *Australian Nursing Journal* 10 (17): 35.

Dregan, A., Stewart, R., and Gulliford, M. (2012). Cardiovascular risk factors and cognitive decline in adults aged 50 and over: a population-based cohort study. *Age and Aging* 42 (3): 338–345. https://doi.org/10.1093/aging/afs/66 (accessed December 2012.

Drewnowski, A. and Warren-Mears, V. (2001). Does aging change nutrition requirements? *Journal of Nutrition, Health and Aging* 5 (2): 70–74.

Dunning, P. and Alford, F. (1993). Dilemmas in the management of the elderly diabetic. A community or medical problem? *Medical Journal of Australia* 3: 158–164.

Dunning, T. and Manias, E. (2005). Medication knowledge and self-management by people with type 2 diabetes. *Australian Journal of Advanced Nursing* 23 (1): 7.

Elias, M., Ceriello, A., Laube, H. et al. (2005). Enteral nutrition support and use of diabetes-specific formulas for patients with diabetes. *Diabetes Care* 28: 2267–2279.

Engle, K. and Hannawa, T. (1999). Techniques for administering oral medications to critical care patients receiving continuous enteral nutrition. *American Journal of Health Systems Pharmacy* **56** (14): 1441–1444.

English, K.L. and Paddon-Jones, D. (2010). Protecting muscle mass and function in older adults during bed rest. *Curr Opin Clin Nutr Metab Care* **13**: 34–39.

Faes, M., Spigt, M., and Olde Rikkert, M. (2007). Dehydration in geriatrics. *Geriatrics and Aging* **10** (9): 590–596.

Fenton, W. and Stover, E. (2006). Mood disorders: cardiovascular and diabetes comorbidity. *Current Opinion in Psychiatry* **19**: 421–427.

Fleming, R. (2002). Report of Federal Department of Health survey into depression in the elderly. *Australian Doctor* **14** (March): 10–11.

Flood, L. and Constance, A. (2002). Diabetes and exercise safety. *American Journal of Nursing* **102** (6): 47–55.

Franco, V., Polanczyk, C., Clausell, N. et al. (2004). Role of dietary vitamin K intake in chronic oral anticoagulation: prospective evidence from observational and randomized protocols. *American Journal of Medicine* **116**: 651–656.

Fried, L., Ferrucci, L., Darer, J. et al. (2004). Untangling the concepts of disability, frailty, and comorbidity: implications for improved targeting and care. *Journal of Gerontology American Biological Science Medical Science* **59**: M255–M263.

Friedman, R. and Kalant, N. (1998). Comparison of long term care in an acute institution and a long term care institution. *Canadian Medical Association Journal* **159** (9): 1107–1113.

Gaughran, F., Walwyn, R., Lambkin-Williams, R. et al. (2007). Flu: effect of vaccine in elderly care home residents: a randomized trial. *Journal of the American Geriatric Society* **55** (12): 1912–1920.

Giannelli, A., Patel, K., and Windham, G. (2007). Magnitude of underascertainment of impaired kidney function in older adults with normal serum creatinine. *American Geriatric Society* **55** (6): 816–823.

Gilbar, P. (1999). A guide to enteral drug administration in palliative care. *Journal of Pain and Symptom Management* **17** (3): 197–207.

Gilden, J., Hendryx, M., Clar, S. et al. (1992). Diabetes support groups improve health care of older diabetic patients. *Journal of the American Geriatric Society* **40**: 145–150.

Goldney, R., Phillips, P., and Fisher, L. (2004). Diabetes, depression and quality of life. *Diabetes Care* **27**: 1066–1070.

Gooberman-Hill, R. and Ebrahim, S. (2007). Making decisions about simple interventions: older people use of walking aids. *Age and Aging* **36** (5): 569–573.

Gradman, T., Laes, A., Thompson, L., and Reaven, G. (1993). Verbal learning and/or memory improves with glycaemic control in older subjects with non insulin-dependent diabetes mellitus. *Journal of the American Geriatrics Society* **41**: 1305–1312.

Graham, J., Christian, L., and Kiecolt-Glaser, J. (2006). Stress, age, and immune function: toward a lifespan approach. *Journal of Behavioral Medicine* **29** (4): 9057–9064.

Gray, L., Woodward, M., Scholes, R. et al. (2002). *Geriatric Medicine*, 2e. Melbourne: Ausmed Publications.

Gregg, E., Mangione, C., Cauley, J. et al. (2002). Diabetes and incidence of functional disability in older women. *Diabetes Care* **25**: 61–67.

Gregg, E., Yaffe, K., Cauley, J. et al. (2000). Is diabetes associated with cognitive impairment and cognitive decline among older women? *Archives of Internal Medicine* **160**: 174–180.

Gross, P.A., Hermogenes, A., Sacks, H. et al. (1995). The efficacy of influenza vaccine in elderly persons. A meta-analysis and review of the literature. *Annals of Internal Medicine* **123** (7): 518–527.

Grossman, T. (2005). Latest advances in anitaging medicine. *Keio Journal of Medicine* **54** (2): 85–94.

Halter, J. (2001). Report of the American Diabetes Association Meeting. *Practical Diabetes International* **18** (7): 251–258.

Haufe, M., Peek, T., and Luijkx, K. (2019). Matching gerontechnologies to independent-living seniors' individual needs: development of the GTM tool. *BMC Health Services Research* **19**: 26. https://doi.org/10.1186/s12913-018-3848-5.

Hong, K., Ngyuen, Y., and Ogden, J. (2004). Understanding HIV and AIDS-Related Stigma in Vietnam. In: *International Center for Research on Women Research Report*. Washington: ICRW.

Howes, L. (2001). Dosage alteration in the elderly – importance of mild renal impairment. *Current Therapeutics* **42** (7): 33–35.

Hu, G., Eriksson, J., Barengo, N.C. et al. (2004). Occupational commuting and leisure-time physical activity in relation to total and cardiovascular mortality among Finnish subjects with type 2 diabetes. *Circulation* **110**: 666–673.

Huang, A.R., Strombotne, K.L., Horner, E.M., and Lapham, S.J. (2018). Adolescent cognitive aptitudes and later-in-life Alzheimer disease and related disorders. *JAMA Network Open* **1** (5): e181726–e181726.

Hudson, H., Daubert, C., and Mills, R. (2000). The interdependency of protein-energy malnutrition, aging, and dysphagia. *Dysphagia* **15** (1): 31–38.

Inouye, S., van Dyck, C., Alessi, C. et al. (1990). Clarifying confusion: the confusion assessment method. *Annals of Internal Medicine* **113** (12): 941–948.

Jackson, L. and Janoff, E. (2008). Pneumococcal vaccination of elderly adults: new paradigms for protection. *Clinical Infectious Diseases* **47**: 1328–1338.

Jennings, P. (1997). Oral antihypoglycaemics: considerations in older patient with non insulin-dependent diabetes mellitus. *Drugs and Aging* **10** (5): 323–331.

Kaffashian, S., Dugravot, A., and Nabi, H. (2011). Predictive utility of the Framingham general cardiovascular risk profile for cognitive function: evidence from the Whitehall 11 Study. *European Heart Journal* **32**: 2326–2332.

Katona, C. (1994). *Depression in Old Age*. New York: John Wiley and Sons.

Keller, H., Østbye, T., and Goy, R. (2004). Nutritional risk predicts quality of life in elderly community-living Canadians. *Journal of Gerontological Association Biological Science Medical Science* **59** (1): 68–74.

Kilvert, A. and Fox, C. (2017). Diagnosis and management of diabetes in older people. *Practical Diabetes* **34** (6): 195–199.

Kirkland, F. (2003). Implementing the NSF for Diabetes through the care of older people. *Journal of Diabetes Nursing* **7** (10): 381–384.

Kirkman, S., Briscoe, V., Clark, N. et al. (2012). Diabetes in older adults: a consensus report. *Journal of the American Geriatric Society* https://doi.org/10.1111/jgs.12035.

Kock, S. and Garratt, S. (2001). *Assessing Older People: A Guide for Health Care Workers*. Eastgardens, NSW, Australia: McLennan and Petty.

Kulminski, A., Ukrantseva, S., Akushevic, I. et al. (2007). Cumulative index of health deficiencies as a characteristic of long life. *Journal of the American Geriatric Society* **55** (6): 935–940.

Lan, C., Lai, J., Chen, S., and Wong, M. (1998). 12-month Tai Chi training in the elderly: its effect on health fitness. *Medicine Science Sports Exercise* **30** (3): 345–351.

Langa, R. (2004). Extent and cost of informal caregiving for older Americans with symptoms of depression. *American Journal of Psychiatry* **161** (5): 857–863.

Lavizzo-Mourey, R., Johnson, J., and Stolley, P. (1988). Risk factors for dehydration among elderly nursing home residents. *Journal of the American Geriatric Society* **36**: 213–218.

Li, F. (2012). Tai Chi and postural stability in patients with Parkinson's disease. *New England Journal of Medicine* **366** (5): 511–519.

Lipscombe, L., Hux, J., and Booth, G. (2005). Reduced screening mammography among women with diabetes. *Archives of Internal Medicine* **165**: 2090–2095.

Logroscino, G., Kang, J., and Grodstein, F. (2004). Prospective study of type 2 diabetes and cognitive decline in women aged 70–81 years. *British Medical Journal* **328**: 548–551.

Maaravi, Y., Berry, E., Ginsberg, G. et al. (2000). Nutrition and quality of life in the aged: the Jerusalem 70-year olds longitudinal study. *Aging* **12** (3): 173–179.

MacKenzie, D. (2019). Rethinking Alzheimer's *New Scientist* (12 February), London.

Martire, L. (2010). Treatment of late-life depression alleviates caregiver burden. *Journal of the American Geriatrics Society* **58** (1): 23–29.

Masters, R., Powers, D., and Link, B. (2013). Obesity and US mortality risk over the adult life course. *American Journal of Epidemiology* https://doi.org/10.1093/aje/kws325.

McAulay, V., Deary, I., and Frier, B. (2001). Symptoms of hypoglycaemia in people with diabetes. *Diabetic Medicine* **18**: 690–705.

McWhirter, J. and Pennington, C. (1994). Incidence and recognition of malnutrition in hospitals. *British Medical Journal* **306**: 945–948.

Medical Research Council (1994). *The Health of the UK's Elderly People*. London: Medical Research Council.

Mehta, K., Pierluissi, E., Boscardin, W. et al. (2011). Clinical Index to stratify hospitalized older adults according to risk for new onset disability. *Journal American Geriatrics Society* **59**: 1206–1216.

Meuleman, J., Brechue, W., and Kubilis, P. (2000). Exercise training in the debilitated aged: strength and functional outcomes. *Archives of Physical Medicine and Rehabilitation* **81**: 312–318.

Middleton, M., Nazarenko, G., Nivison-Smith, I., and Smerdely, P. (2001). Prevalance of malnutrition and 12-month incidence of mortality in two Sydney teaching hospitals. *International Medicine Journal* **31**: 455–461.

Miller, C. (2019). *Nursing for Wellness in Older Adults*, 8e. Philadelphia: Lippincott Williams and Wilkins.

Mitchell, J. (2011). *Oral dosage forms that should not be crushed*. http://www.ismp.org/tools/donot-crush.pdf (Accessed March 2013).

Mooradian, R., McLaughlin, S., and Boyer, C. (1999). Diabetes care for older adults. *Diabetes Spectrum* **12**: 70–77.

Morley, J. and Flood, J. (1990). Psychological aspects of diabetes mellitus in older persons. *Journal of the American Geriatrics Society* **38**: 605–606.

Moyer, A. (2012) Prevention of falls in community-dwelling older adults: US Preventative Services Taskforce recommendations. Annals of Internal Medicine (29 May). www.annals.org (accessed November 2012).

National Health and Medical Research Council (1999). *A guide to the development, evaluation and implementation of clinical practice guidelines*. Commonwealth of Australia: National Health and Medical Research Council.

Nay, R. and Garrat, S. (1999). Sexuality in aged care. In: *Nursing Older People: Issues and Innovations* (eds. R. Nay and S. Garrat), 292–310. Sydney: MacLennan and Petty Pty Ltd.

Novak, D., Uller, M., Rousseaux, M. et al. (2009). Diabetes management in OLDES project. In: *31st annual International Conference of the IEEE*, 7228–7231. Minneapolis, Minnesota, September 2–6: Eng Med Biol Soc.

NPS (National Prescribing Service) (2004). *NPS Service Newsletter*. www.nps.org.au (accessed October 2012).

Oates, D., Berlowitz, D., Glickman, M. et al. (2007). Blood pressure and survival in the oldest old. *Journal American Geriatric Society* **55**: 383–388.

Orford, J., Sesso, H., Stedman, M. et al. (2002). A comparison of the Framingham and European Society of Cardiology coronary heart disease risk prediction models in the normative aging study. *American Heart Journal* **144** (1): 95–100.

Parlente, A. (2012). Antipsychotic use and Myocardial infarction in older patients with treated dementia. *Archives of Internal Medicine* **172** (8): 648–653.

Patel, N., Newstead, A., and Ferrer, R. (2012). The effects of yoga on physical functioning and health related quality of life in older adults: a systematic review and meta-analysis. *Journal of Alternative and Complementary Medicine* **18** (10): 902–917.

Persson, M., Brismar, K., Katzarski, K. et al. (2002). Nutritional status using mini nutritional assessments and subjective global assessments predicts mortality in geriatric patients. *Journal of the American Geriatrics Society* **50** (12): 1992–2002.

Peters, A. and Davidson, M. (1992). Effects of various enteral feeding products on postprandial blood glucose response in patients with type 1 diabetes. *Journal of Parenteral and Enteral Nutrition* **16** (1): 69–74.

Petterson, T., Young, B., Lee, P. et al. (1998). Wellbeing and treatment satisfaction in older people with diabetes. *Diabetes Care* **21** (6): 930–935.

Pharmaceutical Society of Australia, Australasian College of General Practitioners, and Australasian Society of Clinical and Experimental Pharmacologists and Toxicologists (2010). *Australian Medicines Handbook 2010*. Adelaide: Australian Medicines Handbook.

Phillips, P. and Popplewell, P. (2002). Diabetes and dementia. *Medicine Today* **3** (11): 30–40.

Poon, I. and Braun, U. (2005). High prevalence of orthostatic hypotension and its correlation with potentially causative medications among elderly veterans. *Journal of Clinical Pharmacy Therapy* **30** (2): 173–178.

Quayle, S. (2001). Gains of minimising falls: managing the older patient. *Australian Doctor* (July): 43–44.

Ragan, M. and Kane, C. (2010). Meaningful lives: elders in treatment for depression. *Archives of Psychiatric Nursing* **24** (6): 408–417.

Reilly, H. (1996). Screening for nutritional risk. *Proceedings of the Nutrition Society* **55**: 841–853.

Reza, M., Taylor, C., Towse et al. (2002). Insulin improves wellbeing for selected elderly type 2 diabetic subjects. *Diabetes Research and Clinical Practice* **55** (3): 201–207.

Rosenstock, J. (2001). Management of type 2 diabetes in the elderly: Special considerations. *Pulsebeat* (Oct–Nov, 5).

Royal Melbourne Hospital (2002). Project report: The prevention of functional decline in elderly patients, www.rmh.mh.org.au/project-reports/w1/i1017258 (accessed December 2012).

Rutherford, A., Wright, E.D., Hussain, Z. et al. (2004). *DAWN: Diabetes Attitudes, Wishes and Needs – The Australian Experience*. Sydney: Novo Nordisk Australia.

Schwartz, A., Sellmeyer, D., Ensrud, K. et al. (2001). Older women with diabetes have an increased risk of fracture: a prospective study. *Journal of Clinical Endocrinology Metabolism* **86**: 32–38.

Schwartz, A., Vittinghoff, E., Sellmeye, D. et al. (2003). Health, aging, and body composition study diabetes-related complications, glycemic control, and falls in older adults. *Diabetes Care* **3**: 391–396.

Schwartz, A., Vittinghoff, E., Sellmeyer, D. et al. (2008). Diabetes-related complications, glycaemic control and falls in older adults. *Diabetes Care* **31** (3): 391–396.

Shekelle, P. and Vijan, S. (2007). ACOVE: quality indicators for the care of diabetes mellitus in vulnerable elders. *Journal American Geriatric Society* **55** (Suppl S): S312–S317.

Simkin, B. (2004). Even frail elderly patients can benefit from exercise. *Geriatric Times* **3** (4): 331–334.

Simpson, C. (2005). Crushed medications: an emerging guideline. *Australian Nursing Journal* **13** (1): 1) Clinical Update–4.

Sinclair, A. (1995). Initial management of NIDDM in the elderly. In: *Diabetes in Old Age* (eds. P. Funacane and A. Sinclair), 181–201. Chichester: Wiley.

Sinclair, A. (2006). Special considerations in older adults with diabetes: meeting the challenge. *Diabetes Spectrum* **19**: 218–219.

Sinclair, A. (2011). Diabetes care for older people: a practical view on management. *Diabetes and Primary Care* **13** (1): 29–37.

Sinclair, A., Allard, I., and Bayes, A. (1997). Observation of diabetes care in long-term institutional settings with measures of cognitive function and dependency. *Diabetes Care* **20** (5): 778–786.

Sinclair, A., Dunning, T., and Rodriguez-Mañas, L. (2015). Diabetes in older people: new insights and remaining challenges. *Lancet Diabetes Endocrinol* **3** (4): 275–285.

Sinclair, A., Morley, J., Rodriguez, L. et al. (2012). Diabetes mellitus in older people: position statement on behalf of the International Association of Gerontology and Geriatrics (IAGG), the European Diabetes Working Party for Older People (EDWPOP), and the International Taskforce of Experts in Diabetes. *Journal of Applied Research and Clinical Issues* **13** (6): 497–502.

Sinclair, A.J., Hillson, R., Bayer, A.J., and National Expert Working Group (2014). Diabetes and dementia in older people: a Best Clinical Practice Statement by a multidisciplinary National Expert Working Group. *Diabetic Medicine* 31 (9): 1024–1031.

Sinclair, A., Conroy, S., and Bayer, A. (2008). Impact of diabetes on physical function in older people. *Diabetes Care* 31 (2): 233–235.

Smith, G.D. and Kydd, A. (2017). Getting care of older people right: the need for appropriate frailty assessment? *Journal of Advanced Nursing* 73 (1): 3–4.

Sommerfield, A., Deary, I., McAuley, V. et al. (2003). Short term delayed and working memory are impaired during hyperglycaemia in individuals with type 1 diabetes. *Diabetes Care* 26: 390–396.

Speight, J., Brown, J.L., Holmes-Truscott, E. et al. (2011) Diabetes MILES – Australia 2011 Survey Report. Diabetes Australia, Canberra.

Stewart, R. and Liolitsa, D. (1999). Type 2 diabetes mellitus, cognitive impairment and dementia. *Diabetic Medicine* 16: 93–112.

Stressman, J., Hammerman-Rozenberg, R., Maaravi, Y. et al. (2002). Effects of exercise on ease in performing activities of daily living and instrumental activities of daily living from age 70 to 77: the Jerusalem longitudinal study. *Journal of the American Geriatrics Society* 50 (12): 1934–1938.

Szony, G. (2004). Investigating weight loss in the elderly. *Medicine Today* 5 (9): 53–57.

Takata, Y., Ansai, T., Soh, I. et al. (2007). Association between body mass index and mortality in an 80-year-old population. *Journal of the American Geriatrics Society* 55 (6): 913–917.

Testa, M., Simonson, D., and Turner, R. (1998). Valuing quality of life and improvements in glycaemic control in people with type 2 diabetes. *Diabetes Care* 21 (Suppl. 3): c44–c52.

Tiengo, A. (1999). Burden of treatment in the elderly patient: reducing the burden of diabetes. *Diabetes Care* 11: 6–8.

Toraski, C. (2004). Care giving demands increase with depression symptoms in the elderly. *American Journal of Psychiatry* 16: 1857–1863.

Truswell, A. (2003). Nutrient supplements. *Australian Doctor* 21 (March): i–iv.

Tsai, J., Wang, W., Chan, P. et al. (2003). The beneficial effects of Tai Chi Chuan on blood pressure and lipid profile and anxiety status in a randomized controlled trial. *Journal Alternative and Complementary Medicine* 9 (5): 747–754.

UK Prospective Diabetes Study (UKPDS) Group (1998). Intensive blood-glucose control with sulphonylureas or insulin compared with conventional treatment and risk of complications in patients with type 2 diabetes (UKPDS 33). *Lancet* 352: 837–853.

Vaitkevicius, P., Ebersold, C., Shah, M. et al. (2002). Effects of aerobic exercise training in community-based subjects aged 80 and older: a pilot study. *Journal of the American Geriatrics Society* 50 (12): 2009–2013.

van der Velde, N., van den Meiracker, A., Pols, H. et al. (2007). Withdrawal of fall-risk-increasing drugs in older persons: effect on tilt-table test outcomes. *Journal of the American Geriatric Society* 55 (5): 734–739.

Vance, D. (2012). Potential factors that may promote successful cognitive aging. *Nursing Research and Reviews* 2: 27–32.

Verma, S., Luo, N., Subramaniam, M. et al. (2010). Impact of depression on health related quality of life in patients with diabetes. *Annals of Academic Medicine Singapore* 39 (12): 913–917.

Verschoor, R. (2012). GEM unit a plus for older patients. *Australian Nursing Journal* 10 (17): 36.

Victoria Department of Health and Human Services (2013). Improving care for older people program – health service initiatives. https://www2.health.vic.gov.au/hospitals-and-health-services/patient-care/older-people/resources/initiatives (accessed September 2019).

Victoria Department of Health and Human Services (2019). Quality use of medicines. https://www2.health.vic.gov.au/hospitals-and-health-services/quality-safety-service/quality-use-of-medicines (accessed September 2019).

Vidan, M., Bueno, H., Wang, Y. et al. (2010). The relationship between systolic blood pressure on admission and mortality in older patients with heart failure. *European Journal of Heart Failure* 12 (2): 148–155.

Volkert, D., Kreuel, K., and Stehle, P. (2005). Fluid intake of community-living, independent elderly in Germany – a nationwide representative study. *Journal of Nutrition Health Aging* 9 (5): 305–309.

Warren, L., Bacon, W., Harris, T. et al. (1994). The burden and outcomes associated with dehydration among US elderly. *American Journal of Public Health* 84: 1265–1269.

Waszynski, C. (2004). *The Confusion Assessment Method (CAM) Best Practice in Nursing Care of Older Adults (13)*, Revised 2012. New York: New York University.

Weinberg, A.D., Minaker, K.L., and Council on Scientific Affairs AMA (1995). Dehydration: evaluation and management in older adults. *Journal of the American Medical Association* 274 (19): 1552.

Wetzels, R., Harmsen, M., van Weel, C. et al. (2007). Interventions for improving older patients' involvement in primary care episodes. *Cochrane Database of Systematic Reviews* (1): CD004273. https://doi.org/10.1002/14651858.CD004273.pub2.

Wilson, M. and Morley, J. (2003). Impaired cognitive function and mental performance in mild dehydration. *European Journal of Clinical Nutrition* 57 (Suppl 2): S24–S29.

World Health Organisation (1983). Healthy Aging Profiles www.euro.who.int/document/e91887.pdf (accessed December 2012).

World Health Organization (1999). *Guidelines for Older Australians*. Canberra: Commonwealth of Australia.

Young, C. (2004). *Pharmacy Drug Information Paper Prepared in Response to a Personal Enquiry About Administering Commonly Used Diabetes Medications Via Enteral Tubes*. Melbourne: St Vincent's Hospital.

Zembrzuski, C. (1997). A three dimensional approach to hydration of elders: administration, clinical staff, and in service education. *Geriatric Nursing* **18** (1): 20–26.

Zimmerman, S., Sloane, P.D., Williams, C.S. et al. (2007). Residential care/assisted living staff may detect undiagnosed dementia using the minimum data set cognition scale. *Journal of the American Geriatric Society* **55** (9): 1349–1355.

Zuliani, G. (2012). Discharge diagnosis and comorbidity profile in hosptalised older patients with dementia. *International Journal of Geriatric Psychiatry* **27** (3): 313–320.

Key points

- Type 1 and type 2 diabetes both occur in children and adolescents; however, the underlying epidemiology, pathophysiology, and developmental needs are different from adults.
- Type 1 is an autoimmune process with multiple pathways to beta cell destruction (Rewers et al. 2018). Type 2 in children and adolescents is different from type 1 and type 2 in adults. It has a more rapid decline in beta cell function and complications develop earlier.
- A supportive family is an important aspect of diabetes management. Family stress and marital disharmony affect the child's metabolic control.
- Clinicians caring for with children and adolescents with diabetes need to diplomatically assess the family structure and social situation and help the family to support their child.
- Management and education strategies must be applicable to the age diabetes type and developmental stage of the individual.
- Most children have type 1 diabetes, and insulin should not be withheld in these children.
- There is increasing prevalence of type 2 diabetes in children and adolescents and complication risk is often evident at diagnosis or occurs soon after diagnosis, thus a complication assessment should be part of the initial assessment. The rate of change in body mass index (BMI) in childhood predicts adult obesity (Zhang 2019; Zhang et al. 2019).
- Ongoing subclinical cumulative injury to the brain has significant adverse effects in children and adolescents with type 1 and type 2 diabetes.
- Management strategies are different for children with type 1 and type 2 diabetes but both require an appropriate nutritious diet and regular exercise to sustain normal growth and development and psychosocial care.

Rationale

Diabetes management in children and adolescents changes during the various developmental and life transitions that occur as the child grows and develops. Diabetes and its management impacts on the family dynamics and can affect quality of life and mental well-being. Family support is essential if the child is to achieve euglycaemia, independence and psychological wellbeing.

Care of People with Diabetes: A Manual for Healthcare Practice, Fifth Edition. Trisha Dunning and Alan Sinclair.
© 2020 John Wiley & Sons Ltd. Published 2020 by John Wiley & Sons Ltd.

Thus, the family needs support and to be included in education and management decisions. Management plans need to make provision for normal growth and development and a gradual transition to independent self-care and often transition from paediatric to an adult care services, which is often also stressful and often occurs when other major life changes are occurring such as entering university or starting work.

Introduction

The number of children diagnosed with type 1 diabetes is increasing globally and type 2 diabetes in children is an emerging global problem. The incidence of type 1 doubled in the past 10 years by 2–5% (Mayer-Davis et al. 2017). Some 80% of children who develop type 1 have autoantibodies present by age 3. In most countries girls and boys are equally affected by diabetes but the rate is not the same amongst age groups. Diabetes tends to increase with age, peaking around puberty, usually slightly earlier in girls, which is consistent with the earlier onset of puberty. The incidence of type 1 diabetes peaks between five and nine years with a second peak near puberty (Leete et al. 2018). Metabolic progression and changes in c-peptide and beta cell function were discussed in Chapter 1.

A number of forms of diabetes occur in childhood. Type 1 was formerly the most common especially in children <10 years, but the incidence of type 2 in children and adolescents is also increasing. Most are described in Chapter 1 and include:

- Type 1, which accounts for ~98% of diabetes diagnosed in children and results from beta cell destruction leading to absolute insulin deficiency, immune-mediated, or idiopathic (Craig et al. 2009).
- Type 2, which has an increasing prevalence.
- Other specific types:
  - Type 2 diabetes, which mostly occurs in overweight children and adolescents.
  - Monogenic defects of beta cell function, for example, familial diabetes, neonatal diabetes. Neonatal diabetes presents in the first six months of life (Srinivasan and Donaghue 2007; Craig et al. 2009). About 50% have transient neonatal diabetes and insulin treatment is usually not required after about three months, but may recur in the second or third decade.
  - Diabetes as a consequence of diseases of the exocrine pancreas, for example, cystic fibrosis-related diabetes (Chapter 10).
  - Diabetes associated with endocrine diseases such as Cushing's syndrome and hyperthyroidism.
  - Medicine- or chemical-induced diabetes (e.g. chemotherapy, glucocorticoids)
  - Diabetes associated with genetic syndromes such as Down's and Turner's syndromes.

The reasons for the increased incidence of type 1 diabetes in children are relatively unclear. Past and current research suggests type 1 diabetes is most likely triggered at an early age by multifaceted interactions between genetic risk and environmental factors. It is diagnosed by the presence of specific autoantibodies and impaired glucose metabolism and insulin secretion, which develop in an often long prodromal stage.

Past and current research suggests type 1 diabetes in most likely triggered at an early age by multifaceted interactions between genetic risk and environmental factors. It is diagnosed by the presence of specific autoantibodies and impaired glucose metabolism and insulin secretion, which develop in an often long prodromal stage. Various explanations have been proposed; for example, genetic factors such as the *thrifty gene* (Need 1962), the *thrifty phenotype* (Hales and Barker 1992) theories. More recently, the focus has been on environmental changes that could overload the beta cells, which gave rise to the *overload hypothesis* and the *spring harvest hypothesis*, in which genetically predisposed children have an accelerated growth rate and increased body fat during spring.

Likewise, puberty occurs at a younger age. Various environmental triggers such as the decline in breastfeeding, age at which solids are introduced, exposure to foreign antigens early in life that impair the immune system, impact of maternal diet, and the *hygiene hypothesis*, have been implicated (Chapter 1).

The TRIGIR study involved 2160 newborn infants and first-degree relatives with type 1 diabetes and lasted for six to eight months. Human leukocyte antigen (HLA) typing was performed on cord blood or heel prick at birth. All mothers are encouraged to breastfeed, and two weaning formulas were compared: hydrolysed casein and standard cow's milk. The randomised code will be opened when the last recruited child turns 10 years of age (2017) (Akerblom 2011). The study provides important information about the protective effect of breastfeeding and type 1 diabetes.

More recently, omega-3 fatty acids were shown to have a small protective effect in early life due to their anti-inflammatory properties. Likewise, vitamin D metabolism, which modulates the immune and inflammatory systems, could play a role in some genetic diabetes subtypes (McGorm et al. 2018). Early childhood rapid weight gain might accelerate the progression to type 1 diabetes and the development of islet cell autoimmunity (Couper et al. 2009).

Other research shows that rapid changes in BMI are related to rates of changes at different ages during childhood, and the BMI growth curves for adults with and without obesity were evident in early childhood (Zhang 2019; Zhang et al. 2019). However, the strength of the association reduces in ages 5–10 years, then stays stable. These findings highlight the need to start promoting healthy nutrition and activity in early childhood.

The ENDIA and TEDDY studies, which concern the developmental origins of type 1 diabetes, involve several countries. They appear to support the role of the environment in the development of type 1 diabetes. For example, incidence varies around the world: Finland and Karelia, which have the highest incidence, have similar genetic backgrounds. Preconception and pregnancy may also be implicated. For example, research increasingly suggests the father's weight, exercise, and other environmental factors before conception trigger epigenetic changes in sperm that alter the child's metabolic health (Raad et al. 2017).

Rubella, now rare in many parts of the world, is a recognised trigger. Perrett et al. (2019) reported a reduction in the number of young children (0–4 years) diagnosed with type 1 diabetes between 2007 and 2015. The reduction was not reported in other age groups. Infant vaccination for rotavirus was introduced in 2007. The association does not mean there is a definite causal link, but it suggests rotavirus infections may be a risk factor for type 1 diabetes.

Metabolomic biomarkers in the progression to type 1 diabetes in childhood have also been identified. Metabolomics refers to 'a snapshot of all detectable lipids in biological materials and has potential in reflecting genetic and environmental factors contributing to the development of complex diseases, such as type 1 diabetes' (Overgaard et al. 2016). Overgaard et al. studied the progression to seroconversion to onset of type 1 diabetes, using metabolomics in small samples and for short periods of time. Three factors consistently emerged:

(1) Phospholipids are lower at birth in children who develop type 1 diabetes in early childhood.
(2) Methionine is lower in children at seroconversion.
(3) Triglycerides are increased at seroconversion and are associated with microbiome diversity, which suggests the progression of type 1 diabetes is associated with the metabolome and the microbiome.

The microbiome is acquired before and at birth and affects the innate and adaptive components of the immune system. Thus, it may play a critical role in the protection or development of type 1 diabetes. Considerable research is continuing to identify a gut microbiome signal of susceptibility to type 1 diabetes. The infant microbiome is affected by the delivery mode: vaginal or caesarean section, gestational age at birth, feeding and interventions during and after birth, and administration of antibiotics. The microbiome changes rapidly in the first two years of life as the childes nutrition intake and environment expands (McGorm et al. 2018).

Past and current research suggests type 1 diabetes is most likely triggered at an early age by multi-faceted interactions between genetic risk and environmental factors that affect the immune system. It is diagnosed when specific autoantibodies low C-peptide and impaired glucose metabolism and insulin secretion are present. The prodromal stage to impaired insulin secretion can be long.

Recently, researchers recommended checking C-peptide levels after three to five years because it may not be a useful marker at diagnosis due to the 'honeymoon effect' (residual endogenous insulin production); people may be misdiagnosed and actually have type 2 or monogentic diabetes (McCall and Nainggolan 2019). C-peptide should be indictable in type 1 after three to five years. McCall and Nainggolan (2019) assessed C-peptide levels in 757 people with type 1 diabetes of at least three years duration: 13.7% had C-peptide >200 pmol/l. They changed the diagnosis to type 2 diabetes in 27 people and 8 had a new diagnosis of monogenic diabetes.

Diabetes is often misdiagnosed or the diagnosis is delayed in developing regions and under-resourced communities in developed countries, where the symptoms might be attributed to malnutrition or starvation because people do not know the signs and symptoms (Kaufman and Riley 2007). As a consequence, morbidity and mortality rates are high and are compounded by lack of equipment and essential medications. The International Diabetes Federation (IDF) insulin for life programme has a significant impact on the lives and survival of many children in underprivileged countries.

Type 2 diabetes, once rare in children, is increasing (IDF 2002; Sinha et al. 2002; Alberti et al. 2004; Wilmot et al. 2010). Up to 45% of newly diagnosed diabetes in children and adolescents is type 2 (Shaw 2007). Emerging epidemiological data indicate type 2 diabetes mainly occurs in overweight children from specific ethnic groups particularly African Americans, Hispanics, Asians, Native Americans, Indigenous Australians, and Middle Eastern people (Shaw 2007). The increasing prevalence in Asian countries is linked to the increase in Western lifestyles with high-fat diets and reduced exercise (Gill 2007).

Some studies show a link between increasing obesity and high consumption of fructose (Johnson et al. 2007). Fructose appears to affect fat degradation in the liver by inhibiting PPAR-alpha receptor activity, which is lower in humans than rats, and the leptin signalling system, which accelerates fat oxygenation in the liver and reduces fat synthesis (Gressner et al. 2007). Insulin resistance and impaired glucose tolerance and other features of the metabolic syndrome are present in 25% of obese children, which puts them at high risk of type 2 diabetes (Sinha et al. 2002).

In addition, high rates of television viewing and obsession with computer games, an indicator of inactivity, are associated with increased risk of developing diabetes and higher HbA1c (Margeirsdottir et al. 2007; Margeirsdottir 2008; Wilmot et al. 2012). Other possible causes of type 2 diabetes in children include maternal obesity and maternal malnutrition during pregnancy and low birthweight (Wei et al. 2003), and low birthweight associated with 'catch-up growth' (Bhargava et al. 2004), see Chapters 1, 4, and 14.

These findings led to the theory of the Developmental Origins of Health and Disease (DOHaD) (Yajnik 2007). The Scientific Advisory Committee on Nutrition (SACN) (2011) advised against the early introduction of gluten because of a possible link between feeding gluten-containing foods before four months and type 1 diabetes and coeliac disease. Introducing gluten-containing foods after four months and before six months might reduce these risks. The SACN position statement is currently being revised.

Although the onset of type 2 diabetes may be less dramatic than type 1, type 2 diabetes in children is associated with significant risk of dyslipidaemia, hypertension, and polycystic ovarian syndrome, asthma, and obstructive sleep apnoea (Tait 2008; ADA 2019). Cardiovascular disease develops at an early age and is often present at diagnosis (Pinhas-Hamiel 2007) and progression to complications is faster than in children with type 1 diabetes. Significantly, children and adolescents with type 2 diabetes may be at higher risk of microvascular disease, especially nephropathy, than those with type 1 (Alberti et al. 2004; Shaw 2007).

Thus, early identification through comprehensive population health and other screening programmes and effective management of type 2 diabetes in children is imperative to reduce the burden of the disease and the projected health-care costs and should include school-based programmes (Weiss and Caprio 2005; Zimmet et al. 2007). However, the best screening test to use is unclear (Alberti et al. 2004). The IDF introduced diagnostic criteria for the metabolic syndrome in children, which was described in Chapter 1. The ADA released a position statement Evaluation and Management of Youth-Onset type 2 Diabetes (Arisianian et al. 2018) that also addresses these issues.

It is important to differentiate amongst type 1, type 2, and monogenic diabetes because the therapeutic approaches and education required differ amongst the three forms. It may be necessary to measure diabetes-associated autoantibodies such as ICA, GAD, IA 2, and IAA to detect underlying genetic abnormalities. HbA1c might be useful, but the evidence to support HbA1c as a diagnostic tool is still debated (Craig et al. 2009). Measuring fasting insulin and/or C-peptide when the blood glucose is high enough to stimulate insulin release might be useful to diagnose type 2 diabetes in young people (Craig et al. 2009).

Impact of hyper- and hypoglycaemia on brain development and function

The adult brain consumes ~25% of total body glucose utilisation. Daily brain glucose consumption peaks at 5.2 years and varies between 146 and 167 g/day. A stable blood glucose supply is critical to normal brain development and function but glucose variability and dysglycaemia often occur. Ketoacids, altered counter-regulatory hormone levels, and anti-apoptotic neuronal factors (e.g. IGF-1 and C-peptide) could be toxic to the developing brain in type 1 diabetes. Micro- and macrovascular events such as nephropathy and retinopathy can occur within 5–10 years after diagnosis; they are very rare in young children. However, ongoing, subclinical, cumulative brain injury could be a significant effect of type 1 diabetes in childhood and adolescence. See Chapters 6 and 7.

Hyper- and hypoglycaemic fluctuations affect mental efficiency and cognitive function (Gonder-Frederi et al. 2009). A single episode of serious diabetic ketoacidosis (DKA) at diagnosis in young children with type 1 diabetes affects brain growth and cognitive scores (Aye et al. 2019). DKA is associated with clinical and subclinical cerebral oedema at diagnosis and three months after diagnosis, and repeated episodes of DKA has long-term cognitive effects (Jessup et al. 2015) and changes in learning, emotion and concentration, and long-lasting effects on memory in children aged 7–16 years (Ghetti et al. 2010).

Hypoglycaemia increases global cerebral blood flow in people with type 1 diabetes and impaired hypo awareness, but not those without diabetes and those who recognise hypoglycaemiac symptoms and may be neuroprotective (Wiegers et al. 2016).

Some research suggests young people with type 2 diabetes have lower cognitive scores and structural brain changes, but the evidence is sparse (Redel et al. 2019). Deficits are reported in executive functioning and memory, consistent with the findings in adults with type 2 diabetes, and could be associated with abnormalities in brain structure (Cukierman et al. 2005; Redel et al. 2019). Various small brain imaging studies ($n = 5$–20) show:

- Lower frontal lobe in obese children and lower integrity in grey and white matter in obese people
- Lower hippocampus and prefrontal areas in obese people
- Lower caudate thalamus in obese people
- Lower caudate and putamen and lower white matter integrity in obese people
- Lower grey matter and clusters
- Higher grey matter clusters

The mechanisms driving these changers are unknown. Proposed mechanisms include:

- Macrovascular injury affecting blood flow
- Microvascular disease in the brain
- Inflammatory processes and oxidative stress
- Disruption to the hypothalamic–pituitary axis

It is essential to consider neurological effects of both type 1 and type 2 diabetes in children and adolescents when the brain is still developing. For example, limiting hyper- and hypoglycaemia, but specific treatment, apart from managing glycaemia and limiting glucose variability is unknown.

Managing children and adolescents with diabetes

The health-care needs of children and adolescents change as they grow and develop, regardless of diabetes type. Some aspects of care are common to both type 1 and type 2 but there are inherent differences in managing type 1 and type 2. Multidisciplinary team care involving a paediatric endocrinologist, diabetes educator, dietitian, psychologist, and other experts as indicated is essential to achieving optimal outcomes.

A number of management guidelines and position statements are in current use and should be referred to for specific detailed information. These include:

- National Evidence-Based Clinical Care Guidelines for Type 1 Diabetes in Children, Adolescents and Adults (2012) Australian Paediatric Endocrine Group and the Australian Diabetes Society
- ADA position statement Evaluation and Management of Youth-Onset Type 2 Diabetes (Arisianian et al. 2018)
- Standards of medical care in diabetes: special considerations for children and adolescents (ADA 2013; 2019)
- SIGN (2010)
- Nice Guidelines
- Clinical Practice Consensus Guidelines (2009) Compendium International Society for Paediatric and Adolescent Diabetes

Aspects of care that apply to both type 1 and type 2 diabetes in children and adolescents

Where possible, education and stabilisation at diagnosis should occur in an ambulatory setting. However, hospitalisation is necessary in about 30% of newly diagnosed type 1 children (Silverstein et al. 2005). If hospitalisation is necessary, such as for significant ketoacidosis, the time spent in the hospital should be minimised.

The overall aims of management are to provide an individualised education and management plan to achieve an accurate diagnosis. This is important to subsequent management and monitoring.

Differentiating between type 1 and type 2 diabetes at diagnosis is not always straightforward due to the increasing prevalence of obesity, ketonuria, and DKA (Svoren and Wolfsdorf 2005). About one third of adolescents with type 2 diabetes are ketotic and 25% of newly diagnosed people present with DKA. If the diabetes type is not clear, it may be advisable to measure islet cell autoantibodies and C-peptide. Table 1.2 in Chapter 1 depicts the main differences between type 1 and type 2 diabetes, as discussed at the beginning of the chapter. The following are care guidelines:

- Prevent or delay the onset of diabetes-related complications, including short-term complications such as hypoglycaemia, hyperosmolar states, and ketoacidosis. Long-term complications are rare before puberty, but complication screening typically begins around age 10 or earlier.
- Provide a balanced nutritious diet suitable for the growth and development stage of the child (Marks 2019).
- Accept the diabetes by the child and the family.
- Develop a holistic, integrated health plan that includes psychological heath, sexual health, responsible contraception, and planned pregnancy suitable to the age and developmental stage of the young person.
- Measure HbA1c every three to four months. The target should be individualised, working towards HbA1c < 7.5% (53 mmol/mol) without hypoglycaemia. All management should be personalised and developed with the child and their parents where relevant.
- Enable the family and child to gradually take over the diabetes self-care tasks.

- Consider admission to acute care, should the need arise.
- Preventive care includes regular blood glucose monitoring, complication screening, counselling about smoking risks, immunisation according to immunisation schedules, and influenza vaccinations during at-risk periods when the child is >6 months, as well as screening children with type 1 diabetes for other diseases associated with compromised immunity such as thyroid disease and coeliac disease (Chapter 10).
- Screen for macro and microvascular complications and blood pressure, generally commencing between 10 and 12 years. Screening should include monitoring the effects on cognition, eating disorders, and psychological well-being, including diabetes-related distress and depression (Chapter 15) and in susceptible children for drug addiction (Hagger et al. 2016, 2018).
- Facilitate smooth transfer to adult care, which includes a structured familiarisation and education process, which should be a collaborative process between paediatric and adult services (SIGN 2010).
- Sexual health education including safe sex, contraception counselling is an important part of caring for children with diabetes during puberty and adolescence.
- Diabetes service providers and schools/education facilities should work together to ensure the child's diabetes self-care needs can be performed in school and that school staff are knowledgeable about managing hypoglycaemia and disk days and have emergency telephone numbers if needed. Some Australian schools have structured gardening and cooking programmes that focus on preventative heath, healthy eating, and activity.

Almost all guidelines recommend that a knowledgeable and experienced multidisciplinary team provides diabetes care. The child should be involved in developing their diabetes management plan within their capabilities. Disagreements between the family and the child about who is responsible for managing their diabetes and poor adherence are predictors of high HbA (Anderson et al. 1991). The child's involvement in their self-care gradually increases as they mature and their fine motor and problem-solving and coping skill develop.

Regular assessment of general health and diabetes status and how the family is managing is essential because there are major physical, psychological, emotional, spiritual impacts of diabetes, and social differences amongst the growth and development stages. Assessing maturity, sensitive supervision, and enabling the child to gradually take over specific diabetes self-care tasks according to their capability should be factored into a holistic diabetes plan. The family needs to be involved in developing the care plan and monitoring progress.

Educating teachers and other carers is also important and the child should be involved in these activities if appropriate. Diabetes should not preclude the child from attending school excursions and camps but extra precautions will need to be taken, for example, being able to eat on time. Diabetes camps provide an important learning experience and many children who attended camps when they were young help out on diabetic camps, as they grow older. The peer support children and adolescents receive in camps contributes to psychological well-being (ADA 2004c).

Managing type 1 diabetes

Type 1 usually presents with a sudden onset of symptoms, and insulin injections are needed for survival. A well-balanced diet and adequate appropriate exercise are also essential. This usually includes carbohydrate counting using programs such as Dose Adjustment for Normal Eating (DAFNE) (REF) and possible for rat and protein (REF). Referral to a dietitian is recommended. The diet needs to supply essential nutrients and consider the need to manage under- and overeating and their consequences. Obesity is common in children with type 1 diabetes and significantly increases cardiovascular risk (ADA 2019).

Insulin and dietary requirements can change rapidly, especially in children, due to rapid changes in activity levels and growth. Therefore, consistent acceptable blood glucose levels may be difficult to achieve.

Children and their families should receive appropriate education as well as recommendations about healthy eating and exercise. Such education includes recognising and managing hypo- and hyperglycaemia, adjusting insulin for activity and frequent blood glucose monitoring. Many children and families elect to use an insulin pump, including closed loop and hybrid closed-loop systems and or continuous blood glucose monitoring (Chapter 3).

Most children with type 1 diabetes should be treated with basal bolus regimens or continuous subcutaneous insulin infusions (insulin pump). They/family will need to monitor their blood glucose 6–10/day, including preprandial and some postprandial and prebed monitoring. Monitoring is also required during and after exercise and during illness (ADA 2019).

- Newly diagnosed type 1: initial dose ~0.5–1.0 units/kg/day. Lower doses may be required before puberty. Higher doses may be needed after puberty and in DKA. Infants and toddlers require very small doses. Insulin pens that can deliver 0.5 unit doses are available and should be used where possible. Great care and appropriate parental education is required for accurate dilutions.
- Newly diagnosed type 1 is often followed by a honeymoon period once the acute metabolic disturbance is reversed. Endogenous insulin production increases for varying periods up to ~12 months. Insulin doses usually need to be reduced to prevent hypoglycaemia. Insulin requirements increase as the honeymoon phase ends and at the onset of puberty. During puberty, 1.5 units/kg/day are often needed.
- Screen for associated autoimmune diseases such as coeliac disease (Chapter 10), and thyroid disease soon after diagnosis and coeliac disease within two years after diagnosis and again after five years. If the diagnosis is confirmed the child will require a dietary review and a gluten free diet.
- Manage cardiovascular risk: blood pressure to ensure it is within the 90th percentile range for age, height, and gender, if the child is hypertensive the diet and activity should be reviewed and ACEI or ARD medicines at an appropriate dose initiated. Fasting lipids should be measured when the blood glucose is stable and in children 10 years and older and dietary changes implemented if necessary and statins initiated if diet and exercise are not successful. The goal is low-density lipoproteins (LDL) 2.6 mmol/mol (<100 mg/dl) (ADA 2019).
- Annually screen for microvascular complications such as nephropathy, e.g. spot urine at puberty and after age 10; and retinopathy dilated comprehensive eye examination and neuropathic examinations after three to five years of diabetes or after age 10 and at puberty and administering relevant treatment to prevent progression (ADA 2004a,b; 2019).

A supportive and encouraging family is important if the child is to accept diabetes and eventually take over diabetic self-management. The family, in turn, needs support, advice, and encouragement. Good control is associated with a structured supportive family (Johnson et al. 1990; Thompson et al. 2001). Families need to provide appropriate supervision and discipline and maintain a family structure that meets the needs of the child and other family members.

Hypoglycaemia can be unpredictable in children whose activity level and intake and consequently insulin needs can vary enormously from day-to-day and within the day. Insulin need also changes with exercise and pubertal hormone changes. Hypoglycaemia can be difficult to deal with in young children and can manifest as:

- Unaccustomed naughtiness
- Noisy behaviour
- Aggression
- Crying
- Tremulousness

If it is not recognised and treated promptly, the child can become unconscious, which is frightening for the child and those around them (see Chapter 6). Parents often feel safer if they have glucagon available, and some also like it to be available at school if the teacher or school nurse is appropriately educated. Nocturnal hypoglycaemia can be particularly difficult to manage.

Table 13.1 Self-management expectations according to age and stage. (a) Metabolic targets need to be appropriate to the age and stage and revised regularly as the child grows and develops; and (b) recommended HbA1c targets.

key	Key milestones	Management considerations
(a) Developmental stage		
Babies <1 year	The parents are responsible for care. Significant hypoglycaemia risk due to undeveloped catecholamine response.	Family stress. Unrecognised hypoglycaemia, coma, seizures. Nocturnal hypoglycaemia.
1–3 years	The parents are responsible for care. Food refusal is common and increases the risk of hypoglycaemia. Hypoglycaemia may manifest as temper tantrums.	Consistent rules and discipline are important. Blood glucose testing is needed to distinguish normal toddler's behaviour from hypoglycaemia.
3–7 years	Fine motor skills are developing and whilst the parents retain responsibility for providing care they should involve the child in their care.	Involve the child in self-management.
8–11 years	Children are capable of undertaking many diabetes self-management tasks but still require parental guidance and support. They may enjoy diabetes camps and teaching their class about diabetes but care must be taken to ensure these activities do not negatively impact on their difference from nondiabetic children.	Diagnosis at this age often results in mild depression and depression increases with longer duration of diabetes but is different for girls and boys. Depression may be precipitated when the 'honeymoon phase' ends.
Adolescence	Physical, cognitive, and emotional development occurs rapidly. Puberty can affect metabolic control. Diabetes self-care can inhibit independence Most adolescents should be responsible for their self-care but parental support and guidance are still needed.	Poor metabolic control and nonadherence may indicate psychological problems or family conflict. Parental support is still needed but needs to be tactful.
(b) HbA1c targets		
Age range	HbA1c targets	Blood glucose target range
Children <6 years	7.5–8.5%	<6 months, 5–15 mmol/l
6–12 years	<8%	<6 years, 7–12 mmol/l (bedtime)
Adolescents	<7.5%	>12 years, 4–8 mmol/l, 7–10 mmol/l (bedtime)

Australian Paediatric Endocrine Group (2005). But note the imperative to consider the individual child's capabilities and needs.

There may not be any significant long-term effects associated with nocturnal hypoglycaemia, but it can affect mood the following day. The child maybe irritable on waking and might impair recognition of daytime hypoglycaemia (Dunger and Hovorka 2007). If hypoglycaemia is severe and frequent, then diet, exercise, and medication regimen need to be revised and other contributing factors excluded. The parents may learn to use glucagon; see Chapter 6. Table 13.1 depicts the major management strategies according to developmental stage.

Managing type 2 diabetes

Screening for prediabetes and diabetes could commence in at-risk children at puberty or after age 10 and when they are overweight with BMI > 95th percentile for age and gender and other risk factors. The test should be repeated every three years or more frequently, e.g. increasing BMI using fasting plasma glucose or the two-hour glucose after a 75 g glucose load. Pancreatic autoantibodies could be assessed to exclude type 1 diabetes, because overweight and obesity also occur in children with type 1 diabetes (ADA 2019).

- Type 2 diabetes in children is more common in ethnic minorities, and in some countries these might be migrants or refugees who require specific consideration for access to essential treatment and to detect discrimination. Like type 1, they require the support and understanding of teachers and other school staff.

- Management consists of healthy eating and regular physical activity, avoiding smoking. Blood glucose self-monitoring needs to be individualised considering the medicine management regimen. Referral to a dietitian is recommended. The HbA1c target is usually, 7% (53 mmol/mol) or, in high-risk children, <6.5% (48 mmol/mol) if hypoglycaemia can be avoided (ADA 2019). Schwenk (2007) showed an intensive weight management programme consisting of intensive nutrition information, and a structured education programme led to improvements in blood pressure, HDL, and LDL cholesterol, weight loss, and lower BMI compared to controls. However, Schwenk noted the programme was intensive and time consuming. Cost–benefit analysis was not reported.

- Medications are often needed to control fasting and postprandial blood glucose and blood lipids if they are not controlled using lifestyle interventions. Metformin is first-line therapy and may assist with weight loss (Copeland et al. 2005) Weight loss and exercise are central to management but symptoms, weight loss, and persistent hyperglycaemia indicates medications are needed. Insulin (~2 units/kg) may be required initially (Svoren and Wolfsdorf 2005). Metformin could be commenced initially in children with no contraindication such as renal impairment. The recommended starting dose of metformin for children 10–16 years is 500 mg/day, which can be increased to 500 mg DB with further weekly 500 mg increments to a maximum daily dose of 2000 mg, provided there are no contraindications to its use or associated adverse events (Svoren and Wolfsdorf 2005). Alternatively, 500 mg metformin XR can be administered with the evening meal to reduce the gastrointestinal side effects. Bedtime basal insulin such as glargine can be commenced at bedtime if blood glucose is not controlled using metformin.

- Those who present with hyperglycaemic symptoms, weight loss, and hyperosmolar hyperglycaemic states (HHS) or acidosis should be treated with insulin, initially. Prescribing recommendations for glucose-lowering medicines (GLMs) and other guidelines in the relevant country should be followed.

- HbA1c should be measured every three months and treatment intensified if blood glucose and HbA1c targets are not achieved.

- General care such as vaccinations and complication screening (macro- and microvascular disease, sleep disturbance/apnoea, neuropathy, and psychological health) should be part of the comprehensive care plan.

- Assess for nonalcoholic fatty liver disease (NAFLD) at diagnosis and then annually (Chapter 10).

- Like type 1 diabetes, family involvement in the child's care is critical. This can be challenging in some families where one or both parents also have type 2 diabetes and do not adequately self-care. The whole family might benefit from lifestyle counselling, if they agree. Education for the child and parents is essential and should include information about hypoglycaemia if insulin or insulin secretagogus are used (Chapter 5).

The glucagon response might be blunted in adolescents with type 1 diabetes. Inadequate glucagons response is associated with the duration of diabetes but can occur within a month of diagnosis, which means a key protective mechanism against hypoglycaemia is deficient (Gruden et al. 2012). Other factors that can affect hypoglycaemia recognition include environmental factors such as distraction, and genetic makeup, glycaemic control, and age.

During adolescence the hormonal surge at puberty can make blood glucose control difficult. Dietary restrictions and the diabetes self-care regimen can be seen as obstacles to fitting in with peer activities and may be neglected. Achieving independence from the family can be difficult if diabetes is diagnosed at this time.

Social pressure and the emphasis on food that is part of the diabetes management regimen can increase the likelihood of eating disorders. Young people with diabetes fear putting on weight and skip meals and run their blood glucose levels high to avoid weight gain (Dunning 1994). Eating disorders are widespread amongst adolescent girls, and diabetic-specific concerns may contribute to their development. The full range of subclinical and clinical eating disorders may be more prevalent in women with diabetes (Colton 2007). Eating disorders in type 1 diabetes often arise in adolescence and often persist into adulthood (Colton 2007).

Colton distinguished between disturbed eating and eating disorders and found girls with an eating disorder had higher HbA1c and BMI but that the HbA1c was not necessarily higher in the presence of disturbed eating. Health professionals need to be sensitive to social pressures and body image issues and the possibility that an eating disturbance might be present. Screening for disturbed eating is essential and referral for specific counselling might be indicated to avoid long-term nutritional problems and other associated risks such as depression. Children with type 2 diabetes may be at particular risk given the focus on weight loss.

The menarche affects control in girls and thereafter the blood glucose profile often reflects the stages of the menstrual cycle (see Chapter 11). When the child becomes an adolescent, counselling regarding contraceptive and pregnancy are vital. Metabolic control often deteriorates partly due to the increase in growth hormone and reduced insulin sensitivity at puberty. Psychosocial issues such as privacy, body image, and independence also have an impact. Negative feedback about the adolescent's metabolic control and 'nagging' about the risk of long-term complications is unlikely to be effective and may actually result in inattendance.

Polycystic ovary syndrome (PCOS) is associated with insulin resistance and diabetes and often first manifests at menarche. The effects of unpredictable, heavy menstrual bleeding are disabling and place the young woman at risk of iron deficiency anaemia, and tiredness (Legro and Dunaif 1997). Chronic anovulation increases the risk of endometrial hyperplasia and endometrial cancer. Infertility is a consequence and has a negative impact on the young person's self-concept. Early diagnosis and management is important. PCOS often manifests as excess facial hair and irregular periods, see Chapter 14.

Generally, paediatric depression is serious, common, and persistent. It is the second leading contributor to the global disease burden between ages 15 and 44 and recurs in 70% of affected individuals (World Health Organization [WHO] 2004). It is more common in boys before puberty and in girls after puberty. Mood disorders are associated with high morbidity, concomitant diseases, and risk-taking behaviour such as excess alcohol consumption, smoking, and illegal drug use. Children with diabetes are at particular risk and higher rates of depression have been reported in young people with diabetes than the general population (Blanz et al. 1993); thus, regular mental health assessment is essential. Bryden (2002) reported poor clinical outcomes in approximately one third of young people with diabetes, which highlights the need to identify problems early.

Children from single-parent families and families with marital conflict are at increased risk of poor metabolic control (Thompson et al. 2001). Family dysfunction, inadequate treatment adherence, and unacceptable glycaemic control often go hand-in-hand (Lorenz and Wysocki 1991). Unacceptable glycaemic control carries the risk of admissions to hospital with ketoacidosis and the development of long-term diabetic complications (see Chapter 10). Nonadherence is multifactorial and may be a sign of rebellion or forgetfulness. Aggressive antisocial conduct is more likely to result in poor metabolic control whereas emotional problems tend to lead to better glycaemic control (Bryden et al. 2001).

Discrepancies between home blood glucose tests and HbA1c might indicate underlying stress and coping problems. It represents an opportunity to explore factors operating in the young person's life, their feelings about diabetes, and the management regimen and their coping mechanisms (Conrad and Gitelmand 2006). This needs to be undertaken very tactfully using techniques suitable to the child. For example, inviting young children to write a story, poem, or draw a picture about their life with diabetes for the next visit, which can act as the basis for meaningful discussion and/or indicate whether referral for specialist counselling is needed.

An emerging issue that has both positive benefits and negative consequences for young people is their disclosure of personal information on the Internet. Internet support groups can enable young people to anonymously discuss diabetes with peers, access information, and reduce feelings of isolation. However, an analysis of information entered on MySpace revealed that most entries by 16- and 17-year-olds included personally identifiable information, information about personal risk-taking behaviours such as sexual activity and drug and alcohol use, and often included a photograph/s (Moreno et al. 2007).

Table 13.2 Important medicine-related information children need. Information should be provided, using recognised education strategies and quality use of medicines. Quality use of medicines is discussed in Chapter 5.

(1) Children have a right to information about their medicines appropriate to their age, diabetes type, and developmental levels. The information should encompass over-the-counter and complementary medicines as well as conventional medicines be personalised.

(2) Children are innately curious and want to know about their medicines. Health professionals should provide relevant information to the child as well as their parents.

(3) Children should gradually assume responsibility for their medicines management, including keeping a record of the medicines they are taking.

(4) Health professionals, family, and carers should set a good example with respect to medicines use, including safe use, appropriate storage and disposal, and sharps disposal.

(5) Children should be involved in discussions about participating in clinical trials and be given the opportunity to accept or decline participation.

The transfer from paediatric care to adult specialist care can be very stressful.

Transfer should be a planned process between the child, their family and adult service providers. Neglecting the diabetes self-care, not attending appointments, and poor metabolic control are common at this time. Tact and understanding are very important if these young people are not to be lost to adequate medical supervision (Rosen et al. 2003).

Medicine self-management

Managing medicines is an important aspect of self-care that must gradually be assumed by the child. The transition to assuming responsibility for managing diabetes medicines is a key aspect of most diabetes education programmes. However, adolescents are likely to use a range of other medicines; thus, medication management should include age-appropriate information about other medicines including over-the-counter and complementary medicines (CM) as well as diabetes medicines.

Self-initiated over-the-counter medicines use begins early in adolescence: by about 16 years the majority of adolescents have self-prescribed medicines such as analgesics and antipyretics, girls self-prescribe more frequently than boys (Buck 2007). However, adolescents' knowledge about these medicines is often inadequate and, significantly, parental education did not influence medication knowledge.

Medicine education programmes for adults are usually appropriate for children >11 years. A number of medicine education programmes have been developed for younger children (Curry et al. 2006; Gardiner and Dvorkin 2006; Federal Drug Administration [FDA] n.d.). Table 13.2 outlines important information to facilitate the transition to medication self-management.

Other conditions associated with diabetes

Chapter 10 discussed conditions associated with diabetes that are relevant to children and adolescents, such as liver problems, coeliac disease, and cystic fibrosis-related diabetes. Other rare conditions that can occur in young people with diabetes requiring early diagnosis and monitoring include:

- Mauriac syndrome in children with persistently poorly controlled diabetes and is more common in developing countries that do not have access to essential medicines and other products.
- Hypothyroidism due to autoimmune thyroiditis.
- Hyperthyroidism, which is less common than hypothyroidism.
- Lipodystrophy (lipoatrophy and lipohypertrophy), which is less common since human insulin was introduced but does still occur, thus it is important to check insulin injection sites regularly.

- Necrobiosis lipoidica diabeticorum, which typically occurs in the pretibial region.
- Limited joint mobility (LJM), which is an early complication of type 1 diabetes. It is bilateral and usually painless and occurs in the finger and large joints and the skin usually has a tight waxy appearance. LJM is associated with increased risk of retinopathy, nephropathy, and neuropathy. Management consists of monitoring growth and development, screening for specific conditions such as thyroid function tests and routine examination of joints and radiological examination if indicated. Optimising glycaemic control is essential (Kordonouri et al. 2009).

Strategies for enhancing adherence during adolescence

Establishing a therapeutic relationship with the young person is essential so they feel comfortable about discussing issues with health professionals.

Young people with and without diabetes engage in risk-taking behaviour, including not following medical advice, but no more so than adults (Johnson et al. 1990). A management approach that seeks concordance between health professional advice and the young person's behaviour is more likely to be successful (Fleming and Watson 2002).

A range of issues can impact on normal growth and development and some issues have a greater priority than health status for the young person. It is normal adolescent behaviour to think in the short-term, learn from their experience, and experiment. This means that short-term goals are more likely to be effective and can be modified progressively. Young people should be encouraged to discuss their experiences, which can be used as experiential teaching and learning strategies.

Many young people feel vulnerable, and this can be exacerbated by diabetes and the need to take on the responsibility for adult roles and diabetes management. Exploring these concerns and identifying diabetes-related distress and depressive symptoms is essential. Hagger et al. (2018) showed diabetes distress (36%) and depressive symptoms (21%) occurred in children 13–19 years using the Problem Areas in Diabetes-Teen Version (PAID-T). Diabetes distress was associated with high HbA1c, infrequent blood glucose monitoring.

Many young people feel frustrated when they 'do all the right things' and their metabolic control is inadequate. This can lead to decreased motivation and feelings of helplessness and hopelessness, especially if they do not have a supportive family (Kyngas 2000). Focusing on the positive aspects and small gains and not on 'good' and 'bad' control can take the focus off failure. Striving for diabetes balance is more important than control. Metabolic control will be achieved if the individual's life is in balance.

The lack of a consistent and accessible health service and dealing with new health professionals when moving to adult care can be stressful. Collaboration between paediatric and adult services and a planned transition process can overcome some of these problems (Dunning 1994; Department of Health 2001; ADA 2019). The Endocrine Society developed guidelines for managing care transitions for children with type 1 diabetes that can help clinicians support the family during care transition (https://www.endocrine.org/guidelines-and-clinial-praactice-resources/transition-of-care).

Using multiple strategies and consultation techniques that encourage young people to ask questions is more likely to uncover accurate and meaningful information than the consultation where the young person tells the health professional 'what they want to hear' and the health professional does not pick up on relevant cues that things may not be 'all right'. Adherence issues should be discussed in the context of the young person's lifestyle and goals. Adherence can be enhanced by taking these steps:

- Organise a youth-appropriate service.
- See the young person separately from their parents as they mature and begin to take responsibility for their diabetes management.
- Address the broader issues and life priorities and put diabetes into that context.
- Give clear simple instructions and supporting verbal information with written instructions and the availability of telephone advice.

- Utilise family/carers as appropriate.
- Consider the type of questions likely to get honest answers; for example, instead of asking, 'Do you always take your correct dose of insulin?' try, 'What dose of insulin suits you best?' (Fleming and Watson 2002).

Clinician responsibilities in hospital

In addition to the care tasks outlined in specific chapters such as Chapter 1, it is important to:

- Document height and weight on percentile charts.
- Monitor blood glucose four times per day and when the child feels symptoms of hyper or hypoglycaemia. Vary testing times so that some tests are performed two hours after a meal or after activity. Test at night to detect nocturnal hypoglycaemia. Children managed using insulin pumps require more frequent monitoring.
- Test blood ketones if blood glucose is ~15 mmol/l or the child is acutely ill or has a fever.
- Encourage independence and encourage the child to administer their insulin injections and test their blood glucose. This can be an opportunity to assess technique or for the child to learn these techniques.
- Monitor dietary intake and ensure appropriate dietary review by dietitian.
- Ensure diabetic knowledge is assessed.
- Ensure privacy during procedures.
- Avoid admitting adolescents and children to wards with older people, if possible.

Clinical observation

Enuresis is an unusual presentation of diabetes in children.

Ketoacidosis in children

The management of ketoacidosis is described in Chapter 7. Additional issues specific to children follow:

- Cerebral oedema is a very serious medical emergency in children. Monitoring mental status and strict fluid calculations are essential, especially when using IV insulin infusions.
- Headache and/or altered behaviour may indicate impending cerebral oedema. Management includes bolus IV mannitol, nursing with the head of the bed elevated, and fluid restriction.
- Sodium bicarbonate is not usually given in childhood DKA because of the risk of hypokalaemia, cerebral acidosis, and changed oxygen affinity of haemoglobin.
- Monitor sodium levels and adjust IV fluid appropriately as the blood glucose falls. Hyponatraemia can herald impending cerebral oedema.

Complementary therapy use in children

Complementary and alternative medicine (CAM) use in children is a complex issue. There are benefits and risks depending on the age of the child and the therapy used and their capacity to make an informed choice and understand the consequences of the choice to use or not use CAM. Young children with immature livers, developing central nervous systems and immune systems that increases their susceptibility to adverse medicine events: both conventional and CM medicines.

Complementary medicine (CM) cathartic and diuretic medicines may cause electrolyte imbalance and dehydration rapidly in young children. Long-term use may increase the likelihood of acute, chronic, or cumulative adverse effects; others are contraindicated in children

(Woolf 2003). However, therapies such as music, massage, yoga, and meditation have significant health benefits. Most parents/children who use CM do not stop their conventional management regimen but only ~32% inform their conventional health professionals they use CM. Thus, health professionals should ask about CM use and the reasons for using specific therapies on a regular basis.

The reported prevalence of CM use in children generally varies from 2% to 95%, depending on where the information was collected and the underlying condition being treated (Cranswick and Lim 2006; Picciano 2007; Tsao et al. 2007). In Germany, Dannemann et al. (2008) found 42% of a sample of children with type 1 diabetes used at least one CM modality. Significantly, the children did not stop their insulin. Commonly used therapies include:

- Vitamin and mineral supplements.
- Echinacea for treating common childhood illnesses such as URTI or to boost the immune system.
- Massage, with and without essential oils. Massage reduces stress and improves quality in children with type 1 diabetes and their parents providing the massage (Field et al. 1997).
- Yoga.
- Meditation.
- Energy therapies.
- Music therapy.
- Hypnotherapy.

General reasons for using CM include to improve well-being, reduce stress and anxiety, the assumption that CM have fewer side effects, and because the parents have an interest in self-care. Particularly risky therapies are:

- Ear candles.
- Aromatherapy candles.
- Essential oils in vapourisers within reach of small children. Ingesting of even small doses of some essential oils, for example, *eucalyptus* sp. from a vapouriser can cause oral burns and toxicity.
- Moxibustion.
- Case reports indicate Infacalm drops cause hypoglycaemia, drowsiness, and tachycardia in susceptible children.

More information about CM can be found in Chapter 18.

References

ADA (2004a). Nephropathy in diabetes. Position statement. *Diabetes Care* **27** (Suppl. 1): S79–S83.

ADA (2004b). Retinopathy in diabetes. Position statement. *Diabetes Care* **27** (Suppl. 1): S84–S87.

ADA (2004c). Diabetes care in camps. Position statement. *Diabetes Care* **27** (Suppl. 1): S129–S131.

ADA (2013). Standards of medical care in diabetes (position statement). *Diabetes Care* http://www.care. diabetesjournals.org/content/36/Supplement_1.

ADA (2019). Standards of medical in diabetes. Children and adolescents. *Diabetes Care* **42** (Suppl.1): S148–S164.

Akerblom, H. (2011). The trial to reduce IDDM in the genetically at risk (TRIGIR) study: recruitment, intervention and follow up. *Diabetologia* **54** (3): 627–633.

Alberti, G., Zimmet, P., Shaw, J. et al. (2004). The international diabetes federation consensus workshop. Type 2 diabetes in the young: the evolving epidemic. *Diabetes Care* **27**: 1798–1811.

Anderson, B., Auslander, W., Jung, K. et al. (1991). Assessing family sharing of diabetes responsibilities. *Diabetes Spectrum* **4** (5): 263–268.

Arisianian, S., Bacha, F., Grey, M. et al. (2018). Evaluation and management of youth onset type 2 diabetes; a position statement of the American Diabetes Association. *Diabetes Care* **41**: 2648–2668.

Australian Paediatric Endocrine Group (2005). The Australian Clinical Practice Guidelines on the Management of Type 1 Diabetes in Children and Adolescents (www.chw.edu.au/prof/services/endocrinology/APEG).

Aye, T., Mazaika, P., Mauras, N. et al. (2019). Impact of early diabetic ketoacidosis on the developing brain. *Diabetes Care* **42**: 443–449.

Bhargava, S., Sachdev, H., and Fall, C. (2004). Relation of serial changes in childhood body-mass index to impaired glucose tolerance in young adulthood. *New England Journal of Medicine* 350: 865–875.

Blanz, B.J., Rensch-Riemann, B.S., Fritz-Sigmund, D.I., and Schmidt, M.H. (1993). IDDM is a risk factor for adolescent psychiatric disorders. *Diabetes Care* 16: 1579–1587.

Bryden, K. (2002). Turbulent time: the adolescent with Type 1 diabetes. *Journal of Diabetes Nursing* 6 (3): 83–87.

Bryden, K., Pevelr, R., Stein, A. et al. (2001). The clinical and psychological course of diabetes from adolescence to young adulthood: a longitudinal study. *Diabetes Care* 24: 1536–1540.

Buck, M. (2007). Self-medication by adolescents. *Paediatric Pharmacology* 13 (5): 1–4.

Clinical Practice Consensus Guidelines (2009). Compendium International Society for Paediatric and Adolescent Diabetes. http://www.ispad.org/sites/default/files/…/ispad_guidelines_2009.

Colton, P. (2007). Eating disturbance common and persistent in girls with type 1 diabetes. *Diabetes Care* 30: 2861–2862.

Conrad, S. and Gitelmand, S. (2006). If the numbers don't fit … discrepancies between meter glucose readings and haemoglobin A1c reveal stress of living with diabetes. *Clinical Diabetes* 24: 45–47.

Copeland, C., Becker, D., Gottschalk, M., and Hale, D. (2005). Type 2 diabetes in children and adolescents: risk factors, diagnosis, and treatment. *Clinical Diabetes* 23: 181–185.

Couper, J., Beresford, D., Hirte, C. et al. (2009). Weight gain in early life predicts risk of diet autoimmunity in children with first degree relatives with type 1 diabetes. *Diabetes Care* 33 (1): 91–99.

Craig, M., Hattersley, A., and Donaghue, K. (2009). Definition, epidemiology and classification of diabetes in children and adolescents. *Peadiatric Diabetes* 10 (Suppl. 12): 3–12.

Cranswick, N. and Lim, A. (2006). Use of over-the-counter and complementary medicine in children. *Australian Doctor* (21 July), pp. 25–32.

Cukierman, T., Gerstein, H., and Williamson, J. (2005). Cognittive decline and dementia in diabetes – systematic overview of prospective observational studies. *Diabetelogia* 48 (12): 2460–2469.

Curry, H., Schmer, C., and Ward-Smith, P. (2006). Kid Cards: teaching children about their medications. *Journal of Paediatric Health Care* 20: 414–418.

Dannemann, K., Hecker, W., Haberland, H. et al. (2008). Use of complementary and alternative medicine in children with type 1 diabetes mellitus – Prevalence, patterns of use, costs. *Paediatric Diabetes Online* http://www.blackwell-synergy.com/doi/abs/10.111/j.1399–5448.2008.00377.x (accessed April 2008).

Department of Health (2001). *Diabetes National Service Framework: Standards for Diabetes Services*. London: Department of Health.

Dunger, D. and Hovorka, R. (2007). No more nightmares: treatments to prevent nocturnal hypoglycaemia in children. *Diabetes Voice* (May Special Issue): 22–25.

Dunning, P. (1994). Having diabetes: young adult perspectives. *The Diabetes Educator* 21 (1): 58–65.

Federal Drug Administration (FDA) (n.d.). FDA Center for Drug Evaluation and Research. *Medicines in My Home*. http://www.fda.gov/medsinmyhome/MIMH_background.htm (accessed December 2007).

Field, T., Morrow, C., Valdeon, C. et al. (1997). Massage lowers blood glucose levels in children with diabetes. *Diabetes Spectrum* 10: 237–239.

Fleming, T. and Watson, P. (2002). Enhancing compliance in adolescents. *Current Therapeutics* 43 (3): 14–18.

Gardiner, P. and Dvorkin, L. (2006). Promoting medication adherence in children. *American Family Physician* 74: 793–800.

Gill, T. (2007). Young people with diabetes and obesity in Asia: a growing epidemic. *Diabetes Voice* 52: 20–22.

Ghetti, S., Lee, J.K., Sims, C.E. et al. (2010). Diabetic ketoacidosis and memory dysfunction in children with type 1 diabetes. *The Journal of pediatrics* 156 (1): 109–114.

Gonder-Frederil, L., Zrebiec, J., Bauchowitz, A. et al. (2009). Cognitive function is disrupted by both hypo- and hyperglycaemia in school-aged children with type 1 diabetes: a field study. *Diabetes Care* 32 (6): 1001–1006.

Gressner, O., Weiskirchen, R., and Gressner, M. (2007). Evolving concepts of liver fibrogenesis provide new diagnostic and therapeutic options. *Comparative Hepatology* 6: 7. https://doi.org/10.1186/1476-5926-6-7.

Gruden, G., Barutta, F., Chaturvedi, N. et al. (2012). Severe hypoglycemia and cardiovascular disease incidence in type 1 diabetes: the EURODIAB Prospective Complications Study. *Diabetes care* 35 (7): 1598–1604.

Hagger, V., Hendrieckx, C., Sturt, J. et al. (2016). Diabetes distress among adolescents with type 1 diabetes: a systematic review. *Current Diabetes Reports* 16 (1): 9.

Hagger, V., Hendrieckx, C., Cameron, F. et al. (2018). Diabetes distress is more strongly associated with HbA1c than depressive symptoms in adolescents with type 1 diabetes; results from Diabetes MILES Youth-Australia. *Pediatric Diabetes* 19 (4): 840–847.

Hales, C. and Barker, D. (1992). Type 2 (non-insulin dependent) diabetes mellitus: a thrifty phenotype hypothesis. *Diabetelogia* 35: 595–601.

IDF (International Diabetes Federation) Consultative Section on Diabetes Education (2002). *International Diabetes Curriculum: Paediatric and Adolescent Module*. Brussels: International Diabetes Federation.

Jessup, A.B., Grimley, M.B., Meyer, E. et al. (2015). Effects of diabetic ketoacidosis on visual and verbal neurocognitive function in young patients presenting with new-onset type 1 diabetes. *Journal of Clinical Research in Pediatric Endocrinology* 7 (3): 203.

Johnson, S., Freund, A., and Silverstein, J. (1990). Adherence–health status relationships in childhood diabetes. *Health Psychology* **9**: 606–631.

Johnson, R.J., Segal, M.S., Sautin, Y. et al. (2007). Potential role of sugar (fructose) in the epidemic of hypertension, obesity and the metabolic syndrome, diabetes, kidney disease, and cardiovascular disease. *The American Journal of Clinical Nutrition* **86** (4): 899–906.

Kaufman, F. and Riley, P. (2007). Protecting our children worldwide: the first UN-observed World Diabetes Day. *Diabetes Voice* **52**: 9–12.

Kordonouri, O., Maguire, A., Knip, M. et al. (2009). Other complications and associated conditions with diabetes in children and adolescents. *Paediatric Diabetes* **10** (Suppl. 12): 204–210.

Kyngas, H. (2000). Compliance of adolescents with diabetes. *Journal of Paediatric Nursing* **15** (4): 260–267.

Leete, P., Mallone, R., Richardson, S. et al. (2018). The effect of age on the progression and severity of type 1 diabetes: potential effects and disease mechanisms. *Current Diabetes Reports* **18** (115) https://doi.org/10.1007/s11892-018-1084-4.

Legro, R. and Dunaif, A. (1997). Menstrual disorders in insulin resistant states. *Diabetes Spectrum* **10** (3): 185–190.

Lorenz, R. and Wysocki, T. (1991). Conclusions: family and childhood diabetes. *Diabetes Spectrum* **4** (5): 290–292.

Margeirsdottir, H.D., Larsen, J.R., Brunborg, C. et al. (2007). Strong association between time watching television and blood glucose control in children and adolescents with type 1 diabetes. *Diabetes Care* **30** (6): 1567–1570.

Margeirsdottir, H. (2008). Time watching television linked to glucose control in pediatric type 1 diabetes. *Diabetes Care* **30**: 1567–1570.

Marks, K. (2019) Toddler nutrition Healthed Expert monograph 38. www.healthed.com.au.

Mayer-Davis, E., Lawrence, J., Dabelsea, D. et al. (2017). Incidence and trends of type 1 and type 2 diabetes among youths. *New England Journal of Medicine* **376** (15): 1419–1429.

McCall, B. and Nainggolan, L. (2019). C-peptide test should be the norm after type 1 diabetes. Paper presented at the Diabetes UK Professional Conference (7 March), Abstract 8 (P 97).

McGorm, K., Couper, J., and Penna, M. (2018). Developmental origins of type 1 diabetes. *The ENDIA Study* **20** (1): 51–53. www.ogmagazine.org.au/20/1-20/origins-t1-diabetes-endia.

Moreno, M., Parks, M., and Richardson, L. (2007). What are adolescents showing the world about their health risk behaviours in MySpace? *Medscape General Medicine* **9** (4): 9–15.

National Evidence-Based Clinical Care Guidelines for Type 1 Diabetes in Children, Adolescents and Adults (2012). Australian Paediatric Endocrine Group and the Australian Diabetes Society. www.diabetessociety.com.au/position-statements.asp.

Need, J. (1962). Diabetes mellitus: a thrifty genotype rendered detrimental by 'progress'. *American Journal of Human Genetics* **14**: 353–362.

Overgaard, A., Kaur, S., and Pociot, F. (2016). Metabolomic biomarkers in the progression to type 1 diabetes. *Current Diabetes Report* **16**: 127. https://doi.org/10.1007/s11892-016-0820-9.

Perrett, K., Jachno, K., and Nolan, T. (2019). Association or rotavirus with incidence of type 1 diabetes in children. *JAMA Pediatrics* **173** (3): 280–282.

Picciano, M. (2007). Dietary supplement use among infants, children, and adolescents in the United States, 1999–2002. *Archives Pediatric Adolescent Medicine* **161**: 978–985.

Pinhas-Hamiel, O. (2007). Complications of type 2 diabetes in young people – A ticking bomb. *Medical News Today* (30 May). http://ww.medicalnewstoday.com/medicalnews.php?newsid=72100&nfid=crss (accessed June 2007).

Redel, J., Dolan, J., DiFrancesco, M. et al. (2019). Youth onset diabetes and the developing brain. *Current Diabetes Reports* **19**: 3. https://doi.org/10.1007/s11892-019-1120-y.

Raad, G., Hazzouri, M., Bottini, S. et al. (2017). Paternal obesity: how bad is it for sperm quality and progeny health. *Basic and Clinical Andrology* **27** (1): 20.

Rewers, M., Hyoty, H., Lernmark, A. et al. (2018). The environmental determinants of diabetes in the young (TEDDY) Study 2018 update. *Current Diabetes Reports* **18**: 136. https://doi.org/10.1007/s11892-018-113-2.

Rosen, D., Blum, R., Britto, M. et al. (2003). Transition to adult health care for adolescents and young adults with chronic conditions. *Journal of Adolescent Health* **33**: 309–311.

Schwenk, T. (2007). Weight management in overweight children. *Journal Watch* **6** (6): 3.

Scientific Advisory Committee on Nutrition (SACN) (2011). *Joint Statement on timing of introduction of gluten into the infant diet*. www.bsna.co.uk/categories/complementary_feedings/news/index (accessed January 2013).

Shaw, J. (2007). Childhood and adolescent obesity, diabetes and their consequences. *International Diabetes Monitor* **13** (3): 12–16.

SIGN (2010). *Scottish Intercollegiate Guideline Network: National Clinical Guideline*. Edinburgh: SIGN.

Silverstein, J., Klingensmith, G., Copeland, G. et al. (2005). American Diabetes Association Care of Children and Adolescents With type 1 Diabetes A statement of the American Diabetes Association. *Diabetes Care* **28** (1): 186–212.

Sinha, R., Fisch, G., Teague, B. et al. (2002). Prevalence of impaired glucose intolerance among children and adolescents with marked obesity. *New England Journal of Medicine* **346**: 802–810.

Srinivasan, S. and Donaghue, K. (2007). Paediatric diabetes – which children can gain insulin independence? *Medical Journal of Australia* **186** (7): 436–437.

Svoren, B. and Wolfsdorf, J. (2005). Management of diabetes mellitus in children and adolescents. *International Diabetes Monitor* **18** (95): 9–18.

Tait, A. (2008). Obese children at greater risk for perioperative adverse respiratory events. *Anesthesiology* **108**: 375–380.

Thompson, S., Auslander, W., and White, N. (2001). Comparison of single-mother families on metabolic control of children with diabetes. *Diabetes Care* **24** (2): 234–238.

Tsao, J., Meldrum, M., Kim, S. et al. (2007). Treatment preferences for CAM in children with chronic pain. *Evidence Based Complementary and Alternative Medicine* **4** (3): 364–374.

Wei, J., Sung, F., and Li, C. (2003). Low birth weight and high birth weight infants are both at increased risk to have type 2 diabetes among schoolchildren in Taiwan. *Diabetes Care* **26**: 343–348.

Weiss, R. and Caprio, S. (2005). The metabolic consequences of childhood obesity. *Best Practice & Research Clinical Endocrinology & Metabolism* **19** (3): 405–419.

Wiegers, E., Becker, K., Rooijackers, H. et al. (2016). Cerebral blood flow response to hypoglycaemia is altered in patients with type 1 diabetes and impaired awareness to hypoglycaemia. *Journal Cerebral Blood Flow and Metabolism*: 1–8. https://doi.org/10.1177/0271678x16658914.

Wilmot, E., Davies, M., Yates, T. et al. (2010). Type 2 diabetes in younger adults: the emerging UK epidemic. *Postgraduate Medical Journal* **86**: 711–718.

Wilmot, E., Edwardson, C., Achana, F. et al. (2012). Sedentary time in adults and the association with diabetes, cardiovascular disease and death: a systematic review. *Diabetologia* https://doi.org/10.1007/s00125-012-2677-z.

Woolf, A. (2003). Herbal remedies and children: do they work? Are they harmful? *Paediatrics* **112**: 240–246.

World Health Organization (2004). Mood (affective) disorders (F30–F39). In: *International Statistical Classification of Diseases and Health Related Problems*, 2e. Geneva: World Health Organization.

Yajnik, C. (2007). Growth and nutrition in early life and risk of type 2 diabetes. *International Diabetes Monitor* **19** (4): 1–8.

Zhang, T. (2019). Rate of change in childhood BMI predicts adult obesity risk. *Pediatric Obesity* https://doi.org/10.1111/ijpo.12513.

Zhang, Y., Santosa, A., Wang, N. et al. (2019). Prevalence and the Association of Body Mass Index and Other Risk Factors with Prediabetes and Type 2 Diabetes Among 50,867 Adults in China and Sweden: A Cross-Sectional Study. *Diabetes Therapy*: 1–17.

Zimmet, P., Alberti, G., Kaufman, F. et al. (2007). The metabolic syndrome in children and adolescents – an IDF consensus report. *Paediatric Diabetes* **8**: 299–306.

Chapter 14

Women, Pregnancy, and Gestational Diabetes

Key points

- Preconception counselling and family planning should be part of the care of women with diabetes.
- Planning pregnancies is important to manage glycaemia before, during, and after pregnancy to reduce the risks to mother and baby. Only about 50% of women with diabetes plan their pregnancies.
- Diabetes affects women during key life events such as pregnancy where it poses a significant threat to both the mother and the child.
- Women from different cultures and religions may have different views about contraception.
- Gestational diabetes (GDM) can be diagnosed during pregnancy and increases the risk of developing type 2 diabetes in the future for the mother and child.
- Women with, polycystic ovarian syndrome (PCOS) are at high risk of diabetes. PCOS is associated with obesity, insulin resistance, GDM, and infertility.
- Insulin is often required in women with type 2 diabetes during pregnancy and breastfeeding.
- Existing renal disease and retinopathy may deteriorate during pregnancy.
- Diabetes is the most common medical condition complicating pregnancy.
- Adverse maternal and foetal outcomes are still common in many parts of the world.

Rationale

The prevalence of prediabetes, type 1 and type 2, and GDM is increasing globally. Hormonal changes associated with puberty, pregnancy, PCOS, and menopause affect glucose homeostasis and mental well-being. Coordinated care and prepregnancy planning are necessary to ensure optimal outcomes for mother and baby. Planning for an optimal delivery begins in childhood with a healthy lifestyle, general health and sex education, as well as diabetes prevention messages in high-risk families and communities.

Diabetes prevention messages and screening and maternal and child health should ideally be integrated into primary healthcare and general health screening programmes. Diagnostic procedures and criteria should be appropriate to the woman's culture. In some developing countries, birth

Care of People with Diabetes: A Manual for Healthcare Practice, Fifth Edition. Trisha Dunning and Alan Sinclair.
© 2020 John Wiley & Sons Ltd. Published 2020 by John Wiley & Sons Ltd.

attendants, traditional healers, and health-care workers are primary sources of information and care. Working collaboratively with these people and educating them about diabetes is essential (International Diabetes Federation [IDF] 2009).

Diabetes can develop during pregnancy, GDM. Most women without diabetes are screened for diabetes during pregnancy to detect GDM early and manage blood glucose levels to avoid the risks associated with hyperglycaemia for both mother and baby. Women particularly at risk of GDM are those who: have a history of diabetes in the family, had diabetes during a previous pregnancy, or previously delivered a large baby. There is increasing evidence that maternal hyperglycemia has lasting effects on the child and predisposes them to obesity and type 2 diabetes in adolescence and adulthood (IDF 2009; Law and Zhang 2017; AMA 2019).

Polycystic ovarian syndrome

Polycystic ovarian syndrome (PCOS) is common, occurring in 6–10% of women in the reproductive age and 28% of obese women. Of women with PCOS, 75% are overweight or obese. PCOS has long-term health effects, including menstrual irregularities, infertility, GDM, impaired glucose tolerance, insulin resistance, type 2 diabetes, and emotional stress and body image concerns. Thus, early diagnosis and screening women with PCOS for these metabolic changes and evidence of diabetes complications and risk factors at diagnosis and regularly thereafter is essential.

The risk factors for PCOS are shown in Figure 14.1. Making the diagnosis is a process of exclusion and consists of taking a careful family and individual history, and measuring relevant hormone levels such as:

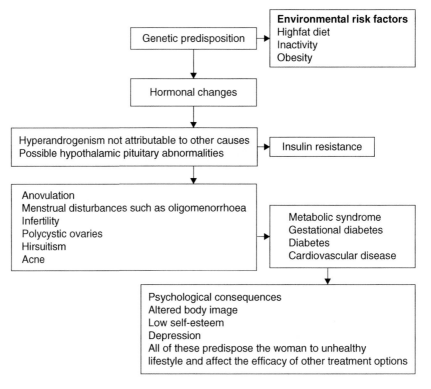

Figure 14.1   Risk factors for polycystic ovarian syndrome (PCOS) and the possible long-term effects. There is still controversy about the diagnostic criteria, and several degrees of severity exist. There is no single diagnostic test: diagnosing PCOS is process of exclusion. Diagnostic criteria include: National Institute of Health (NIH) criteria, which requires oligo-ovulation/anovulation, clinical, and/or biochemical signs of hyperandrogenism and excluding conditions such as congenital adrenal hyperplasia and Cushing's Syndrome; and the Rotterdam criteria, which requires two of the following oligo-ovulation/anovulation, clinical and/or biochemical signs of hyperandrogenism, polycystic ovaries.

- Testosterone: normal <2.4 mmol/l (50–70 mg/dl) in women.
- Sex hormone binding globulin (SHBG): likely to be low in PCOS (normal range 30–90 in nonpregnant women) and is often secondary to insulin resistance and results in higher levels of free testosterone.
- Free androgen index (FAI): likely to be high in PCOS (normal range 1–5%).
- These ranges may differ slightly amongst laboratories.

FAI is a more useful measure than testosterone unless the laboratory can test for free testosterone. Pelvic ultrasound may be indicated to determine whether the ovaries are polycystic and whether the endometrium is thickened if the woman has oligo or amenorrhoea (Rotterdam Consensus Workshop 2004; Teede et al. 2007). Determining follicle-stimulating hormone (FSH), thyroid stimulating hormone (TSH), and beta human chorionic gonadotrophin (HCG) and prolactin levels may be necessary to exclude other endocrine conditions.

Practice points

(1) Living with PCOS can be stressful and affects body image and can lead to depression (Robinson et al. 2016).
(2) Hormone evaluation should be undertaken before prescribing contraceptives.
(3) The risks and benefits of contraceptives should be considered in light of the risks of unplanned pregnancies to the mother and child.
(4) Oral contraceptives (OC) can mask the hormonal changes associated with PCOS.
(5) Each woman should be individually assessed for cardiometabolic risk before commencing contraceptives and monitored according to metabolic and weight targets (Damm et al. 2005; Yildiz 2008; Robinson et al. 2016).

A multidiscipline supportive team approach is important to address the various underlying features of PCOS. Reassurance and education about diet and exercise and weight management aiming to lose 5–10% of weight at diagnosis, the need for regular follow-up is important. The PCOS Association of Australia and National Institute of Health (NIH), amongst other sources, provide useful information about PCOS and its management on their websites. In addition, counselling about fertility may be needed. PCOS is associated with insulin resistance, and usually obesity, therefore blood glucose and lipids should be checked regularly and an oral glucose tolerance test (OGTT) performed if indicated because fasting glucose is not a reliable diagnostic test in PCOS (Teede et al. 2007, 2011) (see Chapter 1). Cardiovascular assessment should be undertaken on a regular basis. Advice about diet and exercise (Chapter 4) are essential, and psychological counselling may be required (Chapter 15).

Weight loss has been demonstrated in women with PCOS consuming the following diets: Atkins, Ornish, Weight Watchers, Zone, and the CSIRO Total Wellbeing Diet (Moran et al. 2003). The woman's food preferences should be considered and the diet should conform to dietary recommendations. One study suggests young women consuming Atkins-type diets are at increased risk of cardiovascular disease (CVD) (Pagona et al. 2012). A prospective study involving 44 000 women predicted Atkins-style diets would be responsible for additional four–five cases of CVD for every 10 000 women per year, which represents a 28% increase in the incidence of CVD. Women with PCOS often try a range of diets and are already at high risk of CVD; thus, sensitive nutrition and activity advice are important.

Metformin may be *added to* the nutrition and exercise regimen if diet and exercise do not control blood glucose. The commencing dose is 500 mg of slow-release metformin daily increasing to 2 g/day. Experts recommend giving metformin at night (Alberti et al. 2007; Teede et al. 2007); although there is evidence to support such a recommendation, metformin is not currently approved for night dosing in some countries. Metformin helps regulate the menstrual cycle and reduce hirsutism and the progression to diabetes by ~50 in high-risk women (Alberti et al. 2007; Teede 2007).

The role of metformin in improving fertility is unclear and it is not first-line fertility treatment. Metformin might be more effective in lean women (DeMaria 2007). Nevertheless, fertility should be discussed with the woman and her family if metformin is commenced because there is a chance of pregnancy. Obesity affects fertility independently of PCOS; thus, losing weight is essential if the woman wants to have a child. Age may also be a factor in low fertility, which declines at around 28 years and falls dramatically after age 35 and falls again after age 40.

Oral contraceptives (OCs) may be indicated to help reduce hirsutism and control menstrual irregularities once other causes of hirsutism are ruled out. For example, low-dose combined OCs such as Ethinyl Estradiol 20 μg increases SHBG and reduces free androgen levels. At higher doses, OC exacerbate insulin resistance (Meyer et al. 2007). Hair removal products or topical antiandrogens such as Vaniqua may be indicated, and cosmetic electrolysis or laser as a last resort. Obesity exacerbates hirsutism, so managing weight will help normalise androgen levels. The risks and benefits of all these options need to be carefully discussed with the woman considering her individual needs and risk profile.

Antiandrogens such as spironolactone 50 mg BD or cyproterone acetate 25 mg daily for days 1–10 of the active OC tablets may be prescribed to enhance fertility. These medicines must be taken with the OC to prevent menstrual irregularities and adverse effects in pregnancy. The regimen takes about six months to be effective. Women who have more than four cycles of antiandrogens per year are at increased risk of endometrial hyperplasia and endometrial carcinoma. The woman should be monitored regularly for these conditions and plan to have a withdrawal bleed every two to three months to reduce these risks.

If endometrial hyperplasia is suspected, transvaginal ultrasound and endometrial biopsy are indicated to confirm the diagnosis, especially if prolonged or irregular vaginal bleeding occurs. Hysteroscopy may be needed to determine whether fibroids or polyps are present. Endometrial hyperplasia sometimes resolves spontaneously. If endometrial hyperplasis atypia is present it may progress to endometrial carcinoma, which is induced by oestrogen and has a relatively good prognosis. Treatment depends on the woman. Intrauterine devices are appropriate if contraception is a goal and to control heavy bleeding. High-dose progestins may be indicated to limit endometrial thickening. The ultrasound and/or biopsy should be repeated after six months of treatment.

Partners and family need to be involved in explanations about PCOS and its effects, management discussions and education programmes where relevant to enable them to support the woman and understand the associated risks. Achievable goals need to be set in consultation with the woman. The effect of having PCOS, its symptoms, and the impact on fertility can generate significant psychological distress, which exacerbates hormonal imbalance, contributes to the diabetes and cardiovascular risk, and reduces quality of life (Coffey and Mason 2003; Wilhelm et al. 2003). Screening tools such as the K10 Profile or Depression Anxiety Stress Scale (DASS) used on a regular basis can help identify the degree and progression of anxiety and depression, are a helpful guide to treatment, and can facilitate early referral for counselling (see Chapter 15). Anxiety and depression need to be treated, preferably with nonmedicine options, because these conditions affect the success of other treatment measures.

Interestingly, Kim et al. (2002) reported lower blood glucose levels and lower odds of developing diabetes in young white and African-American women in the CARDIA study. Insulin levels were higher after adjusting for covariates, but the clinical significance of this finding is unknown. Insulin sensitivity was found to decline in women with PCOS treated with triphasic OCs, but there were no adverse effects on lipid metabolism (Korytkowski et al. 1995). The effects on insulin sensitivity and production might be a consideration in women with the metabolic syndrome, those at risk of GDM, or obese women with type 2 diabetes; however, more research is needed to clarify the clinical implications.

Pregnant women who take antipsychotic medicines are at increased risk of GDM (Boden et al. 2012). The researchers found a twofold risk of GDM among pregnant women on olanzapine and/or clozapine ($n = 169$) 338 on other antipsychotics compared with 350 000 controls. It is not clear whether any of the women had PCOS but the antipsychotic medicine side effects include weight gain, insulin resistance, hyperglycaemia, and hyperlipidaemia, which increase the risk of hyperglycaemia (see Chapter 10), especially when the stress of PCOS and pregnancy are added.

Exercise improves mood and fitness. Women with PCOS report significant body image issues, mood disturbances, depression, reduced emotional well-being, low quality of life and life satisfaction, and a negative impact of PCOS on their sexual self-worth and sexual satisfaction (Janssen et al. 2008). Managing symptoms such as hirsutism, obesity, menstrual irregularity, and low fertility can significantly improve their emotional and sexual well-being. Tailored psychotherapy such as cognitive behavioural therapy or self-help programmes, such as *Mood Gym*, and stress management can be beneficial. If medicines are indicated, those that reduce PCOS symptoms may be useful. For example, SSRIs to control weight but the woman should be warned that these medicines could affect her sleep.

Contraception options for women with diabetes

As indicated, planned pregnancy is vital in women with diabetes; thus, family planning and contraceptive advice is essential. Women with diabetes need specific advice about their contraception options from a qualified expert. The same range of contraceptive methods available to women without diabetes is available to and suitable for women with diabetes, and the same risks and benefits apply (Damm et al. 2005; Broecher and Lykens 2011; Robinson et al. 2016). However, the risks and benefits of each contraceptive option should be discussed with the individual woman with diabetes because extra precautions may apply (e.g. women with hypertension, those at risk of embolism, and those with microvascular disease and CVD). These risks associated with contraceptives may be greater in women with type 2 diabetes (Damm et al. 2005; Robinson et al. 2016). Thus, the benefits and risks need to be carefully considered for each individual woman and include the risk of obesity, CVD, renal impairment, and retinopathy. The WHO (2015) *Medical Eligibility Criteria for Contraception Use* can be helpful.

Important but often overlooked risks are the risks of becoming pregnant and pregnancy-related complications. These risks should be included in the discussion about contraception. Each woman should receive accurate information about the available contraceptive choices, and the partners should be involved in discussions where relevant and possible. Information about safe sex is also important to protect from unwanted pregnancy and sexually transmitted infections (STI). The best way to reduce STIs is to use a barrier method such as male and female condoms and dams. These methods can be used during oral, vaginal, and anal sex.

The following are commonly used contraceptive methods:

- Physical barrier methods include male and female condoms and diaphragms, which are effective contraceptive measure if used correctly, but pregnancy can occur if they are not used correctly. Diaphragms must be left in place for at least six hours after intercourse. Barrier methods are safe for women with diabetes.
- An intrauterine devices (IUD) is a small plastic device with copper or hormones (Mirena) added, which is placed into the uterus. The IUD can stay in place for 5–10 years, depending on the type of device, but can be removed if the woman wants to become pregnant or experiences problems. IUDs are effective contraceptives and are safe for most women with diabetes but hormone-containing IUDs can have a small effect on the hormones that control the menstrual cycle. Copper IUDs are associated with heavier periods.
- Hormonal contraceptives:
  - Oral tablets (OC) and vaginal rings, which are highly effective if used correctly. There are many types of OC with different hormone combinations. While they can be used by women with diabetes, they are not recommended for women at risk or CVD and those who smoke. The mini pill only contains synthetic progesterone and is suitable for women who experience side effects from oestrogen or women when oestrogen-containing OCs are contraindicated. Hormone contraceptive patches are a useful alternative for some women. Vaginal rings contain similar hormones to the combined pill. The ring is inserted into the vagina and stays in place for three weeks, after which time it is removed and another ring inserted after a week.

- Implants and injections, which are very effective. However, they can cause side effects. These methods include: implanon, which is implanted under the skin and lasts for three years. Depo-Provera/Depo-Ralovera are injectable contraceptives that contain progestogen and are effective for 13–14 weeks. Progestin-only contraceptive methods should be avoided while breastfeeding or used with caution (Ringholm et al. 2012, Robinson et al. 2016).
- Sterilisation is mostly a permanent surgical method of achieving contraception. Two methods are available for women: tubal ligation, which is performed under general anaesthetic, and Essure, which involves inserting small coils into the fallopian tubes under local anaesthetic. Male sterilisation, vasectomy, can often be reversed.
- Natural methods include the Billings method and withdrawing the penis from the vagina before ejaculating, but these methods often result in pregnancy.
- Emergency contraception (EC) might be required and is safe for women with diabetes. Emergency contraception involves taking an OC containing progestogen as soon as possible after intercourse and is best taken within 72 hours, but it can be taken up to 120 hours after unprotected sex. Emergency contraception pills prevent 85% of expected pregnancies if taken within the prescribed time following intercourse. EC can be considered in high-risk women with diabetes, providing the woman and her partner are fully informed and are prepared to accept the decision without knowing whether the woman is pregnant.

Concerns have been raised about the effects of OCs on glucose and fat metabolism, which could exacerbate cardiovascular risks. However, several studies suggest OCs do not adversely affect blood glucose or lipid levels, or exacerbate retinopathy or hypertension (Kaunitz 2002) including in women with previous GDM. Other research suggests high-dose combined OC has a small beneficial effect on glucose homeostasis and lipid metabolism, whereas progesterone only OC improves lipid metabolism (Visser et al. 2006). The risks of vascular complications, retinopathy, and rates of thrombolism appear to be low, but progesterone-only preparations cause more irregular bleeding.

Combination OCs, monthly contraceptive injections, vaginal rings, and patches appear to be appropriate for women with diabetes younger than 35 years (Kaunitz 2002; Robinson et al. 2016). These methods might be contraindicated in older women and those with hypertension, and/or micro and macrovascular disease. For these women, IUDs including progesterone-releasing Mirena, progesterone only mini pills, or depo-progesterone (e.g. Depo-Provera) injections or implanon implants may be viable alternatives (Kaunitz 2002).

Trials are currently underway in seven countries, including Australia, to determine the safety and effectiveness of an injectable hormone-based male contraceptive. The contraceptive contains testosterone and progestogen. Other studies have investigated a combination of implanted testosterone and injected progestogen, which did not result in any pregnancies in the men's female partners or affect the men's energy and libido. These studies appear promising, but male contraception is not yet available in Australia.

Practice points

- Contraception is an essential aspect of sexual health (see Chapter 11).
- Contraception appropriateness must be considered for individual women considering her risks and the likely benefits. These include considering the risks of STI and unwanted pregnancies.
- Appropriate contraception choices are likely to change over the lifespan and should be regularly assessed as part of a medicines review and/or complication screening processes.
- Discussions about contraception options should involve both partners where practical, but the decision to include the partner rests with the woman concerned.
- The woman (and her partner) should be given individualised information about the risks and benefits of each contraceptive option so she can make an informed decision.

Pregnancy

Managing diabetes during pregnancy is challenging for the woman concerned and the clinician team. Family support is vital. Hormones released by the placenta predispose the mother to hyperglycaemia and increase the amount of glucose available to the foetus. Insulin sensitivity increases in the first trimester but insulin resistance develops in the second and third trimesters. The placental glucose transporter, GLUT-1, increases the transplacental glucose flux. The activity of GLUT-4 at the maternal cellular level decreases, which means glucose is not utilised by the mother and high levels cross the placenta, where they are utilised by the foetus. This sets the scene for microsomal and foetal abnormalities and makes vaginal delivery difficult and increases the risk of Caesarian section (Hollingsworth 1992; ADA 2019).

The risks are if the HbA1c is high in the first 10 weeks of pregnancy (Guerin et al. 2007), which highlights the value of planning pregnancies and normalising blood glucose levels. If the pregnancy is not planned, it is important to manage blood glucose as soon as possible (<6.5% 48 mmol/mol). Pregnancy enhances insulin sensitivity in the early stages and insulin may need to be adjusted in women using insulin. However, insulin resistance increases in the second and third trimester and insulin doses may need to be increased or insulin commenced.

Prepregnancy counselling is essential to limit risks to mother and baby (Coustan 1997; Australasian Diabetes in Pregnancy Society [ADIPS] 2012) and should commence at puberty and continue in all women of reproductive age as part of overall holistic care (ADA 2019). Women who attend pre-pregnancy counselling have significantly lower risk of major foetal abnormalities (Ray et al. 2001). Women with type 2 diabetes are often overweight, higher parity, and belong to ethnic and minority ethnic groups. However, type 2 diabetes is increasing in prevalence amongst adolescents and unwanted, and unplanned pregnancy rates are high in this age group. In addition, women are delaying childbirth, often until the mid-30s or 40s, which carries age-associated risks, and increases the likelihood that diabetes complications will be present and could affect the pregnancy. For example, age appears to be a significant factor in pregnancy-related MI although MI during pregnancy is rare (Karamermer and Ross-Hesselink 2007).

Coordinated multidisciplinary team care that includes as a minimum an obstetrician, endocrinologist, diabetes educator, dietitian, and paeditrician with experience managing diabetes in pregnancy and GDM is essential to optimal outcomes. Key management strategies include the following:

- Plan the pregnancy.
- Achieve and maintain HbA1c as close as possible to normal before (<6–6.5% 42–48 mmol/mol) in trimester 1 and <6% (42 mmol/mol) in trimester 2 and 3 as long as hypoglycaemia can be avoided/minimised. Noting that HbA1c can be significantly lower in pregnancy due to increased red blood cell turnover (ADA 2019).
- ADA (2019) recommended blood glucose targets are:
  - 5.3 mmol/l (<95 mg/dl) preprandially
  - <7.8 mmol/l (<140 mg/dl) one hour postprandially
  - <6.7 mmol/l (<120 mg/dl) two hours postprandially
  - >6 mmol/l before bed (Lee et al. 2012)
- Regular blood glucose monitoring is essential to achieving optimal outcomes.
- Provide nutrition counselling to optimise the health and inutero growth and development of the baby and match carbohydrate to insulin doses.
- Commence folate supplements (5 mg daily) and refer the woman for a nutritional review.
- Undertake a comprehensive medication review (see Table 14.1). Stop glucose-lowering medicine (GLM) and commence insulin if the woman has type 2 diabetes. Optimise the insulin regimen in women with type 1 diabetes. Insulin analogues confer advantages during pregnancy and may reduce the risk of significant hypoglycaemia. However, not all insulin analogues are approved

Table 14.1   Medication management during pregnancy.

Medication	Management	Potential adverse events
Insulin in women with type 1 and type 2 diabetes and those with GDM if lifestyle strategies do not achieve recommended glycaemic targets.	Dose should be titrated regularly according to blood glucose monitoring pattern to achieve targets and avoid hypoglycaemia. Glargine was been associated with mitogenic activity in a series of papers in 2009 that suggested it should be used with caution in pregnancy (Hirsch 2005) (see Chapter 14). Wu et al. (2017) found long-term use of insulin glargine is associated with increased risk of breast cancer in women with type 2 diabetes and that the risk associated with Insulin detemir remains uncertain. Thus, it is important to following prescribing guidelines and precautions and disclose the potential risk to women. Women with type 2 diabetes and those with GDM may need education about managing insulin and hypoglycaemia as well as reassurance. Insulin doses and dose regimen need to be titrated to the changing blood glucose pattern. Thus, regular blood glucose self-monitoring is essential. None of the currently available insulins appear to cross the placenta. Education about ketone testing should be provided and the sick-day-care plan revised to accommodate pregnancy care during illness and then revised again after the delivery.	Hypoglycaemia, especially nocturnal hypoglycaemia during 6–18 weeks gestation. Significant repeated hypoglycaemia should be investigated to ensure there are no underlying disease processes and monitor foetal growth and development monitored. Death, although rare, does occur (Ter Braak et al. 2002). Weight gain. The low risk of breast cancer associated with long-term use of Glargine should be discussed with the woman. Women with type 1 diabetes and some women with type 2 diabetes are at risk of DKA at lower than usual blood glucose levels. Hypoglycaemia is a significant risk after delivery, thus insulin doses need to be revised.
Oral glucose lowering medicines (GLM) in type 2 diabetes and GDM	Metformin The overall individual risks need to be considered just those associated with pregnancy. Metformin may be indicated in severe insulin resistance (Simmons et al. 2004). There is limited information about dose adjustment during pregnancy and it crosses the placenta. Safety information for the developing baby is unclear. Sulphonylureas Sulphonylureas cross the placenta, but second generation cross to a lesser extent: glipizide 6.6% and glyburide 3.9% (Feig et al. 2007). Thiazolidinediones (TZD) Rosiglitazone crosses the placenta, especially after 10 weeks gestation. Importantly, better outcomes generally occur using insulin (ADA 2019).	A number of studies suggest GLMs do not increase the risk of foetal malformation (Gutzin et al. 2003) and the concentration in breast milk is low (Gilbert et al. 2006). Australasian Diabetes in Pregnancy Study Group (ADIPS 2005) suggested the potential harm from metformin use in pregnancy is outweighed by the benefits. However, long-term data are not available; thus, caution is recommended. The product prescribing recommends changing to insulin during pregnancy. Feig et al. (2007) found no evidence of foetal abnormalities in animal or human studies if the medicines were used in recommended doses, but the studies were small and short term, and these medicines cannot be recommended for use in pregnancy. When a woman with type 2 diabetes becomes pregnant she should be referred urgently to an endocrinologist and GLMs continued until the transfer to insulin to avoid the risk of hyperglycaemia to the foetus (ADIPS 2005).
Antihypertensive agents	ACE inhibitors should be ceased during pregnancy. Methyldopa, Oxprenolol, Clonidine, Labetolol, Prazosin, and Nifedipine can be continued safely (Australasian Society for the Study of Hypertension in Pregnancy 2005). The effects of angiotensin 2 blocker are not known.	ACE, ARB, and statins are potentially teratogenic and should be avoided in sexually active women not using reliable contraception. Some experts recommend not using ACE in women of childbearing age not using reliable contraception (ADA 2019).

Table 14.1 (Continued)

Medication	Management	Potential adverse events
Lipid-lowering agents	Nutrition counselling and regular activity.	Statins have been associated with foetal abnormalities and are contraindicated in pregnancy (Edison and Muenke 2004).
Any other medicine	Check the prescribing information before using. ADA (2019) recommends prescribing low-dose aspirin (50–150 mg/day) for women with type 1 and type 2 diabetes commencing at the end of the first trimester until the baby is born.	Diabetes in pregnancy is associated with increased risk of preeclampsia.

A comprehensive medication review should be undertaken regularly in all people with diabetes, when planning a pregnancy and when the woman becomes pregnant. See also Chapter 5.

for use during pregnancy. Continuous subcutaneous insulin infusion (CSII) appears to be safe. Cease medicines likely to adversely affect the foetus. Metformin and sulphonylurea are not associated with increased risk of congenital malformations or early foetal loss, but they do cross the placenta and are not recommended in pregnancy (SIGN 2010). Commonly used medicines that *may* be contraindicated in pregnancy include:

- Ace inhibitors
- Beta blockers
- Aspirin
- Coumarins
- Calcium channel blockers
- Ace inhibitors have been associated with congenital malformations.
- Statins due to the risk of foetal malformations. However, hypertension should be prevented. Generally, they should not be used whilst breastfeeding.
- Nonsteroidal anti-inflammatory drugs (NSAIDs)
- Caution is required with antidepressants, corticosteroids, and opioids (Gardiner 2002; ADIPS 2012).
- Ask about complementary and alternative medicine/therapy (CAM) use. Women frequently use CAM during pregnancy, particularly supplements such as raspberry leaf, ginger and chamomile tea (Forster et al. 2006). They also use massage and essential oils. Women who use CAM are generally well-informed and likely to take proactive self-care, be well educated, nonsmokers, and primiparous. The proportion of pregnant women with diabetes using CAM is unknown, but CAM use is high in the general population and people with diabetes. Whilst there are many benefits, there are also risks, especially in the first trimester, and for women with renal and liver disease; see Chapters 8 and 10. Some women elect to use complementary approaches (CAM) to pain management during labour or supplement conventional pain management strategies with CAM. Tournaire and Theau-Yonneau (2007) undertook a systematic review of randomised controlled trials, which indicated pain was reduced and women receiving acupuncture and those receiving hydrotherapy required less analgesia. Women were not dissatisfied with conventional pain relief and had different expectations of pain management from health professionals. Strategies such as massage with or without essential oils, which reduce fear also have positive benefits, including reducing lower back pain (Allaire 2001). Combination or single herbal medicines are sometimes used to manage pain (e.g. motherwort). Women sometimes use herbal medicines during the last four to five weeks of pregnancy to prepare the cervix and facilitate delivery (e.g. raspberry leaf in tablet form) and was found to shorten the second stage of labour, and fewer women required forceps deliveries (Simpson et al. 2001). CAM use prior to and during labour should be discussed with the obstetrician and/or midwife. Thus, CAM use should be assessed at regular intervals before and throughout pregnancy, as part of the medicine review.

- Undertake a comprehensive diabetes complication and manage existing disease before pregnancy (e.g. retinopathy requiring laser therapy, CVD). The eyes should be examined through dilated pupils. Women should be aware that preexisting retinopathy could progress during pregnancy. Preexisting CVD can be exacerbated by pregnancy due to haemodynamic changes and increased cardiac output. Delivery places extra demand on the heart (Karamermer and Ross-Hesselink 2007). Significant coronary artery stenosis should ideally be treated prior to pregnancy. The haemodynamic changes gradually return to normal in three to six months (Karamermer and Ross-Hesselink 2007). Kidney function should be checked because women with microalbuminuria are at risk of preeclampsia and microalbuminuria may progress during pregnancy if significant renal impairment is present and require dialysis (Biesenbach et al. 1992; Rossing et al. 2004); see Chapter 8. Some experts regard significant renal impairment to be a contraindication to pregnancy (ADIPS 2012), particularly given a third of women with severe renal impairment die within about 16 years (Rossing et al. 2004). Identify autonomic neuropathy-associated conditions such as gastroparesis, hypoglycaemic unawareness and orthostatic hypotension, which make management more difficult, are distressing for the woman and her family and may put her safety and/or life at risk. Autonomic neuropathy may predispose the mother to intractable vomiting and precipitate metabolic disturbances such as ketoacidosis.
- Assess general health and psychological wellbeing. For example, detect the presence of comorbidities such as thyroid and coeliac disease in women with type 1 diabetes and CVD in type 2 diabetes, which could complicate the pregnancy.
- Undertake an education review of general diabetes knowledge and provide specific pregnancy and childbirth information. Revise home management of emergencies such as sick days/hyperglycaemia and morning sickness.
- Encourage women who smoke to quit and limit alcohol consumption.
- Perform an ultrasound at 18–20 weeks and if necessary; the ultrasound should be repeated to check foetal cardiac status at 24 weeks and foetal growth at 28–30 weeks and again at 34–36 weeks.
- Encourage the woman to eat a healthy well-balanced low GI diet to ensure optimal nutrition for herself and the developing foetus. The carbohydrates need to be spread over the day if problems occur. Foods likely to cause listeriosis should be avoided. Dietitian advice is advisable. Listeriosis can be transmitted from the mother to the foetus and cause miscarriage, stillbirth, premature delivery, or a very ill baby at birth.
- Encourage participation in regular exercise such as 'Preggie Bellies' helps blood glucose control, general fitness, and well-being and mental health.
- Encourage participation in childbirth classes.
- Develop and document a plan for managing insulin during delivery and in the immediate postpartum period.
- Develop a plan for reviewing the mother's glycaemic control after discharge and ensuring the woman has adequate support at home.
- Foster mother–child bonding by providing woman-centred holistic care and supporting the woman and her family to adjust to parenthood and to breastfeed. Monitoring for the 'three-day blues' and postnatal depression is essential. For example, Rasmussen et al. (2007) found women with type 1 diabetes were significantly stressed about the baby's safety if they had a 'hypo' and relied on their mothers and husbands for support. Mutual mother/daughter guilt feelings emerged (the guilt dynamic) where daughters felt guilty about the impact their diabetes had on their mother's lives and mothers felt guilty because their daughters developed diabetes and they could not prevent it. Chapter 15 describes psychological therapy. In addition, many small studies indicate that massage, with and without essential oils, reduces stress, improves sleep for both the mother and baby, facilitates bonding, and is safe (Bongaard 2007). Thus, massage may be a useful nonmedicine option in high-risk groups or could be used in combination with other therapies (Bongaard 2007).
- Specific care of the mother and baby during labour and delivery are specialty areas and outside the scope of this book. Most women should deliver at term and vaginally unless there

are medical or obstetric reasons for earlier delivery/caesarean section. Usually, blood glucose is measure every one to two hours and usual diet and insulin dose maintained. If a caesarean section is needed, the procedure should be scheduled for the morning if possible. The dose of long-acting insulin on the evening prior to the surgery may need to be reduced to reduce the risk of hypoglycaemia after delivery. Women with type 1 diabetes may need an insulin/glucose infusion.

- Women are encouraged to breastfeed. Strategies to reduce hypoglycaemia during breastfeeding include having a snack before or while feeding, avoiding caffeine, drinking plenty of water, and having glucose close by to treat hypoglycaemia early if it occurs. Insulin is not contraindicated in breastfeeding.
- Discuss contraception plans prior to discharge.

Comprehensive assessment should be undertaken every one to four weeks during the first 30 weeks of pregnancy and then weekly until delivery. Routine foetal monitoring should occur and an ultrasound performed to ensure the estimated date of delivery is accurate and develop the delivery plan. In most cases, the women will be able to have a normal vaginal delivery unless there are obstetric complications.

Complications of pregnancy

Complications can be reduced by careful monitoring and proactively managing the pregnancy especially controlling blood glucose and other risk factors. The following maternal complications are possible:

- Early: miscarriage, foetal abnormalities, and difficulty performing ultrasound.
- Hypertension is common and manifests as a range of conditions from mild hypertension to preeclampsia superimposed on chronic hypertension and occurs in 10–22% of pregnancies (Donovan 2012). Hypertension increases the risk of adverse outcomes for mother and baby and increases the possibility that labour will need to be induced or caesarean section will be required because of conditions such as macrosomia, shoulder dystocia. Increased risk of perioperative complications if surgery is required. Some antihypertensive medicines are not recommended during pregnancy, including ACE inhibitors and ARB and diuretics, beta blockers, and calcium challenge antagonists except Nifedipine should be avoided (Donovan 2012). Recommended targets are:
  ○ Pregnant women with chronic hypertension 120/160/80–105 mmHg.
- Hypoglycaemia can have serious consequences in women having epidural anaesthesia because the usual counter-regulatory response is blocked and because pregnant women are more prone to hypoglycaemia. Hypoglycaemia can retard reversal of hypotension in these situations (Marx et al. 1987). However, maternal glucose is often higher during caesarean section than vaginal delivery (Andersen et al. 1998).
- Postpartum: maternal haemorrhage, infection, thrombosis, hypoglycaemia.
- Deterioration in existing diabetes complications, especially renal disease and retinopathy and cardiovascular status. CVD is encountered more frequently because women are older when they begin their families, a family history of cardiac disease, and have often have diabetes for >10 years. In addition, obesity is more common and smoking increases the risk. An ECG should be performed if chest discomfort develops especially if the woman has known cardiovascular risk factors (Karamermer and Ross-Hesselink 2007). Indications of heart disease include:
  ○ Serious or progressive dyspnoea (mild dyspnoea is common)
  ○ Syncope on exertion
  ○ Chest pain/discomfort associated with exertion

The maternal death rate is comparable to nondiabetic women when care is delivered by a qualified, collaborative multidisciplinary team, ~0.5% of pregnancies in the United Kingdom (Chief Medical Officer's Report 2000).

- Urinary incontinence is common in all age groups, especially in women and the risk increases with age (Gorina et al. 2014). The most common cause in women is neuromuscular damage to the pelvic floor during childbirth, which contributes to stress incontinence (Salvatore et al. 2017). Diabetes, age, and overweight are independent risk factors for urinary incontinence and should, which should be included in regular follow-up reviews.

Effects of diabetes on the baby

Consequences of maternal hyperglycaemia for the foetus include macrosomia, foetal distress, and birth injuries, which are largely preventable through good obstetric management and controlling maternal blood glucose levels. After delivery, the baby may develop hypoglycaemia, hypothermia, hypocalcaemia, transient cardiomyopathy, or other problems, depending on the intrauterine conditions during pregnancy, delivery, and gestational age. The baby will need intensive monitoring initially, which might affect the bonding process.

Neonatal hypoglycaemia, defined as blood glucose <2.6 mmol/l up to 72 hours after birth, can cause significant morbidity and death if it is not recognised and treated effectively (Western Australian Center for Evidence Based Nursing and Midwifery 2006). The estimated incidence of newborn hypoglycaemia is between 1 and 5 per 1000 live births, but may be up to 30% in at-risk infants (Hewitt et al. 2005). Hypoglycaemia is often present at birth and is usually transient in babies of nondiabetic mothers. Infants most at risk are:

- <2 kg or >4 kg at birth;
- born before 37 weeks gestation;
- <10th percentile for weight (small for gestational age);
- >90th percentile for weight (large for gestational age);
- retarded uterine growth;
- born to mother with diabetes or GDM;
- those with sepsis (World Health Organization (WHO 1997; Western Australian Center for Evidence Based Nursing and Midwifery 2006).

The maternal and baby's blood glucose levels correlate at birth. Thus, the maternal blood glucose level is the most significant determinant of neonatal hypoglycaemia (Andersen et al. 1998). The signs of hypoglycaemia in the neonate are often nonspecific and include high-pitched crying, hypothermia and poor temperature control, sweating, refusing to feed or poor sucking, exaggerated Moro reflex, irritability, hypotonia, tachyapnoea, tachycardia, cyanosis, and lethargy. All of these signs also occur in other conditions.

Traditionally, hypoglycaemia is diagnosed in the presence of Whipple's Triad: the presence of characteristic clinical signs of low blood glucose, low blood glucose, and resolution of the signs once euglycaemia is reestablished. However, the symptoms are unreliable in neonates, as can be seen from the preceding list. Having a high level of suspicion and blood glucose monitoring is essential. Once hypoglycaemia is corrected, babies are usually able to maintain blood glucose levels with normal breastfeeding on demand. Supplemental formula feeds may be required in the first 48 hours. Babies need to be kept warm and closely monitored in the neonatal nursery until they are stable.

Longer-term effects of maternal hyperglycaemia on the child

Childhood obesity is increasing in many countries, especially in ethnic minorities; see Chapter 1. The factors contributing to childhood obesity and associated consequences (insulin resistance, type 2 diabetes, and diabetic complications) are debated. Genetic and environmental factors play a role (Dornhorst 2003), including the intrauterine environment during pregnancy, which has lasting effects on the child, originally called the Baker hypothesis, and now referred to as the foetal origins hypothesis or the Developmental Origins of Ault Health and Disease (DOHaD) (Armitage et al. 2008). Put simply, the hypothesis states 'exposure to an unfavourable environment during development (either in utero or in the early postnatal period) programmes changes in foetal or neonatal development such that the individual is then at greater risk of developing adulthood disease' (Armitage et al. 2008).

The foetus adapts structurally and functionally to reduced availability of essential nutrients. That is, under intrauterine 'famine' conditions available glucose is diverted to vital organs such as the brain and away from less immediately vital organs such as the pancreas. Insulin resistance develops in peripheral tissues to ensure a constant supply to vital organs and growth (birthweight) is retarded. The combination of reduced beta cell mass and pre-programming insulin-sensitive tissue to be insulin-resistant confers the risk of future diabetes on susceptible individuals (Barker et al. 1993). Low birthweight may be due to inadequate maternal intake and/or placental dysfunction. The association between type 2 diabetes and low birthweight has been demonstrated in a number of population-based studies; however, the risk in developed countries with an adequate food supply is low (Boyko 2000) but may be higher in less-affluent countries.

High birth weight is also associated with future risk of impaired glucose tolerance and type 2 diabetes (Pettitt and Jovanovic 2007), which is likely to be a significant factor as the number of overweight women giving birth increases and they deliver higher birth weight babies. High birth-weight is primarily due to maternal hyperglycaemia. However, starvation and undernutrition also predispose the child to poor health outcomes.

Memory deficits in childhood have also been attributed to poorly controlled maternal diabetes during pregnancy (DeBoer 2007). De Boer suggested inadequate levels of iron and oxygen during development of the hippocampus (memory centre) in utero contributed to the deficits, which were significant by age three and a half. She suggested available iron was used to manufacture haemoglobin and diverted away from the hippocampus, which is a metabolically active part of the brain that requires a lot of iron during prenatal neuronal development. The longer-term implications of De Boer's study are unknown and the research is ongoing. Significantly, the deficits were only noticeable on difficult memory tasks. The findings do underscore the importance of prenatal iron supplements and planning pregnancies.

Gestational diabetes

Gestational diabetes (GDM) refers to carbohydrate intolerance of variable severity that first appears during pregnancy (Rice et al. 2012) and increases the risk in subsequent pregnancies and type 2 diabetes in later life. Law and Zhang (2017) suggested GDM is an early stage in the progression to type 2 diabetes. GDM is the most common metabolic complication of pregnancy. Insulin resistance and hyperglycaemia develop as a result of the hormones produced by the placenta and declining beta cell function. The hormones oestradiol, cortisol, and human placental lactogen rise during pregnancy to ensure that the foetus receives sufficient glucose to grow and develop normally. As a consequence, the mother's cells become more resistant to insulin and the mother compensates by producing more insulin and using fat stores to produce energy for her own needs. GDM may, in fact, represent part of the continuum towards type 2 diabetes.

It is recommended that all pregnant women be screened for diabetes at 24–28 weeks gestation, the time the placenta begins to produce large quantities of diabetogenic hormones, using a 75 g glucose load (Rani and Begum 2016). Diagnostic criteria are fasting venous glucose ≥5 mmol/l, >10 mmol/l at one hour and ≥8.5 mmol/l after two hours. The diagnosis is established if one or more of the three glucose levels are abnormal. These levels were chosen because they are associated with an odds ratio of 1.75 for adverse outcomes compared with mean glucose levels in the HAPO study (HAPO Collaborative 2008). Overt diabetes is present if the fasting glucose is ≥7.0 mmol/l or a random or two-hour glucose is ≥11.1 mmol/l (Rani and Begum 2016).

Women who do not meet the diagnostic criteria for GDM may still have babies with glucose-related macrosomia, respiratory distress, hyperbiluribinaemia, and hypoglycaemia and require admission to neonatal intensive care. Adverse pregnancy outcome such as stillbirth, caesarean section, and preeclampsia can also occur.

Usually the blood glucose returns to normal after the baby is delivered. However, approximately 40% of women with GDM develop type 2 diabetes in later life. In addition, the baby is at increased risk of obesity and type 2 diabetes. In most cases, the OGTT is repeated six to eight weeks after delivery and then on a regular basis, for example, yearly in at-risk women, although many women do not return for follow-up. A National Gestational Diabetes Register was established in Australia in 2011 as a strategy to encourage women to have follow-up screening. Registration is voluntary. Women who elect to join the Register and their nominated doctor are sent reminders to have their glucose checked.

Nilsson et al. (2009) observed women with GDM in Sweden between 1995 and 2005 ($n = 385$) who were tested for beta cell autoantibody markers to determine their risk of developing type 1 diabetes; 6% tested positive for at least one islet cell antibody: ICA, GAD, or IA-2A. These women were followed and autoantibody levels reanalysed. An OGTT was performed in women who did not develop diabetes. Of those women who were autoantibody positive, 50% developed type 1 diabetes and 21% had IFG or IGT, but none had developed type 2 diabetes. The overall sample size in the study was small, but autoantibody testing may be indicated in some women who develop GDM.

Risk factors for gestational diabetes

Gestational diabetes (GDM) can occur in any pregnancy; however, those women at highest risk are categorised as:
- Being obese >12% of ideal bodyweight and/or body mass index (BMI) >35 kg/m^2 and having other features of the metabolic syndrome, see Section 1.6. Overweight can induce chronic low-grade inflammation, which reduces synthesis of xanthurenic acid, ethnicity is associated with the development of prediabetes, GDM and type 2 diabetes (Law and Zhang 2017).
  - Previous GDM
  - Ethnicity, e.g. Indian, Aboriginal, Pacific Islander, Maori, Middle Eastern, and African women
  - Maternal age >40 years, especially if a first-degree relative has diabetes
  - Previous large baby >4500 g at birth
  - PCOS
  - On diabetogenic medicines such as corticostemroids and antipsychotics (ADIPS 2012)

Managing GDM

The following capillary self-monitoring blood glucose targets are generally accepted. However, the blood glucose patterns and the factors that affect blood glucose must be interpreted when making management decisions:

- Fasting ≤5.0 mmol/l
- One hour postprandial ≤7.4 mol/l
- Two hours postprandial ≤6.7 mmol/l (ADIPS 2016)

Diet and exercise are first-line treatment of GDM to control maternal blood glucose and supply essential nutrients for normal foetal growth and development. Generally, low-GI foods are recommended where 40–50% calories come from complex high-fibre carbohydrate, 20% from protein, and 30–40% from unsaturated fats distributed evenly throughout the day. Nutrition counselling by a dietitian is recommended. Insulin is indicated if the blood glucose targets cannot be met.

Calorie restriction can predispose the woman and the foetus to ketonaemia and reduce psychomotor development and IQ between the third and ninth year of age in the child especially during the second and third trimesters (Rizzo et al. 1995). Pregnant women who remain active have a 56% lower risk of developing glucose intolerance and GDM than inactive women (Zhang et al. 2006) and lower risk of type 2 diabetes in the longer term (Ceysens et al. 2006). There are no data for optimal weight gain during pregnancy (Metzger et al. 2007). The Fifth International

Workshop-Conference on GDM (2003) recommended a relatively small weigh increase during pregnancy: ~7 kg for obese women and up to 18 kg in underweight women.

Women at risk of GDM are advised to monitor their fasting and two-hour postprandial blood glucose levels after each meal although there is no objective evidence to support the recommended frequency. CGM may be used to obtain a blood glucose pattern in some women; see Chapter 3.

Insulin will be required during pregnancy if blood glucose cannot be controlled using diet and exercise, generally when the fasting glucose is >5.0 mmol/l on three consecutive occasions, but the duration of time on diet/exercise therapy before commencing insulin is unknown. Buchanan et al. (1994) recommended using insulin if the foetal abdominal circumference is >75th percentile for gestational age on ultrasound. However, a limitation of this method is that it provides a 'snapshot' rather monitoring continuous longitudinal foetal growth and should not be used alone especially given foetal macrosomia is related to maternal blood glucose levels. Insulin analogues are generally used; see Chapter 5 and the starting dose is calculated according to the woman's weight, generally ~0.8 units/kg (nonobese), 0.9–1.0 units/kg (overweight and obese, respectively).

Oral GLMs are contraindicated because they cross the placenta and cause neonatal hypoglycaemia and may have other unknown effects. However, metformin is used in Europe and South Africa and glibenclamide in South Africa without any reported foetal or maternal adverse outcomes. Although most other countries do not recommend GLM use during pregnancy (Metzger et al. 2007) the Metformin in Gestational Diabetes (MiG) (Rowan 2007) set up to compare metformin with insulin on perinatal outcomes suggests metformin is safe in the short term but may be contraindicated if the baby is small, or if the mother has pulmonary oedema or sepsis due to the risk of lactic acidosis; see Chapter 7. Metformin reduces absorption of vitamin B_{12}, but this can be overcome by supplementing with calcium.

Insulin is given as required during labour. Some obstetric units use insulin infusions to control hyperglycaemia, which may be exacerbated by the pain and stress of labour. Frequent blood glucose monitoring is required because insulin requirements fall dramatically after delivery and maternal hypoglycaemia is possible. The baby is prone to hypoglycaemia after delivery and should be monitored closely for 24 hours as indicated in the preceding section.

Encourage breastfeeding. Breastfeeding provides essential nutrition and immunity for the baby. It decreases the risk of obesity and type 2 diabetes in later life in babies of women who develop GDM. Some studies also suggest cow's milk and gluten-containing solid foods should not be introduced before three months of age. Exposure to cow's milk protein may be a risk factor for type 1 diabetes in children with a dysfunctional gut immune system (Luopajärvi et al. 2008). Cow's milk contains different variations of the milk protein casein (A1 or A2), depending on the breed of cattle. Breeds that produce A1 protein in their milk are more common in Europe. Consumption of A1 milk is associated with type 1 diabetes (Laugesen and Elliott 2003). Likewise, gluten is a risk factor for type 1 diabetes-associated autoimmunity in children with a genetic risk of type 1 diabetes (Ziegler et al. 2003). The UNICEF infant feeding guidelines recommend women breastfeed exclusively for six months, introducing solid foods after six months but to continue breastfeeding for up to two years of age.

Perform a follow-up OGTT at 4–12 weeks postpartum. OGTT is preferred because HbA1c can be affected by red blood turnover and blood loss during deliver and because OGG is more sensitive to glucose intolerance (ADA 2019). Follow-up is important because 50–70% of women with GDM develop type 2 diabetes after 15–20 years. They need support to maintain a healthy lifestyle and follow-up every 1–3 years or 4–12 years if the postpartum OGGT is normal.

Type 1 diabetes

As stated, planning the pregnancy and achieving optimal health before becoming pregnant significantly improves outcomes. Insulin requirements vary throughout the pregnancy, and frequent blood glucose monitoring is essential so doses can be adjusted appropriately.

The specific insulin dose depends on individual characteristics. Overweight women may be less sensitive to insulin and may require larger doses than lean women. NovoRapid is approved for use in pregnancy.

Blood glucose testing before and one hour after each meal is ideal to help titrate insulin doses as needed. Insulin requirements usually increases by ~20% in the first 5–6 weeks due to increased levels of progesterone and continues to rise slowly to weeks 9–11, at which time the placenta begins to produce progesterone and ovarian production ceases (Jovanovic 2004).

Progesterone levels may decline temporarily during the switch and consequently insulin requirements can drop especially in lean insulin-sensitive women. Hypoglycaemia risk increases. It may be necessary to perform 3 a.m. blood glucose tests to determine whether hypoglycaemia occurs during the night. Progesterone levels increase again after about 8–10 days. Insulin requirements begin to increase and continue to do so during each trimester. At term when contractions begin, insulin requirements drop because the available glucose is utilised to support uterine contractions, and 3 a.m. blood glucose testing may be required again at this time.

After delivery, insulin requirements generally drop significantly and only very low doses may be needed in the first 24–48 hours and eventually return to prepregnancy requirements. However, breastfeeding women usually require less long-acting insulin because blood glucose is used to produce milk, but they may need more short-acting insulin at mealtimes. Hyperglycaemia may mean extra lactose in breast milk and cause problems for the baby such as diarrhoea and putting on excess weight.

Women with type 1 diabetes may have hypertension as a consequence of nephropathy, or hypertension may develop as a consequence of the pregnancy. Blood pressure must be carefully monitored and controlled to reduce the risk of preeclampsia, progression of renal disease, and retinopathy. Medicines management can be complicated because ACE inhibitors, beta blocking agents, and diuretics are generally contraindicated.

Type 2 diabetes

Women with type 2 diabetes and hyperglycaemia may be commenced on insulin prior to conceiving to optimise blood glucose levels and improve pregnancy outcomes.

Women with type 2 diabetes are usually commenced on insulin during pregnancy. As with type 1 diabetes insulin requirements slowly increase over the course of the pregnancy. However, the typical temporary drop seen about 9–11 weeks in women with type 1 diabetes may not occur because women with type 2 diabetes are generally insulin resistant. Insulin requirements are affected by hormone levels but also by carbohydrate intake and activity levels.

Women with type 2 diabetes should monitor their blood glucose with the same frequency as those with type 1 but are generally less prone to nocturnal hypoglycaemia.

After delivery women who were treated with diet and exercise may be able to resume that regimen but insulin is recommended if the woman decides to breastfeed (ADIPS 2005). OHAs can be used but metformin is present in breast milk and the baby *may* develop hypoglycaemaia. Therefore, regular blood glucose testing may be needed, but could be stressful for the parents.

Practice points

(1) Some women worry about whether injecting insulin into the abdomen can cause or exacerbate stretch marks.

(2) Some women worry about damaging their baby by injecting insulin into the abdomen.

(3) There is no evidence that insulin causes stretch marks, and the needles are not long enough to penetrate into the uterus and damage the baby.

(4) It may be difficult to pinch up a fold of skin during late pregnancy as the skin stretches and tightens. It may be necessary to inject into other sites such as the side of the abdomen or thighs.

Menopause and diabetes

Menopause is a normal life stage for all women as the ability to bear a child ends and levels of oestrogen and progesterone gradually decline. Small amounts of oestrogen are usually still produced. Menopause is complete when menstruation does not occur for 12 months around 51 years of age, although women with type 1 diabetes may experience menopause at an earlier age. However, overweight women with type 2 diabetes may go through menopause later because oestrogen levels do not decline as rapidly in overweight women. Women are living longer; thus, they spend a considerable proportion of their lives in the postmenopausal stage. Older women may develop diabetes as discussed in Chapter 12.

Signs and symptoms of menopause

Some of the symptoms associated with menopause may be associated with normal ageing, others are due to hormonal fluctuations. The signs and symptoms include:

- Mood swings, irritability, anxiety, and depression.
- Difficulty remembering things.
- Increased premenstrual tension.
- Heavier or lighter menstrual flow.
- Hot flushes.
- Changed sexual functioning such as lower libido, vaginal dryness, and recurrent candida infections.
- Susceptibility to UTI.
- Fluctuating and unpredictable blood glucose levels, which adds to the distress associated with menopause. Some women with type 1 diabetes experience more frequent hypoglycaemia. Unexplained hypoglycaemia may be one of the first signs of menopause.
- Sleep disturbance due to hot flushes and/or nocturnal hypoglycaemia.
- Weight gain, especially in type 2 diabetes, which may be associated with reduced activity and may lead to hyperglycaemia.
- Chronic back and joint pain, which can be exacerbated by being overweight.

Managing the menopause

Managing the menopause with women with diabetes is the same as those without diabetes. Maintaining a healthy, active lifestyle is important for all women. A nutrition review may be helpful to ensure adequate nutrition is maintained and limit the risk of common nutritional deficiencies such as calcium and vitamin D and the risk of osteoporosis and fractures. A diet rich in phytoestrogens such as soy products and legumes helps maintain hormonal balance. Limiting alcohol and caffeine helps control hot flushes. A healthy diet and regular exercise control weight and reduces strain on joints, which reduces back pain as well as improving blood glucose utilisation as well as reducing cardiovascular and osteoporosis risk, and improving mental wellbeing.

Regular blood glucose monitoring is important to distinguish menopausal symptoms such as sweating from hypoglycaemia and to guide GLM/insulin dose adjustment. Some overnight testing may be necessary.

A medication review is advisable. Medications, particularly OHA and insulin doses, may need to be adjusted. A through complication assessment is advisable. The risk of CVD increases; thus, lipid-lowering and antihypertensive agents may be needed, if they are not already prescribed.

Hormone replacement therapy (HRT) may improve glycaemic control and lipid levels, depending on the preparations used, and improve cardiovascular risk in younger postmenopausal women (Khoo and Mahesh 2005). Several cardiovascular events are reduced by 34–45% in women aged 50–59 on HRT and with longer use but not those >60 years (Hodis and Mack 2008). However, HRT should not be prescribed to prevent CVD. Diet and exercise, lipid-lowering medicines especially statins, and aspirin may be needed in women with cardiovascular risk factors, but fenofibrate may be contraindicated because of the risk of venous embolism. HRT is increasingly being known as menopausal hormone therapy (MHT) (National Center for Complementary and Alternative Medicine 2008).

The individual benefits and risks need to be considered and carefully explained to the woman. Younger recently menopausal women have fewer risks than older postmenopausal women. Possible adverse events include stroke, venous thrombosis, and breast cancer, but the relative risks are low if HRT is commenced within five years of menopause (WHI study 2002).

HRT may be useful in younger postmenopausal women with type 1 diabetes to prevent osteoporosis, but should be used at the lowest-effective dose. Long-term HRT to prevent osteoporosis is not advisable, but HRT does have a role in managing menopausal symptoms in the short term (Australian Drug Evaluation Committee 2003). Bisphosphonates may be an alternative if HRT is contraindicated (Khoo and Mahesh 2005).

Antibiotics and antifungal agents may be needed to manage UTIs and candida infections but general hygiene, passing urine after sexual intercourse, wearing cotton underwear, eating a healthy diet, and controlling hyperglycaemia are important preventative measures. Cranberry preparations prevent UTIs but may be contraindicated with some medications likely to cause bleeding.

Complementary approaches to managing the menopause

Many women began using CAM to manage menopausal symptoms in 2002 when the findings from the Women's Health Initiative study were released, which questioned the long-term safety of HRT use. At the time many women stopped using HRT and many tried CAM alternatives. The value of using CAM to manage menopausal symptoms is still debated and the long-term benefits of CAM hormone replacement medicines to prevent osteoporosis are unknown. Conventional hormone replacement medicines significantly reduce menopausal symptoms and osteoporotic fractures. Many research trials focus on managing hot flushes and preventing osteoporosis, however, CAM practitioners focus on managing the transition to and through menopause, rather than treating isolated symptoms.

For this and other reasons, CAM therapies continue to be popular with many menopausal women who fear the risks associated with conventional HRT. Australian women of menopausal age are high CAM users (MacLaren and Woods 2001). Popular CAM menopausal treatments include phytoestrogens, herbal medicines, acupuncture, homoeopathy, acupuncture, massage and essential oils, and wild yam cream. Although research shows conflicting results about the benefits of CAM for managing menopausal symptoms they are widely used.

Phytoestrogens

Phytoestrogens are naturally occurring plant compounds, which have a similar chemical composition to but lower potency than oestrogen. Phytoestrogens act at oestrogen receptor sites and may reduce menopausal symptoms but it is not clear whether the effects are due to phytoestrogens or other products in particular foods. Phytoestrogens reduce cholesterol and may have a place in managing cardiovascular risk. They may also improve cognition and increase bone mass. There are three main phytoestrogens:

(1) Isoflavones: found in soy products and beans, for example, lima beans and lentils.
(2) Lignans: found in fruit, vegetables, grains, and seeds such as linseed and flaxseed.
(3) Coumestans: found in sprouted seeds such as alfalfa.

Phytoestrogen should be used with caution by women using medicines that contain oestrogen (e.g. OCs, HRT), and some cancer medicines (e.g. selective oestrogen receptor modulators such as tamoxifen), and women at risk of breast, uterine or ovarian cancer, endometriosis, or uterine fibroids. Women in these categories should seek expert advice rather than self-prescribing.

Herbal medicines

If women choose to use CAM medicines to manage the menopause, they should be clear about their therapy goals and seek the advice of a qualified practitioner. CAM medicines are usually used to manage the symptoms of menopause such as hot flushes, to improve sleep, and maintain well-being. Commonly used medicines include:

- *Hypericum perforatum* (St. John's Wort) effectively reduces anxiety and mild-to-moderate depression (Ernst 1995).
- Vitus agnus-castus (chaste tree) is reputed to be a hormone regulator, but is only useful if other hormones are not being used. It can interact with OC and HRT.
- *Onothera biennnis* (evening primrose) oil has limited evidence to support an effect.
- *Cimicifuga racemosa* (black cohosh) reduces symptoms, including hot flushes. It is a key ingredient in medicines such as remifemin, which has been shown to reduce LH without affecting FSH (Duker 1991). Some studies have not shown any reduction in hot flushes (Newton et al. 2006). There have been case reports of liver damage and hepatitis but no causal association has been proven. However, preparations containing black cohosh may be contraindicated in women at risk of these conditions. Generally, it should not be used longer than six months or during pregnancy and lactation.
- *Angelica sinensis* (dong quai) there is limited evidence that dong quai reduces hot flushes. It interacts with warfarin and may be contraindicated in women using warfarin or the effects on the INR monitored carefully.
- *Panax ginseng or Panax quinquefolius* (ginseng), which may be useful to improve mood, general well-being, and sleep. It does not improve hot flushes. Ginseng has hypoglycaemic properties and may represent a hypoglycaemia risk. However, blood glucose levels are often higher during menopause and the glucose lowering effect may be a beneficial interaction.
- *Piper methysticum* (kava) reduces anxiety, but has been linked to liver damage. Therefore, kava may be contraindicated in women with existing liver disease or those at risk of liver disease.
- *Trifolium pratense* (red clover) red clover contains phytoestrogens and is a key ingredient in CAM medicines such as promensil. Some women report overall benefits but there is limited evidence that it reduces hot flushing.
- Dehydroepiandrosterone (DHEA) occurs naturally in many foods and is often taken as a dietary supplement. DHEA is converted to oestrogen and testosterone in the body. It may reduce the frequency and intensity of hot flushes and improve sexual arousal. Significantly, endogenous DHEA levels decline with age, and many people use DHEA supplements to reduce age-associated symptoms as well as menopause. It may increase the risk of breast and prostate cancer but evidence is lacking. DHEA is sometimes added to bioidentical hormonal compounds such as Biest and Triest, which increased in popularity after the release of the results of the WHI study, which suggested HRT was linked with increased risk of breast cancer (Rossouw et al. 2002).
- Progesterone creams are available by prescription; some formulations contain oestrogen and testosterone. Progesterone declines after menopause due to declining oestrogen levels. However, there is little evidence that progesterone creams reduce menopausal symptoms or improve osteoporosis risk. Only a small amount of progesterone is absorbed from topically applied formulations. *Dioscorea villosa* (wild yam) cream does not contain progesterone, although it was originally marketed in this way because it contains diosgenin, an oestrogen-like compound. Wild yam is an antispasmodic and gentle liver tonic, and CAM practitioners prescribe it for these indications. Progesterone used in conventional pessaries, OCPs, and suppositories is synthesised from diosgenin. However, specific enzymes are required to produce progesterone from diosgenin and these enzymes are not present in the human body. Traditionally, wild yam was taken orally rather than cream, but the cream formulation is a popular self-prescribed menopausal treatment. Progesterone is mainly prescribed to protect the lining of the uterus in women who use oestrogen. Substituting progesterone creams, especially wild yam, for the progesterone component of combined HRT, can increase the risk of endometrial cancer.

Practice points

(1) Women who elect to use CAM to manage menopausal symptoms should do so under the management of a suitably qualified practitioner.
(2) They should advise all their conventional health practitioners if they use CAM.
(3) More research is needed into the benefits of most CAM for managing menopausal symptoms.
(4) CAM medicines used to manage menopausal symptoms can interact with conventional medicines.
(5) Pregnant women need to seek expert advice about using CAM especially CAM medicines and especially in the first trimester.

References

Alberti, G., Zimmet, P., and Shaw, J. (2007). International diabetes federation consensus on type 2 diabetes. *Diabetic Medicine* **24**: 451–463.

Allaire, A. (2001). Complementary and alternative medicine in labour and delivery suite. *Clinical Obstetrics and Gynaecology* **44**: 681–691.

American Medical Association (AMA) (2019). Standards of Medical Care. 14 Management of diabetes in pregnancy. *Diabetes Care* **43** (Suppl. 1): S165–S172. https://care.diabetesjournals.org/content/42/Supplement_1/S165.

Andersen, O., Hertel, J., Schmolker, L., and Kuhl, C. (1998). Influence of the maternal plasma glucose concentration at delivery on the risk of hypoglycaemia in infants of insulin-dependent diabetic mothers. *Acta Paediatrica* **74**: 268–273.

Armitage, J., Poston, L., and Taylor, P. (2008). Developmental origins of obesity and the metabolic syndrome: the role of maternal obesity. *Front Hormonal Research* **36**: 73–84.

Barker, D., Gluckman, P., Godfrey, K. et al. (1993). Fetal nutrition and cardiovascular disease in adult life. *Lancet* **341** (8850): 938–941.

Biesenbach, G., Stoger, H., and Zazgornik, J. (1992). Influence of pregnancy on progression of diabetic nephropathy and subsequent requirement for renal replacement therapy in female type I diabetic patients with impaired renal function. *Nephrology Dialysis Transplant* **7**: 105–109.

Boden, R., Lundgren, M., Brandt, L. et al. (2012). Antipsychotics during pregnancy. *American Medical Archives of General Psychiatry* **69** (7): 715–721.

Bongaard, B. (2007). Is massage beneficial for pregnant women? *Alternative Medicine Alert* **10** (12): 133–136.

Boyko, E. (2000). Proportion of type 2 diabetes cases resulting from impaired fetal growth. *Diabetes Care* **23**: 1260–1264.

Broecher, J. and Lykens, J. (2011). Contraception options for women with diabetes mellitus: an evidence-based guide to safety and counseling American Diabetes Association. *DOS Against Diabetes* (April): 11–18.

Buchanan, T., Kjos, S., and Montoro, M. (1994). Use of foetal ultrasounds to select metabolic therapy for pregnancies complicated by mild gestational diabetes. *Diabetes Care* **17**: 275–283.

Ceysens, G., Rouiller, D., and Boulvain, M. (2006). Exercise for diabetic pregnant women. *Cochrane Database of Systematic Reviews*: CD004225.

Chief Medical Officer (2000). *The Report on the Confidential Enquiries into Maternal Deaths 1997–1999*. London: Her Majesty's Stationery Office.

Coffey, S. and Mason, H. (2003). The effect of polycystic ovary syndrome on health-related quality of life. *Gynecology and Endocrinology* **17** (5): 379–386.

Coustan, D. (1997). Is preconception counselling for women with diabetes cost-effective? *Diabetes Spectrum* **10** (3): 1195–2000.

Damm, P., Mathiesen, E., Clausen, D., and Petersen, K. (2005). Metabolic syndrome and related disorders: Contraception for women with diabetes mellitus. http://www.liebertonline.com. https://doi.org/10.1089/met.2005.3.244 (accessed February 2008).

DeBoer, T. (2007). Maternal diabetes linked to infant memory problems. *Child Neurology* **47**: 525.

DeMaria, E. (2007). Bariatric surgery for morbid obesity. *New England Journal of Medicine* **356**: 2176–2183.

Donovan, P. (2012). Hypertensive disorders of pregnancy. *Australian Prescriber* **35**: 47–50.

Dornhorst, A. (2003). Maternal hyperglycaemia – food for thought. *Practical Diabetes International* **20** (8): 283–289.

Duker, E. (1991). Effects of extracts from *Cimicifuga racemosa* on gonadotropin release in menopausal women and ovariectomised rats. *Plana Medica* **57**: 420–424.

Edison, R. and Muenke, M. (2004). Central nervous system and limb anomalies in case reports of first trimester statin exposure. *New England Journal of Medicine* **350**: 1579–1582.

Ernst, E. (1995). St John's Wort, an antidepressant? A systematic criteria-based review. *Phytomedicine* **2** (1): 67–71.

Feig, D., Briggs, G., and Koren, G. (2007). Oral antidiabetic agents in pregnancy and lactation: a paradigm shift? *Annals of Pharmacotherapy* **41** (7): 1174–1180.

Forster, D., Denning, A., Wills, G. et al. (2006). Herbal medicine use during pregnancy in a group of Australian women. *BMC Pregnancy and Childbirth* **6**: 21.

Gardiner, S. (2002). Drugs in pregnancy. *Current Therapeutics* (October): 31–33.

Gilbert, C., Valois, M., and Koren, G. (2006). Pregnancy outcome after first-trimester exposure to Metformin: a meta-analysis. *Fertility and Sterility* **86** (3): 658–663.

Gorina, A., Schappert, S., Bercovitz, A. et al. (2014). Prevalence of incontinence among older Americans. National Centre for Health Statistics. *Vital Health Statistics* **3** (36): 1–24.

Guerin, A., Nisenbaum, R., and Ray, J. (2007). Use of maternal.

Gutzin, S., Kozer, E., and Mcgee, L. (2003). The safety of oral hypoglycaemic agents in the first trimester of pregnancy: a meta-analysis. *Canadian Journal of Clinical Pharmacology* **10**: 179–183.

HAPO Collaborative Research Group (2008). Hyperglycaemia and adverse pregnancy outcomes. *The New England Journal of Medicine* **358**: 1991–2002.

Hewitt, V., Robertson, R., and Haddow, G. (2005). Nursing and midwifery management of hypoglycaemia in healthy term neonates: a systematic review. *Journal of Evidence Based Healthcare* **3** (7): 169–205.

Hirsch, I. (2005). Insulin analogues. *New England Journal of Medicine* **352**: 174–183.

Hodis, H. and Mack, W. (2008). The beneficial effect of hormone replacement therapy on mortality and coronary heart disease in younger versus older postmenopausal women. *Medscape Obstetrics/Gynaecology & Womens' Health* http://www.medscape.com/viewarticle/569935?src=mp (accessed March 2008).

Hollingsworth, D. (1992). *Pregnancy, Diabetes and Birth*. Philadlephia, PA: Williams & Wilkins.

Australian Drug Evaluation Committee (ADEC) (2003). *Update to ADEC statement on use of hormone replacement therapy*. ADEA (17 October).

Janssen, O., Hahn, S., Tan, S. et al. (2008). Mood and sexual function in polycystic ovary syndrome. *Seminars in Reproductive Medicine* **26** (1): 45–52.

Jovanovic, J. (2004). Answers to questions about pregnancy and diabetes. *Diabetic Mommy*. http://www.diabeticmommy.com/sp-pregnancy-diabetes-bd-faq-answers.html (accessed November 2007).

Karamermer, Y. and Ross-Hesselink, J. (2007). Coronary heart disease and pregnancy. *Future Cardiology* **3** (5): 559–567.

Kaunitz, A. (2002). Contraception for women with diabetes. *Medscape Obstetrics and Gynaecology & Women's Health* **7** (2).

Khoo, C. and Mahesh, P. (2005). Diabetes and the menopause. *Journal British Menopause Society* **11** (1): 6–11.

Kim, C., Siscovick, D., Sidney, S. et al. (2002). Oral contraceptive use and association with glucose, insulin and diabetes in young adult women: the CARDIA study. *Diabetes Care* **25** (6): 1027–1032.

Korytkowski, M., Mokan, M., Horowitz, M., and Berga, S. (1995). Metabolic effects of oral contraceptives in women with polycystic ovary syndrome. *Journal of Clinical Endocrinology and Metabolism* **80**: 3327–3334.

Laugesen, M. and Elliott, R. (2003). Ischaemic heart disease, type 1 diabetes, and cow milk A1 betacasein. *New Zealand Journal of Medicine* **116**: 1168.

Law, K. and Zhang, H. (2017). The pathogenesis and pathophysiology of gestational diabetes mellitus: deducations form a three-part longitudinal metabolomics study in China. *Clinical Chim Acta* **468**: 60–70. https://doi.org/10.1016/cca.2017.02.008.

Lee, J.Y.C., Tsou, K., Lim, J. et al. (2012). "Symptom-based Insulin adjustment for Glucose Normalization"(SIGN) Algorithm: A Pilot Study. *Diabetes Technology & Therapeutics* **14** (12): 1145–1148.

Luopajärvi, K., Savilahti, E., Virtanen, S.M. et al. (2008). Enhanced levels of cow's milk antibodies in infancy in children who develop type 1 diabetes later in childhood. *Pediatric Diabetes* **9** (5): 434–441.

MacLaren, A. and Woods, N.F. (2001). Midlife women making hormone therapy decisions. *Women's Health Issues* **11** (3): 216–230.

Marx, G., Domurat, M., and Costin, M. (1987). Potential hazard of hypoglycaemia in the parturient. *Canadian Journal of Anaesthesiology* **34** (4): 400–402.

McElduff, A., Cheung, N.W., McIntyre, H.D. et al. (2005). Consensus guidelines for the management of type 1 and type 2 diabetes in relation to pregnancy. *Medical Journal of Australia* **183** (7): 373–377.

Metzger, E., Buchanan, T., and Coulstan, D. (2007). Summary and recommendations of the fifth international workshop – conference on gestational diabetes mellitus. *Diabetes Care* **30**: S251–S260.

Meyer, C., McGrath, B., and Teede, H. (2007). Effects of medical therapy on insulin resistance and the cardiovascular system in polycystic ovarian syndrome. *Diabetes Care* **30**: 471–478.

Moran, I., Noakes, M., and Clifton, P. (2003). Dietary composition in restoring reproductive and metabolic physiology in overweight women with polycystic ovarian syndrome. *Journal Clinical Endocrinology and Metabolism* **88**: 812–819.

Nankervis, A., HD, M.I., Moses, R. et al. (2012). *ADIPS Consensus Guidelines for the Testing and Diagnosis of Gestational Mellitus in Australia*. Australasian Diabetes in Pregnancy Society (ADIPS).

National Center for Complementary and Alternative Medicine (NCCAM) (2008). Menopausal Symptoms and complementary health practices nccam.nih.gov/health/menopause/menopausesymptoms (accessed December 2012).

Newton, K., Reed, S., and Lacroix, A. (2006). Treatment of vasomotor symptoms of menopause with black cohosh, multibotanicals, soy, hormone therapy, or placebo. *Annals of Internal Medicine* **145** (12): 869–879.

Nilsson, A., Lagerquist, E., Lynch, K. et al. (2009). Temporal variation of *Ljungan Virus* antibody levels in relation to islet autoantibodies and possible correlation to Childhood type 1 diabetes. *The Open Pediatric Medicine Journal* **3**: 61–66.

Pagona, L., Sandin, S., Lof, M. et al. (2012). Low carbohydrate-high protein diet and incidence of cardiovascular disease in Swedish women: prospective cohort study. *British Medical Journal* (June) https://doi.org/10.1136/bmj.e4026.

Pettitt, D. and Jovanovic, L. (2007). Low birth weight as a risk factor for gestational diabetes, diabetes, and impaired glucose tolerance during pregnancy. *Diabetes Care* **10** (2): S147–S149.

Rani, P.R. and Begum, J. (2016). Screening and diagnosis of gestational diabetes mellitus, where do we stand. *JCDR* **10** (4): QE01.

Rasmussen, B., O'Connell, B., and Dunning, T. (2007). Young women with diabetes using internet communication to create stability during life transitions. *Journal of Clinical Nursing* **1365**: 17–24.

Ray, J., O'Brien, T., and Chan, W. (2001). Preconception care and the risk of congenital abnormalities in the offspring of women with diabetes mellitus: a meta-analysis. *Quality Journal of Medicine* **94**: 435–444.

Rice, G., Illanes, S., and Mitchell, M. (2012). Gestational diabetes mellitus; a positive predictor of type 2 diabetes? *International Journal of Endocrinology* https://doi.org/10.1155/2012/721653.

Rizzo, T., Dooley, S., Metzger, B. et al. (1995). Prenatal and perinatal influences on long term psychomotor development in offspring of diabetic mothers. *American Journal of Obstetrics and Gynaecology* **173** (6): 1753–1758.

Robinson, A., Nwolise, C., and Shawe, J. (2016). Contraception for women with diabetes: challenges and solutions. *Open Access Journal of Contraception* **7**: 11–16. https://doi.org/10.2147/OAJC.S56348.

Rossing, K., Christensen, P.K., Hovind, P. et al. (2004). Progression of nephropathy in type 2 diabetic patients. *Kidney International* **66** (4): 1596–1605.

Rossouw, J., Anderson, G., and Prentice, R. (2002). Writing Group for the Women's Health Initiative Investigators. Risks and benefits of oestrogen plus progestin in healthy menopausal women: principal results from the Women's Health Initiative randomized controlled trial. *Journal American Medical Association* **288** (3): 321–333.

Rotterdam ESHRE/ASRM Sponsored PCOS Consensus Workshop Group (2004). Revised 2003 consensus on diagnostic criteria and long term health risks related to Polycystic Ovarian Syndrome. *Fertility and Sterility* **81**: 19–25.

Rowan, J. (2007). A trial in progress: treatment with Metformin compared with insulin in the Metformin in gestational diabetes study (MiG). *Diabetes Care* **30**: S214–S219.

Salvatore, C., Rademakers, K., DelLancey, J. et al. (2017). Pathophysiology of urinary incontinence, faecal incontinence and pelvic floor prolapse. In: *Incontinence*, 6e (eds. P. Abrams, L. Cardozo and A. Wagg). Anheim, the Netherlands: ISC-ICUD.

SIGN (2010). *Scottish Intercollegiate Guidelines Network*. Edinburgh: SIGN.

Simmons, D., Walters, J., Rowan, J., and McIntyre, D. (2004). Metformin therapy and diabetes in pregnancy. *Medical Journal of Australia* **180**: 462–464.

Simpson, M., Parsons, M., Greenwood, J., and Wade, K. (2001). Raspberry leaf in pregnancy: its safety and efficacy in labour. *Journal of Midwifery and Women's Health* **46**: 51–59.

Teede, H., Hutchison, S., and Zoungas, S. (2007). The management of insulin resistance in polycystic ovarian syndrome. *Trends in Endocrinology and Metabolism* **18**: 273–279.

Ter Braak, E., Evers, I., Erkelens, W., and Visser, G. (2002). Maternal hypoglycaemia during pregnancy in type 1 diabetes: maternal and foetal consequences. *Diabetes Metabolism Research Reviews* **18**: 96–105.

Tournaire, M. and Theau-Yonneau, A. (2007). Complementary and alternative approaches to pain relief during labour. *Evidence Based Complementary and Alternative Medicine* **4** (4): 409–417.

Visser, J., Snel, M., and Van Vilet, T. (2006). Hormonal versus non-hormonal contraceptives in women with diabetes mellitus type 1 and 2. *Cochrane Database of Systematic Reviews* **18** (4): cd003990.

Western Australian Center for Evidence Based Nursing and Midwifery (2006). Management of asymptomatic hypoglycaemia in health term neonates for nurses and midwives. *Best Practice* **10** (1): 1–4.

WHO (2015). WHO Medical Eligibility Criteria for Contraceptive Use. Geneva: 2017. http://www.who.int/reproductivehealth/publication/family.planning/mec-wheel-5th/en.

Wilhelm, K., Mitchell, P., Slade, T. et al. (2003). Prevalence and correlates of DSM-IV major depression in an Australian national survey. *Journal Affective Disorders* **75**: 155–162.

Women's Health Initiative (WHI) Writing Group for the WHI investigators (2002). Risks and benefits of HRT. *Journal of the American Medical Association* **288**: 321–333.

World Health Organization (WHO) (1997). *Hypoglycaemia in the Newborn*. Geneva: WHO.

Wu, J., Azoulay, L., Majdan, A. et al. (2017). Long-term use of long-acting insulin analogs and breast cancer in women with type 2 diabetes. *Journal of Clinical Oncology* **36**: 22. https://doi.org/10.1200/jco.2017.73.4491.

Yildiz, B. (2008). Oral contraception in women with polycystic ovary syndrome. *Seminars in Reproductive Health* **26** (1): 111–120.

Zhang, C., Solomon, C., Manson, J., and Hu, F. (2006). A prospective study of pregravid physical activity and sedentary behaviours in relation to the risk of gestational diabetes mellitus. *Archives of Internal Medicine* **166**: 543–548.

Ziegler, A.G., Schmid, S., Huber, D. et al. (2003). Early infant feeding and risk of developing type 1 diabetes-associated autoantibodies. *Journal American Medical Association* **290** (13): 1721–1728.

Psychological and Quality of Life Issues Related to Having Diabetes

Key points

- The focus of an individualised diabetes management plan should be on achieving a balanced life rather than solely on 'metabolic/diabetes control'. Achieving life balance is an ongoing process of adaptation to changing life circumstances.
- Appropriate social and psychological support is essential to achieving optimal balance and diabetes and general health outcomes.
- Assessing psychological well-being and the individual's social situation and explanatory models should be undertaken at diagnosis and regularly thereafter as an essential part of the diabetes care plan. Assessments should take account of life transitions and their effect on the individual's psychological, spiritual, and physical wellbeing.
- Screening for depression, diabetes-related distress or anxiety, should be considered at the annual review and whenever there are relevant indications. For example, inadequate self-management, including not taking medicines as recommended, the development of complications/comorbidities, the end of the 'honeymoon period' in type 1 diabetes, commencing insulin in type 2 diabetes, eating disorders, and cognitive changes.
- Psychological support is not just the remit of mental health clinicians: most diabetes distress can be managed by diabetes clinicians unless it is severe and/or occurs with other mental health problems. An effective therapeutic relationship with health professionals is as important as other management strategies: in fact, it enables relevant strategies to be considered, shared decisions to be made to achieve personalised care.
- Every individual and relevant others, when indicated, should be involved in developing their diabetes management plan and monitoring the effectiveness of the plan. Thus, their role should be more comprehensive than the usual 'patient experience' and patient satisfaction' surveys. It should encompass their values and individual care goals.
- Quality of life (QOL) is individual, complex, and multifactorial. It encompasses values and life priorities. The latter might change according to life circumstances and experiences.

Care of People with Diabetes: A Manual for Healthcare Practice, Fifth Edition. Trisha Dunning and Alan Sinclair.
© 2020 John Wiley & Sons Ltd. Published 2020 by John Wiley & Sons Ltd.

- Research indicates that diabetes typically has a negative impact on QOL. However, some measures used to assess QOL, like the SF36 and EQ5D, might actually measure health status, not QoL, and often indicate people with T1DM, especially young people with no complications, have similar scores to the general population. These tools usually only show worse scores for people with diabetes when they have complications/comorbidities. In contrast, diabetes-specific measures of QoL such as Audit of Diabetes Dependent Quality of Life (ADDQoL) and Diabetes, Attitudes, Wishes and Needs (DAWN) Impact of Diabetes Profile (DIDP) show negative impact of diabetes for most people living with the condition (Speight 2019 personal communication).
- Labels such as *noncompliant* or *diabetic* are judgmental and should be avoided where possible (Diabetes Australia 2011).

Rationale

Each person with diabetes is unique. People with diabetes focus on being well and living a 'normal' life and, thus, they strive to achieve their definition of life balance. This may be significantly different from a health professional's view of what is important; health professionals are often preoccupied with metabolic control and the prevention of long-term complications. Achieving a balanced lifestyle and good QoL is essential to the physical, spiritual, and psychological well-being of people with diabetes. Yet, achieving such balance and undertaking diabetes self-care for a lifetime is hard, relentless work. Depression is more common in people with diabetes and can impact on their self-care and long-term health outcomes. Health professionals who support people with diabetes to achieve balance are more likely to assist the person to achieve optimal metabolic control for their particular circumstances and social situations than those who focus solely on achieving optimal glycaemia.

Appropriate assessment tools should be used to assess psychological wellbeing and the outcomes of self-care. Many studies use HbA1c as the primary outcome measure of education/psychological interventions, yet psychological factors, self-care, and optimal medicine use are some of the *mediators* of HbA1c; thus, HbA1c is not always an appropriate primary outcome measure (SIGN 2010). Likewise, the clinician as a mediator is rarely measured, except using ubiquitous 'patient satisfaction surveys' that do not encompass highly relevant mediators such as knowledge, beliefs, congruence, ability to develop a therapeutic relationship and cultural competence (Dunning 2013a).

Introduction

People with diabetes are at increased risk of developing various degrees of psychological distress and psychological disorders, including depression and eating disorders (Rubin and Peyrot 2001; SIGN 2010; American Diabetes Association [ADA] 2011). This chapter presents a brief outline of the complex, multifactorial psychological and social aspects of living with a diagnosis of diabetes. A range of factors affect psychological wellbeing and impact on health outcomes, including individual, social and health professional factors (SIGN 2010; ADA 2011, AMA 2019). Such factors include but are not limited to the following:

Individual factors include:

- Age and stage of life, where they are situated in their personal life journey and/or their diabetes journey
- General and diabetes-related attitudes and beliefs, including perceptions of the severity of diabetes
- General health, which changes over time and in different circumstances

- Physical and cognitive capacity, including health literacy and numeracy
- Availability and quality of support, services, and resources
- Available financial, emotional, spirituality, and social resources
- Mental health history

Social factors include:

- Cultural beliefs and customs
- General and diabetes-related attitudes and beliefs
- Family relationships and functioning, including family roles, conflict, inadequate communication skills, and lack of cohesiveness
- Social circumstances including resources
- Religion and culture

Clinician factors

Clinicians can hinder or facilitate effective self-care and wellbeing. Some clinician-related factors are the same as for individuals with diabetes, others are different. Clinician factors include:

- Knowledge and competence in a range of areas.
- Clinical inertia, i.e. the reluctance or inability to intensify medications when clinically indicated. For example, older physicians are less likely to initiate new medicines and follow guidelines (Tung 2011). The same may be true of other health professional groups. Many people with diabetes and inadequate glycaemic management experience significant delay before their treatment is intensified, especially people on glucose lowering medicines (GLMs). The average time to intensifying treatment was three years in a study by Khunti et al. (2016) who indicated clinician 'failure to act' was the main reason for clinical inertia.
- Ability to look beyond diabetes and consider all the factors that could be operating at the time.
- Clinician interpersonal communication skills, especially the key skill of listening, being truly present in an encounter and managing people with diabetes' expectations (Dunning 2013b; Hunt and May 2017).
- Capacity to relate to the individual's distress/suffering on a relevant level: sympathy (understanding the individual's distress, empathy: understanding and feeling another's distress and compassion: understanding and feeling distress and taking steps relieve the distress (Newcombe 2019). Clinicians' own lived experience of having diabetes enables them to relate on all three levels, but it is important that they can maintain empathy but keep enough distance so they can provide evidence-based, experience-informed compassionate care.
- Beliefs and attitudes about diabetes, including about severity, including the unspoken, untrue implication that type 1 diabetes is more serious than type 2; and the unspoken, untrue implication that type 2 diabetes is the fault of the person, who could/should have prevented it.
- Personal health and wellbeing, including whether they or their close family members have diabetes, which type, and where they are situated in their personal life journey and their diabetes journey.
- Setting appropriate/inappropriate examples, e.g. people with diabetes find it difficult to follow 'lifestyle advice' from clinicians who smoke, are overweight, and/or physically inactive because they do not appear to 'practice what they preach'.
- Knowing when to refer an individual for specialist assessment, management, and/or advice.
- Available resources, referral pathways, and support.

Symptoms associated with hyperglycaemia, hypoglycaemia and the focus on diet can mask signs of psychological distress and eating disorders. If present, psychological disorders can interfere with self-care, treatment adherence, including medicine self-management, and exacerbate hyperglycaemia, thus setting up a vicious cycle. Diabetes distress and depressive symptoms affect health outcomes over time, such as the development of complications and life expectancy. Reducing depression does not reduce HbA1c, however, reducing diabetes distress does reduce HbA1c (Fisher et al. 2010). Thus, it is important to differentiate between depression and diabetes distress to offer appropriate support and management.

Furthermore, depression is usually assessed in research that uses questionnaires; there is evidence that such questionnaire scores can be explained in large part by the presence of diabetes distress (Wroe 2001; Gonzalez et al. 2015). Depression is often undetected in older people and is often considered to be part of normal ageing. Approximately 15% of community-dwelling older people experience depressive symptoms and at least 24% of people with diabetes of all ages are depressed (Goldney and Phillips 2004); the incidence rises sharply in older people living in residential facilities (Chapter 12). The second highest suicide rate occurs in men >85 years.

The decision to 'take control of diabetes', which might be better phrased as 'accept diabetes and undertake self-care' is vital (Hernandez 1995). Hernandez found people with type 1 diabetes were initially concerned with being 'normal' and adopted a passive role in their care. The decision to assume personal control often occurred at a turning point in their lives, including feeling betrayed by or not listened to by clinicians, realising that adhering to management regimens would not automatically prevent complications, and clinicians accusing them of 'cheating' or not 'complying' when their blood glucose levels were unstable (Patterson and Sloan 1994). Life and other events can impact on an individual's willingness and ability to undertake self-care, for example age, work, school, religious, cultural, social, and health-related issues. Guidelines include the following:

- Know their body and be able to differentiate usual body cues/symptoms from different or new cues/symptoms. Currently, most diabetes education and management programmes focus on the 'abnormal' and/or assume all people respond in the same way, i.e. the way an 'average person' responds. People gradually learn to recognise and respond to their usual/unusual body cues, e.g. hypoglycaemia. However, diabetes complications such as autonomic neuropathy result in changes that mean the individual no longer experiences the familiar cues, which can be terrifying. Likewise, type 2 diabetes often presents with few symptoms and/or serious complications, which can also be asymptomatic, which affect the individual's perceptions of diabetes and its severity.
- Know how to manage diabetes and have the physical and mental capability and financial and other resources to manage the self-care and problem-solve in a range of situations, especially when they are experienced for the first time.
- Have supportive, constructive relationships with family, friends, and clinicians.
- Encourage positive attitudes, resilience, and adaptive coping mechanisms.
- Encourage clinicians to know the person with diabetes in order to understand their feelings about diabetes, the lessons they learned from living with diabetes, their diabetes explanatory models, and the way they undertake self-care.

Psychological adaptation and maintaining a good QoL depends on a number of factors, including the individual's degree of resilience. Resilience refers to the ability to overcome adversity and not only to rise above it, but also to thrive. It has its foundation in belonging, life meaning, expectations, and happiness. Resilience is at the heart of spirituality, social cohesion, and empowerment (Dunning 2013b). Chronic conditions such as diabetes have a major impact on an individual's life plan, their partner, families, and other relationships. Acquiring coping skills and being resilient can have positive effects on emotional wellbeing and, therefore, on physical outcomes. The constant demands of coping with diabetes is an issue for some people.

Some coping issues for young people with type 1 diabetes encompass:

- Being expected to cope
- Being expected to cope all the time
- Being seen to cope by others
- Having to cope for the rest of their lives
- Having no respite from coping with diabetes (Dunning 1994)

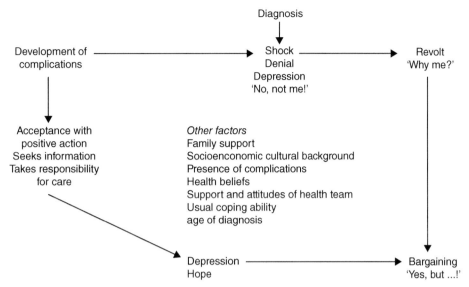

Figure 15.1   Model of the diabetes grief cycle. Not accepting diabetes does not mean the individual does not undertake some or all relevant diabetes self-care.

These issues are important across the lifespan as people with diabetes face life and diabetes-related challenges. Many factors influence how a person reacts to and accepts the diagnosis of diabetes and assumes responsibility for self-care. Reactions to the diagnosis of diabetes are unique to the individual concerned; however, several common reactions have been documented. They include anger, guilt, fear, helplessness, confusion, relief, and denial. Appreciating some of the issues and reactions involved will enable clinicians to better understand the complexity of living with diabetes and enable them to help individuals set achievable goals, develop appropriate coping strategies, and plan appropriate self-care (Skinner 2013).

A period of grief and denial is common. Figure 15.1 shows one model of the 'diabetic grief cycle' loosely based on Helen Kubler Ross's work, associated with death and dying. Lack of knowledge and/or inaccurate knowledge about diabetes, often produces stress and anxiety. The invisible nature of the condition: as indicated; type 2 diabetes and most diabetes-related complications are often present without symptoms (e.g. myocardial infarction (MI), UTI, and retinopathy) can be silent, resulting in disbelief and denial when they are diagnosed. Denial is an appropriate coping mechanism *early* in the course of a condition or complication, and enables people to maintain a positive attitude and come to terms with their altered health status: in the longer term, denial is counterproductive, because it makes it difficult for the person to manage their diabetes and the associated risks.

The person with diabetes needs adequate time to grieve for their perceived losses, for example, loss of spontaneity, lifestyle, having to plan ahead, loss of the respect and love of the people they value (Funnell 2006) and changed body image. However, prolonged denial can inhibit appropriate self-care, cause people to ignore warning signs of other problems and lead to nonattendance at scheduled medical appointments or investigative procedures and/or not seeking advice about health issues, which increases the risk of adverse health outcomes and diabetes complications. Denial can continue for longer than five years after the initial diagnosis in people with type 1 diabetes (Gardiner 1997), but it is not the only explanation for inadequate self-care, which can also indicate severe diabetes distress or 'burnout' from the unremitting demands of living with diabetes. Frequent presentations to hospital or emergency departments could be a signal to clinicians to refer the individual for counselling.

Accepting diabetes involves dealing with some or all of the following:

- Diagnosis, which represents a turning point and change; managing change depends on the individual's resilience and coping strategies.
- Mental and physical pain.
- Hospitalisation or frequent outpatient or doctor visits.
- The health system. This includes clinicians' beliefs and attitudes, and often hospitals and emergency services. These services are not part of the individual's usual care routine.
- Lifelong treatment: 'There are no holidays from diabetes'.
- Body image changes, which can be positive or negative: 'I worry about diabetes all the time' versus 'diabetes helps me be who I am'.
- Friends/family relationships.
- Fluctuating blood glucose levels.
- Emotional stability.
- Loss of independence.
- Societal language, attitudes, expectations, and discrimination, especially in some countries.

The tasks required to maintain acceptable blood glucose ranges are tedious and sometimes painful, despite modern technology in blood glucose monitoring and insulin delivery systems. There are financial costs involved, which can be a burden for some people, e.g. insulin, testing equipment, clinician visits, increased insurance premiums, which add to the stress associated with having a condition most people did not want in the first place.

Clinical Observations

- There are no holidays from diabetes for the person with diabetes.
- The individual has to live with diabetes 365 days a year 24-hours a day, every day for the rest of their life; it is like a job they 'never wanted, and don't get paid for'.
- Some migrant groups 'take holidays' from diabetes when they visit relatives in their home countries. The 'holiday' often includes not taking medicines as prescribed, using complementary medicines (CM) and other complementary therapies, overeating because it is socially expected, and not monitoring their blood glucose.
- Some people regard a hospital admission as an opportunity to have clinicians be responsible for their diabetes care but many worry that some clinicians 'do not know as much about my diabetes as I know'.

Adjustment and spirituality

Managing a chronic condition means straddling two paradigms – the biomedical and the psychosocial – neither of which adequately address spirituality; in the context of this book, spirituality refers to the dimension of self that enables the individual to find value, meaning and purpose in their life. All three are needed to achieve optimal health outcomes. An individual's path through life is influenced by life trajectories and turning points and these include the diagnosis of diabetes, expectations of treatment, and social support. Helping an individual understand their life and diabetes trajectories and identify turning points and transitions is part of holistic care (Dunning 2013b). Spiritual needs are different from emotional needs (Rapport et al. 2019).

Spirituality can be a motivating force that enables the individual to transcend life's challenges, such as the diagnosis of diabetes (Parsian and Dunning 2008). Hodges (2002) described four dimensions of spirituality: each dimension plays a role in the degree of wellbeing an individual experiences:

(1) Finding value, meaning, and purpose in life. Purpose in life is one aspect of wellbeing; happiness or positive affect is another (NHS Scotland 2013). Purpose in life is having something to do, a reason to keep going, for example work and being with grandchildren. Changes

can affect the person' purpose in life and put them at risk of adverse events, e.g. retiring, bereavement after a beloved pet of spouse dies.

(2) Intrinsic values, values are very important; they generally do not change very much throughout the person's life once established, whereas care preferences can change (and often do). See Chapter 17. Values are closely related to meaning and purpose in life. Understanding the person's values can help clinicians and families decide care if the individual is unable to make autonomous decisions and reduces decisional uncertainty (Chapter 17).

(3) Transcendence refers to coming to terms with the challenge/s and adapting to the new situation, e.g. diagnosis of diabetes or a complication.

(4) Spiritual community can be very valuable.

Interestingly, Wolpert (2006) described depression as 'soul loss'. Parsian and Dunning (2008) found a significant association amongst spirituality, being female, higher education, and duration of diabetes (>10 years), lower HbA1c and higher self-concept in young adults with type 1 diabetes when they developed and validated a tool to measure spirituality. Significantly, participants in the study did not consider religion and spirituality to be the same thing; only two respondents who regarded themselves as spiritual used religious practices, mostly prayer, to help them cope.

Over the past 10 years research has demonstrated a link between being affiliated with a religious group and better physical and mental health outcomes, although the association is not clear and may have a cultural element (UK Mental Health Foundation 2006; Gilbert 2007). The connection could be that religion contributes to having a purpose in life and social connectedness or belonging, rather than religion itself. That is, having 'something to do, something to live for and something to hope for' contributes to wellbeing.

Social determinants of health such as education level and income also impact on acceptance, adjustment, and health outcomes and are beginning to inform risk prediction models (Gottlieb and Alderwick 2019). The association between genetics and environment and susceptibility to mental and physical illness, including diabetes, emerged over the past 5–10 years. These changes include changes in the stress reactivity pathway, telomere length, protein expression in the immune system and changes in the volume of the hippocampal, cingulate, and caudate areas of the brain in children and adults. Such research highlights the complexity and inter-related importance of mind and body to a well-functioning 'whole person' and the imperative to provide holistic care (Chapter 2).

Diabetes: reputation and myths

Diabetes has a bad reputation in the community accompanied by many myths, or more correctly, misinformation: for example, 'Eating sugar causes diabetes', and type 2 diabetes is a 'mild form of the disease'. Such misinformation must be discussed and dispelled because it can be associated with self-blame and guilt feelings (Browne et al. 2017).

The perceived severity of diabetes affects the person's mental status. Type 2 diabetes was traditionally considered to be less serious than type 1 diabetes, especially where it is treated without medications, even though type 2 diabetes is associated with progressive loss of beta cell function with consequent insulin deficiency; and complications are frequently present at diagnosis. Clinicians' messages that type 2 diabetes is not or less serious can lead to false hope, and distress and/or depression when medicines, especially insulin, are required (Dunning and Martin 1997, 1999; MILES 2011). Considering the silent, insidious nature of type 2 diabetes and the frequency with which complications are present at diagnosis, type 2 diabetes is hardly 'nothing to worry about'.

In addition, social pressures and ignorance often cause frustration and contribute to sub-optimal self-care, not taking medications at the recommended time, or not following dietary advice. For example, pressure from friends and relatives who say 'a little piece of cake won't hurt you' can be confusing/frustrating for people with type 1 and type 2 diabetes (Newton-John et al. 2017). In some cultures, diabetes changes the individual's perceived 'value' and compromises their acceptance in society generally, acceptability as a marriage partner, and compromises their job prospects (Kreuter et al. 2002). Consequently, diabetes might be denied or hidden. There is an associating between diabetes and diabetes-related distress and depression and some other psychiatric/mental health conditions.

Diabetes-related distress

Clinicians need to mindful of the burden diabetes imposes on people's lives and ask constructive, open-ended questions to help people discuss mental health issues for example: 'What is the hardest thing about living with diabetes for you at the moment?' Focus on successes and support the individual's problem-solving skills, for example, 'How do you think you can manage that?' Involve the family and significant others, if relevant, and with the individual's permission (Speight and Singh 2013) and help them develop emotional resilience and optimism, which are key aspects of empowerment. Importantly, clinicians do not empower people with diabetes: they can help the individual become self-empowered as part of their spiritual journey of becoming.

Useful strategies and screening tool to manage diabetes distress are described in *Diabetes and Emotional Health: A Practical Guide for Healthcare Professionals Supporting Adults with Type 1 and Type 2 Diabetes* (Hendrieckx et al. 2019). Two key screening tools are (Fenwick et al. 2018):

- Problem Areas in Diabetes (PAID)
- Diabetes Distress Scale (DDS)

Quality of life

Quality of life (QoL) is a highly subjective and multidimensional concept concerned with cognitive status, satisfaction, and emotional happiness (Cox and Gonder-Frederick 1992). It has become a major issue in behavioural diabetes research. Poor QoL is associated with neglected self-care and may predict an individual's capacity for self-care. According to life mission theory, people lower their QoL when they are in crisis to survive and adapt. QoL can be increased when the person has the resources to heal (Ventegodt et al. 2003). Healing encompasses *salutogenesis* (Antonovsky 1987) where the individual develops a 'sense of coherence' and develops personally, or in modern terminology, becomes empowered.

Individuals enter a holistic state of healing when:

- Individuals and their health professionals have similar life perspectives and the intent of the health professional is to help the person understand him/herself and take responsibility for their life, and in this case, diabetes.
- They are in a safe environment.
- They have the personal resources.
- They have the will to understand and overcome the crisis and let go of negative emotions and behaviours.
- They and their health professionals have healing intent. There is sufficient holding. Holding is a five-fold process that involves acknowledging the patient and giving them respect, trust, care, and acceptance (Ventegodt et al. 2003; Dunning 2013a).

Four categories of determinants of QoL are described:

(1) Medical: diabetes type, treatment regimen, level of metabolic control and presence of complications. The severity of complications reduces QoL.
(2) Cognitive: acute and chronic blood glucose control and neuropsychological changes can reduce QoL for the person with diabetes and their family. The effect of depression on QoL is greater than the effect of diabetes and is additive to other factors (Goldney and Phillips 2004).

(3) Attitudinal: self-efficacy, locus of control, and social support. People with good support have better QoL and less depression. Empowerment strategies and improving an individual's sense of being in control improve their QoL. This includes considering spirituality, an integral aspect of empowerment.
(4) Demographic: gender, education level, ethnicity, and age. Men report better QoL than women and young people report better QoL than old people. Higher education is associated with better QoL.

Measuring QoL

Most people understand what is meant by 'quality of life' but it is a difficult concept to measure. A number of tools have been developed that measure the general aspects of QoL and are widely used in research because they can compare participants with each other. Diabetes-specific QoL are available. These tools include the generic Health-Related Quality of Life, ADDQoL, DIDP, and the Diabetes Specific Quality of Life. Sometimes a number of tools are used together.

Some of these tools are simple to use and are, or could be, incorporated into the routine diabetes assessments. However, it is important to realise that, although these tools are validated and widely used, they, may not indicate an *individual's* specific QoL. Patient-generated QoL measures developed specifically by the individual may be useful to monitor the QoL issues relevant to the individual (Jenkinson and McGee 1998). The process consists of asking the individual to nominate their top three to five QoL issues, then developing a Likert scale on which the individual rates each issue. The author prefers to us a three point Liker scale ranging from high, do not know unsure to poor because it is easier for people to make choices and still enable them to choose a 'don't know' option if they choose.

Significantly, in the authors' practice pets and being with family consistently rate high as important QoL issues for a wide range of people. The tool can be administered as part of complication screening, when health status changes and during major life transitions.

Measuring QoL may be useful to plan holistic nursing care and address issues of empowerment. It is important to consider individual meaning of QoL and to ask about these individual issues as well as global issues.

Recommendations to encourage mental and physical wellbeing

The following strategies can be used to assist people with diabetes to maintain mental wellbeing:

* Coping strategies including problem-focused coping to deal with or prevent problems and emotion-focused coping to deal with negative emotions (Peyrot and Rubin 2007).
* Enhancing diabetes-specific self-efficacy, which involves encouraging realistic expectations and enhancing motivation by helping people identify their successes and encouraging optimism and realistic expectations. For example, motivational interviewing (Rollnick et al. 1999). High self-efficacy is associated with lower rates of depression (Steunenberg et al. 2007) and spirituality (Parsian and Dunning 2008).
* Improving metabolic control to relieve the effects of hyperglycaemia and fear of hypoglycaemia on mood and QoL.
* Interactive behaviour change technology (IBCT), which includes personal digital assistant tools, person-centred websites, online peer support groups, brain training websites, coaching telephone calls, DVDs, audiotapes, blogs, vlogs, podcasts, apps touch screen kiosks designed to help people maintain independence, can help people improve their diabetes self-care and monitor change (Piette 2007). Some technologies can also be useful to support informal caregivers and wearable technologies can promote activity, for example, pedometers can help people engage in physical activity.
* The Internet enables people to remain anonymous, which is important to some people (Rasmussen et al. 2007a). People need advice about how to assess the veracity of websites because the information is often of low quality, may be misleading and can do more harm than

good. Information technologies do not take the place of human contact and are more effective when combined with human contact (Piette 2007).
- Recognise that psychological issues affect metabolic control and need to be addressed in order to maintain QOL and effective diabetes self-care.
- Provide supportive education and advice, when it is required and tailor education to the individual's needs. An empowerment model of care and a holistic approach are more appropriate for chronic diseases such as diabetes where frequent visits to health professionals are required. Empowerment models seek to involve the individual in decisions about their management and to establish a therapeutic relationship with the individual; see Chapter 16.
- Improve communication. Provide an appropriate environment for consultations, plan for continuity of care, including discharge planning, ask open questions and give the individual the opportunity to ask questions. Ask person-focused questions such as 'What are your concerns today?' put the focus on the individual in contrast to 'What can *I* do for you today?'
- Address complications honestly but optimistically. Foster self-esteem and coping skills. In hospital this may mean allowing the person with diabetes to monitor their own blood glucose and administer their own medications.
- Offer options and help with goal setting.
- Give the message that diabetes is a serious disease and focus on the benefits of managing the condition rather than what will happen if they do not.
- Focus on the person not on their HbA1c; doing the former will help to achieve the latter.
- Acknowledge that it is difficult to live with diabetes.
- Monitor psychological wellbeing as well as physical wellbeing (Bradley and Gamsu 1994).
- Recognise that assistance animals, especially dogs, can have a significant effect on mental wellbeing and safety, e.g. glycaemia assistance dogs (Chapter 6).

As indicated, family and friends often play a key role and assume a large care burden for children and older people with diabetes. The latter can be particularly challenging when the person with diabetes has dementia and/or incontinence. Considering the family care givers' health and wellbeing is important because both these conditions are reasons for placing a relative in an aged care home (Chapter 12). The following tools can be used to assess family carer's stress:

- Diabetes Family Support and Conflict Scale (DFSC).
- Caregiver Strain Index (CSI).

Diabetes and depression

The World Health Organization predicted that depression will be the second major health issue by 2020. Approximately 5.8% of adults experience a depressive disorder (Andrews et al. 1999) and depression accounts for 8% of the non-fatal disease burden. People with diabetes have a higher incidence of depression than the general public and the depression often precedes the diagnosis of diabetes. Depression may be an independent risk factor for type 2 diabetes (Rubin and Peyrot 2001), whilst depression and hopelessness can arise from having a chronic disease (Lustman 1997). Furthermore, it is possible that there is an underlying mechanism causing depression and type 2 diabetes (Eaton et al. 1996; Peyrot 1997; Carnethon et al. 2003; Pouwer and Speight 2014; Silva et al. 2019). Type 2 is associated with increased risk of dementia, neuropsychiatric and mood disorders. Possible mechanisms include molecular mechanisms associated with the neural reward system, neurogenesis, synaptic neuroplasticity, the hypothalamic–pituitary–adrenal axis, tumour necrosis factor (TNFα) and defective insulin signalling in depression (Silva et al. 2019).

Likewise, it is not clear whether depression increases the risk of type 2 diabetes per se or through the associated social determinants of health and consequent lifestyle risk factors such as poor diet, smoking, and inactivity. Carnethon et al. (2003) found depression was associated with lower than high school education in a cohort from the NHANES 1 study ($N = 6910$):

low education was an independent of risk factor for developing diabetes. Carnethon et al. (2003) suggested causal mechanisms for the link could include genetic predisposition, inflammation and activation of the hypothalamic–pituitary–adrenal axis. These factors are similar to those proposed for the association amongst diabetes, cardiovascular diseases, and depression; see Chapters 1 and 8, and the effects on immunity and inflammation (Gottlieb and Alderwick 2019).

Depression could be a component of the insulin resistance syndrome (see Chapter 1). People who are depressed are less likely to perform adequate preventative health self-care, more likely to present to the emergency department, require specialist intervention and exhibit lowered self-worth and physical functioning (Ciechanowski et al. 2000). Diabetes-related distress is also associated with inadequate treatment adherence and high HbA1c amongst people with type 2 diabetes, which is partly mediated by perceived self-efficacy and control over diabetes (Gonzalez et al. 2015).

Relationships amongst these factors could be reciprocal over time and likely involve other constructs such as beliefs about self and the future that can be affected by the way the individual processes information and likely the way information is presented. The relationship between self-efficacy and perceived control and their impact on stressful experiences, adaptation and emotional distress were recognised in the 1980s (Litt 1988).

Adaptation also involves negotiating the expectations of others, which is part of everyday life. It involves balancing normative expectations, and for people with diabetes, clinicians' expectations, with the capacity to act. It is a complex social process that involves the relational aspects of quality/inequality in power and knowledge/expertise known as cognitive authority theory (Hunt and May 2017). The associated burdens of diabetes, self-care, medicines, and managing other people's expectations can overwhelm the individual's capabilities and contribute to diabetes distress and depression.

The course of depression in people with diabetes is chronic and severe and depressive episodes may be particularly severe because of the hyperglycaemia and the neuroendocrine response (Rubin and Peyrot 2001) and the presence of microvascular and macrovascular complications. Thus, depression is associated with increased healthcare costs (Egede et al. 2002; SIGN 2010; ADA 2011, 2019). Cavan et al. (2001) suggested the reasons people with diabetes become depressed might be:

- The heavy disease burden
- The strain diabetes places on relationships, especially family relationships, and especially in some cultures
- Stigma associated with diabetes in the family and the community
- Shock and guilt at the diagnosis that are not adequately addressed and resolved
- Uncertainty of the future
- Loss of control
- Past and current negative experiences with diabetes and with clinicians

Some of these issues may be depression and some could be diabetes-specific distress. The difference between the two states has emerged in past few years. Current research suggests diabetes distress is important in its own right, but can also lead to depression (Gonzalez et al. 2015). Fisher et al. (2014) described distress as being on a continuum and having multiple generic and diabetes-specific causes. It is possible that unrelieved distress or emotional dwelling increases the risk of depression.

Recent research has improved understanding of the interconnections amongst the gut microbiota affect brain function through four main factors:

(1) The direct release of humoral messengers
(2) Actions on the gut
(3) The enteric nervous system
(4) Actions on the immune system

The brain also affects the immune system, the enteric nervous system, and the gut. Teisman (2017) described these four factors as the 'four control arms of behaviour in a superorganism made up of both the animal cells and the microbial colony'. Research involving animal models and human studies suggest the microbiome plays a role in several human diseases, including mood, autism, and schizophrenia (Teisman 2017).

Interestingly, metformin had significant cognitive effects on key cognitive functions: verbal learning, working memory, and executive function (Herath et al. 2016). Metformin primarily acts in the gut: however, it is not clear whether there is any connection to the gut microbiome.

Symptoms of depression

The DSM-5 diagnostic criteria for depression states that the individual must be experiencing five or more of the following symptoms during the same two-week period. At least one symptom should be either depressed mood or loss of interest or pleasure (anhedonia). In addition, the symptoms must cause significant clinical distress or affect the individual's social, occupational, or other important areas of functioning and must not be a result of substance abuse or another medical condition. The criteria include the following:

(1) Depressed mood most of the day, nearly every day
(2) Markedly diminished interest or pleasure in all or almost all activities most of the day, nearly every day
(3) Significant weight changes or reduced or increased appetite nearly every day
(4) Slowing down of thought and reduced physical movement apparent to other people, not only subjective feelings of restlessness or slowing down
(5) Fatigue or loss of energy nearly every day
(6) Feelings of worthlessness or excessive or inappropriate guilt nearly every day
(7) Reduced ability to think or concentrate or make decisions nearly every day
(8) Recurrent thoughts of death and/or suicidal ideation without a specific suicide plan, or a suicide attempt or a specific plan for committing suicide

Inadequate self-care in not a criterion for diagnosing depression; although diabetes distress and depression can be accompanied by reduced confidence and non-adherence to some or all aspects of self-care. Likewise, not all people who neglect their self-care are depressed. Clinicians must check their assumptions before making decisions/diagnoses and suggesting management options (Lustman et al. 1996; SIGN 2010). It is also important to understand the difference between intentional and unintentional adherence (Wroe 2001) and prospective memory slips (Trawley et al. 2018).

Screening for generic psychological distress and depression

A range of screening tools is used. They all have advantages and disadvantages and varying degrees of validity in some settings. Not all are suitable for clinical monitoring because of their complexity and length; some tools cannot be used without permission and some copyright holders require potential users to sign an agreement and pay to use the tools. Commonly used tools include:

- Beck Depression Inventory (BDI)
- Diagnostic and Statistical Manual of Mental Disorders (DSM-V)
- Geriatric Depression Score
- Hospital Anxiety and Depression Scale (HADS)
- Hamilton Depression Rating Scale
- Patient Health Questionnaire (PHQ-9 and PHQ-2)
- World Health Organization Well Being Index (WHO-5) (Bonsignore et al. 2001; SIGN 2014; Halliday et al. 2017; NICE 2018)

Managing depression

'The effectiveness of interventions depends on the context in which it is delivered' (Wilson and Holt 2001; Nilsen and Bernhardson 2019). The way clinicians interact with people with diabetes and deliver care may be more important than the care itself (Balint 1955). Whilst Balint's study is old, its message remains very relevant today and many 'Balint groups' have been established especially in the United States to help clinicians cope with their stress and clinical uncertainties and become more effective carers. A Balint group operates in the Geelong region where the author works.

Managing depression and diabetes is complex. Complexity theories suggest all the circumstances that influence behaviour must be considered (Lancaster 2000), which is certainly true of diabetes and depression where individuals:

- Operate within self-adjusting biochemical, cellular, physiological, social, cultural, and religious systems and where a change in one will result in a change in the others.
- Illness and wellness are part of a continuum, are dynamic and arise from an interaction amongst these factors.
- Physical and psychological health can only be maintained using a holistic model of care that incorporates all of these aspects.

Several guidelines are available and provide detailed information about depression and other mental health disorders, diagnostic criteria, management and information for people with depression, including NICE (2018), SIGN (2014), and ADA (2019) addressed diabetes and depression. Most indicate care needs to be integrated across services and recommend a stepped approach that combines 'counselling' therapies and medicine if/when indicated.

Counselling strategies include cognitive behavioural therapy (CBT), mindfulness-based CBT and problem-solving strategies, interpersonal therapy, motivational interviewing, goal setting, and guided self-determination to reduce self-defeating thought patterns and negative behaviours and improve adherence with management regimens. These therapies can be used alone or with antipsychotic medicines when indicated. CBT strategies require the individual to be able to think rationally and actively participate in their management. Usually, a close working relationship with the therapist is needed and it may take months for the individual to change unhealthy thought/behaviour patterns (Better Health Channel 2007). Thus, therapy is often needed in the long term.

Diet, physical activity, not smoking, and not consuming excess alcohol are important aspects of diabetes prevention and management, including mental health and depression. Clinicians can use counselling strategies in routine care. For example, Elley et al. (2003) showed counselling in general practice effectively increased physical activity and improved QoL over 12 months. In a second study (Elley et al. 2007) found a personalised approach focusing on barriers and facilitators to physical activity, internal motivators, recognising time, physical and psychological limitations, and spiritual benefits as well as the role of significant others, was important. Craike et al. (2017) found that for healthy and overweight people, high amounts of activity were significantly associated with fewer depressive symptoms, while for obese individuals, both moderate and high amounts were associated with fewer depressive symptoms.

Complementary therapies (CM) and self-help programmes with the best evidence for effectiveness in depression are *Hypericum perforatum* for mild-to-moderate depression, exercise, bibliotherapy involving CBT, and light therapy for winter depression. There is limited evidence to support acupuncture, light therapy for SAD syndrome, massage, relaxation therapies, S-adenosyl-L-methionine (SAM-e), folate, or yoga breathing exercises (Jorm et al. 2002). CM medicines should be used under the supervision of a qualified practitioner and clinicians and people with diabetes should be aware of possible adverse events associated with CM use (Chapter 18).

Mental health and type 1 diabetes

About 50% of people with of type 1 diabetes are diagnosed in childhood (Pouwer and Speight 2014) but type 1 diabetes can also be diagnosed in adults and older people (Chapter 1). Diabetes diagnosed in childhood can produce enormous guilt and anxiety for the child and the parents (Rasmussen et al. 2007b). Marital strife is not uncommon and is often exacerbated by the diabetes. The parents must learn how to care for the child at the same time as coping with their own feelings. Inflicting pain on a child (injections, blood tests) is very difficult to do, and such tasks often fall to the mother.

As the child matures and develops they need to assume responsibility for their diabetes self-care. It can be extremely difficult for the parents to 'let go', and, therefore, for the child to achieve independence. Other children in the family may feel deprived of attention. Sweets, the traditional reward for good behaviour, are often withdrawn and may be seen as a punishment.

Some childhood behaviour such as irritability and awkwardness can be difficult to distinguish from hypoglycaemia, making hypoglycaemia management difficult. Hypoglycaemia itself is feared and hated by children and parents and mostly underrated by healthcare staff. It is not unknown for people to deliberately run their blood glucose levels high to avoid hypoglycaemia (Dunning 1994) (Chapter 6). Parents with diabetes may have concerns about passing diabetes to their own children in the future. Support, encouragement and referral for counselling, if necessary, are vital aspects of diabetes care.

Diabetes is the 'perfect' condition for manipulating others and gaining attention. Withholding insulin can result in ketoacidosis, which mobilises the family, friends, and health resources. Hypoglycaemia can have the same effect. Repeated admissions for hypoglycaemia or diabetic ketoacidosis (DKA) need to be investigated carefully and diplomatically.

An individual's response to the diagnosis of diabetes depends on their overall psychological and social adjustment and the availability of structured family support. Fitting diabetes into family life can be difficult and changes with duration of diabetes and the intensity of the treatment regimen (Gardiner 1997). Likewise, major life transitions such as leaving home, starting a new job, going to university, and having a child require readaption (Rasmussen et al. 2007b).

Type 1 diagnosis in older adults can be delayed, inappropriately labelled type 2 and mistreated, which can affect symptoms and well-being. Psychological responses of older people differ from the responses of children and adolescents. The Australian National Diabetes Strategy and Implementation Plan (Diabetes Australia 2016–2020) identified some issues specific to people with type 1 diabetes:

- Dependency, for example, during severe hypoglycaemia and fears of being dependent should they develop complications such as blindness.
- Loss of control, either in the short term, e.g. during hypoglycaemia or in the long term.
- Public confusion about the difference between type 1 and type 2 diabetes. This confusion extends to clinicians as the following quote from a referral for diabetes education indicates: 'He used to have type 2 but the doctor started him on insulin yesterday and he is now type 1. Needs education'.
- Who to tell about their diabetes at work – workmates, friends?
- Restrictions, for example, some sporting activities, jobs, and hassles getting a driver's licence.

Note also the epigenetic and cultural issues that affect survival as well as psychological wellbeing in some cultures discussed earlier in the chapter.

Mental health and type 2 diabetes

Type 2 diabetes is increasingly diagnosed in childhood and adolescence (Chapter 1). The diagnosis of diabetes in later life means the person may need to change behaviours developed over years. Eating patterns often have to be modified. 'Restrictions' are often resented with resultant anger, denial, or neglect. Alternatively, the person may meticulously follow the management plan. Knowledge about possible diabetes-related complications or the development of complications leads to stress, which in turn contributes to elevated blood glucose levels. Relationships with families/spouses may be disrupted; they may become overprotective, resulting in over dependence or rebelliousness. People tend to cope better and manage the self-care more easily if the family is supportive yet encourages independence.

More the 50% of people with type 2 diabetes on insulin report reduced QoL. Insulin has a negative impact, which is greater in younger people with a long duration of diabetes and those from non-English-speaking backgrounds (Rubin 2000; Davis et al. 2001; MILES 2011). Men with type 2 diabetes self-report 'depression', disempowerment, and perceived loss of control (Tun et al. 1990). Hopelessness and depression may be the result of the misapprehension that insulin indicates severe/serious disease (Dunning and Martin 1999). Support and explaining the likely progression to insulin are required early in the course of diabetes, e.g. at, or soon after diagnosis.

Thoolen (2006) in the Netherlands found people with type 2 diabetes experience little diabetes-related anxiety, do not regard diabetes as a serious disease and have high self-efficacy and low levels of self-care in the early years after diagnosis (n = 196). People who had been diagnosed for more than two or three years were more likely to consider diabetes to be threatening to their health. People on intensive treatment reported higher levels of stress and lower self-efficacy. Like other studies, Thoolen's study emphasises the importance of taking a thorough history and considering individual and cultural factors and reactions.

The DAWN study (Funnell 2006) (n = 3432, type 2 and 1672, type 1) demonstrated that diabetes is associated with a number of physical and psychological symptoms such as shock and disbelief 35–55%, anxiety 38% type 1, and 19% type 2. Of these, 51% were concerned about hypoglycaemia, 48% about weight change especially type 2, and the disease getting worse 34%. Despite these concerns many were relieved to have a diagnosis. In the Australian cohort 75% were optimistic about the future, about 25% said they felt burnt out by diabetes and <40% were tired of complying with diabetes self-care. Most agreed diabetes did not prevent them from doing what they wanted to do.

Fifty-two percent of people with type 2 not on insulin worried about having to commence insulin and only 10% thought insulin would help control their diabetes. Li et al. (2008) found a higher rate of major depression in people with type 2 diabetes on insulin than those with type 2 not using insulin and those with type 1 diabetes. These studies suggest insulin has a negative impact on people with type 2 diabetes, despite the clinical observation that many report feeling better once they commence insulin and their control improves. Very similar findings emerged in the MILES study (MILES 2011).

Psychological distress and cardiovascular disease

The effect of negative emotions on physical functioning is not new. William Harvey noted that mental distress affected the heart and impaired its function in 1628. Sound evidence for the link between emotions and cardiovascular disease, particularly MI and stroke, has emerged in the last 10 years, and the risk appears to be comparable to those of other known risk factors such as smoking.

Although the course of chronic heart disease and depression fluctuate, negative emotions have cumulative pathophysiological effects. Diabetes is also linked to higher rates of depression than the general population, and cardiovascular disease is a major long-term diabetes complication. The emotional impact people with diabetes attribute to MI and to diabetes changes with the longer duration of time after the acute MI. In the initial stages, surviving the MI is the major concern; by three to four months, concerns about diabetes begin to re-emerge and predominate by six months (Gujadhur et al. 2003).

Depression may contribute to physical damage by activating key neurohormonal systems as well as other mechanisms (Yusef et al. 2004; Everson-Rose and Lewis 2005; Rozanski et al. 2005). Yusef et al. 2004 showed psychological distress was associated with a 2.5-fold greater risk of acute MI than hypertension, abdominal obesity, diabetes (i.e. the metabolic syndrome; see Chapter 1), and other risk factors in the INTERHEART study ($n = 29\,972$ in 52 countries). The association is evident in a number of other studies (Joost et al. 2004; Lett et al. 2004; Rozanski et al. 2005). Janszky et al. (2007) found admission for depression is associated with increased risk of MI, independent of other risk factors, but the mechanism remains unclear.

Lett et al. (2004) suggested depression could be a marker of a broader issue encompassing a range of factors, such as:

- Negative affect
- Vital exhaustion
- Limited social support
- Personality factors
- Anger
- Hostility
- Negative emotions
- Anxiety

Depression and negative affect appear to predict increased risk of cardiovascular disease (Frasure-Smith and Lesperance 2003). Significantly, optimistic individuals have lower risk of cardiovascular disease than pessimists when other risk factors are controlled for (Giltay et al. 2006; Kubzansky and Thurston 2007). Many researchers and clinicians note that people with heart disease have high rates of depression ranging between 40% and 65% (Januzzi et al. 2000). However, 53% of people have a history of depression prior to having an MI, which suggests depression precedes the MI (Rafinelle 2005; Glassman and Miller 2007).

The effect of negative emotions on cardiovascular disease is currently being explored, for example, specific biomarkers, genetic predisposition, and psychological resilience. Negative emotions may have direct physiological effects by stimulating the hypothalamic–pituitary–adrenocortical axis, affecting the immune response and contributing to inflammation. Psychological distress also affects self-care behaviours, in that highly stressed individuals often smoke, drink excess amounts of alcohol, do not exercise or eat inappropriate foods, neglect self-care, and do not adhere to healthcare regimens, including medicines. Psychological distress occurs on a continuum ranging from normal to pathological (eustress to distress).

However, the cognitive, behavioural, and biological components of psychological distress are the same regardless of where the individual is on the distress continuum. Pathological psychological distress is characterised by intense emotions. There appears to be a dose-dependent relationship between the level of emotion and the degree of risk for cardiovascular disease (Kubzansky 2007).

Holistic diabetes assessment and successful depression management programmes encompass mental health and wellbeing and may include using depression screening tools (Callahan et al. 1994). Despite the success of programmes such as Hospital Admission Risk Programs (HARP), clinical practice guidelines for managing pre-event and psychosocial cardiac risk factors are lacking. Psychosocial and behavioural risk factors are not closely inter-related, and structured integrated management systems are needed and are part of an emerging field of behavioural cardiology (Rozanski et al. 2005).

Psychiatric disorders, diabetes, and antipsychotic medicines

Diabetes and cardiovascular disease are common amongst people with mental health problems, especially schizophrenia largely due to shared genetic factors and particularly lifestyle such as smoking and inappropriate diet and activity (Gouveia and Chowdhury 2013; Mamakou et al. 2018). The prevalence of diabetes amongst people with schizophrenia varies amongst studies but appears to be two- to five-fold higher than the general population (Mamakou et al. 2018). It has been proposed as a causal factor for diabetes due to the higher prevalence in young people with anew diagnosis of schizophrenia not treated with antipsychotic medicines and the fact that genetic studies suggest people with schizophrenia have a genetic predisposition to diabetes (Mamakou et al. 2018).

Antidepressant medicines such as serotonin reuptake inhibitors are commonly used and are effective in people with diabetes (Rubin and Peyrot 1994; SIGN 2010).

Atypical antipsychotic medicines are used because they have fewer extrapyramidal effects, better medicine adherence, and improve QoL (Gouveia and Chowdhury 2013). However, they contribute to weight gain, particularly central adiposity, insulin resistance, and metabolic abnormalities. They have a direct effect on glucose and lipid homeostasis. They have been associated with new onset DKA (Mir and Taylor 2001).

The individual's previous experience with antidepressant medicines and the likely side effects need to be considered. Second generation antipsychotic medications effectively treat a range of psychiatric disorders and offer many benefits over older medications such as chlorpromazine and haloperidol (Wirshing et al. 2002; deVane 2007). However, they have significant side effects – namely rapid weight gain, hyperlipidaemia, and insulin resistance – that can affect metabolic control and increase cardiovascular risk in people with established diabetes and cause hyperglycaemia in people without a diabetes diagnosis; however, there is considerable variability in responses amongst individuals receiving the same medication.

A consensus panel of experts from the American Diabetes Association, American Psychiatric Association, the American Association of Clinical Endocrinologists, and the North American Association for the study of Obesity (2004) recommended the following:

- Assess weight, blood glucose, lipids, and blood pressure before starting antipsychotic medicines or as soon as possible after.
- Actively manage these conditions, if present.
- If weight increases by >5%, consider changing to another antipsychotic less likely to cause metabolic effects.
- Antipsychotics listed in order of those with the most to the least metabolic effects are: Olanzapine, Quetiapine, Risperidone, Ziprasidone, Aripiprazole. These medicines all cause weight gain.
- Institute lifestyle modification to manage weight if possible, which will involve helping the person adhere to advice.

However, people often do not comply with their antipsychotic medicines for various reasons, including the fact that they stifle creativity. For example, the author belongs to a creative writing group that meets monthly to participate in various writing-related activities and read and critique each other's work. At least five members ($n = 20$) disclosed they were prescribed antipsychotic medicines for various reasons and all stated they omit or reduce their medicine doses to maintain a degree of mania, which fuels their creativity. Four of the five developed diabetes and significant weight gain after starting on antipsychotic medicines.

As indicated, depression is a chronic condition, and regular monitoring is essential and must be incorporated into routine care, including in the acute care settings. Care includes identifying and treating underlying physical disorders that contribute to psychological distress and depression, such as hypothyroidism and underlying psychiatric disorders, and referring the individual to appropriate mental health services as soon as possible. Counselling and/or antidepressant medicines may be needed.

Diabetes conversations and language

Terms related to diabetes self-care are often judgmental, prejudiced, and pervasively negative in nature. They are labels best avoided (Diabetes Australia Position Statement on Language 2011; Dickinson et al. 2017; Dunning et al. 2017). 'Failure to comply', e.g. with medication or other clinician recommendations does not necessarily indicate diabetes neglect. In fact, there is no single, specific set of 'rules' for managing diabetes, which are relevant to all people with diabetes or agreed by all clinicians, especially in the current climate of shared decision-making and personalised care. For example, self-adjusting insulin doses is commonplace for people with type 1 diabetes, so compliance to a prescribed dose/timing becomes an irrelevant concept.

Indeed, even if 'adherence' is considered a useful concept, it can be intentional nonadherence or unintentional nonadherence (Horne and Weinman 1999). Nonadherence to recommended management can lead to suboptimal outcomes, diabetes progression and increased health costs. Wroe (2001) and Horne and Weinman (1999) amongst others, describe two forms of non-adherence:

- Intentional nonadherence (e.g. missing medicine dose to suit needs), which is influenced by the person's reasons for deciding to take/not take the medicine or undertake/not undertake other aspects of self-care. These include relevance at the particular time. Thus, intentional no adherence is a form of autonomy and informed decision-making and contrasts with the widely held clinician belief that all nonadherence is deviant and undesirable. It could also be associated with dignity of risk
- Unintentional nonadherence (e.g. forgetting to take medicines), which more strongly associated with demographic and social factors than decisional balance. Factors associated with unintentional nonadherence include age, beliefs about the need for the medicines/treatment, which in turn partly depends on the type amount and relevance of information the individual receives and the design layout and literacy level.

Intentional nonadherence is also described as 'intelligent' or rational nonadherence if the prescription was for a potentially inappropriate medicines where the risk could outweigh the benefit (Naples et al. 2016). Primary nonadherence is defined as not having a written prescription filled and is often due to cost and/or access (Naples et al. 2016).

Research also shows 'forgetting' to take medicines is common in type 1 and type diabetes. Trawley et al. (2018) suggested prospective memory is essential to optimal medicine adherence. They suggested prospective memory errors (slips) could play a role in medicine nonadherence. They found 24% of 220 adults with type 1 diabetes and 23% of 211 with type 2 diabetes forgot to take their medicines at least once in the preceding 14 days. Forgetting was associated with more prospective memory slips, younger age, insulin pump use in type 1, and insulin use in type 2 diabetes.

The latter (forgetting to undertake aspects of care) is probably 'normal' behaviour. Indeed, a recent study (Trawley et al. 2018) shows that 25% of people forget to take their medications due to prospective memory slips. Furthermore, obsessive attention to a self-care routine can impact negatively on QoL and may indicate underlying dominant diabetes-related fears and anxieties that may also warrant attention. It is equally important to recognise that so-called 'nonadherence' can be intentional, as this should naturally lead us to be curious about why this might be. It is important not to dismiss nonadherence as a failing on the part of the person with diabetes, but rather, to establish why a particular behaviour is neglected. Reasons may include:

- Unrealistic expectations on the part of health professionals resulting from lack of knowledge (about the person's goals, capabilities, and social situation) or lack of understanding/appreciation of what it takes to achieve optimal self-care.
- Setting goals focused on the health professional's agenda rather than on the agenda of the person with diabetes.
- Lack of knowledge of what is required.
- Low literacy and numeracy.
- Lack of understanding as a result of poor communication, inadequate or inappropriate information, e.g. with respect to culture, age, the particular environment in which the person lives; see Chapter 16.
- Changes in the colour, size, or shape of medicines, e.g. when given generic medicines instead of nongeneric medicines (Kesselheim et al. 2012)
- Inadequate support from family/friends and the healthcare team.

- Health beliefs and attitudes of the patient, family and health professionals.
- Functional limitations such as low vision and diminished fine motor skills.
- Patient burnout.
- Financial and other resource difficulties.

These factors represent the human side of diabetes.

Modern diabetes education concerns having appropriate conversations with people with diabetes to enable them to make informed decisions about their care, including on a day-by-day basis (Chapter 16). Good conversations include asking pertinent questions and listening to the answers. However, the person is often interrupted within the first 18 seconds, (Ospina et al. 2018; Wood head 2019). Interrupting the individual is not necessarily counterproductive, provided it is done respectfully and appropriately; in fact 'nuanced interruption is essential to clinical communication to keep the conversation on track and elicit essential information' (Mauksch 2017). These interruptions can be described as probing and clarifying questions.

Respectful ways to interrupt include excusing yourself for interrupting, acknowledge the topic being discussed, and explaining the reason for interrupting. Interruptions can be:

- Interrogative – How long have you felt distressed?
- Elaborative – Tell me more about how you are feeling.
- Recompleter – So your distress is stopping you from sleeping?
- Refocus – Let's try to sort out what is happening.

Supplementary questions can include questions such as, 'Is there anything else we need to talk about?' which can help ensure important issues are addressed and set the agenda for future conversations.

What people with diabetes require from clinicians

- To be treated as 'normal'.
- To know what will happen and what to expect.
- To be involved in developing their diabetes care plan and monitoring procedures.
- To be treated as a person, not 'a diabetic'.
- To be trusted, accepted, and not judged.
- To be listened to and have their experience and knowledge of diabetes recognised, valued, and used when planning their self-care including when they are in hospital.
- To have their emotional and spiritual needs met and emotional distress acknowledged and respected when they are in hospital.
- To know how and where to obtain advice and be able to obtain it when they need it (now!).

Supportive encouragement and focusing on positive achievements are far more helpful than 'shame and blame'. Achievable goals should be negotiated with the individual because their expectations/goals will be met rather than health professionals' goals. It is important to recognise that managing diabetes is never easy. Words such as 'good' and 'bad' when referring to blood glucose levels are judgemental terms. Substitute 'high' and 'low' or 'out of your target range'. Some people resent being called 'a diabetic'. It is preferable to say 'a person with diabetes' (Diabetes Australia 2011; Dickinson et al. 2017; Dunning et al. 2017).

Some people express concern about being admitted to hospital, over and above the usual reactions to illness/hospitalisation. They feel abnormal by being singled out for special meals and having labels such as 'diabetic diet' attached to their documentation. They often feel incompetent when they have been caring for their diabetes for years when staff do not believe they are 'hypo' when they ask for glucose or eat sweets or when they are capable of testing their blood glucose and administer their own insulin injections but are not permitted to do so whilst they are in hospital. Some people feel they have failed or health professionals blame them if they are admitted to hospital with a diabetic complication. They 'should have known better' and 'taken more care of their diabetes'. People become frustrated in such circumstances and, as one person said, 'staff bugger it (diabetes management) up in hospital' (Savage et al. 2012). Continuous negative feedback only reinforces that the person is not coping, and learned helplessness can result.

In some circumstances, people are willing for clinicians to act on their behalf as long as the options and the situation are clearly explained (Rapport et al. 2019) or when they cannot decide for themselves. The latter can be stressful for families and clinicians and cause decisional uncertainty. Clearly documented values and advance care plans can reduce some of this distress, especially during critical life-threatening events (Dunning et al. 2018); see Chapter 17.

References

American Diabetes Association (ADA) (2011). Standards of medical care in diabetes. *Diabetes Care* **24** (Suppl. 1): S–561.

American Diabetes Association, American Psychiatric Association, American Association of Clinical Endocrinologists and the North American Association for the Study of Obesity (2004). Consensus development conference on antipsychotic drugs and obesity and diabetes. *Diabetes Care* **27**: 596–601.

Andrews, G., Hall, W., Teeson, M., and Henderson, S. (1999). *The Mental Health of Australians*. Canberra: Mental Health Branch, Commonwealth Department of Health and Aged Care.

Antonovsky, A. (1987). *Unravelling the Mystery of Health: How People Manage Stress and Stay Well*. San Francisco: Jossey-Bass.

Balint, M. (1955). The doctor, his patient and the illness. *Lancet* **1**: 683–688.

Better Health Channel (2007). Cognitive Behaviour Therapy. http://www.betterhealth.vic.gov.au/bhcv2/bhcarticles. nsf/pages/Cognitive_Behaviour (accessed December 2007).

Bonsignore, M., Barkow, K., Jessen, F., and Huen, R. (2001). Validity of the five-item WHO well-being index (WHO-5) in an elderly population. *European Archives of Psychiatry Clinical Neuroscience* **251** (Suppl. 2): 1127–1131.

Bradley, C. and Gamsu, D. (1994). Guidelines for encouraging psychological wellbeing. *Diabetic Medicine* **11**: 510–516.

Browne, J.L., Ventura, A.D., Mosely, K., and Speight, J. (2017). Measuring Type 1 diabetes stigma: development and validation of the Type 1 Diabetes Stigma Assessment Scale (DSAS-1). *Diabetic Medicine* **34** (12): 1773–1782.

Callahan, C., Hendrie, H., Dittus, R. et al. (1994). Improving treatment of late life depression in primary care: a randomized clinical trial. *Journal of the American Geriatric Society* **42**: 839–846.

Carnethon, M., Kinder, L., Fair, J. et al. (2003). Symptoms of depression as a risk factor for incident diabetes: findings from the National Health Nutrition Examination Epidemiologic Follow-up Study. *American Journal of Epidemiology* **158**: 416–423.

Cavan, D., Fosbury, J., and Tigwell, P. (2001). Psychology in diabetes – why bother? *Practical Diabetes International* **18** (7): 228–229.

Ciechanowski, P., Katon, W., and Russo, W. (2000). Impact of depressive symptoms on adherence, function and costs. *Archives of Internal Medicine* **160**: 3278–3285.

Cox, D. and Gonder-Frederick, L. (1992). Major developments in behavioural diabetes research. *Journal of Consulting Clinical Psychologists* **60**: 628–638.

Craike, M.J., Mosely, K., Browne, J.L. et al. (2017). Associations between physical activity and depressive symptoms by weight status among adults with type 2 diabetes: results from Diabetes MILES–Australia. *Journal of Physical Activity and Health* **14** (3): 195–202.

Davis, T., Clifford, R., and Davis, W. (2001). Effect of insulin therapy on quality of life in type 2 diabetes mellitus – the Fremantle diabetes study. *Diabetes Research and Clinical Practice* **52**: 63–67.

deVane, L. (2007). *Antipsychotics and Diabetes*. www.medscape.com.viewarticle/558874?src=mp (accessed August 2007).

Diabetes Australia (DA) (2011). *A New Language for Diabetes: Improving Communication with and About People with Diabetes*. Canberra: DA.

Diabetes Australia National Supply Scheme (2016). Diabetes and Emotional Health handbook and toolkit. https://acbrd.org.au/diabetes-and-emotional-health-handbook-and-toolkit.

Dickinson, J., Guzman, S., Marynuik, M. et al. (2017). The use of language in diabetes education and care. *Diabetes Care* https://doi.org/10.2337/ci17-0041.

Dunning, P. (1994). Having diabetes: young adult perspectives. *The Diabetes Educator* **21** (1): 58–65.

Dunning, P. and Martin, M. (1997). Using a focus group to explore perceptions of diabetes severity. *Practical Diabetes International* **14** (7): 185–188.

Dunning, P. and Martin, M. (1999). Health professional's perceptions of the seriousness of diabetes. *Practical Diabetes International* **16** (3): 73–77.

Dunning, T. (ed.) (2013a). The teacher: moving from good to exceptional, Chapter 5. In: *Diabetes Education: Art, Science and Evidence*, 62–77. Oxford: Wiley Blackwell.

Dunning, T. (ed.) (2013b). Turning points and transitions: crises and opportunities. In: *Diabetes Education: Art, Science and Evidence*, 117–132. Oxford: Wiley Blackwell.

Dunning, T., Speight, J., and Bennett, C. (2017). Language, the 'diabetes restricted code/dialect' and what it means for people with diabetes and clinicians. *Diabetes Educator* 43: 18–26.

Dunning, T., Martin, P., Orellana, L. et al. (2018). *Planning Palliative and End of Life Care with Older People with Diabetes: Information for Health Professionals. Centre for Quality and Patient Safety Research*. Geelong, Victoria: Deakin University Barwon Health Partnership Available at: https://www.caresearch.com.au/Caresearch/Portals/0/Documents/FORPTSFAMILIES/Planning-PC-and-eol-with-older-people-with-diabetes.pdf.

Eaton, W., Armenian, H., and Gallo, J. (1996). Depression and risk for onset type 11 diabetes: a prospective population based study. *Diabetes Care* 19: 1097–1102.

Egede, L., Zheng, D., and Simpson, K. (2002). Comorbid depression is associated with increased health care use and expenditure in individuals with diabetes. *Diabetes Care* 25 (3): 464–470.

Elley, C., Dean, S., and Kerse, N. (2007). Physical activity promotion in general practice. *Australian Family Physician* 38 (12): 1061–1064.

Elley, C., Kerse, N., Arroll, B., and Robinson, E. (2003). Effectiveness of counselling patients on physical activity in general practice: a cluster randomised trial. *British Medical Journal* 326: 1–6. downloaded December 2007.

Everson-Rose, S. and Lewis, T. (2005). Psychosocial factors and cardiovascular diseases. *Annual Review of Public Health* 26: 469–500.

Fenwick, E.K., Rees, G., Holmes-Truscott, E. et al. (2018). What is the best measure for assessing diabetes distress? A comparison of the Problem Areas in Diabetes and Diabetes Distress Scale: results from Diabetes MILES–Australia. *Journal of Health Psychology* 23 (5): 667–680.

Fisher, L., Gonzalez, J.S., and Polonsky, W.H. (2014). The confusing tale of depression and distress in patients with diabetes: a call for greater clarity and precision. *Diabetic medicine* 31 (7): 764–772.

Fisher, L., Mullan, J., Arean, P. et al. (2010). Diabetes distress but not clinical depression or depressive symptoms is associated with glycaemic control in bot cross-sectional and longitudinal analyses. *Diabetes Care* 33 (1): 23–28.

Frasure-Smith, N. and Lesperance, F. (2003). Depression and other psychological risks following myocardial infarction. *Archives of General Psychiatry* 60: 627–636.

Funnell, M. (2006). Diabetes attitudes and wishes and needs (DAWN) study. *Clinical Diabetes* 24: 154–155.

Gardiner, P. (1997). Social and psychological implications of diabetes mellitus for a group of adolescents. *Practical Diabetes International* 14 (2): 43–46.

Gilbert, P. (2007). Spirituality and mental health: a very preliminary overview. *Current Opinions in Psychiatry* 20 (6): 594–598.

Giltay, E., Kamphuis, M., Kalmijn, S. et al. (2006). Dispositional optimism and the risk of cardiovascular death: the Zutphen elderly study. *Archives of Internal Medicine* 166: 431–436.

Glassman, A. and Miller, G. (2007). Where there is depression, there is inflammation…sometimes! *Biological Psychiatry* 62: 280–281.

Goldney, R. and Phillips, P. (2004). Diabetes, depression and quality of life. *Diabetes Care* 27 (5): 1066–1070.

Gonzalez, J., Shreck, E., Psaros, C., and Safen, S. (2015). Distress and type 2 diabetes treatment adherence: a mediating role for perceived control. *Health Psychology* 34 (5): 505–513.

Gottlieb, L. and Alderwick, H. (2019). Integrating social and medical care: could it worsen health and increase equity? *Annals of Family Medicine* 17 (1): 77–81.

Gouveia, C. and Chowdhury, T.A. (2013). Diabetes, schizophrenia and metabolic effects of antipsychotic drugs. *Mental Health Today* (Nov-Dec): 24–27.

Gujadhur, A., Dunning, T., and Alford, F. (2003). Metabolic and cardiac outcomes after acute myocardial infarction. *Journal of Diabetes Nursing* 7 (6): 208–212.

Halliday, J., Hendrieckx, C., Busija, L. et al. (2017). Validation of the WHO-5 as a first-step screening instrument for depression in adults with diabetes; results from diabetes MILES – Australia. *Diabetes Research and Clinical Practice* 132: 27–35. https://doi.org/10.1016/jdiabres.2017.07.005.

Hendrieckx, C., Halliday, J.A., Beeney, L.J., and Speight, J. (2019). *Diabetes and Emotional Health: A Practical Guide for Healthcare Professionals Supporting Adults with Type 1 and Type 2 Diabetes*, 2e. London: Diabetes UK.

Herath, P., Cherbuin, N., Eramuddugolia, R., and Anstey, K. (2016). Effect of diabetes medication on cognitive function: evidence from the PATG through life study. *Biomedical Research International*: 7208429. https://doi.org/10.1155/2016/7208429.

Hernandez, A. (1995). The experience of living with insulin-dependent diabetes: lessons for the diabetes educator. *Diabetes Educator* 21: 33–37.

Hodges, S. (2002). Mental health, depressions and dimensions of spirituality and religion. *Journal of Adult Development* 9: 109–115.

Horne, R. and Weinman, J. (1999). Patients' beliefs about prescribed medicines and their role in adherence to treatment in chronic illness. *Psychosomatic Research* 47: 555–567.

Hunt, C. and May, C. (2017). Managing expectations: cognitive authority and experienced control in complex healthcare processes. *BMC Social Services Research* 17: 459. https://doi.org/10.1186/s12913-017-2366-1.

Janszky, I., Ahlbom, A., Hallqvist, J., and Ahnve, S. (2007). Hospitalization for depression is associated with an increased risk for myocardial infarction not explained by lifestyle, lipids, coagulation, and inflammation: the SHEEP study. *Biological Psychiatry* 62: 25–32.

Januzzi, J.L., Stern, T.A., Pasternak, R.C., and DeSanctis, R.W. (2000). The influence of anxiety and depression on outcomes of patients with coronary artery disease. *Archives of Internal Medicine* 160 (13): 1913–1921.

Jenkinson, C. and McGee, H. (1998). *Health Status Measurement*. Oxford: Radcliff Medical Press.

Joost, P., van Melle, M., Jonge, P. et al. (2004). Prognostic association of depression following myocardial infarction with mortality and cardiovascular events: a meta-analysis. *Psychosomatic Medicine* 66: 814–822.

Jorm, A., Christensen, H., Griffiths, K., and Rodgers, B. (2002). Effectiveness of complementary and self-help treatments for depression. *Medical Journal of Australia* 176: S84–S96.

Kesselheim, A., Misono, A., Shank, W. et al. (2012) Variations in pill appearance of antiepileptic drugs and the risk on nonadherence. http://archinte.jamanetwork.com (accessed December 2012).

Khunti, K., Nikoljsen, A., Thorsted, B. et al. (2016). Clinical inertia with regards to intensifying therapy in people with type 2 diabetes treated with basal insulin. *Diabetes Obesity and Metabolism* 18: 401–409.

Kreuter, M., Lukwago, S., Bucholtz, D. et al. (2002). Achieving cultural appropriateness in health promotion programs: targeted and tailored approaches. *Health Education and Behaviour* 30: 133–146.

Kubzansky, D. and Thurston, C. (2007). Emotional vitality and incident coronary heart disease: benefits of healthy psychological functioning. *Archives of General Psychiatry* 64: 1393–1401.

Kubzansky, L. (2007). Sick at heart: the pathophysiology of negative emotions. *Cleveland Clinic Journal of Medicine* 74 (Suppl. 1): S67–S72.

Lancaster, T. (2000). Effectiveness of interventions to help people stop smoking. *British Medical Journal* 321: 355–358.

Lett, H., Blumenthal, J., Babyak, M. et al. (2004). Depression as a risk factor for coronary artery disease: evidence, mechanisms, and treatment. *Psychosomatic Medicine* 66: 305–315.

Li, C., Ford, E.S., Strine, T.W., and Mokdad, A.H. (2008). Prevalence of depression among US adults with diabetes: findings from the 2006 behavioral risk factor surveillance system. *Diabetes Care* 31 (1): 105–107.

Litt, M.D. (1988). Self-efficacy and perceived control: cognitive mediators of pain tolerance. *Journal of Personality and Social Psychology* 54 (1): 149.

Lustman, P. (1997). The course of major depression in diabetes. *Diabetes Care* 59: 24–31.

Lustman, P., Griffith, L., and Clouse, R. (1996). Recognising and managing depression in patients with diabetes. In: *Practical Psychology for Clinicians* (eds. B. Anderson and R. Rubin), 143–152. Alexandria, Virginia: American Diabetes Association.

Mamakou, V., Thanopoulou, A., Gonidakis, F. et al. (2018). Schizophrenia and diabetes mellitus. *Pyschiatriki* 29 (91): 64–73.

Mauksch, L. (2017). Physicians interrupt patients. *Journal American Medical Association* 318: 93. https://doi.org/10.1001/jama.2107.6489.

MILES (2011). Diabetes Miles Study – Australia. www.diabetesaustralia.com.au/.../12.05.16%20Diabetes%20MILES%20Report.pdf (accessed October 2012).

Mir, S. and Taylor, D. (2001). Atypical antipsychotics and hyperglycaemia. *International Clinical Psychopharmacology* 16: 65–73.

Naples, J., Hanlon, J., Schmader, K. et al. (2016). Recent literature on medication errors and adverse drug events in older adults. *Journal American Geriatrics Society* 64: 401–408.

National Institute for Clinical Excellence (NICE) (2018). Depression in adults: Recognition and management. Clinical guideline [CG90]. https://www.nice.org.uk/guidance/cg90.

Newcombe, S. (2019). *My Diabetes Logbook: Weekly Diabetes Record*. United Kingdom: Simon Newcombe.

Newton-John, T., Ventura, A., Mosely, K. et al. (2017). Are you sure you're going to another one of those? A qualitative analysis of the social control and social support models in type 2 diabetes. *Journal Health Psychology* 22 (4): 1819–1829.

NHS Health Scotland (2013). Mental health and wellbeing. http://www.healthscotland.scot/health-topics/mental-health-and-wellbeing.

Nilsen, P. and Bernhardson (2019). Context matters in implementation science: a scoping review of determinant frameworks that describe contextual determinants for implementation science. *BMC Health Services Research* 19: 189. https://doi.org/10.1186/s12913-019-4015-3.

Ospina, N., Phillips, K., Rodriguez-Gutierrez, R. et al. (2018). Eliciting the patient's agenda: secondary analysis of recorded clinical encounters. *Journal General Internal Medicine* https://doi.org/10.1007/s11606-018-4540-5.

Parsian, N. and Dunning, T. (2008). Spirituality and coping in young adults with diabetes. *Diabetes Research and Clinical Practice* 79 (S1): S121.

Patterson, B. and Sloan, J. (1994). A phenomenological study of the decision-making experience of individuals with long standing diabetes. *Canadian Journal of Diabetes Care* 18: 10–19.

Peyrot, M. (1997). Levels and risks of depression and anxiety symptomatology among diabetic adults. *Diabetes Care* 20: 585–590.

Peyrot, M. and Rubin, R. (2007). Behavioural and psychosocial interventions in diabetes. *Diabetes Care* **30** (10): 2433–2440.

Piette, J. (2007). Interactive behaviour change technology to support diabetes self-management: where do we stand? *Diabetes Care* **30** (10): 2425–2432.

Pouwer, F. and Speight, J. (2014). Psychological Factors and Diabetes Mellitus. Chapter 42. In: *Textbook of Diabetes*, 5e (eds. R. Holt, C. Cockram and B. Goldstein). Hoboken, NJ: John Wiley & Sons https://onlinelibrary.wiley.com/doi/10.1002/9781118924853.ch56.

Rapport, F., Hibbert, P., Baysari, M. et al. (2019). What do patients really want? An in-depth examination of patient experience in four Australian hospitals. *BMC Health Services Research* **19** (38) https://doi.org/10.1186/s12913-019-3881-z.

Rasmussen, B., O'Connell, B., and Dunning, T. (2007a). Young women with diabetes: using internet communication to create stability during life transitions. *Journal of Clinical Nursing* **1365**: 17–24.

Rasmussen, B., O'Connell, B., and Dunning, T. (2007b). Young women with type 1 diabetes' management of turning points and transition. *Qualitative Health Research* **17** (3): 300–310.

Rollnick, S., Mason, P., and Butler, C. (1999). *Health Behaviour Change: A Guide for Practitioners*. Edinburgh, UK: Churchill Livingstone.

Rozanski, A., Blumenthal, J., Davidson, K. et al. (2005). The epidemiology, pathophysiology, and management of psychosocial risk factors in cardiac practice: the emerging field of behavioural cardiology. *Journal of the American College of Cardiology* **45** (5): 637–651.

Rubin, R. (2000). Diabetes and quality of life. From research to practice. *Diabetes Spectrum* **13** (1): 21–23.

Rubin, R. and Peyrot, M. (1994). Implications of the DCCT: looking beyond tight control. *Diabetes Care* **17**: 235–236.

Rubin, R. and Peyrot, M. (2001). Psychological issues and treatments for people with diabetes. *Journal of Clinical Psychology* **57** (4): 457–478.

Savage, S., Dunning, T., Duggan, N., and Martin, P. (2012). The experiences and care preferences of people with diabetes at the end of life. *Journal of Hospice and Palliative Care* **14** (4): 293–302.

SIGN (2014). Clinical Practice Guideline on the Management of Depression in Adults. http://content.guidelinecentral.com/guideline/get/pdf/2560.

SIGN Scottish Intercollegiate Guidelines Network (2010). *Management of Diabetes: A National Guideline*. Erdinburgh, UK: SIGN.

Silva, N., Soares, C., Mumnoz, D. et al. (2019). Insulin resistance as a shared pathogenic mechanism between depression and type 2 diabetes. *Frontiers in Psychiatry* https://doi.org/10.3389/fpsyt.2019.00057.

Skinner, T. (2013). Making choices: setting goals, Chapter 4. In: *Diabetes Education: Art, Science and Evidence* (ed. T. Dunning), 49–61. Oxford: Wiley Blackwell.

Speight, J. and Singh, H. (2013). The journey of the person with diabetes, Chapter 2. In: *Diabetes Education: Art, Science and Evidence* (ed. T. Dunning), 12–24. Oxford: Wiley Blackwell.

Steunenberg, B., Beckman, A., Deeg, D. et al. (2007). Mastery and neuroticism predict recovery from depression in later life. *American Journal of Geriatric Psychiatry* **15**: 234–242.

Teisman, G. (2017). The role of the brain-gut-microbiome in mental health and mental disorders. In: *The Microbiota in Gastrointestinal Pathophysiology* (eds. M.H. Floch, Y. Ringel and W.A. Walker), 389–397. Academic Press https://doi.org/10.1016/B978-0-12-804024-9.00042-2.

Thoolen, B. (2006). Early intensive treatment can negatively affect stress and outcome. *Diabetes Care* **29**: 2257–2262.

Trawley, S., Baptista, S., Pouwer, F., and Speight, J. (2018). Prospective memory slips are associated with forgetting to take glucose-lowering therapies among adults with diabetes: results from the second diabetes MILES_ Australia (MILES-2) survey. *Diabetic Medicine* https://doi.org/10.1111/dm3.13873.

Tun, P., Nathan, D., and Perlminter, L. (1990). Cognitive and affective disorders in elderly diabetics. *Clinical Geriatric Medicine* **6**: 731–746.

Tung, A. (2011). The mystery of guideline non-compliance: why don't doctors do the right thing? *Anaesthesiology* **53**: 1–9.

UK Mental Health Foundation (2006). Making space for spirituality: making space to support service users. www.mentalhealth.org.uk/content/assets/PDF/.../making_space.pdf (accessed October 2012).

Ventegodt, S., Andersen, N., and Merrick, J. (2003). Holistic medicine 111: the holistic process theory of healing. *The Scientific World Journal* **3**: 1138–1146.

Wilson, T. and Holt, T. (2001). Complexity science: complexity and clinical care. *British Medical Journal* **323** (7314): 685–688.

Wirshing, D., Boyd, J., Meng, L. et al. (2002). The effects of novel antipsychotics on glucose and lipid levels. *Journal of Clinical Psychiatry* **63** (10): 856–865.

Wolpert, L. (2006). *Malignant Sadness: The Anatomy of Depression*, 3e. London: Faber & Faber.

Wroe, A. (2001). *Intentional and Unintentional Non-Adherence: A Study in Decision Making*, 355–371. Plenum Publishing Corporation 0160-7715/02/0800-0355/0.

Yusef, S., Hawken, S., and Ounpuu, S. (2004). Effect of potentially modifiable risk factors associated with myocardial infarction in 52 countries (the INTERHEART study): case controlled study. *Lancet* **364**: 937–952.

Further reading

Beck, A. and Beamesderfer, A. (1974). Assessment of depression: the depression inventory. *Medical Problems in Psychopharmacotherapy* 7: 151–169.

Johnson, S. (1980). Psychosocial factors in juvenile diabetes. *Journal of Health Psychology* 9: 737–749.

Lustman, P., Griffith, L., Freedland, K. et al. (1998). Cognitive behaviour therapy for depression in type 2 diabetes mellitus: a randomized controlled trial. *Annals of Internal Medicine* 129: 613–621.

Radloff, S. (1977). The CES-D scale: a self-report depression scale for research in the general population. *Applied Psychiatric Measurement* 3: 151–401.

Rafinelle, C. (2005). Depression, stress and the risk of heart disease. *Psychiatric Times* 22: 11.

Raymond, M. (1992). *The Human Side of Diabetes: Beyond Doctors, Diet, Drugs*. Chicago: Noble Press.

I never teach my students – I only try to provide the conditions in which they can learn.

(Albert Einstein)

It is far more important to **know** what **person** the **disease has** than what **disease** the **person has**.

(Hippocrates and many experts since)

Key points

- The aim is to awaken the healing and learning potential within the individuals with diabetes and help them become empowered active participants in their care. This requires self-knowledge, art and science. Thus, clinicians need to have a personal education pedagogy and/or andragogy. Mine are embodied in the two quotes at the start of the chapter.
- Teaching and learning form an interconnected process that depends on effective communication in a caring relationship. Establishing a caring (therapeutic) partnership with the person with diabetes is important to education, care and shared decision-making.
- Social determinants of health, including economic status, education, access to healthcare and health literacy, are important considerations when providing information in any format. Information must be relevant to the individual's, reading capability, age, culture, life stage, and the current context. This means the design and layout as well as the content.
- Diabetes self-care knowledge and capability should be assessed initially and reassessed regularly.
- Improving self-care may have a greater impact on outcomes than medical strategies.
- All clinicians caring for the person with diabetes must provide consistent information to reduce misinformation and confusion.
- Establishing how people learn is helpful to decide teaching strategies that enhance their learning. People learn different things in different ways.
- Clinicians must reflect in and on their behaviours, capabilities, knowledge and performance to enhance their effectiveness.
- Significant others should be included in the education, where relevant.
- People report better healthcare experiences when they are actively engaged in respective therapeutic relationships.

Care of People with Diabetes: A Manual for Healthcare Practice, Fifth Edition. Trisha Dunning and Alan Sinclair.
© 2020 John Wiley & Sons Ltd. Published 2020 by John Wiley & Sons Ltd.

Rationale

Diabetes education is the cornerstone of diabetes management and is a lifelong, ongoing process. Good communication skills, especially listening, are the basis of effective education. Such skills involve teaching at teachable moments and giving the person information about what they want to know. Yet clinicians interrupt within 11 seconds of asking a question and only address the individual's agenda 40% of the time. Interestingly, the person identifies their agenda within 6 seconds if they are not interrupted (Ospina et al. 2018).

Personalised education and shared decision making that supports personal empowerment and autonomy and enhances self-care capacity, is the most effective teaching method.

A balanced therapeutic relationship between the individual and their clinician/s and other carers is more likely to achieve personalised education. Collaboration and communication and being truly present in the encounter are core elements of good communication and hence teaching and learning (Dunning 2013b, pp. 62–76, Silverman et al. 2018).

Teaching and learning form an integrated process predicated on effective communication, which involves knowing the person with diabetes' story and their explanatory models and clinician self-knowledge. Significantly, people with diabetes' and clinicians' explanatory models, perceptions of diabetes, self-care, medicines, risks and benefits and values and goals are likely to be different (Schwarz et al. 2012). That is, people with diabetes ascribe different, intensely personal, meaning to their diabetes experience and their 'story of illness (diabetes)' often competes with clinicians 'story of disease (diabetes)' (Egnew 2009) and the way they find meaning and purpose in their life with diabetes.

Introduction

Education is an integral part of diabetes self-management. The purpose of diabetes education is to have good conversations to develop a therapeutic relationship to assist the person to do the following:

- Learn about and understand diabetes.
- Make informed choices relevant to their personal situation and the relative risks and benefits of various options for them, based on the best available evidence.
- Successfully integrate diabetes into their self-concept/personhood.
- Incorporate diabetes self-care into their daily lives and achieve a balanced lifestyle.
- Develop effective coping strategies and problem-solving skills.
- Perform diabetes self-care to achieve their care goals and optimum metabolic control.
- Successfully negotiate life transitions and turning points.
- Achieve these aims through shared decision-making.

> Shared decision-making can be defined as 'The conversation that happens between a patient and their healthcare professional to reach a health care choice together'.
> (National Health Service 2014).

Diabetes self-care involves the person with diabetes making constant assessments to inform their decisions and often adjusting their care plan, especially during key life transitions (Rasmussen et al. 2007; Jutterstrom et al. 2012; Dunning 2013c, pp. 117–131). Thus, the simple term 'diabetes self-care' encompasses very complex, inter-related factors that affect each other, and consequently the outcome. Self-care is required for life and is influenced by the individual's social situation and values.

Values refers to the enduring things that give meaning and purpose to a person' life. They are shaped by culture and experience and influence their attitudes, behaviours, and decisions (Sweetland et al. 2017), including end-of-life care (Chapter 17). People value continuity of care and being known by the clinicians caring for them (Steiger 2006).

Health professionals aim to deliver holistic personalised diabetes care, often referred to as patient-centred care. Some people with diabetes object to being referred to as patients, although many refer to themselves as patients and/or diabetics, possibly because clinicians use these words as part of the 'diabetes dialect' (Dunning et al. 2017). Significantly, language and particular words affect people differently; clinicians us many judgmental words; for example, 'noncompliant', 'nonadherent', and 'failed to attend' (Speight et al. 2012; Dickinson et al. 2017; Dunning et al. 2017).

Significantly, the International Alliance of Patient Organisations (IAPO 2007) uses the term 'patients'. IAPO recognised that patients', families' and carers' needs and priorities differ amongst countries and diseases, and described five key principles of patient-centred care:

(1) Respect for patients' unique needs, preferences, values, autonomy, and independence.
(2) Patients have a right and a responsibility to participate as equal partners in health care decisions that affect their lives to the level of their ability and choice. In fact, people who are actively engaged in healthcare decisions report greater satisfaction with care (Alston et al. 2012).
(3) They have a right to be involved in developing health care policy *at all levels* to ensure policies are designed with the patient at the centre of care and address access issues.
(4) Healthcare must consider emotional and non-health factors that affect health such as the social situation, education and employment, and patients must have access to healthcare services relevant to their condition.
(5) 'Accurate, relevant and comprehensive information is essential' to enable people to make informed decisions about their healthcare options and the benefits and risks of specific treatment to them. Information must be in a format suitable to the individual's age, literacy level, gender, culture, and healthcare needs (IAPO 2005).

Holistic personalised education and care is consistent with these principles and has a core aim of preventing diabetes and/or diabetes progression and promoting positive health to achieve the best possible outcomes. Patient education describes the theory and skills the individual needs to learn and encompasses establishing goals to be achieved and conditions in which learning can take place (Redman 2001). Thus, diabetes education is a planned, interactive process using a combination of methods to help people learn relevant information and develop and maintain appropriate health behaviours. Significantly, people who learn to and effectively manage their health and make appropriate lifestyle choices use fewer resources and make more effective use of available resources (Tankova et al. 2001).

Standardised patient education and self-management are important frameworks in which the IAPO principles can be applied. However, some frameworks may have limited effectiveness because they rely on traditional teaching methods, primary and tertiary care is not well-integrated, and the programmes and services often only reach a small number of people (Wagner et al. 2002). Modern communication processes using video, Skype, email, smart phones, and other electronic media make it possible to reach a wider audience.

Standardized education often does not meet the complex needs of people with diabetes who have multiple comorbidities who require comprehensive care, continuity of care and a life course approach (Vainieri et al. 2018). *Relational continuity* (the long-term relationship between clinicians and patients) is associated with overall satisfaction with care and more effective self-management for people with multimorbidities (Vainieri et al. 2018) and maybe a core component of diabetes care and education.

Effective chronic disease management consists of:

- Deciding and delivering care according to evidence-based guidelines and protocols. Designing services and education programmes to suit the target audience, which might be an individual, a small group or a population. It is possible to apply the principles of holist education and care in all settings. Increasingly, advocacy and service design bodies and research funders expect services and education programmes to be co-designed with people *with* diabetes and other key stakeholders.
- Managing medicines according to quality use of medicines principles (Chapter 5) and pharmacovigilance, which includes monitoring medicine effects and use and deprescribing when indicated e.g. in palliative and end of life care (Chapter 17).
- Well-designed services and practices such as appointment systems, follow up procedures, referral processes, Alert systems, and education programmes suitable to the needs of the target population. Well-designed services include provision for continuity of care to enable therapeutic relationships to develop.

- A focus on prevention and supporting people to self-manage and make relevant behaviour changes by using education methods that facilitate conversations that assist the person to become empowered and develop problem-solving and decision-making skills (Anderson et al., 2002a,b; Anderson and Funnell 2005). Ideally a process for identifying people who do not meet goals and target ranges is part of the process.
- Ensuring clinicians are educated, competent and supported to undertake their roles, that they function in an interdisciplinary, collaborative team, and there are clear links amongst service providers and resources. Clinicians may benefit from training in health coaching methods and therapeutic conversations and, as stated, must be reflective practitioners. Programmes such as 'Choosing Wisely' should inform diabetes care conversations (Health Direct 2018). In addition, clinicians have a responsibility to take care of their own health and wellbeing.
- Education programmes that meet the needs of the relevant population and provide opportunities for continuing education for patients and clinicians. A review of >30 randomised controlled trials of diabetes education found only half the education interventions included behavioural components (setting goals, counselling techniques, or problem-solving), only one third assessed psychosocial factors (beliefs, self-efficacy, mastery, or locus of control), and significant improvements in knowledge was only demonstrated in one-fifth of the studies (Knight and Donan 2006). It is not clear whether people with diabetes were involved in designing the programmes included in the review, but that seems unlikely, given the results. These findings suggest most current diabetes education programmes may not be holistic or person-centred, and continue to 'do things for/to people' instead of 'with them', despite the rhetoric.
- Performing accurate clinical and investigative procedures and considering each piece of clinical information and where and how it fits into the whole body of information and the individual's diabetes story, rather than as isolated 'facts'.
- Generating, documenting, and communicating appropriate information including chronic disease registers, referral systems, patient reminders, outcome monitoring, and care planning that encompass continuity of care.
- Undertaking continuous quality improvement and audit processes that include patients in the design as well as the evaluation; not only as the subject of the evaluation. Health professional performance should be measured as part of the evaluation process and encompasses more than 'patient satisfaction surveys' (Dunning 2010).

Generally, the diabetes education literature focuses on the person with diabetes. However, to be an effective teacher, the educator must undertake reflective practice and consider his or her own learning style, teaching style, communication style, beliefs and attitudes, health status, knowledge and competence, and how they can affect the way the clinician interacts with other people. In addition, clinicians need to understand how the person's life environment and the teaching environment can facilitate or be barriers to learning, behaviour change, and/or self-care. Thus, personalised education and care means really understanding people. Generally, peoples' teaching style reflects their preferred learning style, which may not suit the learner. A learning style self-assessment tool can be found on http://www.idpride.net/learning-style-test.html.

Clinical observation

A Finnish equestrienne, who won four Olympic gold medals, was asked: 'What needs to change if things are not working and you are not winning, the horse or the rider'?

She replied: 'The horse takes his cue from the rider. The *rider* has to change and work with the horse to help him achieve to the best of his ability – that's winning, even if you don't win' (Interview during Equitana Australia 2 January 2013).

Thus, the clinician has to work with the person with diabetes. They may have to change if their education and care strategies are not working.

Learning styles

Learning is 'a natural, evolving process originating within the learner and growing from the learner's need to interact with their environment' (MacKeracher 1996). Thus, the learner, not the teacher, is in control of what the learner understands and learns. Learning can occur through experience (experiential) or as a planned process. People learn in different ways (learning style), and the learning style may change over the person's life course, just as teaching styles often change through experience and ongoing learning. Learning style refers to the way an individual processes and uses information. Learning involves using the senses: sight, speech, hearing, and can be active or passive. Usually people use a mixture of learning styles and learn different things in different ways. Children learn differently from adults. One size does not fill all people of all situations. Table 16.1 is a composite overview of learning styles and teaching methods appropriate to each learning style. The table clearly shows that learning is a process not merely an outcome (Kolb 1984) and has important implications for what we measure as 'effective education and care'.

Kolb described four learning styles:

(1) Divergent – emphasises feeling rather than thinking.
(2) Assimulative – values facts and thinking over feeling.
(3) Convergent – like to apply information and hands-on activities.
(4) Accommodative – learn by trial and error/problem-solving.

Other learning theories and learning styles and the cognitive processes and physical factors that affect learning and memory include:

- Neurolinguistic programming (NLP) (auditory, kinesthetic, and visual)
- Multiple intelligence model that consists of eight domains
- Making connections, based on 'jigsaw theory' (Dunning 2013a, pp. 28–40)

Table 16.1 Learning styles and some teaching strategies that can be used to facilitate learning.

Learning style	Learning process	Teaching strategy
Active	Retain information by doing something active.	Teach in group settings.
	Like learning in groups.	Incorporate activities such as demonstrations and return demonstrations.
	Retain information better if they understand how to apply it.	Use problem-based learning, Conversation maps™, the Felt Man, and similar tools and peer education.
Reflective	Prefer to think about things before they act.	Incorporate time for review and reflection.
	Prefer working alone.	Provide short summaries of important information.
		Invite feedback.
		Use decision aid[a] tools such as the Mayo Clinic Diabetes Medication Choice decision aid cards (2009).
Sensing	Like learning facts and solving problems using established methods.	Show how the information relates to their personal situation and the 'real world' in general.
	Like details and are good at memorising facts but may do this and not understand the information.	Use specific examples from the individual's experience. For example, 'You do not eat breakfast but now you are taking insulin at breakfast time. You are at risk of having a hypo. How can we reduce the risk or prevent you from having a hypo?'
	Like hands-on activities.	
	Dislike complications and surprises.	
	Do not like being asked about information that was not covered in education programmes.	
	Practical and careful and like information to be connected to 'the real world'	

(Continued)

Table 16.1   (Continued)

Learning style	Learning process	Teaching strategy
Intuitive	Like to discover possibilities and relationships Like innovation. Are bored by repetition. Are good at understanding new concepts. Usually comfortable with abstract images and statistical information. Are innovative and work quickly but may miss important details and make careless mistakes.	Link theories to facts. Use practical and actual examples using simple facts and figures and graphs. Use creative teaching strategies such as stories, conversation maps and drama.
Visual	Remember best when they see pictures, diagrams, flow charts, films, and demonstrations.	Use visual and verbal information. Incorporate concept and mind maps and/or conversation amps in the teaching. Colour code information for example, 'yellow insulin' or 'purple insulin' to refer to the package colour.
Verbal	Learn best by listening to words.	Use verbal teaching. Give the person tapes to take home. Encourage people to participate and share their stories, e.g. in peer education and group learning.
Sequential	Learn best if a logical step wise or staged approach is used. May not fully understand the material unless they use it. May know a lot about specific topics but have trouble relating them to other aspects of the same subject or to different subjects,	Provide logical material where each piece of information follows the preceding information. Do not move randomly from topic to topic. Give them 'homework' so they can use the information and develop their global learning skills. Explain how the information relates to other information; that is, help the person make connections between what they know and new information.
Global	Learn large amounts of information without seeing connections and suddenly make the connection. May solve complex problems quickly or find innovative ways of doing things once they understand the information. May have problems explaining how they did it.	Paint the big picture first. Explain how topics relate to other topics and to information the person already knows and their experiences.

[a] Decision aids are information documents designed to help people make decisions about their management options. Decision aids are usually used with education and/or counselling. When used in conjunction with counselling, they improve the quality of people's decisions and reduce underuse and overuse of services (O'Connor et al. 2003). Decision aids provide balanced evidence-based information about options in enough detail to help people make an informed decision. They are not 'standard diabetes education information' available from pharmaceutical companies and diabetes associations, but can be used with such information.

People participating in group education programmes are likely to learn in different ways. Therefore, a range of teaching strategies should be used. An individual's preference for one category may be mild, moderate, or strong, but generally a balance of styles results in more effective learning.

A simple self-complete tool that might help health professionals identify an individual's main learning style is shown in Table 16.2. It is also essential to consider whether the person has any sensory changes, e.g. sight and hearing and/or cognitive changes that could influence how education is provided and the environment it is provided in, e.g. if the person usually wears glasses make sure they have them and information is designed to enhance reading, e.g. font size, white space and colour contrast. If they wear hearing aids, make sure they are turned on for verbal teaching.

Table 16.2 A simple tool that can be used to estimate an individual's dominant learning style.

Please put a number in the boxes in the order that best describes how you learn new important information from number 1 to 9. Number 1 is the way you learn best. If you choose the 'other' option please briefly describe how you learn new information.

- Read printed information such as books and pamphlets with a lot of words.
- Read printed information with lots of pictures and diagrams or see models of things.
- Watch videos on YouTube, Facebook, or other electronic media.
- Listen to an audiotape or a lecture.
- Have somebody show you how to do a task such as monitoring blood glucose.
- Talk with other people who have similar problems:
- In a group
- In an Internet chat room
- Individual informal discussion
- Practice using equipment such as injecting insulin or cooking food.
- Other, please describe:...
  ....

Another method is to ask the individual how he or she became competent at a hobby or task they perform regularly.

It is not comprehensive but can be easily and quickly incorporated into routine education and care.

Education and other theories/models

Key education and behaviour theories that can be applied to diabetes education include:

- The health belief model (HBM), which can suggest best content, topics and information sequencing.
- Self-efficacy, the education should build confidence, for example, by ensuring people achieve successes however small and that these are acknowledged.
- Locus of control; if people feel they are not in control they may require more support, for example, coaching and carer/family support.
- Cognitive dissonance theory; design interventions that make people feel unhappy or dissatisfied with their current behaviour and reinforce to prevent relapse.
- Diffusion theory; ensure the intervention is consistent with the individual's belief system and values.
- Stages of change (SOC); design strategies that fit the individual stages and where the individual is at each stage.
- Narrative medicine, which recommends every meeting with a patient, should be treated as the first so that nothing is taken for granted and people are enabled to tell their stories and the health professional seeks meaning in the stories and clarifies their assumptions with the individual. Health professionals have their own stories. Some have diabetes stories that need to be acknowledged but should not take priority and may or may not be disclosed (Bert 2011). Person-centred care is at the heart of narrative medicine.
- Adult education theories; use existing knowledge and problem-solving techniques. A range of other theories can be incorporated into the theories/models listed or used as the basis to develops education programmes such as motivational interviewing, tipping points (O'Connor et al. 2007), nudging (Dunning 2013b, pp. 62–76), and art and drama (Assal and Assal 2013, pp. 98–111).

Diabetes education is a lifelong process, and information needs change as health status changes, new technology and medicines become available, and new models of car and service delivery emerge. Significantly, there is a poor correlation between knowledge and behaviour. Scare tactics and negative information lower mental and emotional wellbeing and might lead to denial and/or nonadherence (Knight and Donan 2006).

On a practical level, diabetes education is often divided into:

- Survival skills – the initial information necessary to begin the self-care journey and be safe at home (described later in the chapter). Given the increasing prevalence of diabetes, survival skills should actually commence before diagnosis and target at risk populations or the whole population. For example, programmes developed by the National Public Health Institute of Helsinki (2007) designed to be delivered in primary care achieved reductions in three key diabetes and cardiovascular risk factors: BMI, waist circumference, and diastolic blood pressure after one year. People who achieved reductions in four or more risk factors had a lower risk of developing diabetes. These findings suggest diabetes educators need to take a population based approach to diabetes education as well as providing individual education and management.
- Basic knowledge – information that builds on survival information and enables the individual to understand diabetes and its management and their role in diabetes management generally, and self-care in particular. A lot of such information is acquired through trial and error.
- Ongoing education – the continued acquisition of new information, including changes in technology and management practices as they emerge. A key aspect of delivering new information is helping the individual decide how it applies to them. That is, the information must be personalised to their particular life context.

Acquiring survival skills and undertaking relevant diabetes self-management usually requires changes in established behaviours. Understanding the individual's readiness to make relevant changes and identifying their personal barriers to change is central to behavioural change interventions. Several models have been developed that attempt to describe the behaviour change processes. These include:

- The HBM (Becker and Maiman 1975).
- Social learning theory (SLT) (Bandura 1986).
- Theory of reasoned action and planned behaviour (TRA) (Ajzen and Fishbein 1980).
- The transtheoretical model of change (SOC) (Prochaska and DiClemente 1983).
- Empowerment model (Funnell and Anderson 2000).
- Coaching models such as the Health Care Australia Coaching Model (Linder et al. 2003; Gale 2007) that are based on positive psychology and focus on helping people form the intention to change and supporting them to make and sustain changes. This is different from telephone or Internet coaching models that aim to help individuals achieve management targets. For example, by prompting them to have various tests or recommending that they ask their doctor about treatment changes (Vale et al. 2003; Young et al. 2007). Peer coaching is widely used in formal processes as evidence for its benefit emerges.
- The ecological model, which focuses on identifying key resources and supporting self-management grounds diabetes self-management in the context of the individual's social and environmental situation (Fisher et al. 2005). It enables the individual's skills and choices to be integrated with the services and support they receive from their social environment, which includes family and friends, health services, and wider community services. The ecological approach determines the impact various factors in the individual's environment have on their self-care ability. The Chronic Care Model and its derivatives is an example of the ecological Model (Wagner et al. 1996).
- Complementary medicine (CM) and Integrative Models (Egnew 2009; Phelps and Hassad 2011) focus on finding the 'doctor within' and enhancing the individual's innate capacity for healing and are also used in conventional care. CM models suggest health professionals are most effective when 'we give the doctor who resides in each patient a chance to go to work' (Schweitzer, in Cousins 2005, p. 78; Dunning 2014). Self-empowerment is at the heart of Schweitzer's statement and narrative medicine underpins these models.

Increasingly, business models are being applied to healthcare, including diabetes education. In particular, marketing strategies and understanding how people make decisions (consumer decision journey) is relevant to diabetes education consultations. Edelman (2012) highlighted the fact that a consumer's journey is complex and iterative through and beyond purchasing a product. Edelman developed a five-point model to highlight the important components of the purchasing journey:

(1) Consider: What products, brands, and prices people have in mind when they think about buying a product.
(2) Evaluate: Consumers collect information from a range of sources including electronic to narrow their choices (and often purchase online).
(3) Buy: Decide what brand to buy and buy it.
(4) Post purchase: Reflect on the buying experience. Their reflections will influence subsequent purchases.
(5) Advocate: Consumers tell other people about the product, brand, and purchasing experiences. We witness many prominent people advertising products in the media, including diabetes products.

Increasingly, diabetes education and care are informed by machine learning/artificial intelligence based on pattern recognition and computational learning theory and involves exploring and constructing algorithms that can learn from and make predictions from data. Likewise, forward-thinking systems models and creative thinking are used to develop novel ideas and ways of working and explain complex systems and the factors encompassed in 'effectiveness' or optimal outcomes.

Practice point

Reflect on how Edelman's model could be applied to diabetes education. In addition, think about the power of marketing and advertising and how it creates expectations. How could diabetes educators use marketing strategies in diabetes education programmes to create realistic expectations and personalise diabetes education and care?

There are several common elements amongst these models: individual behaviours result from perceived benefit of and perceived barriers to change (HBM); expected outcomes and readiness to make changes (SOC); self-efficacy and perceived ability to control the behaviour (SCT); perceptions of social and cultural norms (TRA, Ecological Model); individual innate capacity (doctor within) (CM). Coaching involves helping people identify ways of changing (pathway thinking). In addition, these models all rely on understanding people with diabetes' explanatory models for diabetes and a range of other things, their lived experience of diabetes, and how they negotiate complicated healthcare systems and the associated contradictory language, focus on 'control,' discipline, regular surveillance by a range of clinicians and the need to assume a great deal of responsibility for diabetes care themselves.

Components of effective diabetes management programmes are: high frequency of contact with the person with diabetes, the relationship between the individual and clinicians, especially relational continuity, and the person's ability to adjust treatment with or without health professional approval (Egnew 2009; Pimouguet et al. 2011).

Clinicians need to understand the multiplicity of factors that influence people's explanatory models, including their own influence. For example, type 2 diabetes is frequently described as a 'lifestyle disease', which has a hidden subtext – for example, self-induced disease and blame, media advertising promotes foods such as 'guilt-free chocolate'. The 'voice' in which health professionals seek or deliver information, as well as the actual words they use, affect learning. Three health professional voices have been described:

(1) The 'doctor' voice used when the health professional is seeking information from the patient.
(2) The 'educator' voice used when imparting information to the patient.
(3) The 'fellow human' voice used when encouraging and supporting people.

People with diabetes are more likely to respond to the fellow human voice. They often try to reduce the judgemental connotations inherent within words and conversations by developing their own explanations for diabetes (Dunning 2013a, pp. 78–95).

Communication – having good conversations

Effective communication is central to teaching and learning and the person's role in health-related decision-making. Communication skills are the foundation of most clinical encounters. Good communication fosters a positive therapeutic relationship the (Berman and Chulka 2016). In the context of diabetes education, communication refers to the art of asking 'good' questions, giving the person time to respond and *listening* to the answers. Listening involves being comfortable with silence, which enables the clinician to ask relevant probing and clarifying questions, which, in turn, demonstrates listening and minimises interruptions to arrive at a shared understanding of relevant issues. Importantly, body language must be congruent with spoken language.

However, patients often indicate that clinicians do not listen to them and ask questions that focus on the clinician's agenda (Berman and Chulka 2016). Research consistently demonstrates low patient-clinician concordance about management decisions (Heisler et al. 2003; Parkin and Skinner 2003; Skinner et al. 2007; Schwarz et al. 2012), which clinicians frequently attributed to patients not recalling the content of the consultation. However, Skinner et al. (2007) demonstrated that both patient and clinician recall is poor. Significantly, Skinner et al. found some decisions people with diabetes and clinicians recalled were not evident in recordings of their conversations, and there were discrepancies between the details even when both groups recalled the general topics discussed.

Parkin and Skinner (2003) found people with diabetes were more likely to recall talking about diet and less likely to recall discussing moods or emotions. Conversely, clinicians were more likely to recall discussing mood and emotions. Parkin and Skinner found complete disagreement between patients and clinicians in 19.6% of encounters and about decisions made 20.7% of the time. That is, the 'the two parties seem to recall different consultations.' People with diabetes may forget a great deal of what they are told, but it appears clinicians forget a great deal about what they say.

Likewise, Rushford et al. (2007) found women hospitalised with a cardiac condition recalled receiving information about medication, smoking cessation, and exercise but very few recalled receiving information about resuming gardening, sexual activity, and driving. Obese inactive women only recalled a limited amount of information about diet and activity and only some women with diabetes recalled receiving information about medicines. Older women were least likely to recall advice.

Recent studies of people in hospital show >60% could not name the doctor in charge; 58% did not know why they were in hospital, 67% were prescribed a new medicine but 25% of these did not know they were given a new medicine, 38% did not know they were scheduled for an investigative test on the day the test was scheduled (Wilkins 2012a,b). Similar discrepancies occur in primary care where patients report being interrupted by their doctors within the first 18 seconds when the person begins to talk, doctors underestimate the individual's desire for information, 50% report they are not asked whether they have any questions and 50% leave the consultation unsure about what they are expected to do (Alston et al. 2012). Ospina et al. (2018) found physicians interrupt the individual within 11 seconds of asking a question, whereas patients share their concerns within six seconds if they are not interrupted. Importantly, the person's agenda (concerns) are not addressed 80% of the time.

These studies suggest there is considerable miscommunication and many missed opportunities within clinical encounters for engaging with patients. The reasons for these discrepancies are not clear. However, the more people are told, the more they forget and they tend to recall what they were told first and/or consider important to them. These findings suggest there are many barriers to effective communication, many of which are common to patients and health professionals (see Table 16.1).

Specific strategies to enhance education and promote behaviour change include asking the following questions:

- Is now the 'right' time to address the issue?
- What do I need to know about the person to ask the right questions and address their concerns?
- Does the person have the knowledge and skills to manage their diabetes to best of their ability (including health literacy and numeracy)?
- If not, how can I help them acquire what they need?
- Does the person have access to and/or can he or she identify and use relevant resources and support appropriately?
- Is the individual satisfied with his or her life at the moment? (Schulman-Green et al. 2012).

Other strategies to support behaviour change can include the following:

- Have the individual write down their goals, a strategy used in health coaching, to encourage people to own the decision and to remind them of their behaviour change goals.
- Use written or verbal contracts between patients and health professionals, patients and carers, or health professionals and carers where one or both parties commit to undertaking behaviours. However, there is little evidence that contracts improve adherence or achieve behaviour change (Bosch-Capblanch et al. 2007).
- Blood glucose awareness training (BGATT) has consistently demonstrated improved hypoglycaemia awareness (ability to detect hypoglycaemia) and fewer episodes of severe hypoglycaemia during driving (Cox et al. 2006). It was developed for people with type 1 diabetes, but there is no reason it should not be appropriate to type 2. BGATT was recently made available on the Internet for health professionals and people with diabetes. Likewise, DESMOND and DAFNE show improved self-management for people with type 2 and type 1 diabetes, respectively.
- Peer education programmes were discussed previously. Some organisations have engaged patients to
- Adopting a 'tell [teach]-back-collaborative inquiry' approach (Kemp et al. 2008; Silverman et al. 2018). Many people leave clinical encounters with limited understanding about what occurred in the encounter. Such misunderstanding is associated with high risk of adverse outcomes. Kemp et al. used two video scenarios to assess how people like to receive information. One video showed a doctor explaining a medical condition and its management using three types of inquiry: yes–no (commonly used in health settings), tell-back directive (health professional-centred), and tell-back collaborative (patient-centred and had elements to address patient's feelings). Not surprisingly, people preferred the tell/teach-back collaborative approach. Significantly, the Kalamazoo Consensus Statement developed by communication experts and Silverman et al.'s Calgary Cambridge Model recommend checking for understanding is a core element of communication.

Thus, an empowering education model that encompasses a 'tell/teach-back' collaborative approach enables the individual's explanatory model for diabetes and their personal healthcare needs to be heard, and provides opportunities to negotiate and agree on compromises. Education encounters are often emotional as well as cognitive and rational, and involve reflection and action. Sometimes people have to make difficult management decisions several times a day, which can be stressful and emotionally exhausting. The ecomap and genomap shown in Chapter 2 could help health professionals understand an individual's social environment.

The following issues need to be considered when designing an empowering education encounter:

- Education alone will not change behaviour (World Health Organization (WHO) (2003; Knight and Donan 2006). For example, 28% of people with type 1 diabetes do not have their insulin prescriptions filled or inject the prescribed doses (Morris et al. 1997); only one-third of people with type 2 on monotherapy obtain at least 80% of their prescribed medicines

(Donan et al. 2002), only follow dietary recommendations 50% of the time (Toobert et al. 2000); and only 30% who take out gym membership attend the gym. Likewise, the Internet increases knowledge but does not necessarily change behaviour.

- The individual's feelings, beliefs, and diabetes explanatory models affect their healthcare behaviours.
- Psychosocial situation, coping style, and key relationships.
- Education and literacy level.
- Ability to make informed decisions (the person with diabetes AND health professionals). Therefore, education programmes must have the infrastructure to support the quality of clinical decision-making (O'Connor et al. 2003, 2007; Alston et al. 2012). There is a growing number of diabetes-related clinical decision aids and guidelines that can be obtained from libraries such as the Cochrane Collaboration, Foundation for Informed Decision Making, and the Mayo Clinic. It is interesting that, although key diabetes management guidelines are derived from the same evidence, they often make slightly different recommendations such as treatment targets. The International Patient Decision Aid Standards (IPDAS) Collaboration developed quality criteria concerning essential content, the development process and evaluation processes that can be used to develop diabetes education material, especially when patient decision-making ability is an essential component of care.
- Learning and teaching styles and methods.
- Goals for the session and future life goals.
- Ability to undertake self-care behaviours.
- Satisfaction with the service.

Although current diabetes management and education care models focus on people with diabetes being active participants in their care, and health outcomes are better if the person actively participates, people are not informed about all their options, including the risks and benefits. They may be informed about the option the health professional recommends, and other options 'glossed over' or not discussed (Alston et al. 2012). People, especially those with chronic diseases, want coordinated care, yet only 50% report they receive it (Alston et al. 2012).

People's actual role in and preferences concerning healthcare decision-making is complex. Some people prefer to leave medical decisions to their doctors. Arora et al. (2000) found 58% of patients preferred their doctors to make medical decisions. There was a significant association between older age, lower education and income levels, and male gender and preference for doctor-driven decisions. People with severe cardiac disease and serious diabetes were more likely to adopt a passive role. In contrast, those with clinical or symptomatic depression were more likely to take an active role. People with the lowest coping skills and those who placed a higher value on their health were more likely to leave decisions to their health professionals (Arora et al. 2000).

Many people who choose to use complementary therapies prefer to be active participants in their care (Barnett 2007; Dunning 2007). People choose to use CM because they believe it is more compatible with their philosophies or beliefs about health and illness, their values and their worldview, rather than because they are disillusioned with conventional medicine (Barnett 2007).

The concept of 'patient activation:' activating patients who do actively participate in their care emerged in the past 10 years. A Patient Activation Measure (PAM) was developed and validated by Hibbard et al. (2004), who indicated that activation involves four stages:

(1) Believe the patient role is important.
(2) Have relevant knowledge and competence to act.
(3) Taking action to manage health.
(4) Stay the course, even when stressed.

The implication is that the four stages are patient-related: they are also attributes clinicians should cultivate. Whilst, assessing 'patient activation' is important, the term is also subliminally judgmental and negative. It could be equally or be more important to assess clinicians' competence to engage with patients and enhance their patients' capacity to actively engage in their care.

Teaching: an art and a process

> *Carpe diem* – seize the day (*The Dead Poets Society* 1989).

Effective teaching occurs at a teachable moment. Skilled clinician teachers need to be able to recognise and seize opportunities.

Teaching is a communication process involving planning, implementing, and evaluating information to be learned. Teaching can be delivered individually or in groups and involves:

- Creating an environment in which learning can occur. This includes establishing a relationship with the person and finding their 'doctor within', their innate capacity to address challenges, adapt, and heal (Egnew 2009).
- Assessing learning needs and learning style or styles. The learning needs are used to set goals and plan the teaching. Assessment is an essential first step because patients and clinicians have different ideas about what is important (Woodcock and Kinmonth 2001). Barriers and facilitators to learning and being able to use the information can be identified and the teaching can build on past experience, existing knowledge, and address misconceptions.
- Prioritising learning needs with the individual.
- Setting goals with the individual or group to be achieved that are agreed with the individual or group and are achievable and measurable (Skinner 2013, pp. 49–61).
- Identifying the teaching method most likely to enhance learning and the materials needed to deliver the teaching. This can be as simple as a stick to draw in the sand with or as complex as a sophisticated lecture room. In group settings, a range of teaching strategies need to be used to accommodate different learning styles.
- Delivering the teaching using strategies most likely to facilitate learning.
- Having the insight to teach at teachable moments as the movie *The Dead Poet's Society* portrayed so poignantly.
- Evaluating the outcome. Evaluation is an essential aspect of quality improvement and should not only focus on patient outcomes (knowledge and behaviour). Teacher performance and the overall teaching programme should also be evaluated. There are different forms of evaluation depending on the purpose of the evaluation see recommended reading at the end of the chapter. When planning the evaluation, the data collection process and validity of any tools used need to be considered.

Thus, there is considerable overlap amongst teaching, storytelling, and counselling. In the context of diabetes education where the underlying goal is often to achieve and/or maintain behaviour change, the teacher must find the most effective way to invite the individual to see themselves and their role in a different way and find ways to help the individual help themselves. That is to integrate diabetes into their sense of self and maintain their personhood. Thus, education is a sophisticated form of marketing. It is a challenge selling the product diabetes, with all that entails and the meanings the word holds for individuals and society, to a usually reluctant buyer.

Self-care can be facilitated by co-coordinating self-management activities, recognising that different self-management tasks vary in importance to individuals and at different times in an individual's life, ensuring open, and honest communication with people with diabetes to co-create management plans (Schulman-Green et al. 2012). Health professional training in how to deliver patient-centred education and care may improve performance and patient satisfaction and active engagement in their care (Lewin et al. 2001).

Diabetes education can be delivered individually and is equally effective delivered in groups including initiating insulin (Plank et al. 2004; Yki-Jarvinen et al. 2007). However, people still need to be able to apply the information to their personal situations and have the opportunity to practice relevant behaviours. Group education provides a form of peer support and often helps people feel less alone in the problems they face and feelings about diabetes, which can have positive health benefits. Internet-based education programmes are also effective for younger and older people especially when they are interactive and emphasise behavioural and motivational strategies (Bond et al. 2007).

Health professionals are often also patient advocates; in fact patient advocacy is listed as in *Role and Scope of Practice for the Credentialed Diabetes Educator in Australia* (Australian Diabetes Educators Association (ADEA) 2007) and in similar role descriptions in the UK and US. Specific advocacy actions for diabetes educators and other clinicians and organisations such as Diabetes UK and Diabetes Australia include helping people obtain relevant healthcare, advocating for services, and interceding with other clinicians and services on the individual's behalf. Health advocacy is a complex process and nurses are often hindered in their advocacy by issues such as a sense of powerlessness, lack of support from colleagues, lack of time, and insufficient knowledge and skills (Negarandeh et al. 2006).

Health literacy

The Australian Bureau of Statistics noted that 41% of Australians have inadequate health literacy skills and 59% struggle to understand their health and health choices (Australian Bureau of Statistics 2012). Similar statistics apply in many other countries. Significantly, health literacy encompasses more than the ability to read and write. Considering health literacy and numeracy is essential to the success of person-focused interventions (Coulter and Ellins 2007). Health literacy and numeracy are complex concepts. Nutbeam (2000) defined three levels of health literacy from a risk-factor perspective, where most previous definitions were based on a biomedical perspective of health and ill health. Individuals may not fall neatly into Nutbeam's levels:

Practice points

(1) Listening is an essential element of education and care and heals (Dunning 2013b, pp. 62–76, Silverman et al. 2018).
(2) Diabetes education is not about getting the individual to do what the health professional wants.
(3) Even if the health professional is not trying to control the individual's life, it often feels that way to the person concerned. Most people's instinct is to resist. Core beliefs and values are held more strongly when people feel they have lost control over aspects of their life (Thomas 2001; Speight 2013) and affect readiness and ability to make relevant behaviour changes.
(4) Emotions need to be acknowledged not solved. Health professionals' instinct is to try to solve the problem. The art of teaching is to help the individual find the solution themselves.
(5) Functional health literacy that includes basic reading and writing skills needed to function in daily life.
(6) Communicative/interactive health literacy that includes more advanced literacy and cognitive skills that combine with social skill and enable people to participate in a range of activities and apply information in changing circumstances.
(7) Critical health literacy that encompasses even more advanced cognitive and social skills an individual use to be autonomous and have control over their lives.

More recent definitions of health literacy encompass an asset-based perspective and encompass health system literacy and the individual's ability to understand and interact with the social determinants of health and navigate the health system (de Leeuw 2012), which might also be a requirement of health professionals.

People with low health literacy have poorer health outcomes, less self-care knowledge and self-care skills lower medicine adherence rates, more admissions to hospital and are less likely to engage in healthy eating and exercise (de Walt et al. 2004). In addition, cross-sectional studies indicate poor numeracy skills are common in people with diabetes and might be associated with inadequate glycaemic control as well as low self-efficacy and inadequate knowledge (Cavanaugh and Rothman 2008) and increase the risk of hypoglycaemia (Sarkar et al. 2006, p. 6).

Likewise, Kerr and Varshneya (2012) undertook a confidential online survey of health professionals who provide diabetes education to people with diabetes in the UK, Australia and Germany (*n* = 328). Health professionals believed people with diabetes have trouble with spelling and grammar; find it difficult to understand graphs and tables as well as fractions, decimals and percentages. The health professionals estimated 3–4 people in 10 had difficulty following instructions and felt people struggled to understand the behavioural aspects of diabetes care such as diet and activity advice and managing insulin doses and dose adjustments. Interestingly health professionals scored themselves highly on their ability to effectively meet people with diabetes needs. Thus, it is essential to understand health literacy and numeracy when designing care plans with people with diabetes and when making decisions about their behaviours including risk-taking behaviours.

People with limited health literacy often feel ashamed and try to hide the fact from other people. For example, Parikh et al. (1996) found two thirds of patients had never disclosed their low health literacy to their spouses, more than half had never told their children, and one in five had never disclosed to anybody. Clues to low health literacy include the individual's response to written information, for example, 'I forgot my glasses, I will read it when I get home,' responses to questions about healthcare behaviours, for example, inability to name medicines, actual behaviours, for example, missing appointments or not adhering to medicine regimens. However, these are clues to explore the issue: they are not diagnostic (Davis et al. 1993; Weiss 2007).

Methods of assessing health literacy include:

- Newest Vital Sign (NVS) (Johnson and Weiss et al. 2008) is used to screen for limited health literacy by answering questions about a nutrition label for ice cream.
- Rapid Estimate of Adult Literacy in Medicine (REALM) (Davis et al. 1993) is a word recognition test and is one of the oldest and most widely used health literacy assessment instruments. Variations on the original REAL include a version for adolescents (REALM-Teen), a shorter version than the original 66 questions (REALM-7). Other versions are under development, for example, for dentistry.
- Test of Functional Health Literacy in Adults (TOHLA) is more complex and is often used for research purposes (Parker 1998). It takes ~20 minutes to complete but a shorter version is available that can be completed in 12 minutes. It assesses numeracy as well as literacy.
- National Assessment of Adult Literacy (NAAL) can be used as a population screening tool and identifies four levels of health literacy from basic to proficient (Kutner et al. 2007).
- The eHealth Literacy Scale (eHEALS) is a measure of knowledge, comfort, and skill at using information technology to obtain health information from electronic sources and has been validated with adolescents (Norman and Skinner 2006).
- Nutrition Literacy Scale, which is specific to nutrition.
- Health Literacy Skills Instrument (McCormack et al. 2010), which measures people's ability to obtain and use information and adopts a skills-based approach.

It may be possible to incorporate health literacy assessments into routine clinical practice, but it can be time consuming and patients may not be willing to undergo such testing. If time and resources permit, a health literacy point prevalence survey may provide a guide to the prevalence of the problem in a given target population. It may be more useful to ensure written health information is at grade 8 or 9 level by undertaking various readability and usability tests on the information commonly provided, such as:

- The Simple Measure of Gobbledegook (SMOG).
- CLOZE.
- DISCERN was designed to evaluate the quality of written patient health information (Coulter et al. 1998).

- Fry Readability Graph is commonly used and can be found on the Iowa Department of Health Fry's readability Graph page.
- Gunning FOG can also be obtained from the Iowa Department of Health.
- Material for Informed Choice-Evaluation (MICE) is designed to assess the readability of scientific information for patients (Charnock 1998).
- PMOSE/KIRSCH focuses on material that use lists, charts, and graphs.
- Flesch Reading Ease is used in the Microsoft word grammar checker. However, scores can be 2–3 grades lower than results obtained using valid assessment tools. For example, a score of 7 would most likely be 10 on the SMOG.
- Suitability Assessment of Materials (SAM) was developed by Doak and Doak (Doak et al. 1996) and assesses readability, usability and suitability of materials.

It is very likely that a great deal of information is not at an appropriate literacy level to promote informed health decision-making and may not suit all learning styles. Godolphin et al. (2001) found 50% of the pamphlets on display in doctor's consulting rooms was well below the required level on the DISCERN scale. Generally, people want health information, and if their information needs are met in a form appropriate to their needs, they are more likely to actively participate in their care (Larson et al. 1996; Coulter et al. 1998; McKenna et al. 2003), yet doctors often underestimate people's desire for information and are less likely to provide information for older people (McKenna et al. 2003).

Other design issues are also important, such as colour contrast, font size, font type (sans serif fonts such as Arial and all capital letters are harder to read than serif fonts such as Times New Roman and sentence case), the amount of 'white space,' and the graphics used. Interestingly, a recent study found people taking antiepileptic medicines ($n = 60\,000$) were more likely to miss doses if they were given generic medicine that was a different colour from their usual medicines (Kesselheim et al. 2012).

The *Well-Written Health Information: A Guide. Communicating with Consumers* (Currie, Spink and Rajendran 2000) is useful for assessing many of these parameters for a range of clinical and research purposes.

Clinical observation

The author asked experts to use <u>Currie et al.'s checklist to assess information designed *with* people with diabetes to aid advance care planning and to write to Participant Information and Consent Forms for a research project. The experts found the checklist easy to use, indicated it addresses readability, design features and the evidence used to develop the information.</u>

The digital environment

The digital environment has an increasing role in diabetes education and management and life generally. Having accesses to a wealth of online and cloud-based information expands individual's and group memory capacity and frees up individual's cognitive memory for other purposes such as increasing depth of knowledge in an area of interest (Wegner and Ward 2013). Shared memory is referred to as distributed memory, transactive memory and memory partners. Thus, the human memory is no longer the only or main storage repository for information, including diabetes information.

Wegner and Ward (2013) suggested we may be parts of an 'inter-mind' and will develop new intelligence housed in human brains and internet sites. We no longer need to remember a lot of facts. We do need to know where to find information on the internet, including in the plethora of apps designed to help people manage their diabetes (Chapter 3). Many clinicians recall consultations with people with diabetes who 'consulted Dr Google' before they attended their appointment. Such initiative is laudable and needs to be acknowledged: it can lead to overestimation of actual knowledge and has a powerful effect on beliefs. Significantly, there is a great deal of misinformation on the internet; people with diabetes and families need help to identify reputable websites, and so do many clinicians!

Survival skills

Whilst the preceding information largely addresses the need to consider the mental and social aspects of learning and teaching, there are some tasks that need to be mastered for safe, effective self-care. Survival skills are taught at diagnosis and throughout life as the need arises. The family should be involved whenever necessary if possible. Survival skills education refers to providing minimal information to enable the person to manage their medicines, eat an appropriate diet, monitor blood glucose and ketones, prevent and/or manage hypoglycaemia, safely dispose of used equipment and obtain relevant supplies. Written information can support verbal teaching and is more effective if the health professional gives the information to the individual and points out important information relevant to the individual. However, the individual's specific concerns/questions must be addressed. The person should be able to:

- Demonstrate correct insulin care and administration techniques (if appropriate).
- Know the effect of medications, exercise and food on their blood glucose levels.
- Know the names of their insulin/oral glucose lowering medicines (GLM) (if relevant).
- Demonstrate correct blood glucose monitoring techniques (and blood and ketone testing in type 1 diabetes) and appropriately documenting the results.
- Know the significance of ketones (type 1).
- Recognise the signs and symptoms, causes and appropriate treatment of hypoglycaemia if on insulin or GLMs.
- Know that regular meals containing the appropriate amount of carbohydrate are important.
- Have an emergency contact telephone number if help is required.
- Demonstrate safe disposal of sharps.
- Enrol in the NDSS (in Australia).

Thus, acquiring even the basic diabetes information (survival information) is a significant burden. Significantly, many health professionals do not understand these issues (Dunning 2010; Livingston and Dunning 2010). Dunning et al. (2013c) used the ADKNOWL (Bradley 2003) to determine health professionals' diabetes knowledge in two Australian regional aged care facilities. The response rate was disappointingly low: conversations in follow up interviews with nurses revealed 'the questions were too hard for general nurses'.

This is a major concern considering the ADKNOWL was designed to be used with people with diabetes and clinicians. One expects staff caring for people with diabetes to have *at least* an equivalent level of knowledge about diabetes and its care as people with diabetes, especially when caring for some of the most vulnerable people in society – older people living in aged care homes. It is not surprising many people with diabetes worry that clinicians '*will bugger it* [diabetes care] *up*' when they are in hospital (Savage et al. 2012).

Ongoing education

Education can be continued on an individual basis or in group programmes. Education is a life-long process, thus both methods are usually employed. Survival information should be reviewed and further information given. The person should gradually be able to perform the following depending on their individual care plan:

- Demonstrate appropriate insulin adjustment considering the effects of factors such as food, activity, medicines, and illness on blood glucose as relevant.
- Manage illnesses at home, especially continue insulin/diabetes tablets, continue to drink fluids and test for ketones, especially type 1.

- Recognise the signs and symptoms of hypoglycaemia and treat appropriately.
- Cope in special situations, such as eating out, during travel and playing sports.
- Understand that appropriate complication screening such as foot care will help prevent long-term complications and hospital admissions.
- Know that normoglycaemia and regular examination of the eyes, feet, blood pressure, cardiovascular system, and kidney function can prevent or delay the development of long-term diabetic complications.
- Understand that certain jobs and activities are unsuitable/risky for people with diabetes on insulin, for example, scuba diving or driving heavy vehicles.
- Wear some form of medical alert system identifying them as having diabetes.
- Understand that they should not neglect general healthcare such as mammograms, prostate checks, breast self-examination, regular dental checks, and preventative vaccinations.
- In order to recognise 'abnormal,' for example, hypoglycaemia or signs of a complication, the individual needs to recognise what 'normal' is *for them*. This involves learning to listen to their bodies, interpret body cues, self-diagnose, and make a decision about what to do. They may or may not seek assistance to interpret the body cues. They usually test their theories (legitimisation).

Practice points

(1) Education methods that incorporate behavioural strategies, experiential learning, co-negotiated goal setting, and use reinforcement are more likely to be effective.
(2) Patient satisfaction is a key element of adherence.
(3) Helping the person reflect on events and consider future strategies make education more personal.
(4) The continued therapeutic relationship between the patient and health professional is important to effective education and care.

Empowerment

There is no doubt that diabetes education is essential, but knowledge alone does not predict health behaviour. Social issues, beliefs, attitudes, and satisfaction are some of the intervening variables among knowledge, behaviour, and disease status. These are not constants and they need to be assessed on a regular basis – for example, deciding what is happening at the time, what could/will change, and how will the change affect the individual and their significant others.

Empowerment models of diabetes education are based on shared governance considering the whole person and their life situation and personal environment. These issues are not a new concept. Hippocrates is credited with saying, 'In order to cure the human body it is necessary to have knowledge of the whole'. Likewise, the psychiatrist in T.S. Elliot's play *The Cocktail Party* states that he needs to know a great deal more about the patient than the patient himself could always tell him.

Empowerment models recognise that people with diabetes must, and mostly want to be responsible for their own care. Empowerment is based on three characteristics:

(1) The person with diabetes makes choices affecting their healthcare.
(2) The individual is in control of their care.
(3) The consequences of the choices affect the person with diabetes and they need to take responsibility for their choices.

It is arrogant to think clinicians can empower another person. They can only provide the support and information to empower themselves. Empowerment, then, is a collaborative approach to care where management is co-designed to help the individual make informed choices and maximise their knowledge, skills, and self-awareness. It requires the individual to make deliberate conscious choices, usually several time per day. In reality, most people are *not* disempowered; they make decisions and act on them every day, including deciding to attend or not attend a consultation (Speight 2013).

Empowerment education requires health professionals to accept the legitimacy of an individual's goals even if they result in suboptimal control (Anderson et al. 1996; Skinner 2013, pp. 49–61) and the individual to accept responsibility for the consequences of their decisions. Not everybody is capable of taking control/be empowered. Some people require specific instructions, for example, an individual who has an external locus of control. In addition, stress and anxiety at specific times can impair an individual's ability to take control.

An empowerment model of diabetes education seeks to determine what the person with diabetes wants, and to reach agreement between what should be done and what the individual wants or is capable of achieving, in order to balance the burden of treatment and quality of life (see Chapter 15). Diabetes is only one aspect of people's lives and affects them on many levels:

- Observable, e.g. signs and symptoms of hyper/hypoglycaemia
- Not directly observable, e.g. personhood, self-concept, body image
- Insights into their disease
- Relationships

Special issues

The individual's questions/education needs should be addressed as they arise and planned into teaching programmes as appropriate. Questions/needs may relate to:

- Pregnancy and diabetes
- Sexuality and diabetes
- Exercise
- Diet
- Weight control
- How to manage their medicines
- How to manage sick days and/or hypoglycaemia
- Issues such as diabetes information the person hears or reads in media reports
- Issues that have nothing to do with diabetes, e.g. death of a beloved pet

---

Clinical Observation

It is not absolutely necessary for people with diabetes to have a detailed knowledge about the causes and pathophysiology of diabetes to undertake appropriate self-care and achieve good control.

The clinicians' role in diabetes education

Patient teaching is a recognised independent nursing function and education is a vital part of the diabetic treatment plan. Therefore, teaching patients in acute, aged care, and extended-care facilities is within the scope of professional nursing practice. Some key points should be kept in mind when educating people with diabetes:

(1) Know the aim of diabetes education is autonomy and empowerment.
(2) Consider the psychological and social aspects when discussing diabetes.
(3) Encourage questions and dialogue.

(4) Ask open questions and use active listening.
(5) Teach specific skills and allow the patient time to practice new skills (e.g. insulin administration).
(6) Allow time for patients to discuss difficulties and concerns about diabetes.
(7) Relate new information to the patient's experience.
(8) Make sure the information provided is consistent with the information provided by the diabetes team.
(9) Refer to a diabetes educator when necessary, especially if you do not know the answer.

Although there are many disadvantages to bedside teaching (e.g. noise, distractions, illness, other priorities and concerns, and lack of privacy), it can enable teaching to occur at a 'teachable moment' and effectively reinforce information. The information must be consistent with hospital policies/procedures and the nurse must have the appropriate knowledge in order to teach effectively. Clinicians make a substantial contribution to the health and well-being of the patient by allowing them to participate in decision-making about their care in hospital and to make appropriate decisions at home.

Teaching in the hospital should effectively reinforces the information supplied by the diabetes nurse specialist/diabetes educator, doctor, podiatrist and dietitian. However, ward teaching *must* be consistent with that of the diabetes team and procedures such as insulin technique and blood glucose monitoring performed correctly according to the agreed protocols. Patients are quick to perceive inconsistencies and may become confused or lose faith in the staff if they perceive inconsistencies.

Learning is facilitated when the need/readiness to learn is perceived and immediately applied in a given situation: that is, 'teaching at a teachable moment'. Teachable moments often occur when the ward staff is performing routine nursing care, such as blood glucose tests, or giving injections.

Teaching is nonverbal as well as verbal. In fact, more than 60% of communication is nonverbal. People learn by observation; therefore, the nurse is a role model and care should be taken to perform procedures correctly and to refer questions to another person if they do not know the answer. In this way, formal and informal ongoing education in the ward is possible and desirable. The nurse's own knowledge about diabetes will influence their willingness and ability to participate in patient teaching. Theories of teaching and learning were not traditionally part of the nurse training. This is changing as empowerment in chronic disease management is recognised and accepted along with a focus on preventative healthcare.

Many factors can influence teaching and learning. Some of these are shown in Table 16.3. It is the responsibility of the teacher to ensure that the environment is not distracting. Noise in a busy

Table 16.3 Some common patient and health professional factors that influence teaching and learning.

Factor	Patient	Health professional
Health beliefs	√	√
Social support	√	
Well-being/illness	√	√
Environment	√	√
Knowledge	√	√
Skills	√	√
Time	√	√
Perceived responsibility	√	√
Work priority		√
Perception of teaching role		√
Learning style	√	√

ward can make conversation difficult and hinder learning. The patient should be as comfortable as possible and free from pain and other distractions.

The following basic principles need to be considered when planning a teaching session, whether it is for an individual or a group:

- Know the aim of the session (whose aim?).
- Understand the patient's needs/goals and learning style.
- Objectives should be realistic and achievable.
- The environment must be conducive to learning.
- Ascertain and build on the patient's existing knowledge.
- Relate teaching to patient's own experience.
- Demonstrate the skills to be acquired.
- Provide opportunities for the patient to practice the skill (return demonstration).
- Evaluate the skill and knowledge.
- Provide positive reinforcement.
- Review information before commencing the next teaching session.

It is usual to begin with the simple concepts and proceed to more complex ones.

The Information Sheets at the end of the chapter are examples of information material used in teaching, which is often available in several languages. In some cases, the medical terms may need to be replaced with the patient's words. Blood glucose monitoring is discussed in Chapter 3. Specific patient instruction will depend on the testing system being used and they need to be personalised with the individual and often their family.

Insulin administration

Insulin can be administered using a range of insulin delivery systems including syringes, insulin pens, and insulin pumps. Syringes are not used as often as the other devices in some countries, because other devices offer greater flexibility and portability, reduce dosing errors and are discreet, thus avoiding some of the stigma attached to using syringes. The person should be shown a range of options and helped to choose one that suits them. The short fine needles in use today mean injections are relatively painless – less painful than blood glucose testing.

Insulin should be given subcutaneously (see next section). IM injections, through incorrect technique, cause erratic blood glucose levels because the insulin is absorbed faster than via the subcutaneous route (Vaag et al. 1990). Reusing needles and syringes causes local trauma, microscopic damage to the needle tip and increases the likelihood that the needle will bend and/or break off in the injection site; it should therefore be discouraged. Needles left on insulin pens form a conduit to the outside allowing air to enter the vial and dose inaccuracies (Ginsberg et al. 1994).

These factors may not be an issue in developed countries where needles are supplied under the NDSS scheme, but they still occur in other countries where access is difficult or costly.

Basic guidance for teaching people about insulin delivery systems

The patient should be familiar with the structure and function of the particular insulin device chosen. They must be able to do the following:

- Assemble the device in the correct sequence.
- Load the insulin correctly if necessary.
- Ensure insulin is expelled from the needle after loading the insulin.
- Know when to replace the insulin cartridge/device.
- Know how to inject the insulin according to the particular device chosen.
- Know how to store and transport the device.
- Know the appropriate method of cleaning and maintaining the device.
- Recognise signs that the device may be malfunctioning and know what action to take to remedy the situation.

It is important to discuss with and advise the individual about safe disposal of used equipment, especially sharps disposal at home.

Documenting diabetes education

Documentation was discussed in Chapter 2. Documentation is a legal requirement as well as a method of communication. Documenting diabetes education can be very time-consuming, thus using templates or teaching records that list standard education and make provision for individual differences to be recorded can save time.

Examples of patient instruction sheets appear on the following pages.

Basic example information sheets

These Instruction Sheets are designed for use with a practical demonstration of the procedure/s. They should not be handed out without adequate discussion. *They are examples only*.

The following two information sheets about drawing up insulin in syringes are included because syringes are still used in other countries and in many hospital settings, although most people with diabetes do not use syringes to self-inject in Australia. Likewise, short/rapid acting and Isophane insulins are still used in some places, although premixed insulins are more common in others (Chapter 5).

Example information: managing your diabetes when you are ill: patients with type 1 diabetes

Illness (such as colds and flu) cause the body to make hormones that help the body fight the illness. These hormones usually also cause the blood glucose to go high. High blood glucose levels can lead to unpleasant symptoms like thirst, tiredness, and passing a lot of urine.

By taking some simple precautions, the minor illness can usually be treated at home.

What to do

(1) Tell a family member or friend you are unwell.

(2) Continue to take your insulin. You may need to increase the dose during illness to control the blood glucose and prevent ketones from developing.

(3) Test your blood glucose every two to four hours. Write down the test results.

(4) Test your blood for ketones. If moderate to heavy ketones are detected consult your doctor.

(5) Continue to drink fluids or eat if possible (see recommended food list).

(6) Read the labels on any medication you take to treat the illness because it may contain sugar, sugar substitutes, or other ingredients that cause the blood glucose to go high.

(7) Rest.

(8) Keep the telephone number of your doctor, diabetes clinic, or diabetes nurse specialist/diabetes educator beside the telephone.

When to call the doctor

(1) If you have diarrhoea and/or vomiting.

(2) If ketones develop.

(3) If the blood glucose continues to rise.

(4) If you develop signs of dehydration (loss of skin tone, sunken eyes, dry mouth).

(5) If the illness does not get better in two to three days.

(6) If you feel you need advice.

What to tell the doctor when you call

(1)   How long you have been sick.

(2)   What the blood glucose level is.

(3)   How long the blood glucose has been high.

(4)   The level of ketones in the blood.

(5)   How frequently you are passing urine and how much.

(6)   If you are thirsty, tired, or have a temperature.

(7)   What medications you have taken to treat the illness.

(8)   If you have vomiting or diarrhoea, how frequently and how much.

Food for days when you are sick

It is important to continue to eat and drink. Small frequent meals may be easier to digest.

Suggested foods

- sweetened jelly (not low cal)
- ice cream (1/2 cup)
- custard with sugar (1/2 cup)
- honey (3 teaspoons)
- sugar (1 tablespoon)
- sweetened ice block (one small or 90 ml)
- egg flip – sweetened (similar to eggnog but less creamy 8 oz)
- milk (10 oz)
- Coke, lemonade or other sweetened soft drink (3/4 cup – not low cal)
- unsweetened tinned fruit (3/4 cup)
- orange juice (3/4 cup)
- apple juice (1/2 cup)
- pineapple juice (1/2 cup)
- orange (one medium)
- banana (one small)
- unflavoured yoghurt (100 g or 1/2 carton)
- flavoured (sweetened) yoghurt (200 g or one carton)
- broth or soup

Continuing care

(1)   If the doctor prescribes antibiotics to treat the illness it is important to complete the full course.

(2)   Continue to test for ketones until they show clear for 24 hours.

(3)   Continue to test your blood glucose two to four hourly and record the results until you recover and then go back to your usual routine.

(4)   Go back to your usual food plan when you recover.

(5)   If your insulin has been increased during the illness decrease it again when you recover to avoid hypoglycaemia.

(6)   Develop a sick day management plan.

(7)   Consider writing down a medical history for quick reference in times of illness or in an emergency.

List:

- all the medications you are taking
- past illnesses
- blood group
- date of last tetanus and flu injection
- illnesses that run in the family

This can be worn in an identification tag or be kept with your diabetes record book.

Example information: managing your diabetes when you are ill: patients with type 2 diabetes

Illnesses (such as colds and flu) cause the body to make hormones that help the body fight the illness. These hormones usually also cause the blood glucose to go high. High blood glucose levels can lead to unpleasant symptoms like thirst, tiredness, and passing a lot of urine.

By taking some simple precautions, the minor illness can usually be treated at home.

What to do

(1) Tell a family member or friend you are unwell.

(2) Continue to take your diabetes tablets. This is very important, because the blood glucose usually goes high. In severe illnesses or during an operation, insulin injections may be needed until you recover.

(3) Test your blood glucose every two to four hours. Write down the test results.

(4) Continue to drink fluids or eat if possible (see recommended food list).

(5) Read the labels on any medication you take to treat the illness because it may contain sugar, sugar substitutes or other ingredients that cause the blood glucose to go high.

(6) Rest.

(7) Keep the phone number of your doctor, diabetes clinic, or diabetes nurse specialist/diabetes educator beside the telephone.

When to call the doctor

(1) You have diarrhoea and/or vomiting.

(2) The blood glucose continues to rise.

(3) You develop signs of dehydration (loss of skin tone, sunken eyes, dry mouth).

(4) The illness does not get better in two to three days.

(5) You feel you need advice.

What to tell the doctor when you call

(1) How long you have been sick.

(2) What the blood glucose level is.

(3) How long the blood glucose has been high.

(4) How frequently you are passing urine and how much.

(5) If you are thirsty, tired, or have a temperature.

(6) What medications you have taken to treat the illness.

(7) If you have vomiting or diarrhoea, how frequently, and how much.

Food for days when you are sick

It is important to continue to eat and drink. Small frequent meals may be easier to digest.

Suggested foods

- sweetened jelly (not low-calorie)
- ice cream (1/2 cup)
- custard with sugar (1/2 cup)
- honey (3 teaspoons)
- sugar (1 tablespoon)
- sweetened ice block (one small or 90 mL)
- egg flip – sweetened (8 oz)
- milk (10 oz)
- Coke, lemonade or other sweetened soft drink (3/4 cup – not low cal)
- unsweetened tinned fruit (3/4 cup)
- orange juice (3/4 cup)
- apple juice (1/2 cup)

- pineapple juice (1/2 cup)
- orange (one medium)
- banana (one small)
- unflavoured yoghurt (100 g or 1/2 carton)
- flavoured (sweetened) yoghurt (200 g or one carton)
- broth or soup

Continuing care

(1) If the doctor prescribes antibiotics to treat the illness, it is important to complete the full course.

(2) Continue to test your blood glucose every two to four hours and record the results until you recover, and then go back to your usual routine.

(3) Go back to your usual food plan when you recover.

(4) Develop a sick day management plan.

(5) Consider writing down a medical history for quick reference in times of illness or in an emergency.

List:
- all the medications you are taking
- past illnesses
- blood group
- date of last tetanus and flu injection
- illnesses that run in the family

This can be worn in an identification tag or be kept with your diabetes record book.

Evaluating diabetes education

It is important to evaluate diabetes education delivered to individuals and in education programmes. Likewise, it is important to use appropriate evaluation processes and outcome measures and to value audit, evaluation, and translational research and ensure some ethical oversight is in place. The evaluation method used depends on the aim/s of the evaluation, which might not be the same as the aims of the programme. Systems thinking can help identify which component/s contribute to the effect.

Evaluation typically involves measuring:

- Knowledge change (but knowledge does not necessarily translate into action).
- Biochemical parameters such as HbA1c and lipids: bear in mind that these factors are influenced by a host of interrelated confounding variables and may not be a primary outcome of diabetes education.
- Psychosocial variables (see Chapter 15).
- Satisfaction, recognising high patient satisfaction scores could be an artefact and many satisfaction questionnaires may not ask an appropriate range of questions; PROMs.
- Other outcomes according to the initial nursing assessment.

Programme evaluation is only briefly described here. It is an essential element of diabetes education programmes and should be considered when the programme is *being developed, not planned after the programme has been delivered*. The evaluation method depends on the purpose of the evaluation (aim/s), which will influence the measurement tools and procedures used in the evaluation. In some cases, permission is needed to use copyright tools and some copyright holders charge a fee to use their tools. It is professional courtesy to acknowledge the authors.

Some reasons programme evaluations are undertaken include:

- Cost–benefit/effectiveness to ensure continued funding for the programme
- Determine programme outcomes, bearing in mind it is difficult to interpret the outcomes if the structure and process variables are not considered. Outcomes might be short term or long term.

- Clinician performance should be a component of most evaluation programmes and is usually part of the process variables. Most current patient satisfaction surveys are not adequate to evaluate clinician performance.
- Whether people with diabetes and/or families were involved in designing the programme and its evaluation.
- Needs analysis to determine the characteristics of the target population so the programme can be appropriately planned to suit their need.
- A combination of these broad aims.
- Determine the public health impact of the programme in the short and/or long term: sustainability and scalability.

Glasgow and Osteen (1992) suggested many diabetes education programme evaluations have a narrow focus on HbA1c and knowledge acquisition and do not assess other important variables and do not report important information in research reports and publications readers need to interpret the findings.

Although there has been some improvement in diabetes education evaluation research since 1992, many publications still contain methodological flaws and adopt a narrow focus that does not take account of the many factors and confounders likely to affect the outcome. Glasgow and Osteen recommended assessing outcomes in all relevant aspects of the programme and collecting standardised, objective, and specific measures in each stage of the evaluation and in each of the following categories:

- The social and environment context because these issues impact on people's capabilities e.g.:
  - social support and available community resources;
  - living arrangements;
  - health insurance;
  - organisation of the diabetes clinic or service;
  - time, cost, location, and access to the programme.
- Participant characteristics, which is important to determine whether participants in the programme are representative of the sampling or whole population:
  - description of the target population (sampling population including the approximate size of the population);
  - individual's demographic characteristics;
  - medical history such as diabetes complications and other comorbidities;
  - cognitive functioning;
  - physical functioning especially older people and people with disabilities;
  - measures might include knowledge, attitudes and beliefs, self-efficacy, spirituality, problem-solving ability, health literacy and numeracy, wellbeing and quality of life and metabolic data such as HbA1c, lipids, weight, smoking, and might be measured before and after the programme or at set intervals of time e.g. before, 3–4 months after the programme and again 12–18 months or in the longer term over years.
- Processes:
  - Was the programme delivered as planned?
  - If changes were needed, why were the needed and how did the change affect participants?
  - What did participants think about the programme: content, delivery methods, health professional performance, and the materials used in the programme and may include the parameters listed under participant characteristics?
- Outcomes of the programme, usually also measured before and after the programme:
  - Participation and attrition rates
  - Representativeness of the final sample
  - Changes in diabetes self-care behaviours such as blood glucose monitoring, medicine management, accessing resources, admission to hospital, attending scheduled appointments, morbidity, and mortality

Most importantly, people with diabetes should be involved in designing education programmes, evaluation processes, and quality metrics that are valuable to them (Jones 2013) or the care to be person-centred. Most people want their health professionals to be knowledgeable and competent and to know the care they receive is evidence based, but they value effective communication, empathy, trust, and the health professional being present in the moment.

References

Ajzen, I. and Fishbein, M. (1980). *Understanding Attitudes and Predicting Social Behaviour*. Englewood Cliffs, NJ: Prentice Hall.

Alston, C., Paget, L., Halvorson, G. et al. (2012). *Communicating with Patients on Health Care Evidence*. Washington DC: Washington State Helsink of Medicine of the National Academies.

Anderson, B. and Funnell, M. (2005). *The Art of Empowerment*, 2e. Virginia, USA: American Diabetes Association.

Anderson, R., Funnell, M., and Arnold, M. (1996). Using the empowerment approach to help patients change behaviour. In: *Practical Psychology for Clinicians* (eds. B. Anderson and R. Rubin), 163–172. Alexandria, VA: American Diabetes Association.

Anderson, R., Funnell, M., Burkhart, N. et al. (2002a). *101 Tips for Behaviour Change in Diabetes Education*. Virginia, USA: American Diabetes Association.

Anderson, R., Funnell, M., Burkhart, N. et al. (2002b). *101 Tips for Diabetes Self-Management Education*. Virginia, USA: American Diabetes Association.

Arora, N., Mchorney, C., and Rao, S. (2000). Medical decision-making: who really wants to participate? *Medical Care* **38** (3): 335–341.

Assal, J.-P. and Assal, T. (2013). Role and use of creative arts in diabetes care. In: *Diabetes Education: Art, Science and Evidence* (ed. T. Dunning), 98–115. Chichester, UK: Wiley Blackwell.

Australian Bureau of Statistics (ABS) (2012). Data quoted during the Centre for Culture, Ethnicity and Health forum *Curing the Cultural Barrier: Health Literacy Forum*, Fitzroy Town Hall Melbourne (28 February 2012).

Australian Diabetes Educators Association (ADEA) (2007). *The Credentialled Diabetes Educator in Australia: Role and Scope of Practice*. Canberra: ADEA.

Bandura, A. (1986). *Social Foundations of Thought and Action*. Englewood Cliffs, NJ: Prentice Hall.

Barnett, H. (2007). Complementary and alternative medicine and patient choice in primary care. *Quality in Primary Care* **15**: 207–212.

Becker, M. and Maiman, L. (1975). Sociobehavioral determinants of compliance with health and medical care recommendations. *Medical Care* **13** (1): 10–24.

Berman, A. and Chulka, D. (2016). Assessing effective physician-patient communication skills: 'are you listening to me?'. *Korean Journal of Medical Education* **28** (2): 243–249.

Bert, G. (2011). *Treating with words: Narrative medicine*. ZOE Foundation. http://www.foundazionezoe.it/code/13426/11279 (accessed August 2012).

Bond, G., Burr, R., Wolf, F. et al. (2007). The effects of a web-based intervention on physical outcomes associated with diabetes among adults age 60 and older: a randomised trial. *Diabetes Technology Therapy* **9** (1): 52–59.

Bosch-Capblanch, X., Abba, K., Prictor, M., and Garner, P. (2007). Contracts between patients and health care practitioners for improving adherence to treatment, prevention and health promotion activities. *Cochrane Database of Systematic Reviews* (2): CD004808. https://doi.org/10.1002/1451858.CD004808. pub3.

Bradley, C. (2003). *The Audit of Diabetes Knowledge (ADKnowl) User Guidelines*, 4th draft. Egham, Surrey, UK: Health Psychology Research, Royal Holloway University of London. http://www.healthpsychologyresearch.com/Admin/uploaded/Guidelines/adknowl%20user%20guidelines%20rev24.9.03.pdf.

Cavanaugh, K., Huizinga, M., and Wallston, K. (2008). Association of numeracy and diabetes control. *Annals of Internal Medicine* **148**: 737–746.

Cavanaugh, K. and Rothman, R.L. (2008). Does lower diabetes-related numeracy lead to increased risk for hypoglycemic events? *Annals of Internal Medicine* **149** (8): 594–594.

Charnock, D. (1998). *The DISCERN Handbook: Quality Criteria for Consumer Health Information on Treatment Choices*. Oxford: Radcliffe Medical Press.

Coulter, A. and Ellins, J. (2007). Effectiveness of strategies for informing, educating and involving patients. *British Medical Journal* **335** (7609): 24–27.

Coulter, A., Entwhistle, V., and Gilbert, D. (1998). *Informing Patients: Assessment of the Quality of Patient Information Materials*. London: King's College.

Cousins, N. (2005). *Anatomy of an Illness as Perceived by the Patient*. New York: WW Norton.

Cox, D., Gonder-Frederick, L., Ritterband, L. et al. (2006). Blood glucose awareness training: what is it, where is it, and where is it going? *Diabetes Spectrum* **19**: 43–49.

Currie, K., Spink, J., and Rajendran, M. (2000). *Well-Written Health Information: A Guide. Communicating with Consumers*. Melbourne: Victorian Government Department of Human Services. https://www2.health.vic.gov.au/

about/publications/researchandreports/Communicating-with-Consumers-Series-Volume-1-WellWritten-Health-Information-Guide--July-2000.

Davis, T., Long, S., and Jackson, R. (1993). Rapid estimate of adult literacy in medicine: a shortened screening instrument. *Family Medicine* **25**: 391–395.

Dickinson, J., Guzman, S., Marynuik, M. et al. (2017). The use of language in diabetes care and education. *Diabetes Care* https://doi.org/10.2337/dci17-0041.

Doak, C., Doak, L., and Root, J. (1996). *Teaching Patients with Low Literacy Skills*. Philadelphia, PA: JB Lippincott.

Donan, P., MacDonald, T., and Morris, A. (2002). Adherence to prescribed oral hypoglycaemic medication in a population of patients with type 2 diabetes: a retrospective cohort study. *Diabetic Medicine* **19**: 279–284.

Dunning, T. (2007). *Complementary Therapies and Diabetes: Perfect Partners or Dangerous Liaisons? Integrative Medicine Perspectives*. Sydney: Australasian Integrative Medicine Association (AIMA) Annual Conference, Peppers Fairmont Resort, Blue Mountains.

Dunning, T. (2010). Chronic disease self-management: what do we measure? *Journal of Nursing and Healthcare of Chronic Illness* **2**: 251–253.

Dunning, T. (2013a). Teaching and learning: the art and science of making connections. In: *Diabetes Education: Art, Science and Evidence* (ed. T. Dunning), 28–46. Chichester: Wiley Blackwell.

Dunning, T. (2013b). The teacher: moving from good to exceptional. In: *Diabetes Education: Art, Science and Evidence* (ed. T. Dunning), 62–76. Chichester, UK: Wiley Blackwell.

Dunning, T. (2013c). *Diabetes Education: Art, Science and Evidence*. Chichester, UK: Wiley Blackwell.

Dunning, P., Wellard, S., Rasmussen, B. et al. (2013). *Managing Diabetes Medicines in Regional Residential Aged Care Facilities: Balancing Competing Challenges*. Abstract number ICN 13ENA–2630. Presented at the. Melbourne Australia: International Council of Nurses Conference (18–23 May),.

Dunning, T., Speight, J., and Bennett, C. (2017). The 'diabetes restricted code/dialect' and what it means for people with diabetes and clinicians. *The Diabetes Educator* **43**: 18–26.

Dunning, T. (2014). Overview of complementary and alternative medicine and diabetes. *Practical Diabetes* **31** (9): 381–386.

Edelman, D. (2012). The funnel is dead. The New Consumer Decision Journey. http://www.linkedin.com/today/post/article/2012018110732=1816165 (accessed October 2012).

Egnew, T. (2009). Suffering, meaning and healing: challenges in contemporary medicine. *Annals of Family Medicine* **7** (2): 170–175.

Fisher, E., Brownson, C., O'Toole, M. et al. (2005). Ecological approaches to self-management: the care for diabetes. *American Journal of Public Health* **95** (9): 1523–1535.

Funnell, M. and Anderson, R. (2000). The problem with compliance in diabetes. *Journal of the American Medical Association* **284**: 1709.

Gale, J. (2007). Health psychology meets coaching psychology in the practice of health coaching. www.psychology.org.au/publications/inpsych/health_coaching (accessed December 2007).

Ginsberg, B., Parkes, J., and Sparacina, C. (1994). The kinetics of insulin administration by insulin pens. *Hormone and Metabolic Research* **26**: 584–587.

Glasgow, R. and Osteen, V. (1992). Evaluating diabetes education. *Diabetes Care* **13** (10): 1423–1432.

Godolphin, W., Towle, A., and McKendry, R. (2001). Evaluation of the quality of patient information to support informed shared decision-making. *Health Expectations* **4**: 325–242.

Health Direct (2018). Choosing Wisely Australia. www.healthdirect.gov.au/partners/choosing-wisely-australia.

Heisler, M., Vijan, S., Anderson, R. et al. (2003). When do patients and their physicians agree on diabetes treatment goals and strategies, and what difference does it make? *Journal of General Internal Medicine* **18**: 909–914.

Hibbard, J.H., Stockard, J., Mahoney, E.R., and Tusler, M. (2004). Development of the patient activation measure (PAM): conceptualizing and measuring activation in patients and consumers. *Health Services Research* **39**: 1005–1026. https://doi.org/10.1111/j.1475-6773.2004.00269.x.

International Alliance of Patients' Organisations (IAPO) (2007). *What Is Patient-Centred Healthcare?* 2e. London: UK: IAPO. http://iapo.org.uk/sites/default/files/files/IAPO%20Patient-Centred%20Healthcare%20Review%202nd%20edition.pdf.

International Alliance of Patients' Organisations (IAPO) (2005). *Declaration on Patient-Centred Care*. IAPO http://www.patientsorganisations.org/pchreview.

Johnson, K. and Weiss, B. (2008). How long does it take to assess literacy skills in clinical practice? *Journal of the American Board of Family Medicine* **21**: 211–214.

Jones, K. (2013). Patients need to be involved in quality metrics. Primary care Progress blog (accessed January 2013).

Jutterstrom, L., Isaksson, U., Sandstrom, H., and Hornsten, A. (2012). Turning points in self-management of type 2 diabetes. *European Diabetes Nursing* **9** (2): 46–50.

Kemp, E., Floyd, M., Mc-Cord-Duncan, E., and Lang, F. (2008). Patients prefer the method of 'tell back-collaborative inquiry' to asking for understanding of medical information. *Journal of the American Board of Family Medicine* **21** (1): 24–30.

Kerr, D. and Varshneya, R. (2012). Survey of impact of literacy and numeracy on diabetes patient care. *Practical Diabetes* **29**: 125–168.

Kesselheim, A., Misono, A., Shrank, W. et al. (2012). Variations in pill appearance of antiepileptic medicines. *Archives of Internal Medicine*. https://doi.org/10.1001/2013.jamaainternmed.997.

Knight, K. and Donan, T. (2006). The diabetes educator: trying hard, but must concentrate more on behaviour. *Diabetic Medicine* **23**: 485–501.

Kolb, D. (1984) cited in Arndt, M. & Underwood, B. (eds) (1990)). Learning style theory and patient education. *Journal of Continuing Education in Nursing* **21** (1): 28–31.

Kutner, M., Greenberg, E., Jin, Y. et al. (2007). Literacy in everyday life: Results from the 2003. National Assessment of Adult Literacy. http://nces.ed.gov/pubsearch/pubsinfo.asp?pubid=2007480 (accessed December 2012).

Larson, C., Nelson, E., Gustafson, D., and Batalden, P. (1996). The relationship between meeting patients' information needs and their satisfaction with hospital care and general health status outcomes. *International Journal for Quality in Health Care* **8**: 447–456.

de Leeuw, E. (2012). The political ecosystem of health literacies. *Health Promotion International* **27** (1): 1–4.

Lewin, S., Sea, Z., Entwhistle, V. et al. (2001). Interventions for providers to promote a patient-centred approach in clinical consultations. *Cochrane Database of Systematic Reviews* (4): CD003267.

Linder, N., Menzies, D., Kelly, J. et al. (2003). Coaching for behaviour change in chronic disease: a review of the literature and the implications for coaching as a self-management intervention. *Australian Journal of Primary Health* **9**: 177–185.

Livingston, R. and Dunning, T. (2010). Practice nurses' role and knowledge about diabetes management within rural and remote Australian general practices. *European Diabetes Nursing* **7**: 55–61.

MacKeracher, D. (1996). *Making Sense of Adult Learning*. Toronto: Culture Concepts.

Mayo Clinic (2009). Diabetes Medication Choice Decision Aids Cards. www.mayoclinic.org. news2009-rst/5454. html (accessed December 2012).

McCormack, L., Bann, C., Squiers, L. et al. (2010). Measuring health literacy: a pilot study of a news skills-based instrument. *Journal of Health Communication* **15**: 51–71.

McKenna, K., Tooth, L., King, D. et al. (2003). Older patients request more information: a survey for use of written patient education materials in general practice. *Australian Journal on Aging* **22** (1): 15–19.

Morris, A., Boyle, D., McMahon, A. et al. (1997). Adherence to insulin treatment, glycaemic control, and ketoacidosis in insulin-dependent diabetes mellitus. *Lancet* **350**: 1505–1510.

National Health Service (2014). Shared Decision Making Programme. https://www.england.nhs.uk/wp-content/uploads/2013/08/2sdm-let-stke.pdf.

National Public Health Institute of Helsinki (2007). *The Goal Lifestyle Implementation Trial*. Finland: Helsinki.

Negarandeh, R., Oskouie, F., Ahmandi, F. et al. (2006). Patient advocacy: barriers and facilitators. *BMC Nursing* **5**: 3. https://doi.org/10.1186/1472–6955-5–3.

Norman, C. and Skinner, H. (2006). The eHEALS: health literacy scale. *International Medicine Internet Research* **8**: e27.

Nutbeam, D. (2000). Health literacy as a public health goal: a challenge for contemporary health education and communication strategies into the 21st century. *Health Promotion International* **15**: 259–267.

O'Connor, A., Stacey, D., Entwistle, V. et al. (2003). Decision aids for people facing health treatment or screening decisions. *Cochrane Database of Systematic Reviews* (2): CD001431.

O'Connor, A., Wennberg, J., Legare, F. et al. (2007). Toward the 'tipping point': decision aids and informed patient choice. *Health Affairs* **26** (3): 716–725.

Ospina, N., Phillips, K., Rodriguez-Gutirrez, R. et al. (2018). Eliciting the patient's agenda. Secondary analysis of recorded clinical encounters. *Journal of General Internal Medicine*. https://doi.org/10.1007/s11606-018-4540-5.

Parikh, N., Parker, R., Nuss, J. et al. (1996). Shame and health literacy: the unspoken connection. *Patient Education and Counselling* **17**: 33–39.

Parker, R. (1998). Health literacy: a challenge for American patients and their health care providers. *Health Promotion International* **15** (4): 277–283.

Parkin, T. and Skinner, T. (2003). Discrepancies between patient and professionals' recall and perception of an outpatient consultation. *Diabetic Medicine* **20**: 909–914.

Phelps, K. and Hassad, C. (2011). *General Practice: The Integrative Approach*. Sydney: Elsevier.

Pimouguet, C., Le Goff, M., Thiébaut, R. et al. (2011). Effectiveness of disease-management programs for improving diabetes care: a meta-analysis. *CMAJ* **183** (2): E115–E127.

Plank, J., Kohler, G., Rakovac, I. et al. (2004). Long term evaluation of a structured outpatient education programme for intensified insulin therapy in patients with type 1 diabetes: a 12-year follow up. *Diabetologia* **47**: 1370–1375.

Prochaska, J. and DiClemente, C. (1983). Stages and processes of self-change of smoking: toward an integrative model of change. *Journal of Consulting and Clinical Psychology* **51** (3): 390–395.

Rasmussen, B., O'Connell, D., and Dunning, T. (2007). Young women with type 1 diabetes management of turning points and transitions. *Qualitative Health Research* **17** (3): 300–310.

Redman, B. (2001). *The Practice of Patient Education*. Toronto: Mosby.

Rushford, N., Murphy, B., Worcester, M. et al. (2007). Recall of information received in hospital by female cardiac patients. *European Journal of Cardiovascular Prevention & Rehabilitation* **14** (3): 463–469.

Sarkar, U., Fisher, L., and Schillinger, D. (2006). Is self-efficacy associated with diabetes self-management across race/ethnicity and health literacy? *Diabetes Care* **29** (4): 823–829.

Savage, S., Dunning, T., Duggan, N., and Martin, P. (2012). The experiences and care preferences of people with diabetes at the end of life. *Journal of Hospice and Palliative Nursing* **14**: 293–302.

Schulman-Green, D., Jaser, S., and Martin, F. (2012). Processes of self-management in chronic illness. *Journal of Nursing Scholarship* **44**: 136–144.

Schwarz, P., Felton, A.M., Cobble, M. et al. (2012). Differences in patient and clinician perspectives in T2DM: The MOTIVATE global survey. Poster 966 presented at the European Association for the Study of Diabetes (EASD) Annual Conference (2012), Berlin.

Silverman, J., Kurtz, S., and Draper, J. (2018). *Skills for Communicating with Patients*, 18–19. London, UK: CRC Press.

Skinner, T. (2013). Making choices, setting goals. Chapter 4. In: *Diabetes Education: Art, Science and Evidence* (ed. T. Dunning), 49–61. Chichester, UK: Wiley Blackwell.

Skinner, T., Barnard, K., Craddock, S., and Parkin, T. (2007). Patient and health professional accuracy of recalled treatment decisions in out-patient consultations. *Diabetic Medicine* **24**: 557–550.

Speight, J. (2013). Managing diabetes and preventing complications: what makes the difference? *Medical Journal of Australia* **198** (1): 16–17.

Speight, J., Conn, J., Dunning, T., and Skinner, T. (2012). Diabetes Australia position statement: a new language for diabetes improving communication with and about people with diabetes. *Diabetes Research and Clinical Practice* **97**: 425–531.

Steiger, B. (2006). Survey results: doctors say morale is hurting. *Physician Executive* **32** (6): 6–15.

Sweetland, J., Volmert, A., and O'Neil, M. (2017). *Finding the Frame: An Empirical Approach to Reframing Aging and Ageism*. FrameWorks Institute.

Tankova, T., Dakovska, G., and Koev, D. (2001). Education of diabetic patients – a one year experience. *Patient Education and Counselling* **45**: 139–145.

Thomas, N. (2001). The importance of culture throughout life and beyond. Holistic nursing practice. *The Science of Health and Healing* **15** (2): 40–46.

Toobert, D., Hampson, S., and Glasgow, R. (2000). The summary of diabetes self-care activities measure: results from 7 studies and a revised scale. *Diabetes Care* **23**: 943–950.

Vaag, A., Handberg, M., Lauritzen, J. et al. (1990). Variation in absorption of NPH insulin due to intramuscular injection. *Diabetes Care* **13** (1): 74–76.

Vainieri, M., Querciola, C., Maccari, M. et al. (2018). Reported experience of patients with single or multiple chronic diseases: empirical evidence from Italy. *BMC Health Services Research* **18** (659). https://doi.org/10.1186/s12913-018-3431-0.

Vale, M., Jelinek, M., Best, J. et al. (2003). Coaching patients on achieving cardiovascular health (COACH): a multicenter randomized trial in patients with coronary heart disease. *Archives of Internal Medicine* **163**: 2775–2783.

Wagner, E., Austin, B., and von Korff, M. (1996). Organizing Care for Patients with chronic illness. *The Milbank Quarterly* **74** (4): 511–544.

Wagner, E., Davis, C., Schaefer, J. et al. (2002). A survey of leading chronic disease management programs: are they consistent with the literature? *Journal of Nursing Care Quality* **16** (2): 67–80.

de Walt, D., Berkman, N., Sheridan, S. et al. (2004). Literacy and health outcomes: a systematic review of the literature. *Journal of General Internal Medicine* **19**: 1228–1239.

Wegner, D. and Ward, A. (2013). The internet has become the external hard drive for our memories. *Scientific American* https://doi.org/10.1038/scientificamerican 1213-58.

Weiss, B. (2007). Assessing health literacy in clinical practice. Medscape. http://www.medscape.com/viewprogram/802_pnt (accessed November 2007).

Wilkins, S. (2012a). What's behind the patient satisfaction, doc communication disconnect. Hospital Impact. http://www.hospitalimpact.org/index.php/2012/10/17/p4147#more4147 (accessed December 2012).

Wilkins, S. (2012b). Patient engagement is the holy grail of health care. http://www.kevinmd.com/blog/2012/patient-engagement.holy-grail-health-care.html (accessed January 2012).

Woodcock, A. and Kinmonth, A. (2001). Patient concerns in their first year with type 2 diabetes: patient and practice nurse views. *Patient Education and Counseling* **42**: 257–270.

World Health Organization (WHO) (2003). *Adherence to Long Term Therapies: Evidence for Action*. Geneva: WHO.

Yki-Jarvinen, H., Juurinen, L., Alvarsson, M. et al. (2007). Initiate insulin by aggressive titration and educate (INITIATE). *Diabetes Care* **30**: 1364–1369.

Young, D., Furler, J., Vale, M. et al. (2007). Patient Engagement and Coaching for Health: the PEACH study – a cluster randomised controlled trial using the telephone to coach people with type 2 diabetes to engage with their GPs to improve diabetes care. *BMC Family Practice* **8** (20): 8–13.

Further reading

Broom, D. and Whittaker, A. (2003). Controlling diabetes: moral language in the management of type 2 diabetes. *Social Science and Medicine* **58**: 2371–2382.

DAFNE Study Group (2002). Training in flexible, intensive insulin management to enable dietary freedom in people with type 1 diabetes: Dosage Adjustment for Normal Eating (DAFNE) randomised controlled trial. *British Medical Journal* **325**: 746–751.

Dunning, T. (2013). *Diabetes Education: Art, Science and Evidence*. Chichester, UK: Wiley Blackwell.

Felder, R.M. and Silverman, L.K. (1988). Learning and teaching styles in engineering education. *Engineering Education* **78** (7): 674–681. (The article that originally defined the Felder–Silverman model and identified teaching practices that should meet the needs of students with the full spectrum of styles. The paper is preceded by a 2002 preface that states and explains changes in the model that have been made since 1988).

Makoul, G. (2001). Essential elements of communication in medical encounters: the Kalamazoo consensus statement. *Academic Medicine* **76**: 390–393.

Page, P., Verstraete, D., Robb, J., and Etzwiler, D. (1981). Patient recall of self-care recommendations in diabetes. *Diabetes Care* **4**: 96–98.

Parker, R., Baker, D., Williams, M., and Nuss, J. (1999). The test of functional health literacy in adults (TOFHLA): a new instrument for measuring patients' literacy skills. *Journal of General Internal Medicine* **10**: 537–545.

Partnership for Clear Health Communication (2006). What is Health Literacy? http://www.p4chc.org/health-literacy.aspx (accessed October 2007).

Chapter 17

Managing Diabetes at the End of Life

Dying is a normal part of life. Each person experiences and interprets dying differently.

(Person with diabetes at the end of life).

Dying should be a primary diagnosis

(Hilton et al. 2013).

Key points

- Palliative care can be implemented at any appropriate time throughout the person's life journey with diabetes.
- Palliative care focuses on promoting comfort and quality of life, which encompasses avoiding burdensome monitoring, managing unpleasant symptoms and addressing spirituality and religious cultural needs to help individuals achieve a 'good death', and supporting carers.
- It is essential that the individual and their family are involved in care decisions so that care can be personalised and individualised.
- Proactive planning for palliative and end of life and documenting an advance care plan helps manage uncertainty. Planning could be incorporated into annual diabetes complication screening processes and at other key points in the individual's life journey, e.g. before admission to a care home.
- Advance care plans are documents that describe the person's values, priorities and preferences for future care to be used if the person cannot decide for themselves. They often also name a medical treatment decision-maker (surrogate decision-maker) who can make decisions on their behalf. Clearly documented values help guide such decisions.
- Hyper- and hypoglycaemia contribute to the distressing symptoms associated with end-of-life care, but their presence and significance is often underrecognised.
- Blood glucose monitoring can help identify hypo- and hyperglycaemia and enable appropriate treatment and symptom management.
- The blood glucose range and medicine regimen should be individualised and adjusted as needed, sometimes frequently. Nonmedicine options and deprescribing where possible, should be a priority, especially in the terminal and end of life stages.

Care of People with Diabetes: A Manual for Healthcare Practice, Fifth Edition. Trisha Dunning and Alan Sinclair.
© 2020 John Wiley & Sons Ltd. Published 2020 by John Wiley & Sons Ltd.

- Psychological and spiritual care is central to dignified end-of-life care.
- Care and support must also be available to carers who often derive positive benefits from providing care, but also experience stress from witnessing a loved one suffer, and who may have health issues, themselves.

Introduction

Although life expectancy has increased in the past 20 years, diabetes is associated with significant morbidity and mortality and is among the top 10 leading causes of death globally, along with cancer, lung disease, and cardiovascular disease (McEwen et al. 2006; IDF 2017; World Health Organisation (WHO) 2018). Palliative care, especially at the end of life, focuses on maintaining comfort and quality of life, minimising unpleasant symptoms, providing effective, timely pain management, and providing spiritual and psychological support to the individual and their family.

In order to achieve these goals, the effects of diabetes and its complications on life expectancy and impact at the end of life need to be considered. These include hypo- and hyperglycaemia on comfort and well-being (Diabetes UK 2018; Dunning et al. 2010, 2018). Palliative care is applicable for people with chronic diseases and other life-limiting illnesses and can be used with usual care (the World Palliative Care Alliance (WPCA)/WHO 2014) throughout the illness trajectory (Fjose et al. 2018) if it is consistent with the individual's values and care preferences (e.g. when a person with diabetes develops a complication such as renal disease and/or the disease progresses to end-stage renal disease requiring dialysis).

It is imperative that palliative and end-of-life care is individualised and agreed in consultation with the person with diabetes and their family, when relevant. As indicated, dying is a normal part of the life trajectory. Encouraging people with diabetes to proactively plan for palliative and end-of-life care could and should be part of routine diabetes care and complication screening processes (Dunning and Martin 2018; Dunning et al. 2018). In fact, implementing a palliative approach early could improve people with diabetes' quality of life and disease management (Department of Health and Ageing 2006; Sudore et al. 2012; Diabetes UK 2018).

However, 80% of people are admitted to hospital in the last year of their life, and many spend 30 or more days in hospital (Goldsbury et al. 2015). Significantly, 55% die in hospital, 12% are admitted to intensive care (ICU), and only 24% receive palliative care. Over 20 years ago, Bowling (1983) stated that most people want to die at home but most in hospital for medical reasons. Things have not changed a great deal in that time: most people still want to die at home but 50–70% of people still die in hospital (Sweriessen and Duckett 2014; Dying Matters 2017).

Timely conversations about palliative care, advance care planning, and regarding people having a 'good death' as success rather than seeing death as failure could help many people with diabetes die in their place of choice and without undue suffering.

Explanation of terms: values, life limiting illness, palliative care, terminal care, and end-of-life care

Values

Values refers to the things in a person's life that are important to them and give meaning and purpose to their life. They guide individuals' attitudes, behaviours, and decisions. People consider their values when making important decisions (Witte and Allen 2000). Once values are established, they do not change a great deal throughout life, unlike care preferences, which can and do change, and need to be reassessed on a regular basis.

Life-limiting illness

The term *life-limiting illness* refers to people likely to die in the subsequent 12 months. The Gold Standards Framework Proactive Identification Guidance (PIG) (GSF) (2016) describes indicators for declining life expectancy for cancer, chronic obstructive pulmonary disease, heart failure, renal disease, neurological diseases, frailty, dementia, and stroke. Diabetes is not mentioned in the Gold Standards Framework (GSF) but it is the main underlying cause of renal disease and cardiovascular disease and is associated with some forms of cancer, frailty, and dementia.

Diabetes-related indicators of declining life expectancy include:

- Duration of diabetes and multimorbidity (Botes et al. 2018).
- Glucose variability (high and low blood glucose levels) and rapid reduction in HbA1c (Krinsley 2008; Huang et al. 2011; Iglay et al. 2016).
- Severe hypoglycaemia (Hsu et al. 2012; Cryer 2015; Sicar et al. 2016) especially people on sulphonylureas and insulin with hypoglycaemic unawareness (Chapter 6).
- Lower limb and foot disease (Iversen et al. 2017; Ndosi et al. 2017).
- Polypharmacy (Jyrkkä et al. 2009).
- Comorbid depression (American Diabetes Association 2017) and suicide ideation. The severity of depression influences suicidal ideation. Suicide is twice as common in people >age 74 (Alexopoulos 2005).

Other indicators of declining life expectancy include:

- Decline in health and function.
- Unplanned hospital admissions.
- Symptoms are difficult to manage and the person becomes less responsive to treatment.
- Person chooses not to accept active treatment.
- >10 kg progressive weight loss in the preceding six months.
- Serum albumin <25 g/l (GSF 2016).
- Person relies on carers for support to undertake diabetes self-care and activities of daily living (GSF 2016; Murray et al. 2017).
- Person has declining will to live and self-rated future health, e.g. in five years (Karppinen et al. 2012).

Palliative care

Dying is normal, and it is important to be able to recognise when people are dying. Implementing palliative care signifies a transition from a curative approach to managing comfort and quality of life to achieve a dignified death. It still enables active treatment and usual care. Many older people with diabetes could benefit from combining palliative care into their usual diabetes care.

> An approach that improves the quality of life of patients and their families facing the problems associated with life-threatening illness, through prevention and relief of suffering by means of early identification and impeccable assessment and treatment of pain and other problems, physical, psychosocial, and spiritual.
>
> World Health Organization (WHO) 2005.

Terminal and end-of-life care

Terminal care refers to the last 12 months of life and end of life includes imminent death in a few hours or days. Recognising dying is essential to decide when to act on the individual's advance care directive (ACD) and deliver comprehensive compassionate terminal care

(Palliative Aged Care Evidence (pall*i*AGED) 2019). Dying may be a slow process due to modern technology and treatment (Murtagh et al. 2004), and prognostication is difficult. Signs that the person is entering the terminal stage were described under the GSF indicators of declining life expectancy. Signs the person could be actively dying include being bed-bound, dysphagia, reduced response to stimuli, oliguria, Cheyne-Stokes respirations (the death rattle), and peripheral shutdown.

The specific care will depend on where the person dies (hospital, home, hospice, or aged-care facility). Managing symptoms to promote comfort is important in all settings, including managing pain and stopping unnecessary medicines. Subcutaneous medicine may not be absorbed if the person has peripheral shutdown and other dose forms may be needed. Explaining the signs of death and reassuring the family can reduce stress.

Palliative care outcomes collaborative palliative care stages

Palliative care outcomes collaborative (PCOC) described five stages: stable, unstable, deteriorating, terminal, bereavement (Palliative Care Outcomes Collaborative (PCOC) 2018); see Table 17.1.

General goals of palliative care

The aim of palliative care is to improve quality of life, relieve suffering, and manage distressing symptoms. Palliative care can be used at any time and can complement usual diabetes care. Palliative care should be commenced early for maximum benefit (Murtagh et al. 2004; WHO 2014; Murray et al. 2017). Early palliative care also increases satisfaction with care, function, and life expectancy (Parker et al. 2016). The ethical and legal aspects of care and relevant legislation, polices, and guidelines should be considered when deciding palliative and end-of-life care with people with diabetes to achieve the following broad goals:

- Engage in sensitive and effective communication about the person's disease process, disease course, possible outcomes, and likely prognosis in a timely manner.
- Help the individuals and their family to document their values, care goals and preferences, and the care they do not want to receive in an advance care directive, and appoint a medical treatment decision-maker (sometimes known as a surrogate decision-maker) at an appropriate time.
- Improve and/or maintain dignity, function, independence, and quality of life consistent with the individual's values goals and preferences.
- Provide psychological support to the individual and their family/carers.
- Manage pain and other symptoms.
- In the later stages and during periods of instability, it is important to review management and life goals, provide relevant information, adjust the management and self-care regimens, and make relevant referrals where indicated.
- Achieve a dignified death in the individual's place of choice and according to their values, cultural, spiritual, and religious beliefs and customs.
- Provide support for families during palliative care and after the individual dies.

Advance care planning and advance care directive

Advance care planning refers to the process used to proactively discuss and document an advance care directive that describes an individual's values, goals, and care preferences and the care they would not choose, if they are unable to make an autonomous decision. Various terms and legislation and policies describe these processes in different countries and even within countries. Clinicians need to be familiar with the laws and regulations in the country/organisations where they practice. If planning commences early, it does not need to be hurried or cause undue stress.

Table 17.1 Palliative care outcome collaborative (PCOC) (2018) stages of the dying process and issues health professionals could consider in each stage applied to diabetes.

PCOC stage	Characteristics of the PCOC stage	Brief overview of essential care considerations in addition to managing diabetes
Stable	Includes everybody not in the other four stages. Metabolic status is managed according to an individualised care plan and individualised targets. Symptom burden is managed. Medicines management is reviewed to reduce the medicine burden. The stable period may last for months or years and may become unstable, e.g. during an intercurrent illness such as the flu, or the development/worsening of a complication and then revert to stable.	Undertake a proactive risk assessment for hypo-and hyperglycaemia and their consequences as well as other key risk screening such as cardiovascular risk and malnutrition risk, which can contribute to the symptom burden and affect health status. Determine whether the person has an ACD and other relevant documentation such as a will, enduring power of attorney, or medical treatment decision-maker. Consider future symptom and medicine burden and plan to implement an early palliative approach with the individual and their family/carers. Ensure the person knows how to manage intercurrent illnesses and knows how and when to seek advice early: has a sick-day-care plan that encompasses palliative and end-of-life-care situations. Include family/carers in education sessions.
Unstable	A new, sometimes unexpected, problem or a rapid increase in the severity of existing problem/s such as progression of renal disease or a cardiovascular event occurs and causes metabolic instability. Symptom burden usually increases during the acute episode. Family/carers may need to provide assistance with diabetes self-care and medicine management and other activities of daily living when the person is at home and should be supported to do so in hospitals and hospices.	Decide whether the episode is remediable and treatable or is likely to deteriorate towards the terminal stage. Adjust management plan to manage the metabolic derangement and associated symptom burden and underlying cause. Decide whether the condition can be stabilised or will proceed to the deteriorating stage. If the condition stabilises, review the management plan and future plans for a palliative approach/ care and ACD. Determine family/carers' capacity to care for/ support the individual and whether they need education and support.
Deteriorating	The person's condition rapidly or gradually worsens and they often develop new problems and increased symptom burden. Medicines may be a cause of or contribute to the symptom burden, e.g. when another medicine is prescribed to manage a medicine side effect; thus, pharmacovigilance is essential and deprescribing might be required (Chapter 5).	Refer to dignity therapy programmes if they are available. If indicated, implement the person's ACP. Address the family/carer's needs. Decide when to withdraw treatment.
Terminal and end-of-life care	Terminal often refers to the last 12 months of life and end of life to the last few weeks or days.	Palliative care should be continued to manage symptoms and promote quality of life and a dignified death. Recognise when the person is dying. Follow the person's wishes in their ACD. If there is no ACD, family/carers should be consulted. Arrange for cultural and religious care if relevant and ensure religious conventions regarding treatment of the body after death are adhered to (Healthcare Chaplaincy 2009; The Joint Commission 2010). Support the family/carers and explain what is happening carefully. Declare death compassionately.
Bereaved	The family/carers usually grieve when their loved one dies.	Implement bereavement support or other counselling as needed, for example, their healthcare and risks in the first 12 months, e.g. infections.

ACD = advanced care directive.

People need time to think about these things and consider the risks and benefits for them. Helping them is a rare privilege:

> *Nobody ever asked me about that* [planning for end of life]; *we talk about my diabetes. Thank you for this great gift to me and my family* (person with diabetes documenting her ACD).

Thus, helping people with diabetes develop an ACD is an important aspect of holistic diabetes care because:

> In the absence of a formal visible record of resident's wishes [older people in care homes] places an onerous burden on health care professionals to preserve life, when that may not be the preference of the person or their families.
>
> (Allen and Barnett 2011)

Palliative care and diabetes

Diabetes is prevalent in most countries and is associated with increased morbidity and mortality and some forms of cancer. Likewise, people with diabetes with long-term complications of diabetes such as end-stage renal disease and cardiovascular disease could benefit from palliative care (Emanuel et al. 2004; Burge 2012; Diabetes UK 2018; Dunning and Martin 2018). There is limited research to guide diabetes palliative and end-of-life care due to the vulnerability of people at the end of life and the burden and ethical issues involved in participating in research. Thus, existing guidelines such as Dunning et al. (2010, 2018) and Diabetes UK (2018) are based on the best available evidence and the consensus opinion of experts. These diabetes-specific guidelines can be used with other palliative care guidelines.

Dunning et al. (2010) developed a guiding philosophy as the conceptual framework for their guidelines. The philosophy was derived from the available literature, publicly available narratives written by dying people or relatives, and, significantly, interviews with people with diabetes at their end of life and their families (Savage et al. 2012), and the quality use of medicines framework (QUM) (Department of Health, 2009; National Prescribing Service and Palliative Care Australia 2009) because pharmacovigilance is imperative, especially in palliative and end-of-life situations (Chapter 5).

Key issues in palliative and end-of-life care

Deciding optimal diabetes-related end-of-life care is challenging because of the multifactorial, interrelated issues that need to be considered. Table 17.2 outlines some of these issues concerning diabetes. Diabetes may be the underlying cause of symptoms or contribute to or exacerbate symptoms (Quinn et al. 2006; Dunning 2012). Monitoring blood glucose to detect hyper-and hypoglycaemia can help identify the cause of some symptoms, yet many health professionals regard blood glucose monitoring at the end of life and using glucose-lowering medicines (GLM), especially insulin, as intrusive and inappropriate curative management (Quinn et al. 2006).

However, people with diabetes regard these care aspects as a vital part of appropriate end-of-life care (Savage et al. 2012, Royal College of General Practitioners and Diabetes Australia, 2016). Blood glucose monitoring and using GLMs is consistent with the WHO definition of palliative care and the focus on 'early identification and impeccable assessment'. Likewise, using insulin to reduce hyperglycaemia and its symptoms and risks is consistent with symptom management to promote comfort in palliative care. In this case, insulin is used with palliative intent rather than to achieve tight blood glucose control.

Many people want to die at home and be cared for by their family: but changed family roles mean that is not always possible. Families often prefer hospital/hospice care because 'it preserves personal boundaries of social intimacy' because health professionals deliver care in hospital/hospice settings (Bloomer 2012). Likewise, not all dying people require specialised palliative care

Table 17.2 The relationship between common symptoms encountered in people receiving palliative care, the possible impact on diabetes, and management and/or be diabetes-related.

Common palliative care symptoms	Possible impact on diabetes and its management	May be diabetes-related
Pain (acute/chronic)	Can increase: – Somnolence or confusion/cognitive impairment/ delirium due to pain/analgesic medicines – Risk of hyperventilation – Hyperglycaemia Reduced: – Intake – Mobility – Sleep – Self-care ability – Quality of life	– Peripheral vascular disease – Amyotrophy – Peripheral neuropathy – Myocardial infarction (MI) – Tissue glycosylation (e.g. carpel tunnel syndrome) – Ketoacidosis (abdominal pain)
Depression/anxiety	Can increase: – Fatigue – Lethargy, change in performance status – Risk of diabetic ketoacidosis (DKA), hyperglycaemia hyperosmolar states (HHS) – Social isolation Reduced: – Self-care ability, disinterest, increased risk of hyperglycaemia – Confidence – Inadequate nutrition, increased risk of hypoglycaemia – Communication capacity and self-care – May be suicide risk	– Associated with diabetes, especially hyperglycaemia – Renal disease – Corticosteroid medicines – Hypoglycaemia symptoms can be mistaken for anxiety
Oral pathology (oral and maxillofacial pathology) Mucositis, ulcers, dry mouth	Can increase: – Pain – Dry mouth – Inadequate nutrition, inappropriate weight loss, cachexia, hypoglycaemia if on GLM/insulin Reduced: – Intake – Self-care deficits – Mood	– DKA and HHS may lead to dry mouth, thirst, and clinical dehydration – Risk of dental caries and oral pathology – Risk of hypoglycaemia if on GLM or insulin
Nausea/vomiting	Can increase: – Confusion – Lethargy – Disinterest – Pain/discomfort – Inadequate nutrition → weight loss, cachexia, hyperglycaemia – Hypoglycaemia if on GLM/insulin – Dehydration and electrolyte imbalance – Risk of ketoacidosis/hyperosmolar states Can reduce: – Intake – Energy, depleted energy stores	– May be due to gastric autonomic neuropathy – Renal disease – Hyperglycaemia – DKA, HHS – Medicines: Metformin – Byetta
Delirium	Increased: – Cognitive impairment Reduced: – Ability to communicate and detect signs/ symptoms of hypo/hyperglycaemia – Self-care ability	– May be due to many factors, including hyper- and hypoglycaemia, dehydration, and medicines

(Continued)

Table 17.2   (Continued)

Common palliative care symptoms	Possible impact on diabetes and its management	May be diabetes-related
Sepsis	Can increase: – Pain – Hyperglycaemia – Symptoms, e.g. polyuria	– May be the cause of the admission and may be silent in diabetes, e.g. urinary tract infection (UTI) and MI

Acute dyspnoea	Can increase:
	– Hypoxia contributing to confusion, anxiety
	Reduce:
	– Self-management capacity
		– May precipitate DKA or HHS and increase:
		  ○ Confusion
		  ○ Energy requirements
		  ○ Pain
		– Difficulty interpreting elevated white cell count, which could be caused by hyperglycaemia, sepsis, or other factors
		– Bone marrow failure
		– Reduced:
		  ○ Intake increased DKA, HHS risk
		  ○ Quality of life
		  ○ Wound healing

Diabetes emergencies	– Hypoglycaemia – Hyperglycaemia – DKA and HHS – MI, which is often atypical and/or silent – Renal failure	– Hypoglycaemia – DKA, HHS, lactic acidosis, which contribute to delirium, especially in older people
Oncology emergencies	– Spinal cord compression (corticosteroids) and acute immobility – Superior vena clava (SVC) obstruction (acute dyspnoea and delirium) – High dose of corticosteroids – Febrile neutropenia – Major bronchial obstruction (dyspnoea and use of corticosteroids)	– Hypoglycaemia – DKA, HHS, lactic acidosis

Source: Dunning et al. (2010) with permission
HHS: hyperglycaemic hyperosmolar states. GLM: glucose-lowering medicines.

services, although they could benefit from palliative care to ensure symptoms and pain are managed and ACP are documented (Pesut et al. 2012; Sudore et al. 2012).

Diabetes experts could proactively prepare themselves and people with diabetes and families for palliative care by initiating conversations about advance care planning during regular diabetes assessment, management, and monitoring processes. This does not appear to happen at present. The majority of people with diabetes do not have an ACD or other relevant documents. Likewise, addressing symptom burden and palliative care is not included in most current diabetes management guidelines, exceptions being Diabetes UK (2018) and Dunning et al. (2018). Dunning and Martin (2018) developed three pieces of tailored information for older people with diabetes, families and clinicians, in close consultation with older people with diabetes that can help all parties start conversations.

The Choosing Wisely Program (American Board of Internal Medicine 2012) has been widely adopted globally. It describes five issues that physicians (and other clinicians) and patients should question:

(1) Order diagnostic test to answer specific questions not routinely at regular intervals.
(2) Avoid red blood cell transfusion in patients in ICU with haemoglobin >7 mg/dl who are haemodynamically stable.

(3) Do not use parenteral nutrition in critically ill patients in ICU in the first seven days if they are not malnourished.

(4) Only sedate mechanically ventilated patients if there is a specific reason. If sedation is indicated, clinicians should try to reduce sedation each day.

(5) Life support should be ceased if the patient has a high likelihood of dying and/or severe functional deficits and low likelihood of recovery without discussing palliative comfort care with the family.

Interestingly, there is no suggestion to check whether the person has an ACD before implementing resuscitative therapy. A programme (iValidate) to enhance clinicians competence and willingness to discuss palliative care planning with people in hospital unlikely to benefit from admission to ICU resulted in increased ACDs and fewer people choose recitation as a care goal, but admission rates to ICU did not change (Orford et al. 2019).

People with diabetes often carry a high symptom burden, including acute and chronic pain, fatigue, constipation, nausea, lethargy, insomnia, anxiety, and depression (Sudore et al. 2012). The symptom burden was more prevalent in people with short survival expectancy in Sudore et al.'s study, but was evident in all stages of the diabetes life trajectory (n = 13 71 aged 30–74; mean age 60). Interestingly, Sudore et al. did not report other uncomfortable symptoms associated with hyperglycaemia such as thirst, dry mouth and hypoglycaemic symptoms, which distress people with diabetes (Savage et al. 2012) and contribute to the symptom burden and underlie many of the symptoms Sudore et al. described.

The symptom burden is often overlooked in the imperative to achieve glycaemic and other targets. As indicated, managing symptoms is paramount in end-of-life care but should be considered throughout the chronic disease trajectory, not only at the end of life (Morrison and Meter 2004). Recognising and managing hypo- and hyperglycaemia-related symptoms in a timely manner is important to people with diabetes and can reduce the symptom burden (Savage et al. 2012).

People who are dying expect clinicians to respect 'their ways of being', their dignity and autonomy, and understand time is precious at the end of life. They find waiting for appointments and test results distressing and want some indication of 'how much time they have left' in order to put their affairs in order (Pesut et al. 2012). People also want health professionals to deliver care without being intrusive and work with and support their family carers. In addition, people want some general 'signposts' (cues) to help them recognise when they are entering the deteriorating stage to enable them to make realistic decisions about dying (Pesut et al. 2012; Dunning and Martin 2018). Loss of privacy during the dying process, especially in hospitals/hospices, but also at home, is a concern for some people.

Family and carers worry about their lack of knowledge and skills to undertake diabetes self-care when their loved ones require help, and worry about unnecessarily hastening death or causing discomfort and pain (Dunning et al. 2010). Likewise, carer participants in Pesut et al.'s (2012) study indicated clinicians often overestimate their knowledge and that they 'do not know what questions to ask [clinicians]'. Thus, educating family carers and helping them ask pertinent questions is part of supportive, personalised palliative and end-of-life care.

General management considerations for managing diabetes at the end of life

Diabetes management should be integrated into the overall palliative care plan (or vice versa) and should be a collaborative process among relevant diabetes and palliative care clinicians and other clinicians where relevant:

- Provide individualised personalised care that includes preparing an ACP, identifying cultural, religious, and spiritual beliefs, and customs that influence how palliative care, death and care of the body, and family/carers after death should be managed.

- Communicate with the individual and their family/carers and among health professionals throughout the palliative care journey.
- Identify and manage preexisting diabetes and diabetes complications that affect management decisions, such as medicines choices when renal and liver disease are present and can contribute to pain and discomfort. In addition, corticosteroid-induced hyperglycaemia is common in palliative care situations, in people with preexisting diabetes, and in those with diabetes risk factors (Gannon and Dando 2010; Giovannucci et al. 2010).
- Identify individuals at risk of corticosteroid-induced diabetes when people are admitted to palliative care and/or when steroid medicines are prescribed, detecting diabetes early, and managing diabetes that develops following corticosteroid use (Dunning 1996).
- Identify risk of and developing strategies to reduce episodes of and manage hypoglycaemia, which can be individually or collectively related to GLMs, low hepatic glucose reserves, particularly if the individual is malnourished or has hepatic metastases, renal impairment, or malabsorption due to gastrointestinal disturbance, to anorexia, and cachexia syndrome.
- Choose safe, effective medicines and medicine regimen to achieve optimal glycaemic targets for the individual and the PCOC stage. Renal and hepatic function is often altered and gastrointestinal disturbance and impaired glucose absorption is common, which, along with the prognosis and the individual's care decisions, influences medicine choices. Many oral GLM might be contraindicated and insulin might be a safer, simpler option, but only consensus evidence is available (Australian Diabetes Society (ADS) 2012; Diabetes UK 2018; Dunning et al. 2018).
- Provide adequate nutrition and hydration.
- Avoid diabetes-related emergencies such as ketoacidosis, hyperosmolar states, lactic acidosis, and severe hypoglycaemia (Chapters 6 and 7).
- Decide when to withdraw treatment and activate the Liverpool Care Pathway when the individual is dying (Ellershaw and Murphy 2005).
- Support spiritual growth. Spirituality is difficult to define and is a broader concept than religion, although it might encompass religion, and refers to the transformational process of finding meaning and purpose in life and an inner sense of coherence and resilience (Parsian and Dunning 2009; Koren and Papamiditriou 2013). Spirituality enables people to positively cope with life stressors. Significantly, people can find meaning and purpose in life when they are dying. However, people's spirituality and their connectedness to others can be affected by grief and loss (Puchalski 2011). Spirituality also affects family/carers' ability to cope. The factors that give meaning and purpose to people's lives influences their end-of-life-care decisions. Spirituality should be encompassed in the medical history and regularly evaluated including when there is a change in clinical status. Spiritual distress and depression can overlap and manifest as demoralisation, or people can be depressed and have no hope or become depressed and feel isolated from God (Puchalski 2011). However, people can have spiritual distress without being depressed.

Diabetes-specific considerations

Glycaemic targets

Cardiovascular and renal disease are leading causes of death in people with diabetes; thus, maintaining blood glucose, lipids, and blood pressure within the normal ranges is important to prevent cardiovascular disease and other diabetes complications in the stable phase and improves outcomes in many unstable phases through an individual's journey with diabetes.

Preventing long-term diabetes complications is not a priority of palliative care; however, managing existing complications to manage pain and promote comfort and quality of life and prevent unnecessary admission to hospital is essential.

Opinions differ about the optimal glycaemic target range and blood glucose monitoring frequency in end-of-life care. Targets must be individualised, but generally, aiming for a range between 6 and 11–15 mmol/l (Dunning et al. 2018) and avoiding levels <6 mmol/l and >15 mmol/l

(Diabetes UK 2018) appear reasonable, noting these are consensus targets and there is very little evidence to support them. Likewise, there is no evidence of an optimal HbA1c target, which should be individualised: aiming for ≤8% (64 mmol/mol) might be reasonable, depending on the individual and their health and functional status.

Blood glucose monitoring

Opinions vary about the value of monitoring blood glucose at the end of life: it is important to detect hypo- and hyperglycaemia (because of their effect on comfort and symptom burden), which can be difficult without monitoring blood glucose. Many people with diabetes and their families want their usual blood glucose monitoring regimen continued because it helps them maintain stability at a frightening, uncertain time of life and enables unstable glucose levels to be detected (Dunning et al. 2010; Dunning 2012; Savage et al. 2012). In addition, some people with diabetes and/or their families regard reduced or no blood glucose monitoring as staff 'giving up on them' and feel abandoned.

Some staff are concerned that blood glucose monitoring represents a painful, unnecessary intervention (Quinn et al. 2006), which is interesting, considering the very invasive and painful treatments that are often provided during end-of-life care.

Monitoring frequency should be decided with the individual and according to their end-of-life stage, medicine regimen, and hypo- and hyperglycaemia risk profile. It may not be necessary in the terminal stage.

Hyperglycaemia

Hyperglycaemia causes distressing osmotic symptoms, exacerbates pain, contributes to malnutrition, delirium, and confusion. It reduces mood, problem-solving and decision-making capacity, and quality of life. The symptoms are often attributed to other causes and not appropriately treated. Alternatively, hyperglycaemia can be present without significant symptoms and progress to a diabetes emergency such as ketoacidosis or hyperosmolar states that require urgent care.

Type 2 diabetes is a progressive disease due to loss of beta cell function and declining insulin production and >50% eventually need insulin (Chapter 1). The need may be greater in palliative care situations where medicines and other factors are prohyperglycaemic. Thus, preventing hyperglycaemia can enhance comfort and meet a key palliative care goal. Having an appropriate plan for managing intercurrent illness (sick days) and episodes of hyperglycaemia is as important as an appropriate medicine regimen.

Families/carers may need education about how to recognise and manage hyperglycaemia and what blood glucose levels and symptoms should trigger them to seek clinician. General sick-day management is discussed in Chapter 7, but extra information that encompasses the individuals care goals might be required in palliative situations.

Hypoglycaemia

The risk of hypoglycaemia is increased in palliative situations due to anorexia, malnourishment, liver disease, low glycogen stores, and cachexia syndrome in advanced cancer and a range of other factors (see Chapter 6). Thus, hypoglycaemia risk needs to be considered when deciding medicine management strategies and glycaemic target ranges. Factors that increase hypoglycaemia risk are described in a hypoglycaemia risk assessment tool in Chapter 6, and include:

- GLMs especially sulphonylureas and insulin.
- Medicines can interact with GLMs (see Chapter 5).
- Malnourishment, including cachexia, occurs in 40–90% of the cancer palliative care population.
- Anorexia affects endogenous glucose stores. Some medicine affect appetite and food enjoyment, contributing to the problem.

- Renal and/or liver disease.
- Weight loss.
- Hypoglycaemia unawareness.
- Cognitive impairment and delirium could result from chronic hypoglycaemia, hyperglycaemia, medicines, or dementia.
- Unmanaged pain affects appetite. Adequate pain management is essential and is generally well documented in palliative care plans.
- Fasting for procedures or surgical interventions.
- Health professionals sometimes attribute hypo- or hyperglycaemic coma to other causes such as the dying process.
- Health professional sometimes have incorrect beliefs about an appropriate diabetic diet.

Hypoglycaemia symptoms and management are described in Chapter 6, but symptoms can be atypical, which makes some degree of regular blood glucose monitoring important, especially in high-risk patients.

It is difficult to treat hypoglycaemia when people are anorexic or have nausea or vomiting (McCoubrie et al. 2004; Dunning et al. 2018); thus GLMs are often stopped in people who have hypoglycaemic episodes, which may not be the best management choice because of the resultant hyperglycaemia and its adverse effects. A comprehensive medicine review and managing other underlying hypoglycaemia risk factors is advisable. Educating the individual and family carers (and sometimes clinicians) might also be required, especially if the person's usual hypoglycaemia symptoms change.

The choice of GLM/s, dose and dose frequency needs to be carefully considered and the blood glucose should not fall below 6 mmol/l because of the hypoglycaemia risk (Diabetes UK 2018; Dunning et al. 2018). In addition, dietetic advice can help health professionals and family/carers plan a diet suitable to the individual and provide supplements if necessary to reduce the effects of malnutrition and minimise weight loss.

Medicine management

Pharmacovigilance and adopting a quality use of medicines approach is essential to achieving optimal glycaemic control with minimal risk; see Figure 19.1 and Chapter 5. Pharmacovigilance encompasses proactively monitoring medicines and deprescribing where necessary/possible (Rowett et al. 2012). Pharmacovigilance encompasses QUM, which concerns deciding whether a medicine is needed and selecting medicine options wisely, if a medicine is indicated (National Prescribing Service (NPS) 2009). In addition, medicine choices depend on the prognosis, health status, oral intake, risk profile, and coexisting diseases, as well as the type of diabetes.

Practice points

Insulin:
- Is not a cure for diabetes or any other condition.
- Is essential treatment for people with type 1 diabetes of all ages.
- Is required by most people with type 2 diabetes due to progressive beta cell loss.
- Is an effective way of managing blood glucose levels, including at the end of life, and may be simpler and safer to use than other GLMs and reduce the medicine burden.

Type 1 diabetes

People with type 1 diabetes who are in the stable phase should continue their usual insulin regimens. However, doses should be adjusted if renal disease is present and if weight loss occurs, depending on the eating pattern to avoid hypo- and hyperglycaemia. In the terminal phase, medicines are usually ceased. Generally, basal bolus regimens are used unless contraindicated.

A daily dose of a long-acting insulin analogue and/or small doses of rapid acting insulin when the individual eats might be appropriate in the unstable and deteriorating stages and when nausea, vomiting, and anorexia are present.

However, management in the unstable stage will depend on the likely outcome: recovery and return to the stable phase, or deteriorate. In the former case, an IV insulin infusion might be warranted to manage acute illnesses and during surgical procedures; see Chapters 7 and 9.

Many people use insulin pumps, which enable the insulin regimen to be flexible in changing situations such as palliative care. People who use insulin pumps are very competent at managing their pumps in the stable phase but may need help during other PCOC stages. Basal rates can be set to manage predictable circumstances and to prevent ketosis, and bolus doses can be administered with food or as correctional doses. Health professionals must have the technical expertise and competence to manage insulin pumps, and the advice of expert diabetes health professionals should be sought early.

Blood ketone tests should be performed if the blood glucose is >15 mmol/l, especially if the individual has nausea, vomiting, and signs of dehydration, which could indicate remediable ketoacidosis.

Type 2 diabetes

The individual's GLM regimen can usually be continued in the stable phase, but doses may need to be reduced or insulin initiated to simplify the medicine regimen and/or reduce the risk of hypoglycaemia when the person is at high risk of hypoglycaemia and in the unstable and deteriorating stages. The choice of GLM or GLM combinations depends on the individual's health status and blood glucose pattern. There are different effects of individual medicines within a class, and most have not been systematically evaluated in people receiving palliative care and those at the end of life.

However, gastrointestinal problems and malabsorption syndromes may mean oral GLMs are not absorbed appropriately and will be ineffective.

Metformin

Metformin is the most commonly used oral GLM, especially in overweight people. Renal function needs to be monitored and metformin doses adjusted or the medicine ceased if renal function declines (creatinine >150 mmol/l or eGFR <30 ml/min/1.73 m squared). Metformin might also be contraindicated if the person has risk factors for lactic acidosis (Chapter 7), distressing gastrointestinal symptoms such as nausea and flatulence, and significant weight loss. It contributes to vitamin B_{12} deficiency, which can exacerbate neuropathic pain. The dose usually needs to be reduced or metformin stopped during surgery.

Sulphonylureas

Sulphonylureas are a RED flag for hypoglycaemia.

Sulphonylureas may be contraindicated if renal and/or liver disease is present, if the person is malnourished, and when there is a high risk of hypoglycaemia.

Thiazolididiones

Thiazolididiones are not indicated if liver and/or congestive heart failure is present. They cause oedema, which can cause uncomfortable symptoms. Pioglitazone is contraindicated in people at risk of bladder cancer and people who already have bladder cancer. Some are associated with risk of atypical fractures, especially in women.

Incretins

GLP-1 and DPP-4 analogues may be appropriate, depending on prescribing indications in the relevant country. GLP-1 and sulphonylurea combination increases the risk of hypoglycaemia. GLP-1 often causes nausea and weight loss and may be contraindicated. Both GLP-1 and DPP-4 have been associated with pancreatitis. Thus, they may not be the best choice in people with pancreatic disease and should be stopped if they cause abdominal pain.

Insulin

As indicated, the majority of people with type 2 diabetes eventually require insulin and may already be on insulin when they commence palliative care. Insulin doses are easier to adjust than oral GLMs. Initiating insulin can reduce the tablet burden and simplify the medicine regimen. As indicated, it could be used as a palliative medicine to manage distressing symptoms such as thirst, polyuria, and fatigue.

Sodium-glucose cotransporter-2 inhibitors

There is not enough clinical experience with the sodium-glucose cotransporter-2 inhibitors (SGLT-2) medicines to recommend their use in palliative care situations at present. They are associated with urinary tract and genital infections and polyuria. Some can cause euglycaemic diabetic ketoacidosis (DKA) during surgical procedures, even when the blood glucose is not very high (e.g. dapagliflozin and empagflozin).

Other medicines

Most people with diabetes will also be using antihypertensive and lipid-lowering medicines, and many will be using anticoagulant medicines. The benefits and risks of continuing these medicines need to be considered (Chapters 5 and 8). The gastrointestinal effects of aspirin can be more prominent when the individual is anorexic or using corticosteroids. If these medicines are continued, a proton pump inhibitor or other gastroprotective medicine might be indicated.

Complementary and alternative therapies

Complementary therapies (CM) are discussed in Chapter 18. Many people at the end of life use CM to relieve pain, improve quality of life and manage the spiritual aspects of dying to achieve a good death (free from pain) (Running et al. 2008). CM can also reduce restlessness, agitation, and mental stress. Commonly used CM include:

- Massage, with and without essential oils.
- Music therapy, including thanatology.
- Guided imagery.
- Essential oils in vapourisers, baths or massage.
- Acupuncture.
- Pet therapy: those who know the book, *Making Rounds with Oscar*, by David Dosa (2010) will understand the power of pets at the end of life.
- Meditation.
- Art therapy.
- Reflexology (Horowitz 2009).

However, some CMs can interact with conventional medicines. If they are used, they need to be considered as part of the medicine regimen and monitored in the same way. They should only be used if they are the best, safe evidence-based option.

Nutrition and hydration

People requiring palliative care often have anorexia, cachexia, and dysphagia and at some point will be unable to consume oral food and fluids, which can distress family and carers. Nutrition to sustain energy reserves and provide essential nutrition and fluids needs to be considered on an individual basis and tailored to the palliative care stage. Small, frequent 'meals' (grazing) might be appropriate and acceptable for some people.

People who are actively dying usually do not experience hunger, largely due to the effects of starvation and consequent ketone production; although they may experience thirst. However, thirst is not alleviated by artificial hydration. Comfort care should be provided to manage dry mouth (mouth care) (Kedziera 2001).

The risks and benefits of artificial nutrition need to be carefully considered when it is indicated, including the risk of accelerating death.

Diabetogenetic medicines

Several medicines can cause or exacerbate hyperglycaemia especially antipsychotic medicines, thiazide diuretics and corticosteroids (Chapters 5 and 10). Corticosteroids are an essential part of the management of many disease processes such as haematological malignancies, inflammatory diseases, chronic obstructive pulmonary disease (COPD), allergies and shock, and are commonly used in palliative care to manage symptoms, often dexamethasone or prednisolone.

However, long-term use and high doses of corticosteroids cause hyperglycaemia in people with diagnosed diabetes and predispose people at risk of diabetes to corticosteroid-induced diabetes: incidence of new onset diabetes 2–12% (Donihi et al. 2006; Oyer et al. 2006) and appears to be proportional to the dose, dose form and dose regimen, and duration of treatment (Diabetes UK 2012, 2018). Ocular formulations, inhalers, and topical corticosteroid preparations do not cause diabetes (Donihi et al. 2006). Hyperglycaemia usually occurs when doses of Prednisolone or equivalent medicines exceeds 7.5 mg/day. In contrast, short courses may not cause hyperglycaemia or only have a short-term effect on the blood glucose. The GLM type, dose, and dose frequency might need to be adjusted or GLM commenced in those with a new diagnosis or not using GLMs.

Screening people for diabetes risk factors on admission to palliative care and monitoring blood glucose when people commence corticosteroids will identify corticosteroid-induced hyperglycaemia early and enable treatment to be initiated to reduce the impact on comfort, cognitive function, and other symptoms.

Several mechanisms have been proposed for the diabetogenic effects of corticosteroids:

- Enhance hepatic gluconeogenesis by upregulating key regulatory hormones that contribute to hyperglycaemia such as glucose-6-phoshatase and phosphoenolpyruvate carboxylase (PEPCK).
- Suppress insulin release from the beta cells.
- Induce peripheral insulin resistance by inhibiting production of glucose transporters in adipose and skeletal muscle cells. Insulin resistance and impaired glucose tolerance can occur within 48 hours of commencing corticosteroids.
- Corticosteroids appear to cause both fasting and postprandial hyperglycaemia (Du 2008). However, a morning daily dose tends to cause hyperglycaemia in the late afternoon or early evening.

Practice point

People should be informed they could develop diabetes when they are prescribed oral corticosteroid medicines, especially when they are risk of developing diabetes.

In addition to causing hyperglycaemia, corticosteroids can mask the signs and symptoms of infections, which are often atypical in people with diabetes. The skin can become thin and fragile and prone to tears, especially in older people, which causes considerable discomfort and distress. Corticosteroids also have variable effects on bone formation and reduce calcium absorption from the intestine, which predisposes susceptible individuals to osteoporotic fractures and pain. Mental changes can also occur, ranging from mild psychosis to significant psychiatric pathology. Mild psychological effects may be difficult to distinguish from delirium and other cognitive deficits.

Managing corticosteroid-induced diabetes in palliative care patients

Balancing the benefits of corticosteroid medicines with their effects on glucose homeostasis is multifactorial and challenging and is affected by individual susceptibility, meal schedules, whether dosing is intermittent or continuous and the diabetogenic effects of the individual medicines. The aim is to maintain stable blood glucose, limit glucose variability, prevent ketoacidosis and hyperosmolar states, minimise the risk of hypoglycaemia, and limit the care burden on the individual and their family/carers.

Management consists of monitoring blood glucose, especially in the afternoon, but more frequently if insulin is prescribed, using the lowest effective corticosteroid dose and the least diabetogenic corticosteroid formulation for the shortest possible time, and proactively treating hyperglycaemia. An acceptable blood glucose range is fasting – 6 mmol/l and postprandial <11 mmol/l (Du 2008). People managed using diet may require medicines to manage fasting and/or postprandial hyperglycaemia and its symptoms.

The choice of GLM depends on the person's health status, corticosteroid regimen, and relevant medicine precautions and contraindications (see, e.g. Du 2008; Dunning et al. 2010; Australian Diabetes Society [ADS] 2012; Diabetes UK 2012).

Morning corticosteroid:

- Morning sulphonylurea such as Glipizide OR
- Prebreakfast or BD Isophane insulin
- *BD or TDS* corticosteroid
- BD sulphonylurea uch as Glipizide OR
- Daily long-acting insulin analogue

Bolus doses of rapid acting insulin may be required with some or all meals, depending on the blood glucose and the individual's food intake

GLM doses may need to be reduced if the corticosteroid dose is reduced or ceased. As indicated, blood glucose monitoring is essential to manage GLMs and prevent hypoglycaemia and the associated adverse events, including MI and falls. In addition, large doses of corticosteroid for more than two weeks can induce adrenal insufficiency, which dramatically reduces insulin requirements. The signs of adrenal insufficiency are similar to other palliative care symptoms: increased fatigue, weight loss, nausea, and diarrhoea (Fowler 2009).

Antipsychotic medicines

Depression and anxiety are common in people with diabetes and may occasionally be treated with antipsychotic medicines. Antipsychotic medicines are sometimes used to manage pain associated with peripheral neuropathy, which is a common complication of diabetes, and to manage refractory nausea and delirium (Llorente and Urrutia 2006).

Antipsychotic medicines induce hyperglycaemia. Blood glucose monitoring may be required and oral GLMs or insulin might be required depending on the emerging blood glucose pattern.

Corticosteroid-like antipsychotic medicines should be used for the shortest possible period of time, at the lowest effective dose and using the least diabetogenic medication in the class where possible. People with diabetes and their carers should be informed about the likely effects of corticosteroids and possible effects of antipsychotic medicines on their blood glucose levels and given advice about blood glucose testing and managing hyperglycaemia. Likewise, it is advisable for clinicians to document their advice in the individual's medical record and other relevant documentation.

Supporting family/carers

It is important to inform carers about the person with diabetes' care plan and health status and involve them in decisions where appropriate. Some family carers may require diabetes education if they need to take on the person's usual diabetes self-care tasks such as blood glucose monitoring and administering insulin (Savage et al. 2012). There are positive beneficial effects of care giving, although the stress of witnessing a loved one suffer can be significant (The Joint Commission 2010).

The severity of the individual's distress is the strongest predictor of end-of-life family/carer strain (Fromme et al. 2005). Men are less likely to report caregiver strain than women and use fewer words to describe their strain and distress. Caregiver Strain Index (Hartford Institute for Geriatric Nursing 2013) might be useful to monitor family/carer strain. Dunning et al. Diabetes Australia and Palliative Care Australia (PCA) (2012) published brochures for people with diabetes and family/carers to inform them about diabetes and end of life issues (www.palliativecare. org.au or www.caresearch.com.au).

Health professionals can support family/cares by offering them the opportunity to discuss their concerns and enabling them to express their grief. Enabling family/carers to participate in end-of-life care such as helping with feeds, providing CM and being present, and scheduling rounds to coincide with family/carer visits if possible.

Withdrawing treatment

Withdrawing treatment is an essential aspect of palliative care and peoples' wishes can be documented in ACDs, which help health professionals make decisions about withdrawing treatment. The deteriorating and terminal phases are often key decision points for initiating the Liverpool Care Pathway and withdrawing treatment. Savage et al. (2012) found most people with diabetes do not want unnecessary treatment continued in the terminal phase but they want to be comfortable and die with dignity.

Knowing the prognosis can aid decisions about when to withdraw treatment, but it is difficult to predict prognosis although The Gold Standard Prognostic Indicator (Royal College of General Practitioners 2008) and the PCOC stages (PCOC 2018) are helpful. Factors that indicate limited prognosis include:

- Multiple comorbidities.
- More than 10% weight loss in a short period of time.
- Failure to thrive and/or general decline.
- Serum albumin <25 g/l.
- Reduced performance, e.g. Karnofsky score <50% and requiring significant help to undertake usual activities of daily living and diabetes self-care tasks.
- Will to live, which is a strong predictor of survival in older people regardless of their age, gender, and comorbidities (Karppinen et al. 2012).
- Social factors such as satisfaction and support from family, friends and health professionals might have an important effect on will to live. Will to live could be explored as part of the spiritual history.

GLMs should be stopped when they cause frequent, severe hypoglycaemia associated with other risks such as falls, especially in the deteriorating and terminal phases when the risks outweigh the benefits. However, the discomfort and risks associated with hyperglycaemia need to be considered in light of the prognosis.

There are ethical issues associated with stopping any treatment, even in end-of-life settings (Ford-Dunn and Quin 2004; Ford-Dunn et al. 2006) and the wishes of the patient and their family and ACD, if they are available, must be considered. Family/carers may be concerned about euthanasia and worry that withdrawing food and fluids will cause pain and discomfort. Thus, timely, careful, clear communication is essential.

Diabetes education

Education and support, including bereavement support, is essential for individuals with diabetes, their families, and often health professional carers. Sensitive discussion about the need to adjust medicines and other changes to established self-management routines is essential. In addition, diabetes specialists are in an ideal position to identify regular opportunities of when to begin discussing palliative care and other end-of-life issues.

References

Alexopoulos, G. (2005). Depression in the elderly. *The Lancet* **365**: 1961–1969.

Allen, S. and Barnett, A. (2011). Exploring advanced care planning in rural aged care. *Australian Nursing Journal* **17** (9): 41.

American Board of Internal Medicine (2012). Choosing wisely. http://www.choosingwisely.org/wp-content/uploagds/2017/10/Choosing-Wisely-at-Five.pdf.

American Diabetes Association (2017). Management of common comorbidities of diabetes. http://outpatient.aace.com/type-2-diabetes/management-of-common-comorbidities-of-diabetes.

Australian Diabetes Society (ADS) (2012). *Guideline for Routine Glucose Control in Hospital*. Canberra: ADS.

Bloomer, M. (2012). Care in final days. *Nursing Review* (20 August).

Botes, R., Vermeulen, K., Correia, J. et al. (2018). Relative contribution of various chronic disease and multi-morbididty to potential disability among Dutch elderly. *BMC Health Services Research* https://doi.org/10.1186/212913-017-2820-0.

Bowling, A. (1983). The hospitalisation of death: should more people die at home? https://www.ncbi.nlm.nih.gov/pmc/articles/PMC1059324.

Burge, F. (2012). How to move to a palliative approach to care for people with multimorbidity. *British Medical Journal* **345** https://doi.org/10.1136/bmj.e6324 (Published 21 September 2012).

Cryer, P. (2015). Hypoglycaemia during therapy of diabetes. NCBI Bookshelf. http://www.ncbi.nim.nih.gov/books/NBK279100.

Department of Health and Ageing, Australian Government (2006). Guidelines for a palliative approach to residential aged care. enhanced version. www.nhmrc.gov.au/_files_nhmrc/publications/attachments/ac14.pdf (accessed December 2012).

Department of Health (2009). National Strategy for the Quality Use of Medicines (QUM). Department of Health, Australian Government, Canberra. https://www1.health.gov.au/internet/main/publishing.nsf/Content/nmp-quality.htm.

Diabetes UK (2012). End-of-life care strategy: A strategy document commissioned by Diabetes UK Clinical care recommendations. www.diabetes.nhs.uk/document.php?o=3730.

Diabetes UK (2018). *End of Life Diabetes Care: clinical Care Recommendations*, 3e. www.diabetes.org.uk/professionals/position…management…/end-of-life-care.

Donihi, A., Raval, D., Saul, M. et al. (2006). Prevalence and predictors of corticosteroid-related hyperglycemia in hospitalized patients. *Endocrine Practice* **12** (4): 358–362.

Dosa, D. (2010). *Making Rounds with Oscar*. New York City: Hyperion Books.

Du, L. (2008). Management of steroid-induced diabetes in patients with COPD. *Medscape Diabetes and Endocrinology* (July 17) http://www.medscape.com/viewarticle/458619 (accessed October 2012).

Dunning, T. (1996). Corticosteroid medications and diabetes mellitus. *Practical Diabetes International* **13** (6): 186–188.

Dunning, T. (2012). Managing diabetes at the end of life. *Diabetes Management Journal* **39**: 6–8.

Dunning, T. and Martin, P. (2018). Palliative and end of life care of people with diabetes: Issues, challenges and strategies. *Diabetes Research and Clinical Practice* **143**: 454–463.

Dunning, T., Martin, P., Orellana, L. et al. (2018). *Planning Palliative and End of Life Care with Older People with Diabetes: Information for Health Professionals*. Geelong, Victoria: Centre for Quality and Patient Safety Research, Deakin University Barwon Health Partnership https://www.caresearch.com.au/Caresearch/Portals/0/Documents/FORPTSFAMILIES/Planning-PC-and-eol-with-older-people-with-diabetes.pdf.

Dunning, T., Savage, S., Duggan, N., and Martin, P. (2010). *Guidelines for Managing Diabetes at the End of Life*. Geelong Australia: Centre for Nursing and Allied Health Research.

Dying Matters (2017). Where people want to die. http://www.healthtalk.org/peoples-experiences/dying…/living…/where-people-want-die.

Ellershaw, J.E. and Murphy, D. (2005). The Liverpool Care Pathway (LCP) influencing the UK national agenda on care of the dying. *International Journal of Palliative Nursing* **11** (3): 132–134.

Emanuel, L., Alexander, C., Arnold, R. et al. (2004). Integrating palliative care into disease management guidelines. *Journal of Palliative Medicine* **7** (6): 774–783.

Fjose, M., Eilertsen, G., Kirkevold, M., and Grov, E.K. (2018). Non-palliative care – a qualitative study of older cancer patients' and their family members' experiences with the health care system. *BMC Health Services Research* **18** (1): 745.

Ford-Dunn, S. and Quin, J. (2004). Management of diabetes in the terminal phase of life. *Practical Diabetes International* **21** (5): 175–176.

Ford-Dunn, S., Smith, A., and Quin, J. (2006). Management of diabetes during the last days of life: attitudes of consultant diabetologists and consultant palliative care physicians in the UK. *Palliative Medicine* **20**: 197–203.

Fowler, M. (2009). Pitfalls in diabetes outpatient management. *Clinical Diabetes Journals* **29** (2): 79–85.

Fromme, E., Drach, L., Tollle, S. et al. (2005). Men as caregivers at the end of life. *Journal of Palliative Medicine* **8** (6): 1167–1175.

Gannon, C. and Dando, N. (2010). Dose-sensitive steroid-induced hyperglycaemia. *Palliative Medicine* **24** (7): 737–739.

Giovannucci, E., Harlan, D., Archer, M. et al. (2010). Diabetes and cancer. *Diabetes Care* **7**: 1674–1685.

Gold Standards Framework Proactive Identification Guidance (PIG) (GSF) (2016). www.goldstandardsframework. org.uk/PIG.

Hartford Institute for Geriatric Nursing (2013). Geriatric assessment tools. http://www.hartfordign.org/ publications/trythis/issue14.

HealthCare Chaplaincy (2009). *A Dictionary of Patients' Spiritual and Cultural Values for Health Care Professionals*. New York: HealthCare Chaplaincy http://www.healthcarechaplaincy.org/userimages/doc/ Cultural%20Dictionary.pdf (accessed December 2012).

Hilton, A.K., Jones, D., and Bellomo, R. (2013). Clinical review: the role of the intensivist and the rapid response team in nosocomial end-of-life care. *Critical Care* **17** (2): 224.

Horowitz, S. (2009). Complementary therapies for end of life. *Alternative and Complementary Therapies* **15** (5): 226–230.

Hsu, P., Sung, S., and Cheng, H. (2012). Association of clinical symptomatic hypoglycaemia with cardiovascular events and total mortality in type 2 diabetes mellitus. *Diabetes Care* https://doi.org/10.2337/dc12-0916.

Huang, E., Liu, J., Moffet, H. et al. (2011). Glycemic control, complications, and death in older diabetic patients: the diabetes and aging study. *Diabetes Care* **34**: 1329–1336. https://doi.org/10.2337/dc10-2377.

Iglay, K., Hannachi, H., Howie, P. et al. (2016). Prevalence and co prevalence of comorbidities among patients with type 2 diabetes mellitus. *Current Medical Research and Opinion* **32** (7): 1234–1252. https://doi.org/10.1185/0 3007995.2016.1168291.

International Diabetes Federation (2017). *IDF Diabetes Atlas*, 8e. Brussels, Belgium: International Diabetes Federation http://www.diabetesatlas.org.

Iversen, M., Tell, G., Riise, T. et al. (2017). History of foot ulcer increases mortality among individuals with diabetes. *Diabetes Care* **32** (912): 219302199.

Jyrkkä, J., Enlund, H., Korhonen, M., and Hartikainen, S. (2009). Patterns of drug use and factors associated with polypharmacy and excessive polypharmacy in elderly persons: results of the Kupio 75+ study: a cross-sectional analysis. *Drugs and Aging* **266**: 493–503.

Karppinen, H., Laakonen, M.L., Strandberg, T. et al. (2012). Will-to-live and survival in a 10-year follow-up among older people. *Age and Aging* **41** (6): 789–794.

Kedziera, P. (2001). Hydration, thirst and nutrition. In: *Textbook of Palliative Nursing* (eds. B. Ferrell and N. Coyle). New York: Oxford University Press.

Koren, M. and Papamiditriou, C. (2013). Spirituality of staff nurses: application of modeling and role modeling theory. *Holistic Nursing Practice* **27** (1): 37–44.

Krinsley, J. (2008). Glycaemic variability: a strong independent predictor of mortality in critically ill patients. *Critical Care Medicine* **36** (11): 3008–3013.

Llorente, M. and Urrutia, V. (2006). Diabetes, psychiatric disorders, and metabolic effects of antipsychotic medications. *Clinical Diabetes* **24**: 18–24.

McCoubrie, R., Jeffrey, D., Paton, C., and Dawes, L. (2004). Managing diabetes mellitus in patients with advanced cancer: a case note audit and guidelines. *European Journal of Cancer Care* **14** (3): 244–248.

McEwen, N., Kim, C., Hann, M., and Ghosh, D. (2006). Diabetes reporting as a cause of death: results from the translating research into action for diabetes (TRIAD) study. *Diabetes Care* **29**: 247–251.

Morrison, R. and Meter, D. (2004). Clinical practice palliative care. *New England Journal of Medicine* **350** (25): 2582–2590.

Murray, S., Kendall, M., Moine, S. et al. (2017). Palliatives care from diagnosis. *British Medical Journal* **2017**: 356j878.

Murtagh, M., Preston, M., and Higginson, I. (2004). Patterns of dying: palliative care for non-malignant disease. *Clinical Medicine* **4** (1): 39–44.

National Prescribing Service Ltd and Palliative Care Australia (2009). *Achieving Quality Use of Medicines in the Community for Palliative and End of Life Care: A Consultation Report*. Sydney: National Prescribing Service.

Ndosi, M., Wright-Hughes, A., Browns, S. et al. (2017). Prognosis of the infected diabetes foot ulcer: a 12-month prospective observational study. *Diabetic Medicine* **35** (1): 78–88. https://doi.org/10.1111/dme.13537.

Orford, N., Milnes, S., Simpson, N. et al. (2019). Effect of communication skills training on outcomes in critically ill patients with life-limiting illness referred for intensive care management: a before and after study. *British Medical Journal Supportive and Palliative Care* **9**: e21. https://spcare.bmj.com/content/9/1/e21.info.

Oyer, D., Shah, A., and Bettenhausen, S. (2006). How to manage steroid diabetes in the patient with cancer. *The Journal of Supportive Oncology* **4**: 479–483.

Palliative Care Australia (PCA) (2012). *National Palliative Care Week Survey*. Canberra: PCA.

Palliative Aged Care Evidence (palliAGED) (2019). https://www.palliaged.com.au.

Palliative Care Outcomes Collaborative (PCOC) (2018). https://www.pallcarevic.asn.au/.../palliative-care-outcomes-collaborative-pcoc-website.

Parker, D., Clifton, K., Tuckett, A. et al. (2016). Palliative care case conferences in long-term care: views of family members. *International Journal of Older People Nursing* **11**: 140–148. https://doi.org/10.1111/opn.12105.

Parsian, N. and Dunning, T. (2009). Spirituality and coping in young adults with diabetes: a cross-sectional survey. *European Diabetes Nursing* **6**: 100–1004.

Pesut, B., McLeod, B., Hole, R., and Dalhuisen, M. (2012). Rural nursing and quality end-of-life care: palliative care, palliative approach or somewhere in between. *Advances in Nursing Science* **35** (4): 288–304.

Puchalski, C. (2011). Spirituality is an important component of patient care. WebMD Professional. http://www.medscape.com/viewarticle/738237 (accessed August 2012).

Quinn, K., Hudson, P., and Dunning, T. (2006). Diabetes management in patients receiving palliative care. *Journal of Pain and Symptom Management* **32** (3): 275–286.

Rowett, D., Currow, D., Fazekas, B. et al. (2012). *Prescribing at the End of Life, Pharmacovigilance and Palliative Care*, 2012. Sydney: National Medicine Symposium.

Royal Australian College of General Practitioners (RACGP), Diabetes Australia (DA) (2016-2018). *Diabetes Management in General Practice*. Canberra: RACGP/DA https://www.racgp.org.au/FSDEDEV/media/documents/Clinical%20Resources/Guidelines/Diabetes/General-practice-management-of-type-2-diabetes_1.pdf.

Royal College of General Practitioners (2008). Prognostic Indicator Guidance (version 5), in: National Gold Standards Framework Centre England. http://www.goldstandardsframework.nhs.uk (accessed December 2012).

Running, A., Grant, J., and Andrews, W. (2008). A survey of hospice use of complementary therapy. *Journal of Hospice and Palliative Nursing* **16** (4): 394–312.

Savage, S., Dunning, T., Duggan, N., and Martin, P. (2012). The experiences and care preferences of people with diabetes at the end of life. *Journal of Hospice and Palliative Nursing* **14** (4): 293–302.

Sicar, M., Bhatia, A., and Munshi, M. (2016). Review of hypoglycaemia in the older adult. *Canadian Journal of Diabetes* https://doi.org/10.1015/1.icid.2016.10.004.

Sudore, R., Karter, A., Huang, E. et al. (2012). Symptom burden of adults with type 2 diabetes across the disease course: diabetes and aging study. *Journal of General Internal Medicine* **27** (12): 1674–1681.

Sweriessen, H. and Duckett, S. (2014). Dying well: The Grattan Report. ISBN: 1-925015-81-4.

The Joint Commission (2010). *Advancing Effective Communication, Cultural Competence, and Patient- and Family-Centered Care: A Roadmap for Hospitals*. Oakbrook Terrace, IL: The Joint Commission.

Witte, K. and Allen, M. (2000). A meta-analysis of fear appeals: implications for effective public health campaigns. *Health Education & Behavior* **27** (5): 591–615.

World Health Organization (WHO) (2005). World Health Organisation Definition of Palliative Care. http://www.who.int/cancer/palliative/definition.

World Health Organization (WHO) (2014). Strengthening of palliative care as a component of integrated treatment throughout the life course sixty-seventh world Health assembly April 2014.

World Health Organization (WHO) (2018). Top 10 causes of death. https://www.who.int/news-room/fact-sheets/detail/the-top-10-causes-of-death.

Key points

Modern diabetes management philosophy is consistent with complementary medicine (CM) philosophy, specifically, prevention, the central role of the individual in their care, shared decisions to achieve personalised care.

- The acronym CM encompasses a wide range of therapies as well as herbal medicines. These CM can be used alone or in combination, and in combination with conventional medicine.
- People with diabetes are high CM users and are entitled to unbiased, evidence-based information about the benefits and risks CM.
- CM can work synergistically with conventional care to improve diabetes balance and quality of life; provided the benefits and risks are considered in the context of the individual's health and social situation.
- Many herbal medicines have hypoglycaemic effects. People with diabetes do use glucose lowering herbal medicines; but do not assume every person with diabetes using CM is doing so to manage their blood glucose.
- Herb/medicine and herb/herb interactions and other adverse events can occur.
- Clinicians should ask about and document CM use during routine diabetes assessments, especially when medicines are initiated, when doses are adjusted and prior to surgical and investigative procedures.

Rationale

Complementary medicines (CM) use is increasing, as is the interest in integrative medicine (IM). IM refers to integrating evidence-based CM with conventional care. Some CM can help people with diabetes heal and become proactive, empowered participants in their diabetes management if they used appropriately, within a quality use of medicines (QUM) framework. CM use is associated with both benefits and risks. An essential aspect of any management strategy is making informed decisions *with* the individual about their personal level of risk and tailoring treatment to meet their needs.

Care of People with Diabetes: A Manual for Healthcare Practice, Fifth Edition. Trisha Dunning and Alan Sinclair.
© 2020 John Wiley & Sons Ltd. Published 2020 by John Wiley & Sons Ltd.

CM has both risks and benefits for people with diabetes including those: with cancer, undergoing surgery, having investigations and at the end of life. In fact, we incorporated CM into the second edition of our Guidelines for Deciding Palliative and End of Life Care with People with Diabetes. The information includes a risk benefit analysis and a list of evidence-based resources (Dunning 2001; Dunning and Martin 2019).

Not all CM carry the same level of risk or confer equal benefits. Adopting a holistic QUM approach, including using non-medicine options first when appropriate, can optimise the benefits and reduce the risks. A key aspect of QUM is asking about and documenting CM use. People with diabetes who use CM need written advice about how to manage their CM, including during the surgical/investigative period. People with diabetes who have renal disease and those on anticoagulants and other medicines with a narrow therapeutic index and high risk medicines are at particular risk of adverse events if they use some CM medicines (Dunning 2007).

Introduction

Complementary and alternative medicine (CAM) use is increasing, as people try to manage modern health problems such as chronic lifestyle diseases and depression. When people consider their therapeutic options, they are likely to make choices that are congruent with their life philosophy, knowledge, experience, societal norms, and culture. Depending on these factors people may or may not choose to be actively involved in their care. Many people who use CM regard it as more personalised and holistic than conventional care (Foley and Steel 2017). People with chronic diseases are high CM users.

Understanding these associations is important to understanding an individual's self-care, adherence, and empowerment potential. For example, there is a high correlation amongst health beliefs, spirituality and CAM use (Hildreth and Elman 2007). In addition, there is good evidence that CAM users adopt health-promoting self-care strategies, undertake preventative healthcare (Kelner and Wellman 1997; Garrow and Egede 2006; Foley and Steel 2017) and believe responsibility for their health ultimately rests with them.

CM is used by >50% of the general population in most countries and the rate of use is increasing, particularly by people with chronic diseases, especially women educated to high school level or higher, those with poor health who often have a chronic disease, are employed, and are interested in self-care (Lloyd et al. 1993; MacLennan et al. 1996; Eisenberg 1998; Egede et al. 2002; MacLennan et al. 2002; Grossman et al. 2018). However, there is some evidence that the profile of Cam users is changing and many younger people use CAM (Manya et al. 2012).

The true prevalence of CM use by people with diabetes is largely unknown. Old studies in the general population (Leese et al. 1997; Ryan et al. 1999) found approximately 17% of people with diabetes in diabetic outpatient settings used a range of CAM, particularly herbs, massage, and vitamin and mineral supplements such as zinc. People using CM were satisfied with their chosen therapy even if it 'did not work'. Satisfaction with treatment improves wellbeing (see Chapters 15 and 16). These researchers appeared to assume people used CM to 'control their diabetes', however, the individuals concerned may have had different reasons for using CM from those assumed by researchers and clinicians. Managing blood glucose may not have been their primary aim. The author's experience in a diabetes service suggests that, in many cases, people use CM to maintain health (prevention) as well as to manage conditions such as arthritis, stress, and the unpleasant symptoms of intercurrent illness and diabetes complications, for example, nausea, pain, anxiety, and depression.

More recently, Egede et al. (2002) found that people with diabetes in the US were more likely to use CM than people without diabetics, as were people with other chronic conditions. In particular, people with diabetes over 65 years were the most likely group to use CM. The most commonly used CM was nutritional advice, spiritual healing, herbal medicine, massage, and meditation (see Table 18.1). The high usage rates in people with diabetes are hardly surprising and accord with the established demographics of CAM users. Recently, Dunning and Martin (2019) conducted a point prevalence survey of CM use in a large regional hospital and residential

Table 18.1   Commonly used complementary medicine (CM).

Acupuncture	Meditation
Aromatherapy using essential oils for therapeutic purposes	Music
	Naturopathy
Ayurveda	Nutritional therapies including vitamin and mineral and antioxidant supplements
Chinese Medicine	
Chiropractic	Pet therapy
Counselling (a range of techniques)	Reflexology
	Reiki
Herbal medicine (from several traditions – Indian, Chinese, North American, Australian Aboriginal, Japanese)	Therapeutic Touch
Homoeopathy	Ayurveda and Chinese medicine (use several techniques such as herbs, cupping, moxibustion, essential oils, diet, and exercise)

Many CM are combined, such as aromatherapy and massage. Likewise, traditional medical systems use a range of CM in combination (CM with CM) and different diagnostic techniques instead of or in addition to conventional diagnostic processes, for example, tongue and pulse diagnosis. Often CM is combined with conventional care, formally and informally, in self-prescribed regimens.

aged care facility (400 acute care beds and 410 aged care beds). Respectively, 55% and 38% reported using CM, and significantly, although the majority stated they informed their doctors and nurses, CM use was not document in the medical records audited as part of the study.

Many health professionals, especially nurses and general practitioners (GPs), incorporate CM into their practice to enrich and extend their practice and provide holistic integrated care (Phelps and Hassed 2011; Kotsirilos et al. 2011). Some nurses and GPs who use CM in their practices do not have formal CM qualifications and do not effectively document or monitor the outcomes of CM usage. In addition, they often use CM in their own healthcare. Dunning and Martin (2019) found that 50% of a sample of 37 diabetes nurse specialists/diabetes educators indicated they used CM in their practice, but none had a CM qualification.

There are a great many CMs ranging from well-accepted therapies with an acceptable research basis to 'fringe' therapies with little or no scientific evidence to support their use. The public interprets the term 'CM' differently from health professionals and CM and conventional practitioners and researchers use different definitions, which makes it difficult to compare studies. Several definitions and categories exist. The Cochrane collaboration defined CM as:

> All health systems, modalities and practices and their accompanying theories and beliefs, other than those intrinsic to the politically dominant health system of a particular society or culture in a given historical period. They include all such practices and ideas self-defined by their users as preventing or treating illness or promoting health and wellbeing. The boundaries within and between complementary therapies are not always sharp or fixed.
>
> (Cochrane Collaboration 2000).

National Institute of Complementary Medicine (NICM) defined CM as:

A broad set of health systems, models and accompanying theories and beliefs outside the dominant health system but may be dominant in some cultures to prevent, promote wellbeing. The boundaries between CM and the dominant health system are not fixed. The NICM definition is based on the World Health Organisation definition (2019).

Likewise, several terms are used to refer to CM including complementary and alternative medicine (CM), traditional medicine and non-scientific therapies. These terms are generally understood to mean therapies that are not part of conventional medicine. As the Cochrane

Table 18.2   The information was based on Grossman et al. (2018), Dunn (2019) and Meyers and Vigar (2019).

The following herbal CM shown to reduce HbA1c by at least 0.5% in randomized controlled trials (RCT) lasting ≥3 months, which is similar to many conventional GLMs; however, most CM trials were single studies, small sample sizes, and meta-analyses.

Ayurveda polyherbal formula
Coccinia cordifolia
Zingiber officinale
Aloe Vera
Silymarin
Trigonella foenum-graecum
Traditional Chinese medicine herbs:
Berberine
Fructus mume
Gegen Qinlian
Xiaoke (contains glyburide
Jinlida with metformin
Shen-Qi-Formula with insulin

The following herbal CM had an effect on HbA1c in non-RCTs of short duration:

Panax quinquefolius
Camellia sinesnsi
Mormordica charantia
Salvia officinalis
Vitamins C and E

The following CM and supplements had conflicting effects on HbA1c in trials lasting at least 3 months:

Cinnamon
Zinc
L-carnitine
Magnesium
Coenzyme Q 10
Probiotics

Naturopathic medicine systematic review showed benefits for

Cardiovascular disease, musculoskeletal pain, type 2 diabetes, polycystic ovarian disease, and depression.
Other medicines that can help reduce cardiovascular risk include red rice yeast (which contains the active ingredient from which statins were derived, omega 3 reduce triglycerides. There is increasing evidence for mindfulness therapies e.g. yoga and Tai chi to help manage stress-related issues such as hypertension and sleeplessness.
Others with less evidence include turmeric, co-enzyme Q10.

definition indicates, the status of CM is not fixed and some CM become part of conventional medicine as the evidence base for their safety and efficacy accumulates. See Table 18.2. Interesting, some conventional clinicians do not recommend CM, even when evidence is available. A significant concern is that most CM practitioners are not regulated as stringently as conventional clinicians, although many CM abide by professional standards and regulations (Dunn 2019).

CAM philosophy

The various CAM have a common underlying philosophy. Current diabetes person-centred empowerment strategies that focus on effective professional–patient partnerships, good communication, and preventative healthcare are consistent with this philosophy. CM philosophy embodies the notion that:

- Each individual is unique. Therefore, there is no one 'right' way to manage a person's health problems.
- Balance is important.

- The body has the capacity to heal itself. Healing is not synonymous with treating, managing, or curing. The word is derived from the Anglo Saxon *haelen*, to make whole. Likewise, health is derived from the Anglo Saxon *haelth* from *hal*, which also means to make whole. To achieve healing, all parts and polarities need to be integrated – mind, body, and spirit within the individual's social environment and context.
- Healing occurs by intent. Healing intent is an important component of the therapeutic relationship (Dunning 2013a, pp. 28–48).
- A positive attitude is important to health and wellbeing. Increasing importance is placed on positive psychology, including incorporating it into school curricula. Positivity encompasses resilience, the capacity to overcome adversity and find meaning and purpose in life (transcendence). Thus, resilience is an essential aspect of healing, particularly in chronic diseases (Lloyd et al. 1993; Dunning 2013b, pp. 117–132).
- The client–therapist relationship is a key aspect of the healing process and has a significant effect on outcomes.
- The therapist's role is to support the individual's innate healing potential.
- The mind, body, and spirit cannot be separated – what affects one affects the others (mind–body medicine). The mind–body–spirit model is embodied in Eastern medical philosophy and 'encompasses fundamental and universal elements of well-being' (Chan et al. 2006).
- Illness represents an opportunity for positive change (transcendence) (Bridges 1991).

The following core Hippocratic tenets underpin CM philosophy, particularly naturopathy, but they apply to all healthcare:

(1) *Vis medicatrix naturae* – the healing power of nature.
(2) *Primum non nocere* – first, do no harm.
(3) *Tolle causam* – treat the cause.
(4) Treat the whole person.
(5) *Docere* – the doctor is a teacher.
(6) Prevention is the best cure.

Practice point

Healing does not mean curing. It refers to a process of bringing the physical, mental, emotional, spiritual, and relationship aspects of an individual's self together to achieve an integrated balance where each part is of equal importance and value (Dossey et al. 1998). Disruption to any aspect affects the others, and consequently affects outcomes.

Understanding CM philosophy is important to understanding why people use CM. People seek answers to their health problems that match their existing beliefs and explanatory models. People's health choices are part of their larger life orientation and are not made in isolation from their beliefs and attitudes. They frequently mix and match CM with CM and CM with conventional therapies to suit their needs. Adverse events can arise when due consideration is not given to the potential effects of such combinations, for example, potentially damaging medicine/herb interactions. Alternatively, CM can enhance the effects of conventional medicines, enable lower doses of medicines to be used, reduce unwanted side effects and improve healing rates (Braun 2001).

Integrating complementary and conventional care

QUM is a useful framework for safely integrating health options, including the broad categories of CM and conventional care (see Chapter 5). QUM is congruent with CM philosophy. QUM can be a helpful decision-making framework to achieve optimal heath care including medicines if medicines are indicated. QUM encompasses, prevention, lifestyle strategies, and risk management. Integrated medicine (IM) is a holistic framework that recognises not everybody requires medicines to maintain health.

IM is becoming increasingly popular amongst health professionals, although it was originally consumer-driven (National Centre of Complementary and Integrative Health 2016). CM and IM are not synonymous terms. IM focuses on providing best practice conventional medicine and includes prevention, and emotional wellbeing, thus it might encompass CM. Likewise, QUM is not concerned with either/or choices but with providing holistic care by helping the individual make informed choices about the best way to maintain optional health. IM is defined as:

> The blending of conventional medicine and complementary medicines and/or therapies with the aim of using the most appropriate of either or both modalities to care for the patient as a whole.
>
> (Australasian Integrative Medicine Association (AIMA) 2014)

IM is concerned with wellness and is a flexible approach to responding to the individual and societal factors impacting on healthcare. The specific therapies used in IM depend on the individual, objective evidence for benefit and risk, consideration of alternative choices (QUM), cost/benefit, practitioner experience and knowledge, and/or the need to refer to other practitioners (Kotsirilos et al. 2011; Phelps and Hassed 2011; AIMA 2014).

Significantly, almost 80% of the global population depends on herbal medicines and traditional medical systems (WHO 2002) although the medicines and systems may be different amongst countries and cultures. Migration and refugee displacement through war and natural disasters mean the types of CM available outside the country of origin is increasing. Individuals import some products into their new countries and these products may not be subject to stringent regulatory processes such as good manufacturing practices and other relevant regulations that control many of the system-related risks.

Many health institutions are concerned with regulatory and supply issues as well as benefits, risks, and safe CM use. The degree and processes for regulating CM therapies, products, and practitioners varies from country to country and from therapy to therapy. Frequently there are no formal regulatory processes in place, but some CM professional associations have stringent training and ongoing professional development requirements as part of self-regulation. Some such associations require competence in first aid, for example, the International Aromatherapy and Aromatic Medicine Association.

The safe, effective use of CM, conventional medicine, and/or combination of conventional and CM care involves considering the following issues:

- The importance of asking people about CM use in a non-judgemental manner. Many people (>40%) do not disclose their CM use because clinicians do not ask them about it (Cancer Australia 2010).
- The safety and benefit for the individual based on a collaborative risk assessment and allowing for their personal choices.
- Helping people make informed choices based on understanding the risks and benefits involved when using CM, especially combining CM and conventional care. When the patient is not competent to consent, guardianship issues may arise.
- The clinician/s knowledge and competence to give advice about CM and how to refer to a suitably qualified practitioner if indicated. CM needs to be appropriate to the individual's physical, mental, and spiritual status and selected after considering all the options and after a thorough assessment considering potential interactions with conventional therapies. The continued suitability of CM, like all management strategies, should be reviewed regularly because diabetes is a progressive disease and continued use may be unnecessary or dangerous, e.g. in people with renal and liver disease (see Chapters 8 and 10). Conventional medicine doses should be monitored and may need to be changed.

- Guidelines should be followed where they exist, and consent to use CM is required in some settings. Policies and guidelines need to include processes for communication between CM and conventional practitioners and for collaboration and referral mechanisms to prevent fragmented care (Dunning 2001). Where possible, guidelines should be evidence-based to support best practice. They should not be prescriptive and inflexible.
- Processes for monitoring outcomes and accurately documenting the effects of the therapy should be in place and objective data relevant to the aims of the therapy, should be collected.
- Ensuring that safe, quality products are used is important. Dose variations, contamination and/or adulteration with potentially toxic substances such as heavy metals and animal parts, and unsubstantiated claims made about the product can lead to serious adverse events including irreversible kidney failure (Ko 1998; Bjelakovic and Nikolova 2007). The *Sydney Morning Herald* reported some Chinese medicines confiscated by customs officials contained 'potentially poisonous plants, unlabelled ingredients and bits of endangered animals' concerning pant species included *Aristolochia* species, which have been linked to cancer (Phillips 2012).
- Safety data information should be available where possible and could be included with research papers or medication reference books/electronic databases in a portfolio in areas where CM is used.
- It is important that an accurate diagnosis is made and a thorough health history and assessment are undertaken prior to using any therapy. These considerations are often overlooked, especially when the person with diabetes self-diagnoses and self-treats. Such practices can mask or mimic important symptoms and result in delays in instituting appropriate management and, consequently deteriorating metabolic control.

Practice points

(1) There is an increasing body of scientific evidence as well as a large body of traditional evidence for many CM. However, evidence about the *combination* of CM and conventional medicines is not well documented.

(2) Where there is strong evidence for CM, it should be considered as first-line treatment or used with conventional medicine if there are no contraindications. However, the treatment should not delay other treatment or be offered where the costs outweigh the benefits (AIMA 2014).

(3) It is important to explain the evidence to people seeking to use CM.

(4) Many, but not all, CM have a strong evidence base of traditional use, but this is not the same as 'scientific evidence'. In addition, modern technology has changed the traditional method of manufacturing, administering, and monitoring some CM therapies. Therefore, the traditional evidence base needs to be considered in the light of any such changes.

(5) There are methodological flaws in a great deal of research CM and conventional.

Can Complementary Therapies Benefit People with Diabetes?

Managing diabetes effectively is about achieving balance. To achieve balance, a range of therapies used holistically is usually needed. For example, type 2 diabetes is a progressive, multifactorial disease; thus, a single strategy is unlikely to address the underlying metabolic abnormalities or the consequent effects on mental health and wellbeing. These factors can change over the individual's life course. From a general perspective, and based on the premise people need to be mentally well to achieve physical outcomes including care targets, CM can assist people with diabetes to:

- Incorporate diabetes into the framework of their lives, which encompasses two key aspects of spirituality: transformation and connectedness.
- Accept and manage their diabetes to achieve balance in their lives by reducing stress and depression, which can help them achieve management targets (balance) and reduce hepatic glucose output and insulin resistance. That is, address spirituality, resilience, and coping.
- Develop strategies to recognise the factors that cause stress and methods to manage or prevent stress from occurring.
- Take part in decision-making, increase their self-esteem, self-efficacy, and sense of being in control by improving their quality of life and enabling personal growth and transformation.
- Increase insulin production and reduce insulin resistance, either by the direct effects of the therapy, or by managing stress, or by enhancing the effects of conventional medications.
- Manage the unpleasant symptoms of diabetic complications such as pain and nausea.
- Prevent some associated problems, for example, foot care to maintain skin integrity and prevent problems such as cracks that increase the potential for infection and its consequences.
- Learn and retain information.

Some specific benefits for people with diabetes are shown in Table 18.2 and include the following:

(1) A reduction in blood glucose levels in children being given regular massage by their parents. The parents who reported reduced anxiety levels in themselves (Field et al. 1997). Massage has also been shown to reduce pain intensity, unpleasantness, and anxiety in postoperative patients in the short term, especially in the first four days (Mitchinson et al. 2007). Yoga and meditation reduce features of the metabolic syndrome such as waist circumference, systolic blood pressure, fasting blood glucose, and triglycerides, as well as improve mental health (Agrawal 2007).

(2) Many herbs have been shown to lower blood glucose by various mechanisms, HbA1c and lipids, for example, American ginseng (*Panex quinquefolius*) (Vuksan et al. 2000); Gymnema/gurmar (*Gymnema sylvestre*) (Baskaran et al. 1990), fenugreek (*Trigonella foenum-graecum*) (Sharma et al. 1990, 1996), and chromium picolinate (Finney and Gonzalez-Campoy 1997). These herbs and supplements have primarily been used in type 2 diabetes, but fenugreek has also been shown to lower blood glucose in type 1 diabetes (Sharma et al. 1990). Chromium possibly has a role in reducing insulin resistance. It is excreted in urine at a faster rate in people with diabetes than nondiabetics; thus, a relative chromium deficiency could contribute to insulin resistance (Udani et al. 2006). The evidence for a glucose lowering effect of chromium is confusing and may depend on the formulation used and the dosage. People who use chromium report improved blood glucose levels but the required dose may be higher than that usually used (400 μg): at least 5000 μg chromium picolinate is probably required (Udani et al. 2006). Martin et al. (2006) compared chromium picolinate 1000 μg plus either glipizide or placebo for 24 weeks and reported lower fasting and post prandial glucose, HbA1c less weight gain, and less body fat measured using DEXA (Dual-Energy X-ray Absorptiometry) in the intervention groups. Herbal medicines are also used in diabetes-related conditions such as heart failure *Crataegus species* (hawthorn) (Guo et al. (2008); gastrointestinal reflux (peppermint) (Chaudhary 2007), and CQ-10.

(3) Manage weight. Some CM weight loss medicines and dietary strategies are beneficial, others are associated with significant risks and they should not be self-prescribed or used indiscriminately. Both the FDA in the United States and the AMA in Australia have warned the public about the safety of many weight loss preparations. Weight loss requires an integrated approach that encompasses diet and exercise (see Chapter 4). In particular, products containing ephedra may lead to adverse events (Bent et al. 2003). Einerhand (2006) found conjugated linoleic acid (CLA) led to weight loss from the abdomen in men and women, and

women also lost weight from the thighs. Insulin sensitivity was not affected. The clinical significance of this finding is not clear. CAM therapies frequently used to enhance weight loss include herbal medicines, yoga, meditation, acupuncture, massage, and Eastern martial arts (Sharpe et al. 2007). There is good pooled data to support small weight loss associated with chromium picolinate, but it is not a replacement for diet and exercise.

(4) Remain active. The benefits if tai chi in improving strength, balance, and mood in older people is well documented (Chou et al. 2004). Muscle wasting and reduced strength in the lower limbs is associated with advancing age and can lead to inactivity and contribute to falls. Tai chi can be combined with a healthy diet, resistance training, correcting malnutrition, and controlling blood glucose and lipids. Recent research suggests creatine supplementation may enhance the effects of resistance training but the clinical relevance has yet to be determined (O'sathuna 2007).

(5) Acupuncture can improve the pain of diabetic peripheral neuropathy (Abuaisha et al. 1998). Acupuncture has also been shown to be equivalent to monotherapy at reducing mild to moderate hypertension if it is performed by expert practitioners (Flachskampf et al. 2007). Glucosamine and chondroitin are widely used to manage arthritic and joint pain. There is little evidence that oral dosing contributes significantly to hyperglycaemia.

(6) A range of biofeedback, relaxation, and counselling therapies can reduce stress by attenuating the effects of increased autonomic activity and catecholamine production. Improved mood and reduced blood glucose levels have been reported with biofeedback (McGrady et al. 1991). Exercise also plays a key role. There is good evidence that St John's Wort (*Hypericum perforatum*) effectively improves mild-to-moderate depression and is better tolerated than conventional antidepressants. Recent research suggests it is as effective as paroxetine in moderate to severe depression (Szegede et al. 2005). However, St John's Wort interacts with many conventional medicines; thus, a medication review should be performed before commencing the medicine and its use should be monitored.

(7) Antioxidant therapies receive significant press coverage. There is accumulating evidence that oxidation plays a role in the development of many diseases including vascular disease due to the development of oxidative stress and reactive oxygen species (ROS) (see Chapter 8). For example, O'Brien and Timmins (1999) and Verdejo et al. (1999) suggested antioxidants may delay the progression of retinopathy by increasing blood flow to eyes and kidneys (vitamin E) and/or replenishing vitamin E (vitamin C) and/or improving nerve function (the B group vitamins). A recent study showed Vitamin C lowered blood glucose in people with type 2 diabetes (Mason et al. 2019). Other researchers suggest that free radicals might be markers of disease rather than the cause, and that eliminating them may interfere with normal defence mechanisms (Bjelakovic et al. 2007). Antioxidants are also associated with adverse events and medicine interactions especially in the high doses often used. However, consensus has not been reached about the benefits of using antioxidants, the dose needed, or when in the course of diabetes they should be used.

(8) Prevent illness. For example, cranberry preparations, which prevents bacteria sticking to the bladder wall, can reduce urinary tract infections (UTIs) over a 12-month period, particularly in women who suffer recurrent UTIs (Jepson and Craig 2008). Cranberry juice may also effectively control *Helicobacter pylori* (Zhang et al. 2005).

(9) In 2000 the media reported that baths could help reduce blood glucose levels. The claims have not been substantiated and there could be risks such as postural hypotension, falls, and burns to neuropathic feet if the water is too hot. Faster uptake of injected insulin or reduced stress levels could be methods whereby blood glucose is reduced.

(10) Aromatherapy can be used to enhance wellbeing and relaxation and to reduce stress, which benefits metabolic control. It can also be used for physical conditions such as alleviating pain, reducing blood pressure, improving sleep, and foot care. Aromatherapy may also alleviate stress during procedures such as CAT scans, and post-cardiac surgery (Stevensen 1994; Buckle 1997). Managing stress improves the individual's quality of life and psychological wellbeing. Aromatherapy is beneficial for fragrancing the environment to increase work performance, reduce absenteeism and reduce keyboard errors. In this respect the

benefit is for the health professionals and organisations rather than an individual but it can have a role in diabetes education sessions. Aromatherapy is often combined with music and massage. There is a strong link between touch, aroma, and wellbeing. In aged-care settings, aromatherapy is used to reduce pain, improve sleep, maintain skin integrity, and manage behavioural problems (Thomson 2001). Significantly, difficulty identifying odours may be an early sign of Alzheimer's disease and precedes signs of cognitive dysfunction (Wilson 2007). Wilson showed that every one point decrease in the odour identification score represents an 18% risk of mild cognitive impairment progressing to Alzheimer's disease.

Clinical observation

The powerful effect of odour on physical and mental wellbeing is often overlooked. On a practical level, several media reports in 2001 and 2018 concerning dogs being able to recognise when their owners with diabetes were hypoglycaemic and alert them early enough to enable the person to manage the episode themselves, or to alert another person (Chapter 6). Assistance dogs for visually impaired people are standard therapy and help visually impaired people lead independent lives. Likewise, dogs have alerted individuals or their families to epileptic seizures and horse riding for the disabled is well established in many countries.

Spirituality

Spirituality is a neglected aspect of conventional healthcare and is often confused with religion. The two are quite different, although spirituality may encompass religion and prayer and religion may be used as spiritual tools. Information already presented in this chapter demonstrates that spirituality is central to optimal self-care. There are many definitions of spirituality. Most encompass the following core aspects:

- Positive empowering aspect of being human
- Quest for meaning and purpose in life
- Transcendence
- Holistic perspective
- Connectedness
- Resilience and confidence to turn crises into opportunities for personal growth

Spirituality also has *synergy* at its core — all components work together, and small changes in one component can positively or negatively affect all other components.

These are essential to effective diabetes management. Parsian and Dunning (2008a, 2008b) validated a tool for assessing spirituality and coping in young people with diabetes and demonstrated a significant association amongst spirituality, coping, and lower HbA1c. Females were more spiritual than males and there was no significant association between religion and spirituality. Several other researchers around the world are currently using the tool.

CM and surgery

CM usage is high amongst surgical patients, >51%; especially women aged 40–60 years, and is often used on the advice of friends (Norred et al. 2000; Tsen et al. 2000) (see Chapter 9). There are some well-documented benefits of using CAM to improve the health outcomes of people undergoing surgery. For example, foot massage using essential oils reduced stress and anxiety post CAGS (coronary angiography) (Stevensen 1994) and MRI-associated claustrophobia and stress.

Massage reduced postoperative pain intensity, pain unpleasantness, and anxiety during the first four postoperative days (Mitchinson et al. 2007). Acupuncture and peppermint or ginger tea reduces nausea, and a range of strategies can relieve pain and improve sleep. Prophylactic CQ_{10} prior to cardiac surgery improves postoperative cardiac outcomes (Rosenfeldt et al. 2005).

However, the risks also need to be considered in the context of the individual, the type of procedure and the overall management plan. Significant risks include bleeding, hypo or hypertension, sedation, cardiac dysrhythmias, renal damage, and electrolyte disturbances (Norred et al. 2000). Many conventional medicines need to be adjusted or ceased prior to surgery. There is less information about managing CM medicines in surgical settings but there is a growing body of evidence to suggest that many CAM medicines may also need to be stopped or adjusted before surgery. Thus, it is important for conventional practitioners to ask about CM use, although most do not (Braun 2006).

The following general information is relevant to people already using CAM medicines and those considering using them before or after surgery. People are advised to consult a qualified CM practitioner for specific advice. Self-prescribing is not recommended because many CM medicines require supervised use especially in the context of the complex metabolic and neuroendocrine response to surgery.

Before surgery

People need written information about how to manage CM medicines in the operative period. Conventional health professionals can provide such information if they are qualified to do so. They should refer the person to a qualified CM practitioner if they do not have the relevant information. People also require written instructions about how to manage their conventional medicines as well as any special preparation needed for the surgery or investigation.

Great care is needed if the surgery is major or high risk such as heart, orthopaedic, or neurosurgery, if the person has renal or liver disease, or is very young or elderly. Most people's conventional medication list is unlikely to include CM medicines or supplements, although it should: thus, health professionals should discuss CM use with people during a structured medicines preoperative health assessment.

Some CM medicines such as evening primrose oil, bilberry, cranberry, fish oils, ginger, Gingko, liquorice, guarana, willow bark, meadowsweet, and ginseng need to be stopped at least one week before surgery. St John's Wort and supplements such as vitamin E should be stopped two weeks before surgery, primarily because of the risk of bleeding. Some, such as *Hypericum perforatum* (St John's Wort), may need to be stopped gradually (like conventional antidepressants). However, where CM medicines are the main form of treatment, alternative management may be required to prevent the condition deteriorating and affecting the surgical outcome, for example, glucose lowering herbal medicines.

Some commonly used CM medicines might/do interact with some anaesthetic agents and prolong their sedative effects, others increase the risk of bleeding, some affect blood pressure and the heart rate, others cause changes in the major electrolytes, potassium, calcium and sodium, levels in the blood. Grapefruit juice interferes with the action of some antibiotics such as cyclosporine (and some chemotherapeutic medicines), which may be needed pre- or postoperatively. Not everybody experiences such problems and it is sometimes difficult to predict who will or will not have problems. General safety issues also need to be considered.

Some hospitals have policies about using CM although they may not address surgery, investigations or diabetes specifically. People who wish to continue using CM in hospital should clarify the hospital's policies and procedures with the relevant hospital before they are admitted. Most hospitals do not prescribe or supply CM in Australia.

In addition to managing medicines, achieving the best possible health status before surgery improves recovery afterwards. The preoperative assessment is an ideal time to revise the importance of eating a healthy balanced diet and exercise within the individual's capability to control blood glucose and lipids as well as to support the immune system and enhance wound healing. Most people should continue their usual physical activity unless it is contraindicated to maintain strength and flexibility. Stress management strategies such as meditation, guided imagery, essential oil massage or inhalations, and music can help reduce anxiety and fear about the surgery. Ginger capsules or tablets taken one hour before surgery reduces postoperative nausea (Gupta and Sharma 2001).

The preoperative assessment is also an ideal time to discuss postoperative recovery including pain and sleep management. CM may be a useful alternative to some conventional medicines provided a QUM framework is adopted.

After surgery

A range of CM strategies can be used to manage postoperative pain and most are less likely to cause constipation and drowsiness than pethidine and morphine-based medicines. Alternatively, if these medicines are the best method of managing pain, high-fibre CM medicines such as *aloe vera* juice, probiotics, and psyllium can reduce constipation once oral feeding is allowed. Probiotics also increase bowel health and support natural bowel flora. Peppermint or ginger tea reduces mild-to-moderate nausea. Lymphatic drainage massage is very effective after some surgery to reduce swelling and relieve pain. Valerian, hops, and lavender in a vapourised essential oil blend or massage might promote restful sleep without the side effects of some conventional sedatives.

Some CM products promote wound healing, for example, *aloe vera*, Medihoney, and calendula and could be used depending on the wound. Arnica ointment reduces bruising but should not be used on open wounds. Comfrey poultices are very effective at reducing local oedema and local pain but should not be used on open wounds or taken internally.

After surgery, the person needs information about whether and when it is safe to start using CM again. New conventional medicines might be prescribed or dose and or dose intervals of medicines taken preoperatively might change, for example, anticoagulants, which could influence the choice of CM medicines or the dose. Likewise, some non-medicine CM might need to be used with care such as needle acupuncture and deep tissue massage because they can cause bruising and/or bleeding.

Adverse events

Adverse events encompass safety, which is a complex multifactorial issue (see Table 18.3). Using QUM strategies significantly reduces the risk of adverse events. Adverse events may be general or diabetes specific. CM-conventional medicines interactions can occur at the pharmaceutical, pharmacokinetic. The latter most likely involve changes in medicine absorption, distribution, metabolism, and/or excretion via the cytochrome P450 metabolising enzymes or phase 11 enzymes, especially uridine diphosphoglucuronosyl transferases (UGT) (Nourollahi 2019).

Diabetes-specific adverse events associated with CM reported in the literature include:

- Stopping insulin in a person with type 1 diabetes leading to ketoacidosis (Gill et al. 1994).
- Trauma and burns to neuropathic feet and legs from cupping and moxibustion (Ewins et al. 1993).
- Allergies, drug/herb interactions, and hospital admissions, largely from adulterated traditional Chinese medicine (Biegel and Schoenfeld 1998; Ko 1998).
- Hypoglycaemia following prolonged massage and using herbal therapies.
- Bleeding from herb/anticoagulant interactions (see Table 18.3).
- Kidney and liver damage; see Chapter 8 (US National Library of Medicine 2019).
- Heavy metal poisoning (Keen et al. 1994).

A number of initiatives have been taken to limit some of these problems, for example, in 1991 the World Health Organisation developed guidelines for the safe use, manufacturing

Table 18.3 Medicine-related safety and quality use of CAM and conventional medicines that need to be considered as inter-related factors that impact on outcomes.

Issue	Considerations for practitioners
Health system at global, national local levels	Degree of product regulation including manufacture and marketing Affordability and accessibility of medicines Support for research Adverse event monitoring systems Pre- and post-market surveillance systems including adverse event reporting systems Medicine scheduling systems Marketing processes Methods of communicating important medicine-related information to the public
Practitioner	Education and competence including ongoing professional development Regulation and self-regulatory processes, which includes scope of practice Licences to practice Professional liability insurance Communication, documentation, and referral processes Attitudes towards and beliefs about medicines and CAM
Herbal medicines	Research and development Pre- and post-market testing surveillance Manufacturing practices including herb identification, handling, storing, and infection control procedures, and whether the herb is prepared according to the traditional method Labels Adverse event monitoring including interactions Inappropriate dose and/or dose interval Prescribing to at risk groups Contraindicated
Person with diabetes	Age Physical and mental health status Knowledge Not disclosing herbal medicine use Self-diagnosis and self-treatment, which can delay treating serious problems Storage and handling of medicines Inappropriate use of medicines and CAM Monitoring defined outcomes False hope of cure or control Polypharmacy Cost

The information in this table pertains to type 2 diabetes.

and labelling of plant medicines, the Chinese government introduced strategies for identifying the content of Chinese herbal medicines and global strategies are in place to protect endangered animal and plant species as well as to improve the quality of CAM research. Another initiative, the Convention on International Trade in Endangered Species of Wild Fauna and Flora (CITES) was established in Washington, DC, in 1975 in response to growing concerns that over-exploitation of wildlife through the international trade could contribute to the rapid decimation of many plant and animal species in the world (CITES 2017).

Herb/medicine interactions

There are four main potential mechanisms for herb/medicine interactions. Herbs can:

(1) Induce or inhibit production of liver enzymes, especially the cytochrome P450 system, which reduces or enhances medicine bioavailability.
(2) Induce intestinal D-glycoprotein, which inhibits medicine absorption and metabolism.
(3) Stimulate neurotransmitter production especially serotonin enhancing the effects of some medicines, i.e. they both do the same thing. Others decrease the effects of serotonin-inhibiting medicines (Braun 2001; Braun and Cohen 2015).
(4) Compete with medicines for binding sites on serum protein increasing the amount of free medicine available. People with low serum albumin are especially at risk, for example, the older people and those with malnutrition.

Herb/medicine interactions are a two-way street – alone neither the medicine nor the herb might be a problem, but when used together, the *combination* can be potentially dangerous (see Table 18.4 for an overview of some of the common interactions). However, ingredients in the CM or conventional medicine beside the active ingredient/s might also be responsible for the adverse effects, for example, excipients, preservatives, and contaminants. It should also be noted that liver failure (20–30%) and kidney damage (30%) are recognised serious side effects of readily available conventional medicines, but the benefits are considered to outweigh the risks.

People most at risk of herb/medicine interactions are those who:

• Take medicines with a narrow therapeutic index such as lithium, phenytoin, barbiturates, warfarin, and digoxin and high-risk medicines such as insulin.
• Are at risk of, or have, renal and/or liver damage and therefore, have altered ability to metabolise and excrete medicine.
• Have atopic conditions such as allergies, asthma or dermatitis.
• Are older or are children.
• Take >5 medicines (polypharmacy).
• Use alcohol or drugs of addiction.
• Lack knowledge or consult CM and/or conventional clinicians who lack knowledge about appropriate therapies to use, and/or consult clinicians who do not ask them about CM use.
• Self-diagnosis and self-treat. This can delay seeking medical advice; Failure to tell conventional or CM practitioners about the therapies and medicines they are using increases risk.
• Import products, buy products online, or use products when travelling that are not subject to stringent regulations and good manufacturing practices. The danger of contamination with toxic substances such as heavy metal, pesticides and microbes, conventional medicines, and animal parts from some countries is significant.

People with diabetes are at increased risk because they usually have more than one risk factor present and risk factors could be additive.

How can CM be used safely?

Giving people appropriate advice so they can make informed decisions is an important aspect of nursing care (see Table 18.5). The following information could help clinicians assist people with diabetes to use CM safely and choose therapies appropriate for the problem they want to treat. Patients need to know there could be risks if they do not follow conventional evidence-based

Table 18.4 Commonly used herbs and supplements, their potential interactions, reported adverse events and some management strategies to use should an adverse event occur.

Herb	Potential interactions	Reported adverse events	Management strategies
Echinacea	Hepatoxic medicines, for example, anabolic steroids, amiodarone, methotrexate, ketoconazole Immunosuppressants, for example, corticosteroids, cyclosporine	Allergic reactions especially in atopic people Impairs the action of immunosuppressive drugs Can cause immunosuppression if taken long-term In acute surgery impairs wound healing	Do not use continuously for >8 weeks at a time
Fenugreek	Anticoagulants Oral hypoglycaemic agents (OHA)	Bleeding Hypoglycaemia	Do not use concurrently Monitor Adjust dose of OHA or the herb
Feverfew	NSAIDs, warfarin, offset the herb's effect for migraine and might alter bleeding time	Changed bleeding time	
Garlic	Aspirin Warfarin Cholesterol lowering agents	Risk of bleeding especially when taken with anticoagulants Increased GIT activity Decreased effectiveness of antacids Inhibits platelet aggregation Additive effects	Discontinue seven days before surgery Do not use concomitantly with antacids
Ginger	Antacids Warfarin	Decreased effectiveness of antacids	Do not use at the same time
Gingko biloba	Aspirin Warfarin SSRI MAO inhibitors	Bleeding risk if used with anticoagulants. Can interact with some chemotherapy medicines.	Stop 36 hours before surgery Do not use concurrently
Ginseng Note: there are several species in common use	Corticosteroids Oral contraceptives Warfarin Digoxin Oral hypoglycaemic agents MAO inhibitors and tricyclic antidepressants	Increased risk of bleeding with anticoagulants Suppresses immune system – infections risk Hypoglycaemia Headache Additive effects. Can interact with some chemotherapy medicines.	Stop seven days before surgery Do not use concomitantly with these medicines.
Glucosamine		GIT complaints Allergy if allergic to seafoods Nausea, vomiting abdominal pain Sleepiness Hyperglycaemia	Avoid with seafoods

(Continued)

Table 18.4 (Continued)

Herb	Potential interactions	Reported adverse events	Management strategies
Guar and bulking agents	Antibiotics Alpha-glucosidase inhibitors	Decreased food absorption – hypoglycaemia risk	Do not administer at the same time
Hawthorn	Antihypertensive agents Digoxin Alcohol, Antipsychotics	Hypotension Dizziness Falls	
Kelp (contains iodine)	Thyroid hormones Antithyroid hormones	Altered thyroid function	
Liquorice	Corticosteroids Antihypertensive agents Oral contraceptives Digoxin	Fluid retention Electrolyte imbalance Block oestrogen in contraception Digoxin toxicity	
Slippery elm		Decrease GIT absorption Hypoglycaemia	
St John's Wort	MAO inhibitors SSRI Decreases effect of HIV medications Warfarin Anticonvulsants Activates liver enzyme, hastening drug metabolism and reducing their effectiveness	Alters metabolism of some medicines, for example, cyclosporin, warfarin, steroids Interacts with psychotrophic drugs and can increase their effect Skin allergies	Stop five days before operation Do not use concomitantly. Can interact with some chemotherapy medicines.
Valerian, hops	Anaesthetic agents Barbiturates Hypnotics Antidepressive medicines	Enhance/potentiate the effects of sedatives With long-term use the amount of anaesthetic needed is increased	Withdrawal – symptoms resemble valium addiction Taper dose preoperatively
Tee tree essential oil	Unclear	Rare and conflicting reports of prepubertal gynecomastia in boys	Use with caution and in low doses and not for long periods of time.
Vitamin supplements C and E, B group; often as antioxidants	Vitamin toxicity Niacin	Decreases the beneficial effects of statins on HDL levels	
Zinc	Increased HbA_{1c} in Type 1 Type 1 diabetes		
Magnesium, calcium, iron			Can interact with some chemotherapy medicines.

Many of these interactions are theoretical, others are well documented. When considering the likelihood of an interaction, the total individual situation and medication regimen must be considered. In addition, although 'medicine interactions' is usually used to denote negative interactions, the term itself is objective and non-judgmental. Many interactions may actually be beneficial and it is just as important to document these.
Source: Data from Braun and Cohen (2015).

Table 18.5 Advice health professionals can provide to people with diabetes to help them use complementary medicine (CM) safely.

- Consider what you want to achieve by using CM.
- Decide on your general life and health goals and your diabetes care goals.
- Select a therapy or therapies that is likely to achieve these goals.
- Learn all there is about it/then so you can use the therapy from an informed perspective.
- Consult reputable practitioners for example a member of a professional association that has training standards and requires practitioners to keep up-to-date.
- Buy products from reputable sources that comply with good manufacturing and regulatory processes and are stored appropriately before purchase. Be wary of importing other medicines or buying on the Internet.
- Read labels carefully, e.g. look for Aust L or Aust R on the label in Australia, which means the product is approved by the body that regulates medicines.
- Australia, Canada, UK, US, and some other countries have medicine approval processes that encompass CM
- Have a correct diagnosis before using any therapy. Inform conventional and complementary practitioners about all the therapies you are using and understand there may be risks associated with not following evidence based conventional care.
- Monitor the effects against the health goals you set.
- Keep a list of all the CM medicines and therapies you use, update it regularly and make sure your CM and conventional health professionals have a copy.
- Realise that some CM may take longer to show an effect than conventional medicines.
- Do not stop conventional medicines without consulting your doctor or diabetes educator. CM medicines may need to be adjusted or stopped temporarily before surgery, illness, investigations, and changes in conventional medicines. You should seek advice in these circumstances.
- Seek advice quickly if any of the following occur: hypo or hyperglycaemia, mental changes, abdominal pain, skin rashes, nausea, vomiting, diarrhoea, falls.

diabetes management practices. They should not be made to feel guilty or lacking in judgement if they choose to use CM. People can be advised to:

- Develop a holistic health plan and decide what they hope to achieve by using CAM and use a therapy that is best suited to achieve these goals. For example, to reduce stress: use massage, counselling, or time-line therapy.
- Find out as much about the therapy as they can before using it. Seek information from unbiased sources and be wary of information they find in chat rooms on the Internet and advertising material.
- Consult a reputable practitioner, for example, a member of the relevant professional association, and buy products from reputable sources that are approved. Have labels that meet labelling standards and can provide relevant safety data.
- Store and maintain products appropriately and consider safety issues if children and confused elderly people are part of the household. This also applies to storing products in healthcare settings.
- Ensure the condition for which the person wants to use CM is correctly diagnosed before they treat it; otherwise, appropriate treatment could be delayed and the condition deteriorate.
- Be aware that there are risks if they do not follow conventional evidence-based diabetes management recommendations.
- Be aware that they should not stop or change recommended conventional treatments without the advice of their doctor.
- Inform all practitioners, conventional and complementary, about the therapies they are using so the health plan can be coordinated.
- Some CM should not be used continuously for long periods because it can have cumulative effects.
- Take extra care if they are old, very young, pregnant, breastfeeding, have kidney or liver damage, or are using a lot of other treatments, because these people are at increased risk of adverse events.

- Seek advice about how to manage the therapy if they need surgery or an investigative procedure, especially if radio contrast media are required (see Chapters 3 and 8), or they are starting any new conventional treatment.
- Seek advice quickly if any of the following occur:
  ○ Hypo/hyperglycaemia
  ○ Mental changes
  ○ Abdominal pain
  ○ Skin rashes
  ○ Nausea, vomiting, diarrhoea
- Monitor the effects on their diabetes, for example, blood glucose, lipids, and HbA1c, as well as their response with respect to the reason they chose the therapy, for example, to manage pain.

Clinician responsibilities

Clinicians have a responsibility to respect people's choices and not to be judgemental about the choices they make. They also have responsibilities to their employer, other patients, visitors, and staff. Clinicians can use CM as part of holistic care but they have a duty of care to practice at the level of their education and competence and use safe therapies. The following general advice applies. Specific information about individual CM should be sought before using CM or giving advice about it.

- Reflect on own attitudes towards and beliefs about CM.
- Be sensitive to the philosophical and cultural views of people with diabetes and be aware that they may perceive risks and benefits differently from health professionals.
- Follow guidelines for using CM where they exist – for example, those of the NMC in the UK. In Australia the state nurse registering authorities, the Australian Nursing Federation, and the Australian College of Nursing have all produced guidelines for nurses using CM (McCabe 2001).
- Ensure CM practitioners are appropriately qualified and competent if you decide to use, recommend, or refer a person with diabetes to a CM practitioner.
- Look for evidence of safety and efficiency but do not be too quick to accept or reject 'evidence'.
- Communicate the risks and benefits to people with diabetes and their families/carers. If the person chooses not to follow advice, documentation should outline the information that was given.
- Develop a portfolio of evidence for reference in clinical areas where CM is used.
- Consider the effect of CM on other staff, visitors and patients, for example, vapourising essential oils, playing music.
- Know how to contact the Poisons Advisory Service in the area.
- Have mechanisms in place to clean and maintain any equipment needed, for example, aromatherapy vapourisers. Processes should be in place to deal with any CAM products the patient brings with them.
- Document appropriately, in the same manner as conventional treatment, the type, dose and duration of the therapy, condition it is used for, advice given, expected outcome, actual outcome and report any adverse events.
- Reliably report suspected or actual CM adverse events (see Table 18.6).
- Use CM within the philosophy of QUM and prescribe, administer, document, and monitor within that philosophy. Ask about CM. People are not always willing to disclose such information, and skilled questioning may be required. Questions should be asked in a framework of acceptance. The person has a responsibility to disclose. Clinicians can make it easier for them to do so.
- Value the clinician–patient relationship as an essential aspect of the healing process.

Table 18.6   Scale for assessing the likelihood of a complementary medicine (CM)-conventional interaction and information that should be included in a report.

Interpreting the score[a]:

0–3: Insufficient information to be able to assessed/attribute the event CAM use.

4–7: Interaction is possible but other explanations for the event need to be excluded.

8–10: Interaction is likely.

(1)   The health history is well documented.

(2)   The person has:
   (a) renal disease
   (b) liver disease
   (c) atopic conditions
   (d) significant alcohol or illegal drug use
   (e) is very young or elderly

(3)   The AE[b] was associated with using a CM medicine or therapy.

(4)   The medication regimen is documented and includes conventional medicines, CM medicines, and over-the-counter medicines and doses and dose frequency.

(5)   Alternative explanations for the event are excluded.

(6)   The AE is adequately described, for example, time of onset of symptoms in relation to taking the medicine, what actually happened, what else was occurring at the time the event occurred.

(7)   The time between taking the medicine and the onset of the event is reasonable considering the medicine usual action profile.

(8)   The reaction resolves when the CM medicine is stopped.

(9)   The sequence of events is consistent with an AE.

(10)   The event recurs when the medicine is used again.

---

[a] One point is allocated to each of the following criteria.

[b] AE: adverse event. The event should be noted in the individual's health history and an adverse event report forwarded through the relevant process in the country of origin. In Australia reports go to the Adverse Drug Reactions Advisory Committee (ADRAC) on the 'blue' reporting form (www.tga.gov.au/adr/bluecard.pdf). In the US, suspected interactions can be reported via the MedWatch program (http://www.fda.gov/medwatch/how.htm). In the UK reports can be submitted on the yellow card to the Medicines and Healthcare Products Regulation Agency (MHRA) and the Commission Human Medicine (CHM) (www.yellowcard.gov.au) (Fugh-Berman and Ernst (2001) and the websites cited above).

Identifying quality health information on the internet

Many people gain information about CM from the media. Generally, the media and pharmaceutical bodies are careful to only make medium to general level claims consistent with regulations. They often rely on information published in quality peer-reviewed conventional journals often as meta-analysis or systematic reviews or presented at conferences and frequently use 'experts' to promote their message. These experts should declare any conflict of interest, which is increasingly required in publications but is not common in other media.

However, the media also specialises in telling storeys and sensationalising information, therefore, clinicians may need to verify the source of the information and be wary of sites that quote 'experts' to gain credibility. In addition, the media often reports 'exciting breakthroughs' but the product may not actually be available for many years.

When accessing Internet information, carefully scrutinise the site – the quality and reliability varies a great deal. Nonsponsored sites are likely to be more objective. Questions to ask include:

• What is the name of the individual or organisation that produced the site? Information produced by reputable organisations is likely to be more reliable than that produced by individuals.

• What are their credentials?

• Are their links to other sources I can use to verify the information?

• Is the information presented in an objective way, and does it discuss a range of options and their benefits and risks?

- Is the discussion comprehensive, or does it only discuss one or two options, all available from one manufacturer; i.e. is the information actually advertising/marketing?
- Is the site clearly selling products? As a general rule of thumb, if the site is selling or promoting a product and has a number of glowing testimonials from 'happy, satisfied customers', be wary, and check the information through another source.
- Is there evidence that the information has been verified in any way, e.g. is there a list of peer-reviewed references or links to other reputable sites?
- Is any conflict of interest declared?

Various guidelines have also been developed to evaluate Internet health information but some may not be applicable to CM (Cooke and Gray 2002). The following are examples that might be useful when assessing the reliability of Internet information:

- Biome Evaluation Guidelines
- Sandvik Score
- European Commission Guidelines
- Discern instrument, which was developed for use by the general public
- eHealth Code of Ethics

The following processes are commonly used to grade evidence into a hierarchy according to the quality of the science:

- JADAD score (formulated for CAM)
- National Health and Medical Research Council levels of evidence
- Cochrane Data base process
- Joanna Briggs Center for Evidence Based Nursing

Other factors to consider are the advertising codes of relevant countries.

Self-reflection

(1) How will you respond to a person with diabetes who asks you about taking a Chinese herbal medicine to control his blood glucose?
(2) What will you do when a person with diabetes and end-stage renal failure elects to use herbal medicine?
(3) How would you advise a person with diabetes who asks you if she can use aromatherapy to help her sleep?

Clinical observation

A young Aboriginal man from Central Australia was studying research methods at a university. At the same time, he was being educated about traditional tribal practices. He fractured his tibia and fibula playing football. It was a simple fracture, but he became depressed and the bones were not mending as well as expected.

The young man's mother took him to consult with the tribal elders. On his return, the doctor said to the mother, 'That won't cure him, you know'. The mother replied, 'No, but it will put him in a frame of mind to accept your medicine. That will work now'.

Recommended resources

Cochrane Library complementary and alternative medicine. http://www.cohranelibrary.com/topic/complementary%20alternative%20medicine.

Braun, L. & Cohen, M, (2015) *Herbs and Natural Supplements: An Evidence-Based Guide*. 4 vols. 1 and 2 Churchill Livingstone, Chatswood, Sydney.

NICM health information, www.nicm.edu.au/health_information, and fact sheets: information for consumers www.nicm.edu.au/health_information/information_for_consumers.

References

Abuaisha, B., Boulton, A., and Costanz, J. (1998). Acupuncture for the treatment of chronic painful diabetic peripheral neuropathy: a long-term study. *Diabetes Research and Clinical Practice* **39** (2): 115–121.

Agrawal, R. (2007). Yoga improves sense of well-being, reverses changes in metabolic syndrome. *Diabetes Research and Clinical Practice* **78**: e9–e10.

AIMA (2014). Best practice for integrative medicine in Australian medical practice. http://dx.do1.org/10.1016/j.aimed.2013.12.001.

Australasian Integrative Medicine Association (AIMA) (2014). www.aima.net.au.

Baskaran, K., Kizar, A., Radha, K., and Shanmugasundaram, E. (1990). Antidiabetic effect of leaf extract from *Gymnema sylvestre* in non insulin-dependant diabetes mellitus patients. *Journal of Ethnopharmacology* **30** (3): 295–300.

Bent, S., Tiedt, T., Odden, M., and Shipak, M. (2003). The relative safety of ephedra compared with other products. *Annals of Internal Medicine* **138** (6): 468–467.

Biegel, Y. and Schoenfeld, N. (1998). A leading question. *New England Journal of Medicine* **339**: 827–830.

Bjelakovic, G., Nikolova, D., Gluud, L.L. et al. (2007). Mortality in randomized controlled trials of antioxidant supplements for primary and secondary prevention: systematic review and meta-analysis. *Journal of the American Medical Association* **297**: 842–857.

Braun, L. (2001). Herb – drug interactions: a danger or an advantage? *Diversity* **2** (6): 31–34.

Braun, L. (2006). Use of complementary medicines by surgical patients. Undetected and unsupervised. *Proceedings of the Fourth Australasian Conference on Safety and Quality in Health Care*, Melbourne.

Braun, L. and Cohen, M. (2015). *Herbs and Natural Supplements: An Evidence-Based Guide*, 4e vols. 1 and 2. Chatswood, Sydney: Churchill Livingstone.

Bridges, W. (1991). *Transitions: Making Sense of Life's Changes*. Reading MA, USA: Addison Wesley.

Buckle, J. (1997). *Clinical Aromatherapy in Nursing*. London: Arnold.

Cancer Australia (2010). Complementary and alternative therapies. https://canceraustralina.gov.au/publications-and-resources/position-statements.

Chan, C., Ng, S., Rainbow, T., and Chow, A. (2006). Making sense of spirituality. *Journal of Clinical Nursing* **15**: 822–834.

Chaudhary, S. (2007). Peppermint oil may relieve digestive symptoms, headaches. *American Family Physician* **75**: 1027–1030.

Chou, K., Lee, P., and Yu, E. (2004). Tai Chi on depressive symptoms amongst Chinese older patients with depressive disorders: a randomized clinical trial. *International Journal of Geriatric Psychiatry* **19** (11): 1105–1107.

Cochrane Collaboration (2000). Complementary medicine field. http://www.cochrane.org/.../topic-list-cochrane-complementary-medicine-field-related-reviews-cochraneorg (accessed November 2012).

Convention on International Trade in Endangered Species of Wild Fauna and Flora (CITES) (2017). The CITES species. http://www.cites.org/eng/disc/species.php.

Cooke, A. and Gray, L. (2002). Evaluating the quality of internet based information about alternative therapies: development of the BIOME guidelines. *Journal of Public Health Medicine* **24**: 261–267.

Dossey, B., Keegan, L., Guzzetta, C., and Kolkmeier, L. (1998). *Holistic Nursing: A Handbook for Practice*. Gaithersburg, Maryland US: Aspen Publications.

Dunn, E. (2019). Are unnecessarily tying ourselves up in knots over CAM? Medical Observer. www.medicalobserver.com.au/workwise/are-we-unnecessarily-tying-ourselve-up-in-knots.

Dunning, T. (2001). Developing clinical practice guidelines. In: *Complementary Therapies in Nursing and Midwifery* (ed. P. McCabe), 37–48. Melbourne VIC: Ausmed Publications.

Dunning, T. (2007). Quality use of medicines: does the concept apply to complementary medicines? *The Australian Diabetes Educator* **5**: 20–49.

Dunning, T. (2013a). Teaching and learning: the art and science of making connections, Chapter 3. In: *Diabetes Education Art Science and Evidence* (ed. T. Dunning), 28–48. Chichester: Wiley-Blackwell.

Dunning, T. (2013b). Turning points and transition crises and opportunities, Chapter 8. In: *Diabetes Education Art Science and Evidence* (ed. T. Dunning), 117–132. Chichester: Wiley-Blackwell.

Dunning, T., Chan, S.P., Hew, F.L. et al. (2001). A cautionary tale on the use of complementary therapies. *Diabetes in Primary Care* 3 (2): 58–63.

Dunning, T. and Martin, P. (2019). Guidelines for deciding palliative and end of life care with people with diabetes. Centre for Quality and Patient Safety Research, Barwon Health and Deakin University (trisha.dunning@deakin.edu.au).

Egede, L., Xiaobou, Y., Zheng, D., and Silverstein, M. (2002). The prevalence and pattern of complementary and alternative medicine use in individuals with diabetes. *Diabetes Care* 25: 324–329.

Einerhand, S. (2006). CLA weight loss debate continues. *WebMD Health News* (2006). http://www.webmd.com/.../news/20060522/cla-weight-loss-debate-continues (accessed December 2012).

Eisenberg, D. (1998). Advising patients who seek alternative medical therapies. *American Journal of Health Medicine* 127 (1): 61–69.

Ewins, D., Bakker, K., Youn, M., and Boulton, A. (1993). Alternative medicine: potential dangers for the diabetic foot. *Diabetic Medicine* 10: 980–982.

Field, T., Hernandez-Reif, M., LaGreca, A. et al. (1997). Massage lowers blood glucose levels in children with diabetes. *Diabetes Spectrum* 10: 237–239.

Finney, L. and Gonzalez-Campoy, J. (1997). *Dietary Chromium and Diabetes: Is there a Relationship?* 6–8. Clinical Diabetes.

Flachskampf, F., Gallasch, J., Gefeller, O. et al. (2007). Randomized trial of acupuncture to lower blood pressure. *Circulation* 115 (24): 3121–3129.

Foley, H. and Steel, A. (2017). The nexus between patient-centred care and complementary medicine: allies in an era of chronic disease? *Journal of Alternative and Complementary Medicine* 3: 158–163.

Fugh-Berman, A. and Ernst, E. (2001). Herb – drug interactions: review and assessment of report reliability. *British Journal of Clinical Pharmacology* 52: 587–595.

Garrow, D. and Egede, L. (2006). Association between complementary and alternative medicine use, preventative care practices, and use of conventional medical services among adults with diabetes. *Diabetes Care* 29: 15–19.

Gill, G., Redmond, S., Garratt, F., and Paisley, R. (1994). Diabetes and alternative medicine: cause for concern. *Diabetic Medicine* 11: 210–213.

Grossman, L., Roscoe, R., and Shack, A. (2018). Complementary and alternative medicine for diabetes. *Canadian Journal of Diabetes* 42: S154–S161. https://doi.org/10.1016/jcjd.2017.10.023.

Gupta, Y. and Sharma, M. (2001). Reversal of pyrogallol-induced gastric emptying in rats by ginger (*Zingiber officinalis*). *Experimental and Clinical Pharmacology* 23 (9): 501–503.

Guo, R., Pittler, M., and Ernst, E. (2008). Hawthorn extract for treating chronic heart failure. *Cochrane Database of Systematic Reviews* (1): CD005312. https://doi.org/10.1002/14651858.CD005312.

Hildreth, K. and Elman, C. (2007). Alternative worldviews and the utilization of conventional and complementary medicine. *Sociological Inquiry* 77 (1): 76–103.

Jepson, R. and Craig, J. (2008). Cranberries for preventing urinary tract infections. *Cochrane Database of Systematic Reviews* (1): CD001321. https://doi.org/10.1002/14651858.CD001321.pub4.

Keen, R., Deacon, A., Delves, H. et al. (1994). Indian herbal remedies for diabetes as a cause of lead poisoning. *Postgraduate Medicine Journal* 70: 113–114.

Kelner, M. and Wellman, B. (1997). Health care and consumer choices: medical and alternative therapies. *Social Science and Medicine* 45: 203–212.

Ko, R. (1998). Adulterants in Asian patent medicines. *New England Journal of Medicine* 339: 847.

Kotsirilos, V., Vitetta, L., and Sali, A. (2011). *An Evidence-Based Guide to Integrative and Complementary Medicine*. Chatswood NSW, Australia: Churchill Livingstone.

Leese, G., Gill, G., and Houghton, G. (1997). Prevalence of complementary medicine usage within a diabetic clinic. *Practical Diabetes International* 14 (7): 207–208.

Lloyd, P., Lupton, D., Wiesner, D., and Hasleton, S. (1993). Choosing on alternative therapy: an exploratory study of sociodemographic characteristics and motives of patients resident in Sydney. *Australian Journal of Public Health* 17 (2): 135–144.

MacLennan, A., Wilson, D., and Taylor, A. (1996). Prevalence and cost of alternative medicine in Australia. *The Lancet* 347: 569–573.

MacLennan, A., Wilson, D., and Taylor, A. (2002). The escalating cost and prevalence of alternative medicine. *Preventative Medicine* 35 (2): 166–173.

Manya, K., Champion, B., and Dunning, T. (2012). The use of complementary and alternative medicines among people living with diabetes in Western Sydney. *BMC Complementary Medicines* 12: 1–5.

Martin, J., Wang, Z., Zhang, X. et al. (2006). Chromium picolinate supplementation attenuates body weight gain and increases insulin sensitivity in subjects with type 2 diabetes. *Diabetes Care* 29 (8): 1826–1832.

Mason, S.A., Rasmussen, B., van Loon, L.J. et al. (2019). Ascorbic acid supplementation improves postprandial glycaemic control and blood pressure in individuals with type 2 diabetes: Findings of a randomized cross-over trial. *Diabetes, Obesity and Metabolism* 21 (3): 674–682.

McCabe, P. (ed.) (2001). *Complementary Therapies in Nursing and Midwifery*. Melbourne: Ausmed Publications.

McGrady, A., Bailey, B., and Good, M. (1991). Controlled study of biofeedback assisted relaxation in type 1 diabetes. *Diabetes Care* **14** (5): 360–365.

Meyers, S. and Vigar, V. (2019). The stare of the evidence for whole-system, multi-modality naturopathic medicine: a systematic scoping review. *Journal of Alternative and Complementary Medicine* **25** (2): 141–168.

Mitchinson, A., Kim, H., Rosenberg, J. et al. (2007). Acute postoperative pain management using massage as an adjuvant therapy: a randomized trial. *Archives of Surgery* **142** (12): 1158–1167.

National Centre of Complementary and Integrative Health (2016). Complementary, alternative or integrative health: what's in a name? National Institutes of Health (NIH) US Department of Health and Human Services. https://ncch.nih.gov/health/integrative-health.

US National Library of Medicine (2019). Kidney diseases. MedlinePlus. www.nlm.nih.gov/medlineplus/kidneydiseases.html.

Norred, C., Zamudio, S., and Palmer, S. (2000). Use of complementary and alternative medicines by surgical patients. *American Association of Nurse Anesthetists Journal* **68** (1): 13–18.

Nourollahi, F. (2019). Five things to know about alternative therapies and cancer. https://www.medscape.com/viewarticle/909044_print.

O'Brien, R. and Timmins, K. (1999). Trends. *Endocrinology and Metabolism* **5**: 329–334.

O'sathuna, D. (2007). Creatinine and resistance training for older adults. *Alternative Medicine Alert* **10** (11): 121–124.

Parsian, N. and Dunning, T. (2008a). Validation tool to assess spirituality and coping in young adults with diabetes. In: *Proceedings of the 3rd International Congress of Complementary Medicine Research, (ICMR)*. Sydney, Australia: ICMR.

Parsian, N. and Dunning, T. (2008b). Spirituality and coping in young adults with diabetes. *Proceedings of the 7th International Diabetes Federation Western Pacific Region Congress, (IDFWPR)*. IDFWPR, Wellington, New Zealand.

Phelps, K. and Hassed, C. (2011). *General Practice: The Integrative Approach*. Chatswood NSW, Australia: Churchill Livingstone.

Phillips, N. (2012) Bits of black bear found in Chinese medicines. *Sydney Morning Herald* (13 April), p. 24.

Rosenfeldt, F., Marasco, S., Lyon, W. et al. (2005). Coenzyme Q10 therapy before cardiac surgery improves mitochondrial function and in vitro contractility of myocardial tissue. *Journal of Thoracic and Cardiovascular Surgery* **129**: 25–32.

Ryan, E., Pick, M., and Marceau, C. (1999). Use of alternative therapies in diabetes mellitus. In: *Proceedings of the American Diabetes Association Conference (ADA)*. San Diego, CA, USA: ADA.

Sharma, R., Raghuram, T., and Rao, N. (1990). Effect of fenugreek seeds on blood glucose and serum lipids in type 1 diabetes. *European Journal of Clinical Nutrition* **44**: 301–306.

Sharma, R., Sarkar, A., and Hazra, D. (1996). Use of fenugreek seeds powder in the management of non insulin-dependent diabetes mellitus. *Nutrition Research* **16**: 1331–1339.

Sharpe, P., Blanck, H., Williams, J. et al. (2007). Use of complementary and alternative medicine for weight control in the United States. *The Journal of Complementary and Alternative Medicine* **13** (2): 217–222.

Stevensen, C. (1994). The psychophysiological effects of aromatherapy massage following cardiac surgery. *Complementary Therapies in Medicine* **2** (1): 27–35.

Szegede, A., Kohnen, R., and Dienel, A. (2005). Acute treatment of moderate to severe depression with hypericum extract WS 5570 (St John's Wort): randomized controlled double blind non-inferiority trial versus paroxetine. *British Medical Journal* **330** (7490): 503.

Thomson, S. (2001). Complementary therapies in aged care. In: *Complementary Therapies in Nursing and Midwifery* (ed. P. McCabe), 257–275. Melbourne: Ausmed Publications.

Tsen, L., Segal, S., Pothier, M. et al. (2000). Alternative medicine use in presurgical patients. *Anesthesiology* **93**: 148–151.

Udani, J., Kavoussi, B., and Hardy, M. (2006). Chromium for type 2 diabetes mellitus and weight loss. *Alternative Medicine Alert* **9** (7): 78–82.

Verdejo, C., Marco, P., Renau-Piqueras, J., and Pinazo-Duran, M. (1999). Lipid peroxidation in proliferative vitreoretinopathies. *Eye* **13** (Part 2): 183–188.

Vuksan, V., Stavro, M., Seivenpiper, J. et al. (2000). Similar postprandial glycaemic reductions with escalation of dose and administration time of American ginseng in type 2 diabetes. *Diabetes Care* **23**: 1221–1226.

Wilson, R. (2007). Difficulty identifying odours may herald mild cognitive impairment. *Archives of General Psychiatry* **64**: 802–808.

World Health Organization (WHO) (2002). *Traditional Medicine Strategy 2002–2005*. Geneva: WHO.

World Health Organization (WHO) (2019). Global Report on Traditional and Complementary Medicine. WHO, Geneva. https://apps.who.int/iris/handle/10665/312342;jsessionid=2D797767ADF9C2EC092CCB0B8B05EDBE.

Zhang, L., Ma, J., and Pan, K. (2005). Efficacy of Cranberry juice on *Helicobacter pylori* infection: a double-blind randomized placebo-controlled trial. *Helicobacter* **10**: 139–145.

Index

Page numbers in *italics* refer to figures.
Page numbers in **bold** refer to tables.

A1c-derived average glucose equivalent, 79, 80
A1 protein, milk, 457
Abasaglar, 139
Abbott Libre Freestyle meter, 73
abdomen, insulin injections in pregnancy, 458
abdominal fat, 96
abdominal massage, 270
abdominal obesity, 98, *see also* central obesity
   on adipokines, **95**
   waist circumference, 11, 13, 18, 98
abdominal pain
   emergency surgery, 292
   ketoacidosis, 75, **207**
Aboriginal and Torres Strait Islanders
   erectile dysfunction, 377
   type 2 diabetes in children, 21
abscesses, oral, 328
absorption
   insulin, factors affecting, 69, **145**
   medicines and food, **104**
      antacids on, **105**
   vitamin B_{12}, metformin on, 124
acanthosis nigricans, 20
acarbose, 14, **121**, 189
acceptance of diabetes, 472
acceptance of medicines, 163
accidents *see* crashes
ACCOMPLISH trial, 159
acetoacetate, 74
acetone, 74
acidosis, *see also* lactic acidosis
   ketoacidosis, 207
Acorus calamus, 324
action plan, chest pain, 235
action profiles, insulin, 142
activation (patient activation), 51, 502
active learning style, **495**
activities of daily living, 392
acupuncture, 551
   cancer, 314
   for pain, 265
   smoking cessation, 319

acute complications, 36
adaptation, 477
adaptive triage process, 387
addiction, **316**
   alcohol, 320–322, 330
   nicotine, 318
adherence (term), 483–484
adherence to medicines
   adolescence, 437–438
   education, 164
   person-centred empowerment model, 164
   questionnaires on, 165
adhesive capsulitis, shoulder, 345
adipocyte-derived protein, **227**
adipokines, **95**, 330
adiponectin, **95**, **227**
adipose tissue, 97
   abdominal, 96
adjustable gastric bands, **102**, 293
ADKNOWL, 507
admission to hospital
   children and adolescents, 430
   indications, 202, 280
   readmissions after surgery, 283
adolescence, **433**, 434–435
   adherence to medicines, 437–438
   dementia risk, 395
   glucagon, 434
   hypoglycaemia, 192, 434
   indigenous Australians, 21
   metabolic syndrome, 13–14
   obesity, 96
   over-the-counter medicines, 436
   sex and, 373, 376
adrenaline, **183**
   deficit, 185
   surgery and, **282**
adrenal insufficiency, 538
adrenergic symptoms *see* catecholamines; sympathetic
      symptoms
adulteration, complementary medicines, 549
advance care plans, 523, 526–528, 530, 531

advanced driving classes, 358
advanced glycation end-products, 222, **387**
    dementia, 401
adverse events, 162
    complementary medicine, 554–556, **557–558**
        scores and reporting, **561**
advocacy, 504
aerobic lactic acidosis, 215
Afrezza (insulin), 137
aged-care facilities
    aromatherapy, 552
    complementary medicine, 545
    malnutrition, **403, 404**
    sexual health in, 375
    suboptimal care, 392–393
ageing, 386, *see also* older people
    foot, **266**
    theories, **387**
Agency for Healthcare Research and Quality,
        checklists, 23
age-related macular degeneration *see* macular
        degeneration
age-related weight gain, 100
AIDES method, 163
airway, **285**
alanine aminotransferase, 329
alarm systems, insulin pumps, 143
albumin, *see also* microalbuminuria
    glycated, 24
    herb/medicine interactions, 556
    life expectancy decline, 525
    nutritional deficiency, 91, 405
    urine levels for renal disease, 245
albumin–creatinine ratio, *see also* microalbumin–
        creatinine ratio
    target values, **31**
albumin–creatinine urine test, 245
albuminuria, *see also* microalbuminuria
    antiretrovirals, 343
    omega-3 fatty acids and, 255
alcohol, 107
    addiction, 320–322, 330
    adverse effects, 154
    on blood lipids, **93**, 154
    hypoglycaemia, 107, 193, 322
    interactions with medicines, **105**, 130
    limits, **31**, 94
    lipid estimations and, 81
    liver disease, 331
    older people, 404
    swabbing with, 73
aldose reductase, 223
    inhibitors, 260
algorithms, insulin in type 2 diabetes, 132, *133*, 134
alkaline phosphatase, foot disease, 258
allergy, insulin, 149–150
ALLHAT (trial), 154
alpha fibres, peripheral neuropathy, 260
alpha-glucosidase inhibitors, 117, **121**, 126–127
    medicine interactions, 130
    rapid-acting insulin analogues and, 137
α-interferon, 330

α-lipoic acid, 260
alternate-day steroid regimens, 349
alternative medicine *see* complementary medicine
Alzheimer's disease, 400–401
    gum disease, **396**
    odour identification, 552
Amadori reaction, 79
Amanita muscaria, 324
ambulance services, hypoglycaemia, 177
American Diabetes Association
    on oral glucose tolerance test, 22
    on SMBG, 66
Ames hypothesis, 387
aminophylline, topical, 103
amlodipine, **158**
amputations, 255, 256, 258, 266
anabolism, *10*
anaemia
    coeliac disease, 334
    renal disease, 248
anaerobic exercise, 33–34
anaerobic lactic acidosis, 215
anaesthesia, 289
    epidural, hypoglycaemia, 453
analgesics, 39
ancestral diets, on microbiome, 92
andropause, 377
Angelica sinensis (dong quai), 461
angina pectoris, 226
angiotensin-II antagonists, **161**, 230
angiotensin-converting enzyme inhibitors, 158–159,
        160, 230
    medicine interactions, **129**
    myocardial infarction, 233
    pregnancy and, **450, 451**
    renal disease, 247
angiotensinogen, **95**
angiotensin receptor blockers (ARBs)
    renal disease, 247
    teratogenesis, **450**
Anglo-Scandinavian trial (ASCOT), 154
anhedonia, 478
1,5-anhydroglucitol, 24, 238
animal insulins, 137
animals, continuous blood glucose monitoring, 74
anion gap, **204**
annual reviews, 83
anorexia, renal disease, 249
Antabuse (disulfiram), 322
antacids, on food absorption, **105**
antiandrogens, 446
antibiotics
    foot disease, 257–258
    gastroparesis, 269
    grapefruit juice and, 299
anticellulite preparations, 103
anticoagulants, sulphonylureas and, **189**
anticonvulsants, for peripheral neuropathy, **259**
antidepressants, *see also* tricyclic antidepressants
    metabolic effects, 350
antihypertensives, 158–159, **160–161**, 229–230, 235
    clinical trials, 154

combined with statins, **157**
    hypotension, 158, 233
    pregnancy, **450**, 453
anti-inflammatory properties, insulin, 131
antioxidant chain, 221–222
antioxidants, 88, 222, 387, 551
antiplatelet agents, 159–161
antipsychotics, 350, 483, 538
    cardiovascular effects, **351**
    dementia, 415
    medicine interactions, **129**
    polycystic ovarian syndrome, 446
    screening, 14
antiretrovirals, 342, 343
antiseptics, foot disease and, 263
antithrombotic agents, 229
anxiety
    cardiovascular disease, 232
    end of life, **529**
    polycystic ovarian syndrome, 446
aphrodisiacs, 379
apidra, 137
apolipoprotein A-1 mimetic peptides, 156
appetite, haemodialysis, 249–250
appointments, 411
arnica, 299, 554
aromatherapy, 551–552
arrhythmias, antipsychotics, 350
arthropathy, *see also* limited joint mobility
    haemochromatosis, 332
    on sexual health, 374
artificial intelligence (AI), 40
    retinopathy, 241
artificial pancreas, 41
ascorbic acid, 222, 551
ASCOT (trial), 154
Ashwaganda capsules, 319
aspart, 137
ASPEN (clinical trial), 155
aspirin, 159, 229, 236
    gastric effects, 536
    macular degeneration, 161
    pregnancy, **451**
    retinopathy, 241, 297
assessment
    caregivers, **393**
    cognitive decline, 398
    diabetic ketoacidosis, 206–207
    driving, 357
    frailty, 394
    hypoglycaemic unawareness, 186
    Internet information, 561–562
    learning needs, 503
    people with diabetes, 61–85
assistance dogs
    guide dogs, 242, 243
    medical, 42, 552
atenolol, side effects, 158
atherosclerosis, 225
Atkins-type diets, 445
atorvastatin
    clinical trials, 154–155

ocular effects, 241
atrial fibrillation, 224, 226
at-risk groups, 26
attention-seeking, 480
attitudes of clinicians, 469
atypical antipsychotics, 483
atypical diabetes, **9**
atypical myocardial infarction, 232, *see also* silent
    myocardial infarction
atypical presentations, 391
AUDIT, alcohol dependence screening, 322
AUSLAN (Australian sign language), 344–345
Australia
    diagnostic criteria for ketoacidosis, **204**
    National Prescribing Service, 414
Australian Diabetes Society, on driving, 350
Australian Nutrition Screening Initiative, 405
autoantibodies, 429
    gestational diabetes, 456
    islet cell antibodies, 82
autoimmune markers, type 1 diabetes, **5**
autoimmunity, 15
    islet cell antibodies, 82
    transient, 2, **6**
    treatments directed at, 29
autonomic neuropathy, 37, 266–270, **389**
    blood pressure, 78, **268**
    cardiovascular disease, **227**, **268**
    foot disease, 265
    hypoglycaemia, 192, 470
    pregnancy, 452
    sexual health, **268**, 269, 375
    silent myocardial infarction, 226
    sleep disturbance, 340
    surgery and, 287
Avandamet, **120**

bacteria, *see also* microbiome
    foot infections, 257
    oral disease, 328
Baker hypothesis, 454–455
Balint groups, 479
bandages, foot care, 262
banding (gastric), **102**, 293
bariatric surgery, 101–103, 293, 331
barrier methods, contraception, 447
basal bolus insulin dose regimens, 142–143
    hypoglycaemia risk, 356–357
    type 2 diabetes, 132, **133**
basal insulin (long-acting insulin analogues), 137, 138,
    139, 141
basal secretion, insulin, 118
baths, 551
BD regimens
    insulin, 141–142
    misunderstood, 163
bed, people confined to, low vision, 242–243
bed rest, older people, 417
bedside teaching, 510
bedtime blood glucose, nocturnal hypoglycaemia, 187
bedtime insulin, type 2 diabetes, 132
bedwetting, 15, 206

Beers Criteria (American Geriatrics Society), 414
behaviour change
    interactive technology, 475
    strategies for, 501–502
behaviour change models, 498
behaviour theories, diabetes education, 497
bereavement, **527**
Berlin Initiative Study 2 equation, 245
β_2-adrenergic agents, 189
beta blockers, 130, 158, 230
    hypoglycaemia and, 182
    myocardial infarction, 233
beta cells, 18
    antibodies, 82
    decline, *16*, 130
    transplantation, 150, 327
beta-hydroxybutyrate, 74, 75
BGATT *see* blood glucose awareness training
bicarbonate
    children, 438
    diabetic ketoacidosis, **204**, 209
    hyperosmolar hyperglycaemic state, 213
    lactic acidosis, 216
    before radiological procedures, 247
biguanides, 117, 118–124
    cancer care, 312
    combined with sulphonylureas, **120**
    contraindications, 124
bile acids, 329
bile acid sequestrants, **157**, 331
Billings method, contraception, 372
binge eating, 18
BioChaperoned peptide insulins, 137
biofeedback, 551
biopsy
    coeliac disease, 335
    kidney, 250
    mastopathy, 333
biosimilar insulins, 139
biota *see* microbiome
biphasic insulins, 138–139, 141
birth weight, 455
black cohosh, 461
black liquorice, interactions with
        medicines, **105**
bladder cancer, pioglitazone, 14, 125, 310, 311
bleeding, complementary medicine, 298
blood glucose, *see also* oral glucose tolerance test;
        variability
    artificial nutrition, 305
    cognitive deficit, 398
    corticosteroids on, 347
    equations, 184
    factors affecting, 69
    fasting for religious observances, 360
    fasting levels *see* fasting plasma glucose; impaired
        fasting glucose
    herbal medicines, 550
    home testing record, 409–410
    inaccuracies, 72
    ketones on levels, 75
    meters *see* meters

monitoring, 64–74
    aids for low vision, 242
    artificial nutrition, 309
    children, 432
    children and adolescents, 438
    continuous (CGM), 68, 73–74, 144–145
    corticosteroids, 68, 349
    cystic fibrosis, 337
    effectiveness, 65
    end-of-life care, 528, 533
    for GLM use, 118
    home, 410
    in hospital, 202, 438
    tedium, 472
    myocardial infarction, 226
    neonates, 454
    nocturnal hypoglycaemia, 187
    post-prandial *see* post-prandial plasma glucose
    pregnancy, 458
    random, 22
    strokes, 237
    target values
        corticosteroids and, 538
        end-of-life care, 532–533
        gestational diabetes, 456
        myocardial infarction, 231
        pregnancy, 449, 455
        surgery, 283
    technique, 71–72, 79
    24-hour profile, 253
blood glucose awareness training (BGATT), 501
    driving, 357
blood pressure, 78
    autonomic neuropathy, 78, **268**
    cardiovascular risk reduction, 235
    diastolic, 225
    measurement, 229–230
    target values, **31**, 228, 230, 246
        older people, 413
blood urea nitrogen, 82, 91, 405
blood vessels, metabolic syndrome, 12
Blue Steel (food supplement), 379
blurred vision, 297
body mass index, 11, 99
    children and adolescents, 433
    diabetes in children, 427
    exercise on, 108
    gestational diabetes risk, 456
    macular degeneration, **240**
    malnutrition, 405
    prediabetes, **4**
    renal disease, 244
    target values, **31**
bolus injection, *see also* basal bolus insulin dose regimens
    continuous subcutaneous insulin infusion with, 143
bolus secretion, insulin, 118
bone mineral density, 346
bots (chatbots), 40
bowel preparation, fluid balance, 294, 295
brain
    diabetic ketoacidosis, 205, 210
    foetus, 455

glucose homeostasis, 183
hyperglycaemia, 429
hypoglycaemia, 193, 194, 429
microbiome and, 88, 477–478
type 2 diabetes, 429
brain-centric model, 10
breakfast, 90
breast
  cancer, 309–310
  mastopathy, 333
breastfeeding, 453, 457
  insulin, 458
  TRIGIR study, 427
Brief Medication Questionnaire, 165
brittle diabetes, 211, 326–327
bronchospasm, beta blockers, 158
bulking agents, adverse effects and interactions, 558
bupropion SR, **321**
burettes, 148
business models, 498–499
Bydureon, 127

caesarean section, 453
caffeine
  on hypoglycaemia, 182
  interactions with medicines, **105**
calamus, 324
calcific medial stenosis, renal failure, 246
calcium, cancer care, 314
calcium channel blockers, **160**
calcium-regulated potassium channels, 222
calcium score, 228
caloric intake, 90, 404
camps, 431
canagliflozin, **122**, 128
cancer, 309–315
  bladder, pioglitazone, 14, 125, 310, 311
  emergencies, **530**
  endometrial, 309, 446
  inhaled insulin, 137
  insulin analogues, **450**
  liver, 330
  lung, inhaled insulin, 137
  risk factors, 310
  screening in renal disease, 248
  smokeless tobacco, 320
  tobacco smoke, 316–317
cannabis, **323**, 324
cannabis (medical), 323–324
cannulae, oral glucose tolerance test, 25
capillary blood glucose, 72, 202
capillary refill, 288
capsaicin, **260**
carbamazepine, for peripheral neuropathy, **259**
carbohydrates
  complex, 94
  for hypoglycaemia, 190–191
  intake measurement, 92
  on lipids, **93**
  renal disease, 249
  target intake, 90
carcinogens, tobacco smoke, 316–317

cardiac markers, 226–228
cardiac risk calculators, 226–228, 234–235
CARDIA study, 446
cardiovascular disease, 37, 220, 223–237
  adolescence, 13
  Atkins-type diets, 445
  autonomic neuropathy, **227**, **268**
  children, 428, 432
  complementary medicine on risk, **546**
  distress on, 481–482
  driving, **354**
  exercise preventing, 107
  falls, 413
  hypoglycaemia, 194, 224
  illegal drugs, 324–325
  metabolic syndrome, 12, 14
  older people, **389**
  pregnancy, 452, 453
  risk factors, 98, 234–236
    cardiac risk calculators, 226–228, 234–235
  smoking, 316
  thiazolidinediones and, 125
CARDS (clinical trial), 154–155
caregivers, 417–418
  assessment, **393**
  depression in older people, 400
  end-of-life care, 531, 538–539
  medicine-related nonadherence, 163
  strain, 539
  stress measurement, 476
care models, 30, 53–55
care plans
  documentation, 57
  older people, 401–410
carotid artery stenosis, 236
carpal tunnel syndrome, 345, **355**
casein, 457
casts (plaster), 258, 264
catabolism, *10*, 405
catecholamines, *see also* sympathetic symptoms
  hypoglycaemia, 224
  surgery and, **282**
Caverject, 378
CB$_1$ (endocannabinoid), 96–97
CEL mutation, **16**
central catheters
  care of, 308
  parenteral nutrition, 307
  renal disease, 248
central obesity, 11, *see also* abdominal obesity
  waist circumference, 11, 13, 18, 98
central sleep apnoea, 340
cereals, interactions with medicines, **105**
cerebral oedema
  children, 211, 438
  diabetic ketoacidosis, 210, 211
  insulin infusions, 148
cerebrovascular disease, 236–237
Champix (varenicline), **321**
Chantix (varenicline), **321**
Charcot's deformity, 256, 257
Charter of Aged Care Rights, 375

charting by exception, 56
chatbots, 40
checklists
    advance care planning, 506
    Agency for Healthcare Research and Quality, 23
    Hydration Assessment, 405
cheese effect, **351**
cheiroarthropathy, 345
chemotherapy
    herbal medicines and, 314
    side effects, 315
chest pain, action plan, 235
children, 425–442, *see also* infancy
    cerebral oedema, 211, 438
    diabetic ketoacidosis, 205, 210, 438
    hypoglycaemia, 177, 182, 192, 432–433
    massage, 439, 550
    maternal hyperglycaemia on, 454–455
    metabolic syndrome, 13–14, 428
    obesity, 96, 428, 454–455
        brain, 429
    passive smoking, 316
    prevalence of diabetes, 3
    sexual health, 376
    surgery, 283
    type 1 diabetes, 426, 480
        management, 431–433
    type 2 diabetes, 6, 425, 428, 430
        indigenous Australians, 21
        management, 433–436
Chinese medicine *see* traditional Chinese medicine
chlorpropamide, surgery and, 287
cholesterol
    bariatric surgery and, 102
    dietary fats on, **97**
    nutritional deficiency, 405
    renal disease risk, 245
    target values, **31**, 81, 154
cholesterol ester transfer proteins, 156
cholestyramine, **105, 157**, 269
Choosing Wisely programmes, 65, 530–531
chromium, 550
chronic hypoglycaemia, 182, 186
cimetidine, on PDE-5 inhibitor levels, 378
Cimicifuga racemosa (black cohosh), 461
cirrhosis, 330
cisapride, 269
cisplatin, 315
citalopram, **351**
citrus fruits, interactions with medicines, 129
Clarke method, assessment for hypoglycaemic
        unawareness, 186
claudication, management, **264**
climate change, 28
clinical inertia, 67, 134, 410, 469
clinical trials, 116
    lipid-lowering agents, 154–155
clinician factors, 469–472
clinicians, *see also* health professionals
    attitudes of, 469
    clinical inertia, 67, 134, 410, 469
    complementary medicine and, 560–561

in diabetes education, 499, 509–512
    education of, 43, 494
    patient activation and, 502
    performance, 42–43
clonidine, **129, 259**
clopidogrel, 159
clozapine, **129**, 350, 446
coaching by telephone, 236
coaching models, 498
COACH protocol, 236
cocaine, **323**
Cochrane review, on diabetes prevention, 26–27
Cockcroft-Gault equation, 244
coeliac disease, 334–336, 432
coenzyme Q10, 222, 230, 298, 553
cognitive authority theory, 477
cognitive behavioural therapy, 479
cognitive decline, assessment, 398
cognitive deficit, *see also* dementia
    diabetic ketoacidosis, 205, 429
    driving, 353, **355**
    hypertension, 235
    hypoglycaemia, 178, 193, 194
    odour identification, 552
    older people, 395–398
cognitive effects, metformin, 478
cognitive reserve, 395, **396**
coincidence model, cardiovascular disease, 232
collaborative inquiry (tell-back), 501
colonoscopy, 295
colour contrast, 243
colour perception, **390**
combination oral contraceptives, 448
comfrey poultices, 299, 554
commercial weight loss programmes, 100, 101
communication, 52–53, 54, 500–502
community services, stabilisation of diabetes,
        151–153
comorbidities, *see also* illnesses (intercurrent)
    geriatric syndromes, 394–395
complementary medicine (CAM), 543–565
    cancer care, 313–314
    cardiovascular disease, 230
    children, 438–439
    definitions, 545–546
    depression, 479
    end-of-life care, 536, 544
    hypoglycaemia, 189
    integrating with conventional care, 547–549
    liver disease, 331–332
    menopause, 460–462
    philosophy, 546–547
    pregnancy, 451
    prevalence of use, 544–545
    reasons for choosing, 502
    renal disease, 254–255
    safety, 548, 549, 556–560
    self-healing capacity, 498
    for sexual problems, 379
    smoking cessation, 319
    surgery and, 281, 284, 287, 298–300, 552–555
    weight reduction, 103, 550–551

complex carbohydrates, 94
complexity, 220–221
compliance (term), 483–484, *see also* nonadherence
complications
    diabetes, 36–37, 211, 221, 339, *see also* long-term complications
    pregnancy, 37, 453–454
compresses, gastroparesis, 270
computer games, 428
concordance, medicine-related, 162
confidentiality, 57
confocal microscopy, retinopathy, 241
conformational switching, insulin, 3
Confusion Assessment Method, 396–398
conjugated linoleic acid, 550–551
consciousness
    dehydration, 288
    diabetic ketoacidosis, 210
consequence model, cardiovascular disease, 232
consumer decision journeys, 498–499
contamination, complementary medicines, 549
continuous ambulatory peritoneal dialysis, 251–254
continuous blood glucose monitoring (CGM), 68, 73–74, 144–145
continuous positive airway pressure, 341
continuous subcutaneous insulin infusion (CSII), 143–144
    surgery and, 292
contraception
    men, 372–373, 448
    polycystic ovarian syndrome, 445, 446
    women with diabetes, 447–448
contrast-induced nephropathy, 247, 297
contrast media *see* iodinated contrast media
conversation model, 53
conversations, 485, 492, 494, 500–502
coronary artery calcium score, 228
coronary care units, length of stay, 231
coronary risk equivalent, 226
correction doses, 146
corticosteroids, 347–350
    adverse effects, 537
    blood glucose monitoring for, 68, 349
    cancer care, 313, 315
    diabetes from, 348, 537–538
    foot disease, 257
    hyperglycaemia, 347, 532
    increase for illness or surgery, 350
    medicine interactions, **129**
    skin, 312, 349
cortisol, **183**, 267
    obstructive sleep apnoea, 340
costs, 472
    insulin pumps, 144
cough, ACE inhibitors, 159
coumarin derivatives, **189**
coumestans, 460
counselling, 479
    decision aids, **496**
    prepregnancy, 449
    sexual, 380–383

counter-regulatory response, 178–179, **183**
    driving, 356
    older people, 416
    reduction, 185
    Somogyi effect, 143, 188
cow's milk, 3, 15, 457
C-peptide, 81–82
    children, 428
    latent autoimmune diabetes in adults, 17
    neuropathy, 260
cracks, foot disease, **264**
cranberry formulations, 411, 460, 551
crashes
    driving, 352–353
    hypoglycaemia, 356
Crataegus monogyna (WS 1442), 230, **558**
C-reactive protein, 12
    macular degeneration, **240**
CREATE (trial), on depression, 232
creatine kinase, 156
creatine supplements, 551
creatinine, 78, 91, 246
    diabetic ketoacidosis, 209
    glomerular filtration rate *vs*, 244
    older people, 78, 246, 250, 392, 405
creatinine clearance, 82
creativity, antipsychotics on, 483
crude weight, 99
crushing of medicines, 309, 407, 408, 414, 415
cyproterone, 446
cystatin-c, falls, 413
cystic fibrosis, **7**, 336–338
cystitis, 380
cytokines, 12

daily injection, insulin, 141, *142*
    multiple (MDI), 67, 392
daime (hoasia), 324
dairy diet, 101
dairy products, 92, **105**
damage theories of ageing, **387**
Daonil, **119**
dapagliflozin, on liver, 331
DARTS study, hypoglycaemia, 177
data protection, 41–42
dawn phenomenon, 143, 188
DAWN study, 481
day–night dip, blood pressure, 235
daytime sleepiness, 236, **285**
De Boer, T., on *in utero* iron deficiency, 455
decision aids, 51, **496**, 502
decompensation, ketoacidosis, 205–206
degludec, 132, 137, 138
dehydration, **207**
    delirium, 396
    fasting, 359
    hyperosmolar hyperglycaemic state, 212, 213
    older people, 399–400
    signs, 288
dehydroepiandrosterone, 461
delirium, 396–398, **529**

dementia, 395–398, 400–401, *see also* Alzheimer's disease; cognitive deficit
    antipsychotics, 415
    hypoglycaemia, 194
    multi-infarct, 236, *see also* vascular dementia
    nutrition, 406
    odour identification, 552
denial, 471
denosomab, 346
dental care, 252, 329
dependence, *see also* addiction
    alcohol, 322
DE-PLAN, diabetes prevention, 28
Depo-Provera/Depo-Ralovera, 448
depression, 12, **397**, 476–479, 483
    adolescence, 437
    in Alzheimer's disease, 401
    cardiovascular disease and, 232, 481–482
    children, **433**
    end of life, **529**
    insulin on, 481
    on life expectancy, 525
    management, 479
    older people, 400, 470
    polycystic ovarian syndrome, 446
    postnatal, 452
    on sexual health, 374, 376
    St John's wort, 551
    symptoms, 478
derived NGSP units, haemoglobin A1c, 80
desaturase enzymes, **97**
detemir (Levemir), 137
    weight gain, 135
developing regions, 428
    pregnancy, 443–444
developmental origins of adult health and disease (DOHaD), 12, 454–455
dextrose
    for hypoglycaemia, 191
    PEG, 306
    surgery, 288
Diabetes Control and Complications Trial, hypoglycaemia, 175
Diabetes Prevention Program, 26
Diabetes Prevention Study (DPS), 27
diabetes-related distress, 470, 474, 477
    adolescence, 437
    cardiovascular disease and, 482
Diabetes Training and Treatment Program, German, 92
diabetic ketoacidosis, 199, 204–212
    abdominal pain, 75, **207**
    assessment, 206–207
    brain injury, 429
    children, 205, 210, 438
    decompensation, 205–206
    diagnostic criteria, 204
    differential diagnosis, 206
    eating disorders, 89, 211
    emergency surgery, 293
    euglycaemic, 128, 211–212
    follow-up, 210
    signs and symptoms, **205**, *206*

    treatment, 207–211
        complications, 211
    type 2 diabetes, **6**, 430
Diabex, **120**
diacylglycerol, 222
Diaformin, **120**
diagnosis, 22–26
dialysis, 250–254
Diamicron MR, **119**
diaphragms (contraceptive), 447
diarrhoea, 340
    alpha-glucosidase inhibitors, 127
diastolic blood pressure, 225
didanosine, 343
diet, 88–95, *see also* foods
    cancer care, 311, 314
    cardiovascular risk reduction, 235
    children, 431
    coeliac disease, 335–336
    cystic fibrosis, 337
    factors affecting change, 103–107
    gastroparesis, 269
    gestational diabetes, 456
    goals, 95
    histories, 90
    hypoglycaemia risk, 356
    illnesses, **203**
    macular degeneration, **240**
    menopause, 459
    older people, 404
    polycystic ovarian syndrome, 445
    pregnancy, 452
    renal disease, 248–250
    role in management, 31
    smartphone apps, 41
    smoking cessation, 319
    type 2 diabetes prevention, 27
    weight reduction, 100–101
dietary recall, 100
DIGAMI protocol, 233
DiGEM (trial), 65
dignity, 52
1,25-dihydroxyvitamin D, levels and diabetes, 348
Dioscorea villosa (wild yam cream), 461
diosgenin, 461
dipeptidyl peptidase-4 inhibitors (DPP-4 inhibitors), 117, **121**, 127, 535–536
dipsticks, microalbumin, 78
dipyridamole, 159
disabilities, 55–56, *see also* functional ability
disposable insulin devices, 139
distress *see* diabetes-related distress
disturbed eating, eating disorders *vs*, 435
disulfiram, 322
diuretics, **160**
    with ACE inhibitors, **160**
    medicine interactions, **129**
DIY looping, 76
docosahexaenoic acid, albuminuria and, 255
documentation, 55, 56–58
    diabetes education, 512–515
    patient-held records, 409–410

dogs
  continuous blood glucose monitoring, 74
  guide dogs, 242, 243
  hypoglycaemia detection, 42, 194, 552
  medical assistance dogs, 42, 552
dong quai, 461
dopamine pathway, smoking, 318, 319
dosages, *see also* basal bolus insulin dose regimens;
      top-up doses
  insulin, 137
  insulin infusions, 147
  misunderstood, 163
  writing prescriptions, 149
Dose Adjustment for Normal Eating, 92, 144
DPS (Finnish Diabetes Prevention Study), 27
dressings, foot care, 262, 263
driving, 350–359
  assessments, 357
  hypoglycaemia, 178, 352–353, **354**, 355–357
  after laser therapy, 296
  stopping, 402
drug abuse, **316**
drug dependence/addiction, **316**
drugs (illegal), 322–326
dry mouth, 328
dry skin, foot disease, **264**
duloxetine, cardiovascular effects, **351**
duodenal tubes, 306
Dupuytren's contracture, 345
  driving, **355**
durometers, **264**
dying, 525–526, **527**, 531
  hospital patients, 524
dysphagia
  older people, **388**, 405
  stroke management, 237
dyspnoea, end of life, **530**

eating disorders, 18, 89, 434–435
  diabetic ketoacidosis, 89, 211
eating disturbance, eating disorders *vs*, 435
echinacea, 439, **557**
e-cigarettes, 320
ecological model, 498
ecomaps, 56–57
ecstasy, **323**
Edelman, D., on consumer decision journeys, 498–499
Eden Alternative, 402
Edinburgh Hypoglycaemia Scale, 356
education, 491–521, *see also* school education
  adherence to medicines, 164
  cardiovascular disease, 234
  children, 432
    medicines, 436
  of clinicians, 43, 494
  continuous ambulatory peritoneal dialysis, 254
  diabetic ketoacidosis, 208
  driving, 358–359
  end-of-life care, 539–540
  evaluation of, 515–517
  on fasting, 359–360
  foot care, 262

on hypoglycaemia, 184–185, 190
illness prevention, 200–201
older people, 408–409
for people with hearing loss, 344
on person-centred care, 55
on sexual health, 380
stabilisation of diabetes, 166–167
eHealth Literacy Scale, 505
eicosapentaenoic acid, albuminuria and, 255
elderly people *see* older people
electronic blood glucose meters, 55
emergencies, cancer, **530**
emergency contraception, 448
emergency departments, people with diabetes in, 279–280
emergency surgery, 292–293
empagliflozin, 128
empathy, 469
empowerment, 474
  education, 492, 507–508
empowerment model *see* person-centred
      empowerment model
endangered species, 555
ENDIA study, 427
endocannabinoids, 96–97
end-of-life care, 311, 313, 523–542
  complementary medicine, 536, 544
  diabetogenic medicines, 537–538
  medicine management, 534–536
  nutrition, 536–537
  renal disease, 254
  withdrawal of treatment, 539
endometrial cancer, 309, 446
endometrial hyperplasia, 446
endothelial lipase inhibitors, 156
endothelium, cardiovascular disease, **227**
ENRICH (trial), on depression, 232
enteral nutrition, 304–309, **404**
  formulations, 406–407
  older people, 406–408
environmental causes, diabetes in children, 426–427
epalrestat, 260
ephedra, 103, 324, 550
epidural anaesthesia, hypoglycaemia, 453
epigenetics, 11, 12
equations
  blood glucose balance as, 184
  renal disease, 244–245
ErecAid®, 379
erectile dysfunction (ED), 377–380
  booklet on, 383
errors *see* mistakes
erythropoesis-stimulating medicines, renal disease, 248
escitalopram, **351**
essential oils, 298
  cancer care, 314
  children, 439
  foot care, 263
  liver damage, 332
Essure, 448
estimated A1C, 74
estimated GFR, 77–78, 245
  SGLT-2 inhibitors and, 118

ethinyl oestradiol, 446
ethnicity
    gestational diabetes risk, 456
    macular degeneration, **240**
Euglucon, **119**
euglycaemic ketoacidosis, 128, 211–212
Euphasia superba, omega 3 fatty acids, 94
EURODIAB sub-study 2, 15
Europe, United States *vs*, dairy products, 92
evening primrose oil, 461
evidence base
    assessment, 562
    complementary medicine, 549
examination (physical), 78
    foot, 262
    obstructive sleep apnoea, 341
exanatide, **122**, 127
exception, charting by, 56
exchanges, carbohydrates, 92
exercise, 32–36, 100, 107–108
    on blood glucose, 69
    cancer care, 314
    depression and, 479
    hypoglycaemia, 35, 36, 108, 183, 187, 192, 415
    older people, 415–416
    pregnancy, 452
    strategies, 108
    targets, **31**
    type 2 diabetes prevention, 27
exercise books, home blood glucose testing, 410
exercise capacity, 107
Exubera, 137
eye disease, 237–243, *see also* retinopathy
    pregnancy, 452
    procedures, 295–297
ezetimibe, 156, **157**

falls, 412–414
    autonomic neuropathy, 270
    corticosteroids, 349
    driving crash risk, 352
    hypoglycaemia, 190, 194, 412, 413
    prevention, 414, 417
    prevention programmes, 414
    risk factors, 352
false negatives
    haemoglobin A1c, **81**
    ketones, 75
false positives, haemoglobin A1c, **81**
families, 476
    diabetes in children, 425–426, 431, 432, 434, 480
    end-of-life care and, 528, 538–539
    type 2 diabetes, 481
fasting, 297, *see also* catabolism
    hypoglycaemia, 192, 359
    for investigative procedures, 294
    ketones, 75
    meaning of word, 292
    precautions, 79
    religious observances, 359–360
    surgery, children, 283
fasting hyperglycaemia, 359
    morning, 143, 188

fasting plasma glucose, 22, 118, *see also* impaired
        fasting glucose
    gestational diabetes, **7**
    HbA1c with, 24
    older people, 392
    prediabetes, **4**
    target values
        corticosteroids and, 538
        ranges, 31, **33**
    type 1 diabetes, **5**
    type 2 diabetes, **6**
fat (abdominal), 96
fat (dietary), 93
    diets compared, 92
    renal disease, 249
    type 2 diabetes prevention, 27
    types, **97**
fathers, diabetes in children, 427
fatigue
    antihypertensives, 158
    radiotherapy, 312
    sleep disturbance, 340
fatty liver disease, 330
fears, hypoglycaemia, 134, 193
Federal Study of Adherence to Medications in the
        Elderly, 164
fed state (anabolism), *10*
fenugreek, 550, **557**
fertility, 446
FeSS protocol, stroke management, 237
fever, stroke management, 237
feverfew, **557**
fibrates, **157**, 230
    VA-HIT (trial), 155
fibre intake
    on blood lipids, **93**
    complementary medicine, 299
    on glycaemic index, 93
    interactions with medicines, **105**
    type 2 diabetes prevention, 27
fibroblast growth factors, 10
fiction, 53
fine needle aspiration biopsy, mastopathy, 333
Finnish Diabetes Prevention Study (DPS), 27
fish oil supplements, 101
5As approach, smoking cessation, 318–319
fizzy drinks, PEG tube clearance, 308
flash blood glucose monitoring, 73
Flatbush diabetes, **9**
flatulence, alpha-glucosidase inhibitors, 127
Flesch Reading Ease (readability test), 506
flexor tenosynovitis, 345
flora *see* microbiome
flowcharts, 57
flucloxacillin, foot disease, 258
fluid balance
    bowel preparation, 294, 295
    diabetic ketoacidosis, 209
    dialysis, 252–253
    for investigative procedures, 294
    surgery, 288, 289
fluid intake, 404
fluid resuscitation

hyperglycaemia, 202
hyperosmolar hyperglycaemic state, 214
illnesses, **203**
fluid retention, beta blockers, 158
fluorescein angiography, 295–296
fluorine-18 fluorodeoxyglucose, 294
flushing, insulin infusions, 147
flu vaccination, 402
fly agaric, 324
foetal origins hypothesis, 454–455
foetus, macrosomia, 456, 457
folic acid, 222, 449
fonts, readability, 506
food absorption
    antacids on, **105**
    medicines affecting, **104**
food additives, 106–107
food consumption measurement, 99–100
food frequency questionnaires, 100
food labels, 106–107
food records, 99–100
foods, *see also* diet
    coenzyme Q10, 222
    for hypoglycaemia, 191
    interactions with medicines, **105**
    sugar-free, 104–105
    takeaway, 90
food supplements, 222, 405–406
    for erectile dysfunction, 379
foot, 262
    ageing, **266**
    not to prick, 69
foot disease, 255–259, 263–265
    risk factors, 260–261, *265*
    wound management, 263–265
foot ulcers, 255, 263, **264**
    hyperosmolar hyperglycaemic state, 214
    swabs, 258
forearm, blood glucose, 71
Forestier's disease, 345
forgetting to take medicines, 484
fractures, 346
    falls, 412
    hypoglycaemia, 190, 194
    immunosuppressants, 257
    SGLT-2 inhibitors, 128
    thiazolidinediones, 126
fragrant oils, 314
frailty, **286**, **389**, 394
    assessment, 394
    blood glucose, 305
    fractures, 346
    HbA1c target levels, 392
Framingham risk calculator, 229, 234–235
Framingham Study, 155
    on cognitive function, 395
free androgen index, polycystic ovarian syndrome, 445
free fatty acids, 18, *35*
    heart failure, 224
    liver disease, 330
    myocardial infarction, 231
free radicals, 551, *see also* reactive oxygen species
frequency of assessment, 62

frequency of SMBG, 65–66, 67–68
frizzled proteins *see* secreted frizzled-related protein 4
fructosamines, 24, 81
fructose, 104–105, 428
fucoxanthine, 101
functional ability, older people, 392–395
functional neuroimaging, hypoglycaemia, 186
funding, *see also* subsidisation, insulin pumps, 144

gabapentin, for peripheral neuropathy, **259**
GAD antibodies, 82
gadolinium, 247
gait speed, 394
galectin-3, 245
gamification, 40
gamma-linolenic acid, 94
garlic, adverse effects and interactions, **557**
Garvan Fracture Risk Calculator, 346
gastric bypass surgery *see* bariatric surgery
gastric stasis, **207**, 269, 270
gastrointestinal tract
    autonomic neuropathy, 267, **268**, 269, 270
    brittle diabetes, 326
    effects of surgery, 282, **285**
    investigative procedures, 295
    neuropathy, 340
    regurgitation, 287
gastrostomy, 306
    care of tubes, 308
GCK mutation, **16**
gemfibrozil, 158
gender differences
    cerebrovascular disease, 236
    renal disease risk, 246
general practitioners
    barriers to optimal treatment, 43
    complementary medicine, 545
    incentive schemes, 411
generic medicines, 506
genetics, 29, 426
genetic testing, coeliac disease, 335
genograms, 57
genomaps, 56–57
geriatric evaluation units, 402
geriatrics *see* older people
geriatric syndromes, 394–395
German Diabetes Training and Treatment
        Program, 92
gestational diabetes, 7, 21, 444, 455–458
    type 2 diabetes after, 19
ghrelin, 97
GIK (glucose, insulin, potassium and fluids), 146
ginger
    interactions, **557**
    nausea, 554
gingivitis, 328
Ginkgo biloba, **557**
ginseng, 461, **557**
glargine, 137
    pregnancy, **450**
    type 2 diabetes, 132
    weight gain, 135
gliadin, 334

glibenclamide, **119**, 124
  pregnancy, 457
gliclazide, **119**
Glimel, **119**
glimepiride, **119–120**
glipizide, **119**
  pregnancy, **450**
glitinides, 117
  cancer care, 311
global learning style, **496**
Global Monitoring Framework, 28–29
glomerular filtration rate, 77–78, 245
  creatinine *vs*, 244
  sodium-glucose cotransporter-2 inhibitors and, 118
glucagon
  adolescence, 434
  for hypoglycaemia, 191, 194–195
glucagon (intrinsic), 175, **183**
  deficit, 185
  surgery and, **282**
glucagon-like peptide-1, 127
glucagon-like peptide-1 agonists (GLP-1 agonists),
      117, **122**, 127, 535–536
glucometer (term), 73
gluconeogenesis, 204
Glucophage, **120**
glucosamine, adverse effects, **557**
glucose
  in dialysate fluid, 251
  homeostasis, 3–10
    brain, 183
    oral contraceptives, 448
  for hypoglycaemia, 191
  levels *see* blood glucose
glucose-dependent insulinotropic peptide, 127
glucose, insulin, potassium and fluids, intravenous
      infusions, 146
glucose-lowering medicines (GLM), 117–129, *see also*
      specific drugs
  alcohol and, 322
  antiretrovirals and, 343
  cancer care, 312, 313
  cancer risk, 310
  cardiovascular benefits, 230
  corticosteroids and, 538
  end-of-life care, 528, 535, 539
  enteral nutrition, 407–408
  exercise and, 33
  hypoglycaemia, 177, 356, 413, 416, 534
  with insulin, 130, 130–134
  on kidney, 246
  pregnancy, **450**, 457
  surgery and, 281, 286–287, 291
glucose-responsive insulins, 137
Glucovance, **120**
GLUT-1, 449
GLUT-4, *19*, 449
glutamic acid decarboxylase (GADA), 17
glutathione peroxidase 1, **227**
gluten, infancy, 428, 457
gluten-sensitive enteropathy (coeliac disease),
      334–336, 432
glyburide, pregnancy, **450**

glycaemic index (GI), 92–93
glycaemic load (GL), 93
glycated albumin, 24
glycated haemoglobin *see* haemoglobin A1c
glycogen, *35*
  autonomic neuropathy on conversion, 267
glycopyrrolate, 269
glycosuria, 64, 76, 128
  diabetic ketoacidosis, **207**
  euglycaemic ketoacidosis, 211–212
glycosylation, proteins, 222
goji berries, 379
Gold method, assessment for hypoglycaemic
      unawareness, 186
Gold Standards Framework, life-limiting illness, 525
gout, 345
grandchildren, malnourished mothers, 12
grapefruit juice
  antibiotics and, 299
  interactions with medicines, **105**, 129, 553
grief cycle, diabetic, 471
group education, 503
growth hormone, **183**
guar, adverse effects and interactions, **558**
guide dogs, 242, 243
guidelines
  complementary medicine, 549, 560
  cystic fibrosis, 336
  depression, 479
  diabetes management, 31, 43, 62
    children and adolescents, 430
    listed, **63**
  diet, 92
  driving, 351
  haemoglobin A1c, 80
  Internet, 562
  older people, 62, 391
    sexual health, 375
  palliative care, 528
  statins, 155
  surgery, 289, 290–292
guilt dynamic, 452
gum, nicotine, **321**
gum disease, Alzheimer's disease, **396**

Haemaccel, 148
haemochromatosis, 330, 332–333
haemodialysis, 250–251
  nutrition, 249–250
haemoglobin, monitoring, 248
haemoglobin A1c, 32, 79–81
  acceptance as test, 23
  advantages, 23
  assay methods, 79–80
  blood glucose *vs*, 72
  cancer risk, 309
  children, 429, 430, **433**, 434
  complementary medicine, **546**
  cystic fibrosis, 337
  estimated, 74
  factors affecting results, **81**
  gestational diabetes, 21
  haemodialysis, 251

microvascular disease risk *vs*, 221
monitoring, for GLM use, 118
older people, 392
as outcome measure, 468
postpartum, 457
renal disease risk, 245
surgery and, 283
target values, **33**, 80, 228–229, 392, **433**, 434
  pregnancy, 449
thiazolidinediones on, 125
type 1 diabetes, **5**
type 2 diabetes, **6**
urological complications, 339
hallucinogens, 322, **323**
Hashimoto's thyroiditis, 327
hawthorn *see Crataegus monogyna*
Hawthorne effect, 65
healing (term), 547
health behaviour tracking systems, 41
health histories
  diet, 90, 91
  foot assessment, 261–262
  holistic personalised care, 55–58
  sexual health, 380–381
health literacy, 504–507
Health Literacy Skills Instrument, 505
health professionals, *see also* clinicians
  complementary medicine, 545
  diabetes knowledge, 507
  performance, 42–43
  'voices', 499
hearing loss, 343–345
heart failure, 223, 224
  thiazolidinediones and, 125–126
Heart Protection Study, 154
heavy vehicles, driving crash risk, 352
Helicobacter pylori, 12
heparin, 159
  interaction with tobacco smoke, 317
hepatocellular carcinoma, 330
herbal medicines, *see also* complementary medicine
  chemotherapy and, 314
  on glucose levels, 550
  on haemoglobin A1c levels, **546**
  interactions with conventional medicines, 556, **561**
  menopause, 460–461
  pregnancy, 451
  with psychoactive properties, 324
  renal disease, 254–255
  smoking cessation, 319
  surgery and, 287
Hero (food supplement), 379
hexosamine pathway, 223
HFN-4A mutation, **16**
high-density lipoproteins, 153–154
  adolescence, 13
  choice of lipid-lowering agents, 158
  metabolic syndrome, 11
  prediabetes, **4**
  target values, **31**, 81, 154
hippocampus, 455
hirsutism, 446
histories *see* health histories

HIV/AIDS, 342–343
HNF1B mutation, **16**
HNFIA mutation, **16**, 22
hoasia, 324
holding (attitude to person with diabetes), 474
holidays, 472
holistic personalised care, 49–60, 151–153,
    492–493, *see also* person-centred
    empowerment model
  assessments, 78
  complementary medicine, 544, 550
  defined, 51–52
  insulin in type 2 diabetes, 135
  medicines, 116
  puerperium, 452
holistic state of healing, 474
home blood glucose testing record, 409–410
home OGTT, 23
homocysteine, **227**
HonCode logo, 103
honeymoon cystitis, 380
honeymoon period, type 1 diabetes, 432
hormone replacement therapy
  menopause, 459–460
  oestrogens, 225
  testosterone, 375, 378, 379
hospital patients, 39, 201–202, *see also* admission to hospital;
    bedside teaching; emergency departments
  adverse medicine-related events, 162
  children and adolescents, 438
  complementary medicine, 553
  dying, 524
  exercise, 35
  foot disease, 256
  glucose monitoring, 67–68
  hyperglycaemia, 67, 69, 202
  hypoglycaemia, 184
  leaving hospital, 291
  malnutrition, **404**
  myocardial infarction, 231
  psychological aspects, 485–486
  sliding scales, 146
  stabilisation of diabetes, 150–151
  undernutrition, 89
Humalin 30/70, 139
Humalog Mix 25, 138
  confusion of dose with number, 139
Humalog Mix 50, 139
human dignity, 52
human insulin, 137
Hydration Assessment checklist, 405
25-hydroxyvitamin D, 15
hygiene
  blood glucose meters, 71
  foot, 262
hyperbaric oxygen, 265
hyperglycaemia, 37, 199, 200, 202–204
  alcohol, 107
  brain, 429
  cancer, 315
  cardiovascular disease, **227**
  causing complications, 221
  corticosteroids, 347, 532

hyperglycaemia (*cont'd*)
cystic fibrosis, 337
diabetic ketoacidosis, **207**
driving, **354**
enteral nutrition, 305
exercise, 35
fasting, 359
morning, 143, 188
foot disease, 265
hospital patients, 67, 69, 202
insulin infusions, 149
mimicking infections, 39
morning, 143, 188
myocardial infarction, 231
older people, 388, 391
after organ transplantation, 8
palliative care, 533
prednisolone, 537
prevalence, 3
ranges in hospital, 67
on renal function, 247–248
self-monitoring to detect, 66
on sexual health, 375
on sleep, 341
as stress response, 26
surgery and, 284
top-up doses and, 145–146
type 2 diabetes, 18–19
Hypericum perforatum see St John's wort
hyperinsulinaemia, 12, 17
hyperkalaemia, renal disease risk, 245
hypernatraemia, 209
hyperosmolar hyperglycaemic state, 199, 212–214, *215*
emergency surgery, 293
surgery, 282
hyperostosis, 345
hypertension, 225, **227**
adolescence, 13
children, 432
cognitive deficit, 235
macular degeneration, **240**
metabolic syndrome, 11
prediabetes, **4**
pregnancy, 453–454, 458
proteinuria, 77
renal disease and, 245–246
type 2 diabetes, 20
hypertonic dehydration, 399
hypertriglyceridaemia, prediabetes, **4**
hypoglycaemia, 175–198, *see also* nocturnal
hypoglycaemia
adolescence, 192, 434
alcohol, 107, 193, 322
alert glucose level, 67
alpha-glucosidase inhibitors, 127
autonomic neuropathy, 192, 470
brain, 193, 194, 429
breastfeeding, 453
cancer care, 312
cardiovascular disease, 194, 224
causes, 183–184
children, 177, 182, 192, 432–433
coeliac disease, 336

defining, 179–182
dogs detecting, 42, 194, 552
driving, 178, 352–353, **354**, 355–357
in emergency departments, 280
end-of-life care and, 532
epidural anaesthesia, 453
exercise, 35, 36, 108, 183, 187, 192, 415
falls, 190, 194, 412, 413
in families, 480
fasting, 192, 359
fears, 134, 193
grading, 176, 179, 356
on haemoglobin A1c levels, 80
insulin in type 2 diabetes, 135–136
ketone monitoring after, 75
management, 190–191, 194–195
menopause, 459
neonatal, 454, 457
nocturnal *see* nocturnal hypoglycaemia
older people, 182, 186, 192, 391, 416
palliative care, 533–534
prevention, 184–185
prolonged, 191–192
psychological effects, 193
recognition, 182
risk assessment, *180*, 184, 192–193
self-monitoring to detect, 66
sensor augmented pumps detecting, 76
on sexual health, 375
signs, **181**
sulphonylureas, 124, 181, 183, 191, 356
surgery and, 284
symptoms, 178, **181**
thiazolidinediones, 126
venesection, 333
Hypoglycaemic Awareness Questionnaire, 187
hypoglycaemic unawareness, 177, 185–187
driving, 357
in hospital, 184
prevalence, 185–186
hypo junkies, 194
hyporeninaemic hypoaldosteronism syndromes, 159
hypotension
antihypertensives, 158, 233
falls, 413
haemodialysis, 250–251
hyperosmolar hyperglycaemic state, 213
postural, 233, 267, 269, 359, 413
hypothermia, 195, 206, 416
hypotonic dehydration, 399, 400

IFCC reference system, HbA1c, 80
illegible prescriptions, 149
illnesses (intercurrent), 39, 303
corticosteroids increase, 350
diabetic ketoacidosis, 205
in emergency departments, 279–280
hyperosmolar hyperglycaemic state, 212–213
information sheets on, 512–515
insulin, 204
lactic acidosis, 214
management, **203**
prevention, 200–201

self-care, 202
  prevention, 201
IMAGE, diabetes prevention, 28
immobility, 386
  bed rest, 417
immunity, left brain activity, 417
impaired fasting glucose
  gestational diabetes, 21
  metabolic syndrome, 11
Implanon, 448
implants, contraceptive, 448
incentive schemes, general practitioners, 411
incontinence, 206, 338–340, 454
incretins, 127–128
  cancer care, 312
  end-of-life care, 535–536
Index of Sexual Life, 380
indicator plaster neuropad, 261
indigenous Australians
  erectile dysfunction, 377
  type 2 diabetes, children, 21
Infacalm drops, 439
infancy, 11, 12, **433**
  feeding, autoimmunity, 15
  gluten, 428, 457
  microbiome, 427
infections, 200
  corticosteroids and, 349
  foot, 257–259
  hyperglycaemia mimicking, 39
  hyperosmolar hyperglycaemic state, 213
  menopause, 460
  older people, 411
  renal disease, 251
  renal replacement therapies, 252
  rotavirus, 427
  on sexual health, 374
  SGLT-2 inhibitors, 128
  theories of ageing, **387**
  urinary tract, **285**, 338, 411
    cranberry formulations, 411, 460, 551
inflammation, 12
  insulin on, 131
  overweight, 456
influenza, 201
information sheets, 512–515
inhaled insulin, 137
  interaction with tobacco smoke, 317
inhaled nicotine, **321**
INITIATE study, NovoMix 30, 132
injection
  insulin, 140–141
    devices for low vision, 242
    intramuscular, 511
    pregnancy, 458
  penile, 378
INS mutation, **16**
instruction sheets, 512–515
instrumental activities of daily living, 392
insula, 318
insulin, 136–139, 534, *see also* basal bolus insulin
    dose regimens; intensive insulin therapy;
    specific types e.g. glargine, degludec

absorption, factors affecting, 69, **145**
action profiles, 142
administration, 511–512
alcohol and, 322
allergy, 149–150
artificial nutrition and, 309
cancer care, 311, 312, 313
children, 432
  type 2 diabetes, 434
corticosteroids and, 349, 538
cystic fibrosis, 337–338
delivery systems, required knowledge,
    511–512
end-of-life care, 528, 534–535, 536
enteral nutrition and, 408
exercise and, 33
fears, 134
glucose-lowering medicines with, 130, 130–134
hyperosmolar hyperglycaemic state, 214
hypoglycaemia risk, 356
in illnesses, 204
impaired response, 326
infusions, 146–149
  blood glucose monitoring, 68
  diabetic ketoacidosis, 209, 210
  hyperosmolar hyperglycaemic state, 214
  lactic acidosis, 216
  mistakes, 148–149
  myocardial infarction, 147, 233
  stroke management, 237
  surgery, 288
injection, 140–141
  devices for low vision, 242
  intramuscular, 511
  pregnancy, 458
for investigative procedures, 294
for latent autoimmune diabetes in adults, 17
mixing, 141
myocardial infarction, 231, 232–233
overdoses, 191
parenteral nutrition, 307
patients on dialysis, 253–254
peritoneal dialysis, 251
postnatal, 458
postoperative, 290
pregnancy, 449–451, 457–458
pumps *see* insulin pumps
quality of life and, 411–412, 481
regimens, 141–143
renal disease, 248
resistance *see* insulin resistance
short-acting *see* short-acting insulin
starting, 151–153, 166–167
  type 2 diabetes, 131–136
storage, 139
sulphonylureas with, 118, 130
surgery, 286, 288, 290–291, 292
tobacco smoke and, 317
transformation products, 139
type 2 diabetes, 21, 36
  starting, 131–136
types of, 136–139
insulin/glucose infusions, 231, 286

insulin (intrinsic), 136
   autonomic neuropathy on secretion, 267
   effect pathways, *19*
   release, 3, *10*, 18, 118
   secretagogues, 117
   surgery and, **282**
   type 1 *vs* 2 diabetes, 20
insulinoma, 181
insulin pumps, 143, 144
   children, 432
   end-of-life care, 535
   sensor augmented, 76
   surgery and, 288, 292
insulin resistance, 17–18, 37
   corticosteroids, 537
   cystic fibrosis, 337
   depression and, 477
   foetus, 455
   insulin infusions, 148
   liver disease, 330
   metabolic syndrome, 11–12
   older people, 392
   pregnancy, 449, 455
   type 1 diabetes, 14
insulin transformation products, 139
insulin-treated diabetes (term), 36
integrated care planning, 411
integrated medicine, 543, 548
intensification, medicines, 67–68, 469
intensive care, diabetic ketoacidosis, 209
intensive insulin therapy
   diabetic ketoacidosis, 209
   heart failure, 224
   for hyperglycaemia, 202
   hypoglycaemia, 176, 184
   mortality, 229
   renoprotection, 248
intensive weight management programme, 434
intent, healing by, 547
intentional nonadherence, 484
interactive behaviour change technology, 475
interdisciplinary teams, 30–31
interference, support *vs*, 418
interleukin-6, **95**, **227**
intermediate-acting insulin, 138
   action profiles, *142*
   mixing with short-acting insulin, 141
International Alliance of Patient Organisations,
      on patient-centred care, 493
International Patient Decision Aid Standards
      Collaboration, 502
Internet, 40, 41, 506–507
   assessing information, 475–476, 561–562
   sexual information, 383
   support based on, 54
interpersonal relationships, measurement
      tools, 381
interpretations of illness, 51
interrupting, in conversations, 485, 492, 500
intracavernosal therapy, 378
intramuscular injection, 140, 511
intrauterine devices, 447

intravenous infusions, *see also* infusions *under* insulin
   care of lines, 308
   diabetic ketoacidosis, 209
   hyperosmolar hyperglycaemic state, 214
   for hypoglycaemia, 191
   insulin/dextrose, surgery, 286
   parenteral nutrition, 307
   radiography and, 294, 295
intravenous trolleys, 208
intuitive learning style, **496**
investigative procedures, 293–295
iodinated contrast media, 234, 247, 295,
      297–298
   biguanides and, 124
iodine-rich foods, interactions with medicines, **105**
IRE1α (cow's milk), 3
iron
   deficiency in utero, 455
   overload, 332
   vegetarian diets and, 92
ischaemic heart disease, 223, *see also* myocardial
      infarction
ischaemic preconditioning, 199
islet cell antibodies, 82
islet cell transplantation, 150, 327
isoflavones, 460
isophane insulin, type 2 diabetes, 132
ISO standards, blood glucose meters, 70
isotonic dehydration, 399, 400
iValidate (programme), 531

jargon, 52
jejunal tubes, 306
Jianpi Wenshen recipe, 331
judgmental words, 493, 499

Kaplan, H., on sexual response, 373
kava, 461
kelp, **558**
ketoacidosis *see* diabetic ketoacidosis
ketoconazole, on PDE-5 inhibitor levels, 378
ketones, 74–75
   blood levels, **64**
      children in hospital, 438
      DKA, **204**
      end-of-life care, 535
      illnesses, **203**
      monitoring, 68, 74–75
   corticosteroids and, 68
   pregnancy, 75, 456
   urine, 74, 75, 280
ketosis-prone type 2 diabetes, **9**
Kivexa (antiretroviral), 343
koalas, continuous blood glucose monitoring, 74
Kombiglyze, **122**
krill, omega 3 fatty acids, 94

labels
   complementary medicines, 559
   foods, 106–107
   medicines, 163
   tobacco, 320

labile diabetes (brittle diabetes), 211, 326–327
labour, 452–453
  insulin, 457
  pain, complementary medicine, 451
lactate
  cancer, 315
  in dialysate fluid, 251
lactic acidosis, 199, 214–216
  biguanides, 123
  iodinated contrast media, 297
  surgery and, 287
lactose, breast milk, 458
lamotrigine, **259**
language, power of, 52, 483–486, 492–493, 499
laparoscopic adjustable gastric banding,
    102, 293
large baby, gestational diabetes risk, 456, 457
laser therapy, eye, 296–297
latent autoimmune diabetes in adults (LADA), **7**,
    15–17, 131, 132
  insulin deficiency, 36
  older people, 391
leakage, from injection sites, 140
learning capacity, older people, 403, 409
learning needs, assessment, 503
learning style, 494, 495–497
  estimation tool, **497**
left brain activity, immunity, 417
lens (eye), 136, 239
leptin, **95**
  signalling system, 428
Levemir *see* detemir
lidocaine patches, **260**
life balance, 467–490
life expectancy, *see also* longevity
  indicators of decline, 525
life-limiting illness, 525
life mission theory, 474
lifestyle disease, type 2 diabetes as, 499
life support, end-of-life care and, 531
lignans, 460
limited joint mobility, 437
linolenic acid, 94
lipid-lowering agents, 153–158, 230
  monitoring, 157–158
  nonadherence, 162
  side effects, 156–157
  trials, 154
lipids
  bariatric surgery and, 102
  carbohydrates, alcohol and fibre on, **93**
  cardiovascular disease, **227**
  cardiovascular risk reduction, 235
  children, 432
  diabetic ketoacidosis, **207**
  fructose on, 104–105
  liver disease, 330
  target values, **31**, 81, 154, 432
lipodystrophy, 436
liquorice, **105, 558**
liraglutide, 127
lispro, 137

listening, 500
listeriosis, 452
literacy (health literacy), 504–507
lithium, cardiovascular effects, **351**
liver disease, 329–332
  hepatocellular carcinoma, 330
  metabolic syndrome, 12
  nicotine, 320
  thiazolidinediones, 126, 331
Liver-X receptor agonists, 156
lixisenatide, **122**, 127
long-acting insulin analogues, 137, 138,
    139, 141
longevity, *see also* life expectancy; mortality
  overweight on, 11, 392
  smoking on, 317
long-term complications, 37, 219–277, *see also*
    cardiovascular disease
  pathogenesis, 221–223
look-alike medicine alert policies, 139
looping (DIY looping), 76
low-density lipoproteins, **227**
  target values, **31**, 81, 154, 228
    children, 432
low-dose insulin infusion, 147
low-energy meals, 100
lower limbs
  amputations, 258, 266
  autonomic neuropathy, **268**
  macrovascular disease, 257
  neuropathy, 255, 256
  older people, 411
lozenges, nicotine, **321**
lung cancer, inhaled insulin, 137

machine learning, 40
macrosomia, foetus, 456, 457
macrovascular disease, 37, 220, 221, *see also*
    cardiovascular disease
  blood glucose monitoring on, 65
  driving, **354**
  exercise preventing, 107
  hypoglycaemia, 194
  lower limbs, 257
  screening, 261
macular degeneration, 238, 239, **240**
  aspirin, 161
macular oedema, thiazolidinediones, 126
maculopathy, 238
magic mushrooms (*Amanita muscaria*), 324
magnesium
  surgery and, 282
  type 2 diabetes prevention, 27
magnetic resonance imaging, 294
  foot disease, 258
malabsorption, causes, 403
Malmberg et al., DIGAMI protocol, 233
malnutrition, 88–90, 304–305
  bariatric surgery and, 102
  older people, 403–408
  pregnancy, 12
  renal disease, 249–250

management, 29–36
    aims, 31–32, 38–39
    children, 431–436
    guidelines, 43, 62
        listed, **63**
    hypoglycaemia, 190–191, 194–195
    illnesses (intercurrent), **203**
    medicines, 113–173
    obesity, 100–103
    with other illnesses, 39
manipulation (psychological), 480
MAP-kinase, 3, *19*
marijuana *see* cannabis
marketing strategies, 498–499
massage, 550
    abdominal, 270
    children, 439, 550
    puerperium, 452
    surgery and, 552–553
Masters, W. and Johnson, V., on sexual response, 373
mastopathy, 333
maternal hyperglycaemia, 454–455
maternal mortality, 453
maternal obesity, 12, 19, 428
maturity onset diabetes of the young, **8**, 21–22
    single gene disorders, **16**
Mauriac syndrome, 436
meal replacements, 100, 101
meals, low vision, 243
medical assistance dogs, 42, 552
medical records, 55, 57–58
Medicare, coverage for HbA1c tests, 23
medicines, *see also* adherence to medicines
    appearance, 163
    artificial nutrition and, 309, 407–408
    cardiovascular disease, 228–230
    causing hyperosmolar hyperglycaemic state, 213
    causing lactic acidosis, 215
    causing weight gain, 96
    children, 434, 436
    cognitive deficit, 398
    diabetogenic, **8**, 201, 537–538
    driving, 353, 357–358
    end-of-life care and, 532
    enteral nutrition, 407–408
    for erectile dysfunction, 378
    erectile dysfunction from, 377
    food and, 104, **105**
    generic, 506
    glucose-lowering *see* glucose-lowering medicines
    hearing loss from, 344
    herbal *see* herbal medicines
    intensification, 67–68, 469
    interactions, 129–130
        complementary medicine, 299, 554–561
        foods, **105**
        grapefruit juice, **105**, 129, 553
        hypoglycaemia, 189
        illegal drugs, 325
        tobacco smoke, 317
    liver disease, 331
    management, 113–173

menopause, 459
    on nutrition, 104, **403**, 415
    OGTT and, 24
    older people, 250, 414–415
    palliative care, 534–536
    for peripheral neuropathy, **259–260**
    pharmacovigilance, 414–415, 534
    pregnancy, 449–451
    for retinopathy, 241
    self-management, 161–165
    self-monitoring (SMBG) for, 66
    for smoking cessation, 320, **321**
    for weight reduction, 101
meditation, 550
Mediterranean diet, 27
megestrol acetate, 342
meglitinides, 117, **120**, 125
memory
    children, 455
    diabetic ketoacidosis, 429
    factors affecting, 409
    prospective errors, 484
    shared (Internet), 506–507
MEMs containers, 165
men
    contraception, 372–373, 448
    sexual health, 377–380
menopause, 459–462
Men's Sheds, 322, 378
menstruation, 376
mental health, *see also* depression
    cardiovascular disease, 232
    corticosteroids, 350
    older people, assessment, **393**
    smoking, 317, 319
    type 1 diabetes, 480
    type 2 diabetes, 480–481
metabolic acidosis, **207**, *see also* lactic acidosis
metabolic burnout, **387**
metabolic syndrome, 10–14
    children, 13–14, 428
metabolomics, 427
metered-dose spray, insulin, 137
meters
    blood glucose, 66, 69–72
        electronic, 55
    for ketones, 75
metformin, 117, 118–124
    AIDS patients, 343
    alcohol and, 130
    on blood lipids, 156
    cancer risk and, 310
    children, 434
    cognitive effects, 478
    in combinations, **120**
    end-of-life care, 535
    hypoglycaemia risk, 356
    with insulin, 130, 131
    iodinated contrast media, 297
    lactic acidosis, 216
    latent autoimmune diabetes in adults and, 17
    metabolic syndrome, 14

on microbiome, 88
polycystic ovarian syndrome, 445–446
pregnancy, **450**, 451, 457
SGLT-2 inhibitors with, **122**
surgery and, 287
vegetarian diets and, 92
methionine, 427
metoclopramide, 269
mexiletine, for peripheral neuropathy, **259**
Micral-Test dipstick test, 78
microalbumin–creatinine ratio, 78
microalbuminuria, 243, 244, 245, 247
hypoglycaemia, 192
microvascular disease, **227**
pregnancy, 452
tests for, 77–78, 245
microbiome, 88, 305, 427
ancestral diets on, 92
brain and, 88, 477–478
micronutrients, ageing, 387
microvascular disease, 37, 220, **227**
blood glucose monitoring on, 65
children, 428, 432
driving, **354**
exercise preventing, 107
foot, 257
HbA1c and, 221
hypoglycaemia, 194
mid-arm circumference, 405
migration, type 1 diabetes, 15
milk
cow's, 3, 15, 457
interactions with medicines, **105**
milk thistle, 314, 319
mind–body–spirit model, 547
mind–body therapies, 314
Minidiab (glipizide), **119**
Mini Nutritional Assessment, 405
mini pill (contraceptive), 447
minor surgery, 287
misinformation, 473–474
sexual health, 374
mistakes
insulin infusions, 148–149
medicine-related, 162
mitochondrial function, 221, 222
mixed insulins, 139
biphasic insulins, 138–139, 141
mixing
blood glucose samples, 79
insulins, 141
Mixtard 50/70, 139
mobilisation, after amputations, 266
Modification of Diet in Renal Disease, e-GFR, 77
monoamine oxidase inhibitors
cardiovascular effects, **351**
foods interacting, **105**
sulphonylureas and, **189**
monoclonal antibodies, diabetes prevention, 29
monogenic syndromes, **16**, 426, *see also* maturity
onset diabetes of the young
neonatal diabetes, 8, 426

monounsaturated fatty acids, **97**
mood, hypoglycaemia, 179
Morisky Scale, 165
morning hyperglycaemia, 143, 188
mortality, 221, *see also* longevity
cardiovascular disease, 231
hyperosmolar hyperglycaemic state, 212, 213
intensive insulin therapy, 229
lactic acidosis, 214
maternal, 453
metabolic syndrome, 13
type 2 diabetes, weight on, 95–96
motivational interviewing, 103
multi-infarct dementia, 236, *see also* vascular
dementia
multimorbidity, 220
multiple daily insulin injections (MDI), 67, 392
musculoskeletal disease, 345–347
driving, **355**
mushrooms, magic (*Amanita muscaria*), 324
myocardial infarction, 220
distress, 481
extension, 233
hospital treatment, 231
hyperglycaemia, 231
hyperosmolar hyperglycaemic state, 213
insulin, 231, 232–233
insulin infusions, 147, 233
invasive treatment, 231
pregnancy, 449
risk in renal disease, 234
risk of diabetes, 225
rosiglitazone, 126
SGLT-2 inhibitors on, 128
silent, 226, 231 *see also* atypical myocardial
infarction
myocardium, 225–226
myositis, statins, 156
myths *see* misinformation

narrative competence, 53
narrative medicine, 497
nasal sprays, nicotine, **321**
nasogastric tubes, 208, 306, 308, 407
National Assessment of Adult Literacy, 505
National Gestational Diabetes Register, 456
National Health Service, guidelines for surgical
patients, 289
National Institute of Health criteria, polycystic
ovarian syndrome, *444*
National Prescribing Service, Australia, 414
nausea, 282, 308
acupuncture, 314
cancer care, 311
complementary medicine, 298, 299
end of life, **529**
ginger, 554
glucagon, 195
necrobiosis lipoidica diabeticorum, 437
needles, 140, 141
reusing, 511
neonatal diabetes, 8, 426

neonates
    hypoglycaemia, 454, 457
    large baby, gestational diabetes risk, 456, 457
    maternal hyperglycaemia, 454–455
    microbiome, 427
nephrogenic systemic fibrosis, 247
nephropathy, 77–78, 244, *see also* renal disease
    children, 432
    contrast-induced, 247, 297
    driving, **354**
neuroglycopaenia, **181**, 194
neurology, glucose homeostasis, 10
neurons, glucose-excited and glucose-inhibited, 183
neuropathy, 37, 220, 255–266, **389**, *see also*
        autonomic neuropathy
    driving, **355**
    gastrointestinal tract, 340
Newest Vital Sign (health literacy measure), 505
Nicorette, **321**
nicotine
    addiction, 318
    replacement therapy, 320, **321**
nicotinic acid, **129**, 156, **157**, 230
nifedipine, medicine interactions, **129**
night dosing, metformin, 445
night smoking, 317
nitrates, topical, **260**
nitroprusside reagents, drug interactions, 75
nocturnal hypoglycaemia, 187–189
    blood glucose monitoring for, 68
    children, 433
noise, 344, 345
nonadherence, 113, 162–165, 483–484, 501–502
    hypoglycaemia and, 184, 193
    monitoring, 165
nonalcoholic fatty liver disease (NAFLD), 330
nonalcoholic steatohepatitis, 330
noncompliance *see* nonadherence
non-nutrient food components, on blood lipids, **93**
non-nutritive sweeteners, 106
nonsteroidal anti-inflammatory agents, renal disease, 248
noradrenaline, **183**, **282**
normality, 470
normoglycaemia
    bariatric surgery, 102, 293
    as target, 67
NovoMix 30, 138
    confusion of dose with number, 139
    type 2 diabetes, 132
NRLP3 inflammasome, 3
nucleoside reverse transcriptase inhibitors (NRTI), 343
numeracy, 505
nurses
    autonomic neuropathy, 270
    brittle diabetes, 327
    complementary medicine, 545
    diabetic ketoacidosis, 209–210
    diet and, 89
    as role models, 510
    self-care and, 82–83
    stabilisation of diabetes in hospital, 151
nursing history, sexual health, 380–381

nursing notes, 57–58
Nutbeam, D., on health literacy, 504
nutrition, 87–112, *see also* diet; enteral nutrition;
        malnutrition; parenteral nutrition; undernutrition
    ageing and, 387
    coeliac disease, 335–336
    end-of-life care, 536–537
    liver disease, 331
    medicines and, 104, **403**, 415
    neonates, 455
    older people, **388**, 403–408
    renal disease, 248–250
    signs of deficiency, 91
    smoking cessation, 319
    stress, 98–99
    surgery and, 282
nutritive sweeteners, 106
nuts, 229

oatmeal, interactions with medicines, **105**
obesity, 87, 95–103, *see also* abdominal obesity;
        central obesity
    cardiovascular disease and, **227**
    children, 96, 428, 454–455
        brain, 429
    diseases from, 98
    gestational diabetes risk, 456
    macular degeneration, **240**
    management, 100–103
    maternal, 12, 19, 428
    pathogenesis, 96–99
    polycystic ovarian syndrome, 444
    renal disease, 243, 244
    research, 29
    sarcopenic, 394
    stress, 98–99
    surgery and, 282, **286**
    type 2 diabetes, 18
        management, 100–103
    waist circumference, 11, 13, 18, 98
obesity paradox, 96
observations, diabetic ketoacidosis, 209–210
obstructive sleep apnoea, 340–341
    driving, **355**
    erectile dysfunction and, 378
octreotide, 191
odour control, foot care, 262, 263
odours, 552
oedema, thiazolidinediones, 125
oestrogens, 225
olanzapine, 350, 446
older people, 385–424
    basal bolus insulin dose regimens, 143
    brittle diabetes, 211
    care planning, 401–410
    creatinine, 78, 246, 250, 392, 405
    depression, 400, 470
    driving ability, 353
    driving crashes, 352
    factors affecting metabolic control, 410–417
    Federal Study of Adherence to Medications in the
        Elderly, 164

foot disease, 256
glargine, 132
guidelines, 62, 391
   sexual health, 375
hearing loss, 343, 344
hyperosmolar hyperglycaemic state, 214
hypoglycaemia, 182, 186, 192, 391, 416
myocardial infarction, 231
oral health, 328
overall care, 417–418
overweight, 98
renal disease, 250
sexual health, 375, 376, 411
surgery, 283–284
top-up doses, 145
type 1 diabetes, 480
weight gain, 100
omega-3 fatty acids, 93–94, **97**, 158
   albuminuria and, 255
   supplements, 405–406
omega-6 fatty acids, 93–94, **97**
omega-9 fatty acids, 93–94, **97**
one-stop appointments, 411
1-2-3 study, NovoMix 30, 132
online disease management, 40
opioids, 39
   illegal, **323**
   for peripheral neuropathy, **260**
OptimAAPP (smartphone app), 41
OPTIMISE (trial), 42
oral contraceptives, 447, 448
   polycystic ovarian syndrome, 445, 446
oral glucose tolerance test, 22
   adolescence, 13
   cystic fibrosis, 337
   gestational diabetes, 7, 21
   information sheet, 25
   method, 24–25
   polycystic ovarian syndrome, 445
   postpartum, 457
   pregnancy, 455, 456
   self-administered, 23
oral health, 328–329
   on cognitive reserve, **396**
   end of life, **529**
   on nutrition, **403**, 405
   renal replacement therapies, 252
oral insulin, 137
Oral-Lyn, 137
orange juice, interactions with medicines, **105**
orlistat, 14
orthostatic hypotension, 233, 267, 269, 359, 413
osmolality, dehydration, 399
osteoarthritis, 345
osteomyelitis, 258
osteoporosis, 346–347, 348
   corticosteroids, 257, 349
   hormone replacement therapy for, 460
   SGLT-2 inhibitors, 128
otelixizumab, 29
outpatients, stabilisation of diabetes, 151–153, 166–167

overactive bladder, 339
overdoses, insulin, 191
overload hypothesis, 426
over-the-counter medicines, adolescence, 436
overweight, 95–103
   inflammation, 456
   on longevity, 11, 392
   macular degeneration, **240**
   menopause, 459
oxidative tissue damage, 88, 221–222, 387
oxygen desaturation index, 341
OzDAFNE (education programme), 144

pain, *see also* abdominal pain
   cancer care, 311
   chest pain, action plan, 235
   complementary medicine, 299
     labour, 451
   end of life, **529**
   foot disease, **264**, 265
   peripheral neuropathy, 259–260
palliative care, 523, 524, 525–532
   hyperglycaemia, 533
   hypoglycaemia, 533–534
   medicines, 534–536
   renal disease, 254
Palliative Care Outcomes Collaboration, stages of dying, 526, **527**
Panax spp. (ginseng), 461, **557**
pancreas
   artificial, 41
   cancer, 309
   injuries, **9**
   transplantation, 150
     foot fractures, 257
papillopathy, 239
Paracelsus, quoted, 113
parenteral nutrition, 304–305, 307
   blood glucose monitoring, 68
   end-of-life care and, 531
parents *see* families
partners
   management of erectile dysfunction, 380
   sexual history, 381
passive smoking, 316
passivity, 502
patient (term), 493
patient activation, 51, 502
patient-centred (term), 50, 492–493
patient-held records, blood glucose testing, 409–410
patient noncompliance *see* nonadherence
PAX4 mutation, **16**
peanuts, 229
Pederson–Bjergaad method, 186
pedometers, 108
penile injections, 378
penile prosthetics, 378–379
pen needles, 141
pennyroyal, 332
people with diabetes
   assessment and monitoring, 61–85
   documentation by, 58

percutaneous endoscopic gastrostomy, 306
    care of tubes, 308
periodontal disease, 328–329
peripheral neuropathy, 37, 220, 255–266, **389**
    defined, 259
    driving, **355**
    medicines for, **259–260**
peritoneal dialysis, 251–254
permission-giving, PLISSIT model, 382
peroxisome proliferator-activated receptor γ agonists
            see thiazolidinediones
person-centred empowerment model, 31, 54–55,
            476, *see also* holistic personalised care
    adherence to medicines, 164
person-centredness, defined, 50
pets, 403, 411, 536
Peyronie's disease, 377
pH
    diabetic ketoacidosis, **204**, 209
    hyperosmolar hyperglycaemic state, 213
    lactic acidosis, 216
pharmacovigilance, 414–415, 534
phenytoin, **129**, 415
phosphate binders, 246
phosphodiesterase type 5 inhibitors, 378
phospholipids, 427
photocoagulation, eye, 296–297
phototherapy, foot disease, 263
physical activities of daily living, 392
physiotherapy, diabetic ketoacidosis, 210
phytoestrogens, 460
pioglitazone, 117, **121**, 125
    cancer risk, 310, 311
    metabolic syndrome, 14
Piper methysticum (kava), 461
PK C epsilon, 20
placenta, glucose flux, 449
plasminogen activator inhibitor-1, **95**, 223
plaster casts, 258, 264
plastic, insulin binding, 147
plate waste methodology, 100
PLISSIT model, 382
pneumonia, 201
point-of-care HbA1c tests, 23
polycyclic aromatic hydrocarbons, 316
polycystic ovarian syndrome, 443,
            444–447
    thiazolidinediones, 126
polyol pathway, 222–223
polypharmacy, 113, 116, 162–163
    surgery and, **285**
polysomnography, 341
polyunsaturated fatty acids, **97**
polyuria, SGLT-2 inhibitors, 128
Porphyromonas gingivalis, **396**
portions, carbohydrates, 92
positivity, 547
positron emission tomography, 294
postoperative care, 289–290
    complementary medicine, 299, 554
postoperative ketosis, 212
post-prandial hypotension, 413
post-prandial plasma glucose, 118, *see also* anabolism

cardiovascular disease prediction, 231
cystic fibrosis, 337
meglitinides on, 125
morbid, 3
older people, 392
reducing, 67
target values, **31**
    corticosteroids and, 538
type 1 diabetes, 5
type 2 diabetes, **6**, 18
post transplantation diabetes, 8
postural hypotension, 233, 267, 269, 359, 413
potassium
    diabetic ketoacidosis, **207**, 209
    surgery and, 282
potassium channels, 222
potatoes, 15
PPAR-alpha receptor, 428
prandial insulin, 131, 137, *see also* rapid-acting insulin
            analogues
pravastatin, clinical trials, 155
prayer, 314
prayer sign, 345
prealbumin, 405
prediabetes, **4**, 10–11
    HbA1c with fasting plasma glucose, 24
predictors, nocturnal hypoglycaemia, 187
prednisolone, 313, 349, 537
prefilled disposable insulin devices, 139
pregnancy, 449–455, *see also* gestational diabetes
    complications, 37, 453–454
    developing regions, 443–444
    glucose-lowering medicines, **450**, 457
    hypoglycaemia, 182
    insulin, 449–451, 457–458
    ketones, 75, 456
    malnutrition, 12
    planning of, 443
    progesterone levels, 458
    proteinuria, 246
    retinopathy, 239, 452
    self-monitoring (SMBG), 66
    sweeteners, 106
    weight gain, 456–457
preoperative care, 284–289
    complementary medicine, 298–299, 553–554
prepregnancy counselling, 449
prescriptions, illegible, 149
pressure off-loading, foot disease, 258
pressures, social, 473
prevalence of diabetes, 1, 2–3
prevention
    of diabetes, 26–29
        models, 28
    falls, 414, 417
    hypoglycaemia, 184–185
    illnesses (intercurrent), 200–201
previsit record books, 410
priapism, 378
primary nonadherence, 484
primary prevention, 116
probenecid, **189**
probiotics, 299

problem lists, 56
procoagulant state, 12
proformas, insulin in type 2 diabetes, 132
progesterone
    creams, 461
    pregnancy, 458
progestin-only contraceptives, 448
progestogen, male contraceptive, 448
prognosis, end-of-life care, 539
programmed theories, ageing, **387**
programme evaluation, diabetes education, 515–517
prolonged hypoglycaemia, 191–192
prolonged QT interval
    antipsychotics, 350
    SSRIs, **351**
prospective memory errors, 484
PROSPER (clinical trial), 155
prostate cancer, 309, 315
prostatectomy, incontinence, 339
prostheses, limb, 266
protease inhibitors, HIV-1, 342
protein(s)
    glycosylation, 222
    plasma levels, 405
protein 13-kinase, 3, *19*
protein (dietary)
    inadequate intake, 91
    intake target, 94, 404
    renal disease, 249
    surgery and, 282
protein kinase C, *see also* PK C epsilon
    inhibitors, 260
    isoforms, 222
proteinuria, 244, 245
    hypertension, 77
    pregnancy, 246
pseudogout, 345
psychological effects, hypoglycaemia, 193
psychological issues, 467–490
psychological review, diabetic ketoacidosis,
        210, 211
psychosis, corticosteroids, 350
puberty, diabetes incidence, 426
public health programmes, weight reduction, 100
purchasing journeys, 498–499
purpose in life, 472–473

QRS complex, tricyclic antidepressants, **351**
quality control, blood glucose meters, 70–71
quality of care, 42
quality of life, 467–468, 474–475
    insulin and, 411–412, 481
    measurement tools, 475
    older people, 411–412
quality use of medicine framework (QUM), 114–116
    complementary medicine, 544, 547–548
questionnaires
    on adherence to medicines, 165
    food frequency, 100
    Hypoglycaemic Awareness, 187
    sexual health, 381
questions for person-centred care, 54–55
Quetelet's Index *see* body mass index

radiography, *see also* iodinated contrast media
    foot disease, 258
    intravenous infusions and, 294, 295
radiotherapy, 312
Ramadan, 359
ramipril, 158–159
random plasma glucose, 22
random urine tests, microalbumin, 78
rapid-acting insulin analogues, 142, *see also* prandial
        insulin
    alpha-glucosidase inhibitors and, 137
    mixing with other insulins, 141
Rapid Estimate of Adult Literacy in Medicine, 505
reactions (allergic), insulin, 149–150
reactive oxygen species, 221–222, *see also* free radicals
readability tests, 505–506
readmissions, after surgery, 283
REALM (Rapid Estimate of Adult Literacy in
        Medicine), 505
reboxetine, cardiovascular effects, **351**
recall, conversations, 500
red blood cell transfusions, end-of-life care and, 530
red clover, 461
red rice yeast, **546**
reflective learning style, **495**
reflective practice, 494
refrigeration, insulin, 139
regulations, 62
    complementary medicine, 548
rehabilitation
    amputations, 266
    cardiovascular disease, 234
relational continuity, 493
relative hypoglycaemia, 189
relatives, *see also* families
    type 2 diabetes patients, 15
religion, 473
religious observances, fasting, 359–360
remifemin, 461
remote monitoring, 40
renal artery stenosis, ACE inhibitors, 159
renal biopsy, 250
renal disease, 243–255, **390**
    from chemotherapy, 315
    myocardial infarction risk, 234
    risk factors, 245–246
    smoking, 316
    stages, **244**, 249
renal failure, 246–248
    hyperosmolar hyperglycaemic state, 213
    lactic acidosis, 216
    pregnancy, 452
renal function
    glucose-lowering medicines on, 246
    hyperglycaemia on, 247–248
    metformin, 535
    monitoring, 77–78
    older people, 392
    pregnancy, 452
    sodium-glucose cotransporter-2 inhibitors, 246
renal threshold, 64, 76
    self-monitoring to establish, 66
    24-hour urine glucose, 68

reporting, adverse events, **561**
resilience, 470, 547
resistance training, 416, 551
resistance vessels, 222
respiratory tract
    effects of surgery, **285**
    smoking, 316
retinopathy, 237–243, 295
    aspirin, 241, 297
    children, 432
    driving, **354**
    pregnancy, 239, 452
    smoking, 239, 316
    thrombolytic agents and, 234
retirement, smoking cessation, 318
rice, 27
rifampicin, on PDE-5 inhibitor levels, 378
rimonabant, 97, 156
road traffic accidents *see* crashes
robots, 40–41
rosiglitazone, 117, **121**, 125, 126
    in combinations, **120**
    metabolic syndrome, 14
    pregnancy, **450**
ROSSO study, 65
rotavirus infection, 427
Rotterdam criteria, polycystic ovarian
        syndrome, *444*
Roux-en-Y procedure, **102**
rubella, 427
ruboxistaurin, 222
ruminant fat, 92
ruvastatin, 155

SADHART (trial), on depression, 232
safety
    complementary medicine, 548, 549, 556–560
    medicines, 161–162
    older people, 412–415
sage, 324
salicylates, 159
saline
    diabetic ketoacidosis, 209
    hyperosmolar hyperglycaemic state, 214
    stroke management, 237
    surgery, 288
salivary glucose, 24
salt, 94, 404
    interactions with medicines, **105**
    renal disease, 249
salutogenesis, 474
Salvia divinorum, 324
samples, blood glucose, 72
    mixing, 79
Sanchis, J., cardiac risk assessment, 232
sarcopenia, **286**, **389**, 394
saturated fats, 27, **97**
saw palmetto, 332
saxagliptin, **121**, 127
schizophrenia, 482–483
    microbiome and, 88
school education, 431
    depression and, 476–477

Schwenk, T., intensive weight management
        programme, 434
SCI-DC (foot disease screening), 261
Scientific Advisory Committee on Nutrition, on gluten, 428
screening
    adolescence, 14
    AIDS patients, 342
    alcohol dependence, 322
    anxiety, 446
    cancer, 310, 315
        in renal disease, 248
    children, 428, 430, 431
    coeliac disease, 335
    depression, 446, 478
    diabetes-related distress, 474, 478
    dialysis patients, 252
    dysphagia, stroke management, 237
    foot disease, 261
    indigenous Australians, 21
    liver disease, 330–331
    metabolic syndrome, 14
    nutrition, 89, 90–91
        tools, 91
    obesity affecting, 96
    older people, 393–394
    oral glucose tolerance test, 22
    prediabetes, **4**
    pregnancy, 455
    renal disease, 243, 245
    retinopathy, 240–241
    type 2 diabetes, 26, 28
secondary prevention, 116
second-hand smoke, 316
secretagogues, of insulin, 117
secreted frizzled-related protein 4, 20
security of data, 57
sedation
    end-of-life care and, 531
    falls, 412
sedentary time, 19, 107, 229
selective serotonin reuptake inhibitors, cardiovascular
        effects, **351**
self-care, 82–83, 470, 492, *see also* person-centred
        empowerment model
    depression and, 478
    documentation, 58
    driving, 353–355
    illnesses, 202
        prevention, 201
    older people, 409–410
    renal replacement therapies, 252
self-efficacy, diabetes-specific, 475
self-help programmes, weight reduction, 100
self-help websites, smoking cessation, 319
self-management
    children, **433**, 436
    medicines, 161–165
self-monitoring (SMBG), 62, 64, 65–67
    aims, 66
sensation, testing, 261
sensing learning style, **495**
sensor augmented pumps, 76
sepsis, end of life, **530**

sequential learning style, **496**
serotonin, herb/medicine interactions, 556
serotonin and norepinephrine reuptake inhibitors,
    cardiovascular effects, **351**
serotonin reuptake inhibitors, 101, 483
sex hormone binding globulin (SHBG), 29
    polycystic ovarian syndrome, 445
sexual counselling, 380–383
sexual development, 373
sexual health, 371–384
    autonomic neuropathy, **268**, 269, 375
    children and adolescents, 431
    measurement, 381–382
    misinformation, 374
    older people, 375, 376, 411
sexually transmitted diseases, 372
sexual response, 373
shared decision-making (SDM), 50–51, 492
shift work, 340
shock, dehydration, 288
short-acting insulin, 138
    action profiles, *142*
    mixing with intermediate-acting insulin, 141
    nocturnal hypoglycaemia, 188
shoulder adhesive capsulitis, 345
shoulder–hand syndrome, 345
sibutramine, 101
SIGN guidelines, cystic fibrosis, 336
sign language, 344–345
sildenafil, 378
silent diseases, 39
silent myocardial infarction, 226, 231, *see also*
    atypical myocardial infarction
Silymarin (milk thistle), 314, 319
simulators, driving, 353
simvastatin, ocular effects, 241
single gene disorders *see* monogenic syndromes
sitagliptin, 127, 128
    in combinations, **120**
sitting time (sedentary time), 19, 107, 229
situational sexual problems, 374
skin
    cancer care, 312
    corticosteroids and, 312, 349
    older people, **390**
sleep disturbance, 340–341
    complementary medicine for, 299
    driving, **355**
    erectile dysfunction and, 378
    insulin resistance, 12
    statins, 156
    stroke risk, 236
sleeve gastrectomy, **102**
sliding scales, 145, 146, 288
slippery elm, adverse effects, **558**
slow-wave sleep, 340
smart insulins, 137
smartphone apps, 41
smokeless tobacco, 320
smoking, 20, 316–320
    cessation, 317–320
        medicines for, 320, **321**
    coeliac disease, 334

foot disease, 260
    hypoglycaemia and, 182
    macular degeneration, **240**
    retinopathy, 239, 316
soap, foot care, 262
social aspects, 473
social dignity, 52
sodium (levels)
    children, 438
    dehydration, 399
sodium-glucose cotransporter-2 inhibitors, 117–118,
    122, 128–129
    end-of-life care, 536
    euglycaemic ketoacidosis, 212
    on kidney, 246
    on liver, 331
    surgery and, 287
    urinalysis and, 280
soluble fibre, 27
Somogyi effect, 143, 188
sorbitol, 106
    in polyol pathway, 222–223
sore throat, postoperative, 290
specific gravity, urine, 209
spirituality, 32, 51, 472–473, 532, 552
spironolactone, 446
spot albumin–creatinine urine test, 245
spring harvest hypothesis, 426
squeezing, blood glucose sampling, 72
stabilisation of diabetes, 150–153
    outpatients, 151–153, 166–167
standardized education frameworks,
    493, 494
standard protocols, 58
standards
    blood glucose meters, 70
    haemoglobin A1c, 80
stat doses, 145–146
statins, 154–157, 230
    ocular effects, 241
    side effects, 156
    teratogenesis, **450**, **451**
stavudine, 343
steatohepatitis, 332
    nonalcoholic, 330
stem cells, 29
sterilisation, 448
steroids *see* corticosteroids
stevia, 106
St John's wort, 298–299, 461, 551
    adverse effects and interactions, **558**
    stopping before surgery, 553–554
stockings, 269
storage, insulin, 139
stories, narrative medicine, 497
stress
    on blood glucose, 69
    cardiovascular disease, 235
    complementary medicine, 550
    hypoglycaemia, 188
    on immunity, 417
    nutrition and obesity, 98–99
stress incontinence, 339

stress response, 12
    hyperglycaemia as, 26
    with other illnesses, 39
    surgery, 281–282
strokes, 236–237
structured SMBG, 65
stump care, 266
subsidisation
    insulin pumps, 144
    test strips, 65
substance use, 315–326
sudden hearing loss, 344
sugar
    for hypoglycaemia, 190
    intake target, 94
sugar-free foods, 104–105
suicide, 525
Suitability Assessment of Materials (readability test), 506
sulphonamides, **189**
sulphonylureas, 117, **119**, 124
    alcohol and, 130
    combined with biguanides, **120**
    end-of-life care, 535
    fasting, 359
    hypoglycaemia, 124, 181, 183, 191, 356
    with insulin, 118, 130
    latent autoimmune diabetes in adults and, **7**, 17
    medicine interactions, 189
    pregnancy, **450**, 451
support garments, 269
supportive care
    cancer, 310
    palliative, 254
support programmes, smoking cessation, 319
surgery, 280–293
    complementary medicine, 281, 284, 287, 298–300,
        552–555
    corticosteroid increase, 350
surveys, patient satisfaction, 54
survival skills, 498, 507–508
swabs, foot ulcers, 258
swallowing difficulties
    medicines, 414–415
    on nutrition, 405
sweating, **268**, 269
sweeteners, alternative, 105–106
swimming, 416
sympathetic symptoms, *see also* catecholamines
    hypoglycaemia, **181**, 182
sympathy, 469
symptom burden, 531
synergy, 552
syringes, 139, 141, 511
    medicines via enteral tubes, 407
Systematic Coronary Risk Evaluation, 235

tablet failure (term), 131
tachycardia
    hyperosmolar hyperglycaemic state, 213
    marijuana, 324
    tricyclic antidepressants, **351**
tachypnoea, hyperosmolar hyperglycaemic state, 213

tai chi, 108, 416, 551
takeaway foods, 90
target intake
    carbohydrates, 90
    protein (dietary), 94, 404
    sugar, 94
targets, weight reduction, 89
targets (regulatory), 62
target values, 31, 67–68
    blood glucose *see under* blood glucose
    blood pressure *see under* blood pressure
    haemoglobin A1c, **33**, 80, 228–229, 392, **433**, 434
        pregnancy, 449
    lipids, **31**, 81, 154, 432
Taxus celebica, 255
teachable moments, 510
teach-back collaborative inquiry, 501
teaching, 503–504, 510–511
teaching strategies, 495
technology, 40–42, 54, 475, *see also* Internet; meters
    continuous blood glucose monitoring (CGM), 68,
        73–74, 144–145
    diabetes education, 499
    health information, 55
    hypoglycaemia prevention, 185
TEDDY study, 427
tee tree, **558**
telehealth consultations, 40
telephone coaching, 236
television viewing, 107, 428
tell-back collaborative inquiry, 501
teplizumab, 29
teratogenesis, **450**
    statins, **450**, **451**
terbutaline, 189
terminal care, 525–526
terminology (language), power of, 52, 483–486,
    492–493, 499
Test of Functional Health Literacy in Adults, 505
testosterone, 188
    on diabetes risk, 12
    levels, 378
    male contraceptive, 448
    polycystic ovarian syndrome, 445
    replacement, 97
    supplements, 375, 378, 379
test strips
    for ketones, 75
    subsidisation, 65
    technique, 71–72
theory of mind, 53
therapeutic relationships, 152
thiamine, for lactic acidosis, 216
thiazides, 233
thiazolidinediones, 117, **121**, 125–126
    AIDS patients, 343
    cancer care, 312
    corticosteroids and, 348
    end-of-life care, 535
    latent autoimmune diabetes in adults and, 17
    liver disease, 126, 331
    pregnancy, **450**

thioredoxin-interacting protein, 3
third world *see* developing regions
thirst
   end-of-life care, 537
   older people, **390**
three-talk model, 51
three-way adaptors, 148, *149*
thrombolytic agents, 233, 234
thrush, vaginal, 376
thyroid disease
   children and adolescents, 436
   Hashimoto's thyroiditis, 327
TIAs (transient ischaemic attacks), 236
time of day, insulin in type 2 diabetes, 131
tolerance of uncertainty, 50
Toll-like receptor 4, 12
toolkit, diabetes prevention, 28
topical creams, weight reduction and, 103
topical nitrates, **260**
top-up doses, 145–146
torcetrapib, 156
touch, older people, 375
traditional Chinese medicine
   contaminated products, 549
     on liver, 331
     renal disease, 255
traffic accidents *see* crashes
transcendence, 473
transcranial magnetic stimulation, 320
transdermal patches, nicotine, **321**
trans fatty acids, **97**
transformational model of change, insulin in type 2
     diabetes, 135
transforming growth factor-β_1, 223
transient ischaemic attacks (TIAs), 236
transplantation
   diabetes after, **8**
   islet cells, 327
   pancreas, 150
     foot fractures, 257
Treat-to-Target study, 132
triage process, adaptive, 387
triamcinolone, intravitreal, 241
triceps skin fold, 405
tricyclic antidepressants
   cardiovascular effects, **351**
   peripheral neuropathy, **259**
Trifolium pratense (red clover), 461
trigger-bolster hypothesis, 15
trigger finger, 345
TRIGIR study, 427
triglycerides, 153–154
   adolescence, 13
   cardiovascular disease, **227**
   choice of lipid-lowering agents, 158
   diabetes in children, 427
   metabolic syndrome, 11
   target values, **31**, 81
Trizivir (antiretroviral), 343
troponins, 231
T-score, bone mineral density, 346
tubal ligation, 448

tuberculosis, 341–342
TUG, frailty assessment, 394
tumour necrosis factor-alpha, **95**
tunnel vision, 296
TV viewing, 107, 428
24-hour blood glucose profile, 253
24-hour urine, 245
Two-Cal®, 406
type 1 diabetes, 2, **5**, 14–15
   beta cell decline, *16*
   blood glucose monitoring, 68
   children, 426, 480
     management, 431–433
   coeliac disease, 334
   end-of-life care, 534–535
   hypoglycaemia, 177
   information sheet on illnesses, 512–513
   mental health, 480
   osteoporosis, 346
   pregnancy, 457–458
   prevention, 29
   sexual health, women, 376
   type 2 diabetes *vs*, **20**, 480
   urological complications, 339
type 2 diabetes, 2, **6**, 17–21
   alcohol, 322
   beta cell decline, 130
   children, 6, 425, 428, 430
     indigenous Australians, 21
     management, 433–436
   cognitive deficit, 429
   dementia, 395
   end-of-life care, 535
   hyperosmolar hyperglycaemic state, 212
   hypoglycaemia, 177
   hypoglycaemic unawareness, prevalence, 185
   information sheet on illnesses, 514–515
   insulin, 21, 36
     starting, 131–136
   as lifestyle disease, 499
   mental health, 480–481
   neuropsychiatric effects, 476
   obesity, 18
     management, 100–103
   pregnancy, 458
   prevention, 26–29
   seriousness, 473
   sexual health, women, 376
   smoking on, 317
   type 1 diabetes *vs*, **20**, 480
   weight on mortality, 95–96

UKPDS risk calculator, 229
ultrasound, pregnancy, 452
unawareness *see* hypoglycaemic unawareness
uncertainty tolerance, 50
unconscious patient, hypoglycaemia, 191–192
undernutrition, 88–90
   infancy, 11, 12
under-resourced communities, 428
   pregnancy, 443–444
underweight, 95

unintentional nonadherence, 484
United Kingdom, diagnostic criteria for
    DKA, **204**
United Kingdom Prospective Diabetes Study,
    hypoglycaemia, 175
United States
    diagnostic criteria for DKA, **204**
    Europe *vs*, dairy products, 92
unmyelinated C-fibres, peripheral neuropathy, 260
unwashed fingers, 69
uppers (illegal drugs), 322, **323**
urea (blood urea nitrogen), 82, 91, 405
urethral medicines, 378
urinary incontinence, 338–339, 454
urinary tract
    autonomic neuropathy, **268**, 269
    infections, **285**, 338, 411
        cranberry formulations, 411, 460, 551
urine albumin, target values, **31**
urine glucose, 22, 62–64
    24-hour, 68
    monitoring, 76–78
    SGLT-2 inhibitors, 128
urine ketones, 74, 75, 280
urine output, diabetic ketoacidosis, 209
urine-to-creatinine ratio, 77
U/s (confusing prescriptions), 149

vaccinations, 201
    older people, 402, 417
    rotavirus, 427
vacuum devices, penile, 378–379
vaginal dryness, 375, 376
vaginal rings, 447
vaginal thrush, 376
vagus nerve, on insulin secretion, 267
valerian, **558**
values (personal), 473, 492, 524
vaping, 320
vardenafil, 378
varenicline, **321**
variability of blood glucose, 66, 221, 327
    CGBM monitoring, 73
    cystic fibrosis, 337
    on sexual health, 376
vascular dementia, 400–401, *see also* multi-infarct
    dementia
vascular insufficiency, screening, 261
vascular resistance, obesity, **286**
Vassa (Buddhist Lent), 359
vegan diet, 92
vegetables, interactions with medicines, **105**
vegetarian diets, 27, 92
venesection, 333
venlafaxine
    cardiovascular effects, **351**
    peripheral neuropathy, **259**
verbal learning style, **496**
Veterans Affairs, VA-HIT (trial), 155
vildagliptin, 127, 128
vision, 237–243
    blurred, 297

driving, **354**
    insulin in type 2 diabetes, 136
    after laser therapy, 296
    resources for loss, 241–242
    sudden loss, 240
    treatment, 295–297
visual estimation, food intake, 100
visual learning style, **496**
vitamin(s)
    deficiencies
        medicines increasing, **105**
        vegetarian diets, 92
    supplements
        cancer care, 314
        renal disease, 249
vitamin B$_{12}$, metformin on absorption, 124
vitamin C, 222, 551
vitamin D, 15, 20
    1,25-dihydroxyvitamin D, 348
vitamin E, 298, 551
vitamin K, low intake, 405
vitus agnus-castus, 461
voices of health professionals, 499
vomiting
    cancer care, 311
    end of life, **529**
    enteral nutrition, 308
    ketosis, 212
    surgery and, 282

waist circumference, 11, 13, 18, 98
waist–hip ratio, 18, 99, 244
walking, 416
walking aids, acceptance, 409
warfarin, 159, 161
    cranberry formulations and, 411
warm-up periods, blood glucose sensors, 144
water-soluble fibres, 93
websites, 41
    smoking cessation, 319
weight
    measurement, 99
        artificial nutrition, 308
weight gain
    age-related, 100
    antipsychotics, 483
    beta blockers, 158
    causes, 98–99
    insulin in type 2 diabetes, 135
    medicines causing, 96
    pregnancy, 456–457
weight loss, *see also* weight reduction
    cancer, 315
    life expectancy decline, 525
    older people, 405
Weight Management Industry Code of Practice, 103
weight reduction, 89, 98, 100
    adjustable gastric bands, 293
    commercial programmes, 100, 101
    complementary medicine, 103, 550–551
    diet, 100–101
    exercise on, 108

intensive management programme, children, 434
  medicines for, 101
  older people, 392
  polycystic ovarian syndrome, 445
  programmes, 100
  type 2 diabetes prevention, 27
Well-Written Health Information, 506
white adipose tissue, 97
white cell counts, diabetic ketoacidosis, 210
wild yam cream, 461
will to live, 539
withdrawal of treatment, end-of-life
        care, 539
withdrawal symptoms, nicotine, 318
women, 443–465
  AIDS patients, screening, 342
  antipsychotics, 350
  cardiovascular disease, 226
  sexual health, 373, 376
  stress incontinence, 339
  strokes, 236

World Health Organization
  Fracture Risk Calculator (FRAX), 346
  on oral glucose tolerance test, 22
  sexual health
      defined, 372–373
      measurement manual, 382
wound management
  complementary medicine, 299, 554
  foot disease, 263–265
writing prescriptions, dosages, 149
WS 1442 (*Crataegus monogyna*), 230, **558**

yaje (hoasia), 324
yoga, 550
young people, 2

Ziagen (antiretroviral), 343
zidovudine, 343
zinc
  adverse effects, **558**
  deficiency, 159

Printed and bound by CPI Group (UK) Ltd, Croydon, CR0 4YY

27/10/2024